Eukaryotic Cell Function and Growth

Regulation by Intracellular
Cyclic Nucleotides

NATO ADVANCED STUDY INSTITUTES SERIES

A series of edited volumes comprising multifaceted studies of contemporary scientific issues by some of the best scientific minds in the world, assembled in cooperation with NATO Scientific Affairs Division.

The series is published by an international board of publishers in conjunction with NATO Scientific Affairs Division

A Life Sciences	Plenum Publishing Corporation
B Physics	New York and London
C Mathematical and Physical Sciences	D. Reidel Publishing Company Dordrecht and Boston
D Behavioral and Social Sciences	Sijthoff International Publishing Company Leiden'
E Applied Sciences	Noordhoff International Publishing Leiden

Eukaryotic Cell Function and Growth

Regulation by Intracellular Cyclic Nucleotides

Edited by

Jacques E. Dumont

Institute of Interdisciplinary Research
University of Brussels Medical Schools
Brussels, Belgium

and

Barry L. Brown and Nicholas J. Marshall

Institute of Nuclear Medicine
The Middlesex Hospital Medical School
Thorn Institute of Clinical Sciences
London, United Kingdom

PLENUM PRESS • NEW YORK AND LONDON
Published in cooperation with NATO Scientific Affairs Division

Library of Congress Cataloging in Publication Data

Nato Advanced Study Institute on Regulation of Function and Growth of Eukaryotic
  Cells by Intracellular Nucleotides, Wépion, Belgium, 1974.
  Eukaryotic cell function and growth.

  (NATO advanced study institutes series: Series A, Life sciences; v. 9)
  "Lectures presented at the NATO Advanced Study Institute on Regulation of Func-
tion and Growth of Eukaryotic Cells by Intracellular Nucleotides held in Wépion,
Belgium, September 23–October 1, 1974."
  Includes bibliographies and index.
  1. Cellular control mechanisms–Congresses. 2. Cyclic nucleotides–Congresses. I.
Dumont, Jacques E., 1931-   II. Brown, Barry L., 1941-   III. Marshall,
Nicholas J., 1944-   IV. Title. V. Series.
QH604.N37 1974   574.8'761   76-10784
ISBN 0-306-35609-0

Lectures presented at the NATO Advanced Study Institute on
Regulation of Function and Growth of Eukaryotic Cells by
Intracellular Nucleotides held in Wépion, Belgium, September 23–
October 1, 1974

© 1976 Plenum Press, New York
A Division of Plenum Publishing Corporation
227 West 17th Street, New York, N.Y. 10011

Printed in the United States of America

Preface

The day it rained in Wépion ......

   The NATO Course on Regulation of Function and Growth of Eukaryo-
tic Cells by Intracellular Cyclic Nucleotides was organized in
Wépion (Belgium) from September 23 to October 1, 1974, by L. Birn-
baumer (Chicago), B.L. Brown (London), R.W. Butcher (Worcester),
J.E. Dumont (Brussels), M. Paiva (Brussels) and G. Van den Berghe
(Louvain), under the benevolent and most efficient aegis of
Dr. T. Kester (NATO, Brussels).

   The formula of the Course was inspired by the Gordon Conference with its combination of a pleasant, friendly and easygoing
atmosphere together with a solid and critical scientific diet
offered in the morning and evening, the afternoon being free. For
these reasons, the meeting was located in a pleasant motel in
beautiful surroundings by the side of the Meuse river, in the
country, but close to the town of Namur. Everything, absolutely
everything, from swimming to tennis, to horse riding, was available
to make the afternoons agreeable and to facilitate social contacts.
As we said in the announcement "The weather is often, but not
always, very good at that time of the year". On the Sunday we
arrived in Wépion the sun shone brightly ... at the end of the
afternoon it began to rain ... and our arrival proved to be the
signal to start rain for the next four months. Already, after
one week in Wépion, the radio was proudly announcing that all
records had been broken and that Belgium had replenished its badly
depleted water reserves ...

   Despite this drawback the general opinion was that the Course
had been a success. The audience came from many countries :
Belgium, Canada, France, Germany, Italy, Israel, Netherlands,
Norway, Portugal, Switzerland, United Kingdom and United States.
It was formed of a rather unusual mixture of chemists, bio-
chemists, physicists, mathematicians, biologists and morphologists,
and physicians, amongst others, working on a wide variety of pro-

blems ranging from purely clinical to totally fundamental ones.
Some of the participants, as well as some lecturers like ourselves,
felt they had a deep but far too narrow experience in one part of
the field and wanted to broaden their outlook : others wanted to
get at the very bottom of one specialized area. We hope we catered
for all tastes, and all departed satisfied.

The Course was designed to be a Course, i.e. "to be" didactic
and to cover for an unspecialized audience the subject in breadth
and in depth. However, it was well understood that to give the
talk the flavour of the most recent research, each speaker would
make full use of his own results. In fact, while some talks were
very instructional, others were more oriented as presentations of
personal results. On the whole the balance is reflected in this
book.

The formula of the Course was to have a long session with
4 talks in the morning and a short session with 2 talks at the
beginning of the evening. Each talk was supposed to last 35 to
45 minutes with the rest of the hour left for questions and discussion. Most of the speakers respected this rule. The organizers
stated in the programme : "We would greatly appreciate if this
Course is not confused with a church service, where a few authorities
deliver the gospel without discussion or questions. The talks
should be a <u>critical</u> evaluation of present knowledge and we would
expect that issues be discussed, changes of interpretation and
discrepancies be brought forward and the unknown pointed out, at
least in the discussion, in a friendly and relaxed atmosphere.
The chairman's job will be to approach this ideal." Thanks to the
chairmen (L. Birnbaumer, B.L. Brown, R.W. Butcher, J.D. Corbin,
N. Crawford, J.E. Dumont, J.H. Exton, J.G. Hardman, K.D. Hepp,
C. Jacquemin, R. Kram, J. Nunez, J. Otten, G.A. Robison, G. Schultz,
G. Van den Berghe, M. Vaughan), this ideal was approached. After
each talk there were first questions for information and then sometimes very acute discussion. Few issues, disagreements or discrepancies were shunned and in general the audience felt they had
received a sound and critical evaluation of the field. After a
slight lag period, questioning increased exponentially - a goal
difficult to achieve in Europe and even elsewhere. A great part
of the merit for this atmosphere should be attributed to R.W. Butcher
(Worcester) who, from the very beginning, decided he would not let
anything unclear, incomprehensive, debatable or incorrect pass.
By doing this he greatly contributed to the success of the Course,
and we express our gratitude.

As this field and the Course owed so much to the Nashville
School, it was quite fitting that the Course began by a talk by
R.W. Butcher on the life and philosophy of E.W. Sutherland and
ended up with the announcement that the highest Belgian Scientific

Award, the Francqui Chair for 1974, had been attributed to J.G.
Hardman.

We should like to thank NATO Advanced Study Institute which
sponsored and supported the Course, the Caisse Générale d'Epargne
et de Retraite and the Fonds National de la Recherche Scientifique
which support most of the Belgian research presented at the meeting,
and Boehringer Pharma, S.A., and Sandoz, S.A. which helped to defray
some of the expenses. The programme of the Course was set up with
Drs. L. Birnbaumer, B.L. Brown, R.W. Butcher and G. Van den Berghe,
who also organized the sessions and the discussions with us. Our
thanks to them for having made the Course so stimulating. This
Course could not have been a success without the organizational
prowess, and artful public relations of Mrs. Ch. Borrey who, with
the help of Mrs. D. Legrand and Miss M. Opdenberg, carried most
of the burden of administrative and secretarial work. We extend
our thanks to these ladies. We would also like to thank all the
researchers of the Institut de Recherche Interdisciplinaire en
Biologie Humaine et Nucléaire who organized the sessions and
helped with the organization. Of course, lastly and not least,
our thanks to Mrs. F. Morent who typed this book.

                    J.E. DUMONT   M. PAIVA

Contents

CONTENTS

CONTENTS

INTRODUCTION: A COMMEMORATION OF EARL W. SUTHERLAND, JR.

Reginald W. Butcher
Department of Biochemistry
University of Massachusetts Medical School
Worcester, Massachusetts 01505, U.S.A.

It seems most appropriate that the introduction to the course and to the proceedings which derived from it should start with a few words about Earl W. Sutherland, Jr., who discovered cyclic AMP and thus in a real sense provided the initial impetus for our gathering. However, it is impossible to properly evaluate or even describe the contributions which he made to our understanding of control systems in living organisms. It will be more for future generations to judge his greatness than those of us who write or read these words.

Nonetheless, even a cursory listing of his accomplishments is most impressive. Standing first among them, of course, is research, signalled by the discovery of cyclic AMP. However, many other entries, although seemingly less dramatic are very important. An early example was the identification of phosphorylase as the rate-limiting step in glycogenolysis when the whole concept of regulatory enzymes was only dimly perceived. Another, and one of great significance, was the demonstration of the chemical nature of phosphorylase activation. Shortly thereafter with Henion he reported that liver and muscle phosphorylases differed with respect to immunological properties although they catalyzed the same reaction. This was, to my knowledge, the first demonstration of isozymes.

One of the most striking things about Sutherland's research was that he, at least to the best of my recollection, never made an error in the strategy of his research. This is, there were many crossroads along the trail from his initial interest in the hyperglycemic effect of the catecholamines to the identification of cyclic AMP as the heat stable factor responsible for phosphorylase activation in homogenates, yet he never took a wrong turn. This was partially because he had a very clear sense of the question he was asking: *"How do hormones act?"* Thus, he resisted taking any sideroads which might lead him to other (albeit interesting) answers. As a matter of fact, he often said that one of the most difficult decisions in science was what not to do. However, this is only one of the several reasons for his successes.

Another very important ingredient was his scientific intuition. Along with an intense curiosity about all things biological, he had a knack of sensing how things might work in a living cell. Occasionally he might be startled by a new development in our understanding of biological functions, but he could always rationalize the value of the function in terms of survival value to the organism (if the observation was valid). As an example, he had a clear concept of allosteric enzymes and effector interactions long before the formal theories were enunciated. His conceptualisation was less elegant than allosterism because he referred to effectors as "quirking" enzymes. However, it was perfectly logical to him that effectors could interact at sites distinct from the active sites of key enzymes and alter their activities.

Another characteristic of Earl Sutherland, and one which was legendary to all of us who were privileged to work with him, was his memory. Long after I had forgotten even doing experiments (the results of which I had told him about) he could come up with the actual numbers. This could involve the span of five or ten years. I think he worked very hard on his memory and made a conscious effort to remember those things which he considered important. As a matter of fact, we all came to know a far-away look in his eyes which meant that he wasn't particularly interested in what we were talking about — probably because he considered it irrelevant — and would change the subject as quickly as possible. Fortunately, he never seemed to remember things he was told during such incidents.

Not unexpectedly, since Earl did seem to be able to direct himself down the proper scientific road at every crossing, he had a highly disciplined mind. Whenever confronted with a decision of any moment, he would write down a list of pros and cons on a piece of yellow legal-sized paper. His lists of pros and cons were extremely interesting, for they were free of bias. That is, he was sufficiently disciplined and sufficiently objective that his pros and cons were unweighted by any preconceived notion about what his decision should be. An enjoinder which he dispensed frequently and freely upon his younger associates was that, *"You should never fall in love with your hypothese"*, and this was a precept he lived by. Indeed, one is struck by the fact that science in general would be far better off if this attitude towards hypotheses could be maintained by all of us.

Earl tried to maintain as much independence as possible. This was not so much a state of being but a state of mind, for he wanted to avoid the plague of commitments and anxieties which seemed to debilitate so many scientists. I think this had much to do with his giving up a departmental chairmanship and his move to Vanderbilt in 1963. It also, at least in part, explains why he sometimes allowed mail to go unanswered for weeks or even months. It was not that he was unkind nor unfeeling, because he was a kind and considerate man, most especially to his junior colleagues. Rather, he wanted to keep his mind clear and his memory bank as free of extraneous material as possible so that he could concentrate upon his science. While this may be of little consolation to those who waited months for an answer to a letter, it is a fact. He simply wanted to retain his independence and his concentration on research, free of distractions, to the best of his ability.

Dr. Sutherland was a very pleasant and easy-going man to work for. He was amiable and informal, and always willing to spend time with other scientists, especially younger ones, when available. During all of the time I was in his group, I never heard him speak critically of or to any of his people. Indeed, he always went out of his way to praise those who were productive and he would omit mention of those who were not.

Earl also had a deep and abiding commitment to open scientific communication. This was consistent with his view of science; that is, that is should be an open society of talented individuals seeking new truths about nature. Therefore, there were no withheld items of data, either internally or externally, in his group. This was not because he was lacking in competitive spirit, because he was fiercely competitive. However, above all he was very curious and he wanted to understand how things worked. Since that could only occur with all available information, secrets were anathema to him.

Finally, Earl was a master at writing experimental protocols. He had a clear sense of the controls needed to prove or disprove a particular point, so much so that his experiments were almost always free-standing.

These then, were some of the attributes which went into the making of what I consider a quintessential man of science. As an individual he was considerably more complex than he was as a scientist, and as he saw more of the world, he became more pessimistic. As a rationalist, he felt that it should be possible to solve human problems by the application of human intelligence, just as he had brought his intelligence to bear upon the problem of catecholamine-induced hyperglycemia. As a matter of fact, for

the last several years of his life, he felt that he might be
able to make a substantive contribution to solving problems
such as the maldistribution of resources and food, population
overgrowth, and most particularly, tribal antagonisms. However,
the more he watched and thought, the more pessimistic he became
about there being rational solutions to the problems of mankind
and indeed, the entire planet. He tried to hide his pessimism,
but it became increasingly obvious to those of us who knew him
well. Nonetheless, his pessimism notwithstanding, one is struck
by the feeling that those attributes which made him a successful
scientist would have equipped him marvelously for such an under-
taking. This conviction makes his loss all the more tragic, for
in times like these, an effective rationalist would be of
inestimable value.

       A meeting such as this NATO course would have been very
dear to Earl's heart, because it embodies the best in science;
that is, open communication between individuals of different
nationalities and backgrounds, all dedicated in the search of
truth. Dr. Sutherland bequeathed us not only his oeuvre but also
his open rationality. Therefore, we can best commemorate him
by assisting in the development of a new generation of scientific
rationalists.

CELL FRACTIONATION BY CENTRIFUGATION METHODS

Maurice Wibo

International Institute of Cellular and Molecular
 Pathology, and Université de Louvain
Avenue Hippocrate, 75
B-1200 Brussels, Belgium

Contents

INTRODUCTION

To many investigators, cell fractionation is a tool, which provides them with a preparation of a given subcellular component, endowed with functional properties that form the matter of sophisticated studies. However, the complexity of such subcellular preparations is not always clearly recognized, sometimes leading to erroneous conclusions. Our purpose is to discuss briefly some of the major difficulties likely to arise in cell fractionation, from its very first step, homogenization of tissue, to its final step, analysis of the fractions obtained and determination of their composition in terms of subcellular entities. A detailed treatment of this subject will be found in several reviews (de Duve, (1), (2), (3)).

1

HOMOGENIZATION

Homogenization markedly influences the outcome of the whole
cell fractionation process. Its aim is to disrupt cells, while
preserving their components as much as possible in their "native"
state. The numerous mechanical devices which have been used will
not be reviewed here (see, for instance, Hughes and Cunningham,
(4); Mathias, (5)). Little progress has been made recently in
this field, which is still largely empirical. Each material poses
a particular problem. Resistance to breakage depends on the amount
of connective tissue present, but is a common feature of isolated
cells (Dingle and Barrett, (6)). The fragility of the organelles
may also vary from tissue to tissue.

The choice of the suspension medium is another important
matter for the success of fractionation. Except in special cases,
the homogenization medium should protect organelles sensitive to
hypotonicity, and minimize aggregation and adsorption artefacts.
Isotonic sucrose is the basic and most common medium, since saline
solutions often cause agglutination of the organelles. In spleen
homogenates, however, aggregation was avoided by using 0.2 M KCl
(Bowers, Finkenstaedt and de Duve, (7)).

The quality of an homogenate can be judged on morphological
and biochemical criteria. Phase contrast microscopy easily esta-
blishes the degree of cell disruption and discloses aggregation
artefacts. The structural preservation of cell components is partially accessible to electron microscopic observation, but more
deeply and more easily to biochemical investigations on various
structure-linked properties, such as enzyme latency. It is known
that many particulate enzymes localized within the matrix of the
particle display little activity towards added substrates as long
as the particles have suffered little damage. The barrier
restricting the access of the enzymes to these substrates is the
membrane of the organelle (Figure 1). Usually, the membrane is
impermeable to both the enzyme and the substrate. For instance, β-
glycerophosphate cannot pass through the lysosomal membrane (Berthet
et al, (8)) and is not acted upon by the lysosomal acid phosphatase.
It is well known also that the inner mitochondrial membrane is impermeable to the pyridine coenzymes and to the substrates of various
dehydrogenases of the mitochondrial matrix, which display a high
degree of structure-linked latency in well-preserved mitochondria
(Bendall and de Duve, (9)). Less frequently, the membrane is
permeable to the substrate, but the diffusion of the latter from
the surrounding medium becomes the rate-limiting step of the reaction. Such is the case of the catalase activity in rat liver
peroxisomes (de Duve, (2)). As a result of the high catalase
concentration within the peroxisome matrix, the average concentra-
ation of H_2O_2 is much lower than in the surrounding medium, which

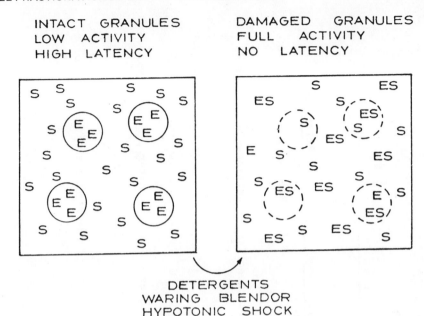

Figure 1 *Schematic representation of the mechanism of*
enzyme latency.
S = substrate,
E = enzyme,
ES = enzyme-substrate complex.

decreases the measured activity to the same extent, since the catalase reaction follows first order kinetics.

In practice, it is an easy matter to determine, usually in the presence of a suitable detergent, the "total" activity of the enzyme, and to compare it with the "free" activity, displayed by non-treated preparations, under conditions which preserve the organelles, particularly from osmotic disruption. Some latent enzymes used to check the state of preservation of the host particles in rat liver homogenates are listed in Table I.

Ultimately, homogenization will be evaluated in the light of the results of fractionation. If the aim is to purify one kind of subcellular component, or to preserve some delicate function, the procedure has to be adapted accordingly, even at the expense of

TABLE I Some structurally latent enzymes of rat liver homogenate

Enzyme	Subcellular localization	Reference
Malate dehydrogenase Glutamate dehydrogenase	Mitochondrial matrix	Bendall & de Duve, 1960
Sulfite cytochrome c reductase	Intermembrane space of mitochondria	Wattiaux-De Coninck & Wattiaux, 1971
Lysosomal hydrolases	Lysosomal matrix	Wattiaux & de Duve, 1956
Catalase	Peroxisomal matrix	de Duve, 1965
Nucleoside diphosphatase *	Endoplasmic reticulum vesicles	Ernster & Jones, 1962

* *This enzyme appears to be loosely bound to the matrix side of the membrane of ER vesicles (Kuriyama, 1972)*

other requirements. For example, Neville (10) prepared liver plasma membranes by grinding the tissue in hypotonic medium, which leads to osmotic breakage of sensitive organelles such as mitochondria and lysosomes.

FRACTIONATION METHODS

Cell fractionation by centrifugation methods makes use of differences in size and density between subcellular components. When these are submitted to a centrifugal field in a liquid column, they move at a speed, $\underline{v}$, which is given by the Svedberg equation :

$$\underline{v} = \frac{\phi \, (\ell_p - \ell_m)}{f} \, \omega^2 \underline{x} = \underline{s} \omega^2 \underline{x}$$

where ϕ is the particle volume, ℓ_p the particle density, ℓ_m the density of the medium, $\underline{f}$ the frictional coefficient, $\omega^2 \underline{x}$ the centrifugal field, and $\underline{s}$ the sedimentation coefficient.

Fractionation can be achieved in two ways. Either ℓ_m is everywhere lower than ℓ_p and particles will separate according to their rate of sedimentation. Or particles travel through a medium the density of which increases markedly with radial distance, so that they finally reach a zone where $\ell_p = \ell_m$, and stop. In practice, the first method, designated differential centrifugation, separates particles mainly on the basis of size; the second one, called isopycnic centrifugation or density equilibration, rests only upon differences in particle density.

Differential Centrifugation

According to the classical method of differential centrifugation, particles of decreasing size and density are extracted successively from the initial homogenate, as a result of centrifugation runs performed for increasing times at increasing rotational speeds. The original procedure, developed by Schneider and Hogeboom (11), divided the liver homogenate into four fractions : nuclear, mitochondrial, microsomal and supernate. Later, it was found useful to separate a "light mitochondrial" (L) fraction, intermediate between the "heavy mitochondrial" (M) and the microsomal (P) fractions, which is enriched in peroxisomes and lysosomes (de Duve *et al*, (12)). From glandular tissues, it is customary to isolate a special fraction containing mostly secretory granules (Siekevitz and Palade, (13)).

Following these methods, the pellets obtained at each stage contain not only all the particles with a sedimentation constant

sufficient to bring them from the meniscus to the bottom of the
tube, but also smaller particles initially present near the pellet
region. It is thus essential to wash each sediment once or several
times. The method is somewhat tedious and a more efficient procedure, known as rate-zonal centrifugation, has been put forward
(Figure 2). The particles are loaded on top of a shallow density
gradient, the upper density limit of which is lower than the
density of any of the particles. The gradient serves only to
stabilize the system against convections. The centrifugal field
applied is such that particles are incompletely sedimented at the
end of the run. Particles with different sedimentation coefficients
separate from each other in the gradient and are recovered in distinct fractions.

Rate-zonal centrifugation in fixed-angle and in swinging-bucket
rotors meets with a number of difficulties : swirls arising when
rotors are started, or stopped, and convections caused by the non-

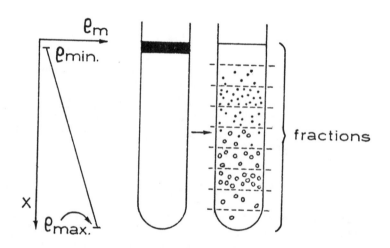

DIFFERENTIAL SEDIMENTATION
Gradient : shallow, $\varrho_{max.} < \varrho_{p\ min.}$
Centrifugation :→incomplete sedimentation
Parameter : sedimentation constant

DENSITY EQUILIBRATION
Gradient : steep, $\varrho_{max.} > \varrho_{p\ max.}$
Centrifugation : prolonged, high speed
Parameter : equilibrium density

Figure 2. The two kinds of density gradient centrifugation.

ideal geometry of the centrifugation cell (Anderson, (14) ;   de Duve,
Berthet and Beaufay, (15)). These extrinsic sources of artefact are
suppressed in zonal rotors, which are equipped with sector-shaped
compartments of high capacity, and which can be filled and emptied
while running (Anderson, (16)). However, the amount of material
that can be layered on top of the gradient is still severely limited
by zone spreading. Indeed, when particles penetrate the upper part
of the gradient, the density of that part becomes higher than that
of the underlying zone. Owing to the density inversion, droplets
of liquid carrying particles move towards denser parts of the
gradient, until density equilibrium is restored. As a consequence,
the particle zone spreads through the gradient by convection, to
an extent which increases with the amount of particles.

   It should be stressed that zonal rotors can hardly resolve
the homogenate into its many different components in a single run
on the basis of sedimentation rate only. One can easily calculate
that the sedimentation coefficients of liver nuclei, mitochondria,
and microsomes are of the order of, respectively, 100, 1 and 0.03
nanoseconds in 0.25 M sucrose. This spectrum is too wide to allow
simultaneous separation of the three classes of particles by
differential centrifugation.

                           Density Equilibration

   Differential centrifugation, which separates the homogenate
into classes of particles differing largely in size, is usually
applied as a preliminary step in cell fractionation. Further
resolution of the fractions obtained can be achieved by density
equilibration (Beaufay *et al*, (17), (18), (19)); Amar-Costesec *et
al*, (20)).

   Following this method (Figure 2), the particles are layered on
a steep density gradient, since the uppon density limit of the
gradient must exceed the density of any of the particles. Centrifugation is prolonged until particles reach the level of their
equilibrium density. This often takes a long time, since $\underline{v}$
diminishes as the particles travel through the gradient, owing to
the decrease of the buoyancy term ($\ell_p - \ell_m$), and to the increase of
viscous drag, with radial distance. To shorten the centrifugation
time, it is thus advisable to decrease the radial distance which
must be travelled by the particles in the gradient. A rotor (E-40)
particularly suitable for isopycnic centrifugation of subcellular
components was constructed by Beaufay (Beaufay, (21);   Leighton *et
al*, (22)). It combines in its ring-shaped cell a small radial
depth (1 cm) with a convenient capacity (50 ml). At 35,000 rpm

density equilibration of microsomal fractions is nearly obtained in
3 hours, as compared with 12 to 15 hours in a SW-39 rotor (Beaufay
et al,(19)).

Another advantage of a small radial depth of the gradient is
the reduction of the hydrostatic pressure to which the particles are
submitted. Mitochondria are indeed disrupted by the hydrostatic
pressure generated in high-speed rotors (Wattiaux, Wattiaux-De
Coninck and Ronveaux-Dupal,(23)). Other subcellular components are
also markedly affected by hydrostatic pressures of the order of, or
below, those produced in some centrifugation systems (Figure 3).
The pressure, $\underline{p}$, generated at the radial distance $\underline{x}$ by the centrifugal field is given by :

$$\underline{p} = \int_{\underline{x}_o}^{\underline{x}} \omega^2 \ell \underline{x} \, d\underline{x}$$

where $\underline{x}_o$ is the radial distance at the meniscus. Assuming, for the
sake of simplicity, that the density ℓ of the liquid column is constant, one obtains :

$$\underline{p} = \frac{1}{2} \omega^2 \ell (\underline{x}^2 - \underline{x}_o^2)$$

It can be computed that, at 40,000 rpm, the centrifugal force would
develop 1720, 660 and 120 $kg.cm^{-2}$ at the periphery of SW 41 Ti, SW
39 (Beckman), and E-40 rotors respectively, if they are filled up
with water. These differences illustrate the marked influence of
the rotor shape on the pressure attained.

Isopycnic equilibration is usually performed in a concentration
gradient of sucrose in water. Non-ionic macromolecular solutes,
such as glycogen or Ficoll, have also been used as gradient-
forming substances. These latter cause minimal osmotic shrinkage
of the particles and do not permeate biological membranes. Thus,
their concentration has little effect on the density of subcellular
particles, contrary to the effect of sucrose concentration.
Organelles poorly separated in a sucrose gradient may dissociate
from one another in a gradient made of a macromolecular solute.
Experimental studies on the behaviour of the organelles in various
media has led to models describing physically the particles in terms
of dry matrix, sucrose space, osmotic space and hydration water
(de Duve, Berthet and Beaufay, (15); Beaufay and Berthet, (24),
Beaufay et al, (18)).

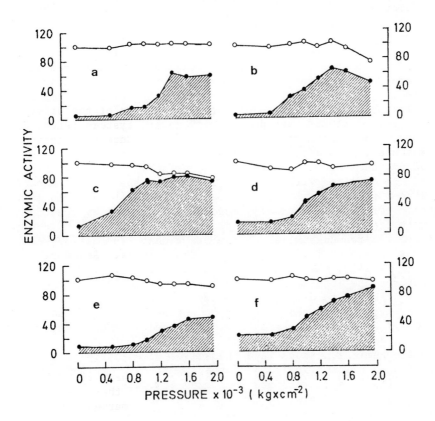

Figure 3. Decrease of enzyme latency induced by compression. Liver homogenates free from soluble proteins were submitted to various pressures during 30 minutes at 3.5° C. Free (•-•-•) and total (o-o-o) activities are given in per cent of the total activity in the untreated sample :

(a) malate dehydrogenase;
(b) sulfite cytochrome c reductase;
(c) catalase;
(d) N-acetyl-β-glucosaminidase;
(e) nucleoside diphosphatase;
(f) acid phosphatase.

From Bronfman and Beaufay (1973)

ANALYSIS OF THE FRACTIONS AND INTERPRETATION OF THE RESULTS

Complete separation of the various populations of subcellular components often cannot be achieved, owing to their great polydispersity and to the non-ideal conditions under which centrifugation experiments are carried out. Accordingly, the composition of the fractions obtained must be quantitatively assessed in terms of subcellular components.

At first sight, morphological evaluation of the fractions would seem ideal for this purpose. However, the minuteness of the material that can be conveniently examined under the electron microscope is too often overlooked. Assuming a section thickness of 50 nm, the volume of material shown in Figure 4 is less than 1 μm^3, as compared with 5,000 μm^3, for one hepatocyte. According to Weibel *et al*, (25)), there are 150,000 hepatocytes in 1 mg of liver. Moreover, the usual procedures of packing by centrifugation used in the processing of cell particles for electron microscopy do not provide random samples of the fractions. In this respect, a filtration method is preferable (Baudhuin, Evrard and Berthet, (26)). Finally, the distinctive morphological features of some cell structures are lost by homogenization. For instance, it becomes hardly possible to distinguish between smooth microsomal vesicles arising from the smooth endoplasmic reticulum, the plasma membranes, the Golgi apparatus, or the outer mitochondrial membrane.

Biochemical methods lend themselves more easily to quantitative and unbiased analysis of the fractions. It is known that many particulate enzymes are localized essentially in one kind of cell structure and are, in first approximation, homogeneously distributed among the population of host-particles (postulate of biochemical homogeneity; de Duve *et al*, (12)). Accordingly, the amount of marker enzyme is a measure of the amount of the corresponding organelle in the fraction. Let RSA_i be the relative specific activity $(RSA)^*$ of a marker enzyme of subcellular component A in a given fraction i, a be the percentage of the protein of the homogenate contributed by A, and A_i be the percentage of the protein of fraction i accounted for by A. Then it is easily shown that

$$A_i = a \times RSA_i$$

----

*
  *The relative specific activity of an enzyme in a fraction is the
  ratio of its specific activity in the fraction to that measured
  in the homogenate. Taking the specific activity in the homogenate
  as 1 eliminates one source of variation between enzymes and
  experiments.*

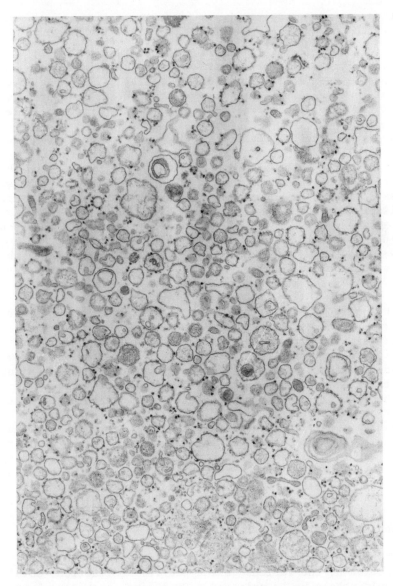

Figure 4. Microsomal fraction isolated from rat liver. Particles were packed by centrifugation on a Millipore filter. The whole thickness of the pellicle appears on this micrograph, taken from a section cut perpendicularly to the surface of the pellicle. Since the filtration procedure produces no heterogeneity along the surface of the pellicle, the picture gives a representative view of the microsomal fraction. Rough vesicles (carrying ribosomes) and smooth vesicles are easily recognized. Magnification : 30,000 x.

Ideally the value of $\underline{a}$ should be obtained from the $\underline{RSA}_p$ of the
marker enzyme in a completely purified preparation, p, of component
A, in which obviously $\underline{A}_p$ = 100. In practice, the value of $\underline{a}$ can be
estimated without complete purification (Leighton *et al.*, (22)).
If reasonably purified preparations are not available, one can
sometimes rely on morphometric data (Beaufay, (27)). As an example,
the contribution of various types of membranes to the protein content of the rat-liver microsome fraction is reported in Table II.

The postulate of biochemical homogeneity is not rigorously
obeyed in all cases. For example, liver lysosomes exhibit a
marked enzymatic heterogeneity (Beaufay *et al.*, (18)) , and the
ratio of glucose 6-phosphatase to NADPH cytochrome c reductase
increases with the ribosome load of the microsomes derived from
endoplasmic reticulum (Amar-Costesec *et al.*, (28); Wibo *et al.*,
(29); Beaufay *et al.*, (19)). Liver plasma membranes can be broken
down into parts differing in enzymatic content (Evans, (30);
Thinès-Sempoux, (31)). Consequently, the amount of these subcellular components should preferably be estimated on an average
basis from several marker enzymes.

Obviously, the validity of such calculations depends also on
more trivial points, such as the absence of modification of enzyme
activity as a result of the fractionation. In this respect, it is
essential to assay the enzymes in all fractions obtained from the
homogenate, in order to establish a balance sheet. If the sum of
the activities recovered in the fractions is appreciably different
from the activity of the homogenate, this fact should be taken into
account in the conclusions drawn. Whenever possible, it is
preferable to rely on marker enzymes firmly bound to the membranes,
since damage to the particles can lead to the release of matrix
enzymes and to their adsorption on other subcellular components.
In many cases, disruption of particles should be avoided as much
as possible : breakage of lysosomes and peroxisomes, for example,
gives rise to membranous ghosts for which we have no valuable
marker at the present time, and which can contaminate purified preparations of other cellular membranes.

When a complex tissue forms the starting material, the relative
contribution of the various cell types to the fractions obtained
should ultimately be established. Promising in this respect are
various methods which have been devised recently to separate and
purify a given cell type, for example parenchymal cells in the case
of liver (Berry and Friend, (32)).

TABLE II : Biochemical analysis of the microsomal fraction from rat liver

Market enzyme	Subcellular component (A)	RSA in microsomes *	$\frac{\#}{a}$	$\frac{A \text{ in}}{\text{microsomes}}$
Glucose 6-phosphatase	Endoplasmic reticulum	3.9	20	78
NADPH cyt. $\underline{c}$ reductase		3.5		
5'-Nucleotidase	Plasma membranes	2.5	3	7.8
Alk. phosphodiesterase I		2.7		
Cytochrome oxidase	Mitochondria	0.25	20	5
Galactosyltransferase	Golgi apparatus	4.3	1	4.3
Monoamine oxidase	Detached outer mitochon-drial membranes (?)	1	3	3
Acid phosphatase	Lysosomes	0.93	0.7	0.5
N-Acetyl-β-glucosami-nidase		0.50		
Catalase	Peroxisomes	0.31	2.5	0.8

* Calculated from Amar-Costesec et al.(1974 a). The lower RSA of NADPH cytochrome $\underline{c}$ reductase, as compared to glucose 6-phosphatase, is due to the occurrence of NADPH cytochrome $\underline{c}$ reductase activity in the final supernatant.

The protein contents of endoplasmic reticulum, mitochondria, and peroxisomes were estimated by Leighton et al. (1968); those of plasma membranes, Golgi apparatus and lysosomes by, respectively, Thinès-Sempoux (unpublished results), Wibo (unpublished results) and Beaufay (1969).

CONCLUSION

In conclusion, cell fractionation, like any chemical fractionation, should be conducted with analytical rigour. A variety of
sophisticated separation techniques have been applied with success
to the purification of most subcellular components. Too often
however, the fractions obtained are hastily equated to their main
component, and little attention is paid to their still complex
cytological origin. Indeed, most preparations remain appreciably
contaminated by minor components, which can account for some of
their biochemical and functional features. It is thus important to
analyze carefully the subcellular fractions with the help of a
complete battery of marker enzymes.

The author wishes to thank Dr. H. Beaufay for the substantial
improvements he suggested for this paper. The author is Chargé de
Recherches of the Belgian Fonds National de la Recherche Scientifique.

REFERENCES

(1)   DE DUVE, C., (1964) Principles of tissue fractionation, J.
      Theoret, Biol. 6, 33

(2)   DE DUVE, C., (1965) The separation and characterization of
      subcellular particles, Harvey Lect. Ser. 59, 49

(3)   DE DUVE, C., (1967) General Principles, in "Enzyme cytology"
      (D.B. Roodyn, ed.), 1, Academic Press, London

(4)   HUGHES, D.E., and CUNNINGHAM, V.R., (1963),Methods for dis-
      rupting cells, Biochem. Soc. Symp., 23, 8

(5)   MATHIAS, A.P., (1966), Separation of subcellular particles,
      Brit. Med. Bull. 22, 146

(6)   DINGLE, J.T., and BARRETT, A.J., (1969), Some special methods
      for the investigation of the lysosomal system, in "Lysosomes
      in biology and pathology", vol. 2, (J.T. Dingle and H.B. Fell,
      eds.), 555, North Holland Publishing Co., Amsterdam

(7)   BOWERS, W.E., FINKENSTAEDT, J.T., and DE DUVE, C., (1967),
      Lysosomes in lymphoid tissue. I. The measurement of hydrolytic
      activities in whole homogenates, J. Cell Biol. 32, 325

(8)   BERTHET, J., BERTHET, L., APPELMANS, F., and DE DUVE, C.,
      1951, Tissue fractionation studies, II. The nature of the
      linkage between acid phosphatase and mitochondria in rat liver
      tissue, Biochem. J. 50, 182

(9)   BENDALL, D.S., and DE DUVE, C., (1960), Tissue fractionation
      studies. 15. The activation of latent dehydrogenases in mito-
      chondria from rat liver, Biochem. J. 74, 444

(10) NEVILLE, D.M. Jr., (1960), The isolation of a cell membrane
      fraction from rat liver, J. Biophys. Biochem. Cytol. 8, 413

(11) SCHNEIDER, W.C., and HOGEBOOM, G.H., (1950), Intracellular
      distribution of enzymes. V. Further studies on the distri-
      bution of cytochrome c in rat liver homogenates, J. Biol.
      Chem. 183, 123

(12) DE DUVE, C., PRESSMAN, B.C., GIANETTO, R., WATTIAUX, R., and
      APPELMANS, F., (1955), Tissue fractionation studies. 6.
      Intracellular distribution patterns of enzymes in rat-liver
      tissue, Biochem. J. 60, 604

(13) SIEKEVITZ, P., and PALADE, G.E., (1958), A cytochemical study
      on the pancreas of the guinea pig. I. Isolation and enzymatic
      activities of cell fractions, J. Biophys. Biochem. Cytol. 4,
      203

(14) ANDERSON, N.G., (1956), Techniques for the mass isolation of
      cellular components, in "Physical techniques in biological
      research", Vol. 3 (G. Oster and A.W. Pollister, eds.) 299,
      Academic Press, New York.

(15) DE DUVE, C., BERTHET, J., and BEAUFAY, H., (1959), Gradient
      centrifugation of cell particles. Theory and applications,
      Progr. Biophys. Chem. 9, 325

(16) ANDERSON, N.G., (1966),The development of zonal centrifuges
      and ancillary systems for tissue fractionation and analysis,
      Nat. Cancer Inst. Monogr. 21

(17) BEAUFAY, H., BENDALL, D.S., BAUDHUIN, P., WATTIAUX, R. and
      DE DUVE, C., (1959), Tissue fractionation studies, 13.
      Analysis of mitochondrial fractions from rat liver by density
      gradient centrifuging, Biochem. J. 73, 628

(18) BEAUFAY, H., JACQUES, P., BAUDHUIN, P., SELLINGER, O.Z.,
      BERTHET, J., and DE DUVE, C., (1964), Tissue fractionation
      studies, 18. Resolution of mitochondrial fractions from rat
      liver into three distinct populations of cytoplasmic
      particles by means of density equilibration in various
      gradients, Biochem. J. 92, 184

(19) BEAUFAY, H., AMAR-COSTESEC, A., THINES-SEMPOUX, D., WIBO,
      M., ROBBI, M., and BERTHET, J., (1974), Analytical study of
      microsomes and isolated subcellular membranes from rat liver.
      III. Subfractionation of the microsomal fraction by isopycnic
      and differential centrifugation in density gradients, J. Cell
      Biol. 61, 213

(20) AMAR-COSTESEC, A., WIBO, M., THINES-SEMPOUX, D., BEAUFAY, H.,
      and BERTHET, J., (1974 b), Analytical study of microsomes
      and isolated subcellular membranes from rat liver. IV.
      Biochemical, physical, and morphological modifications of
      microsomal components induced by digitonin, EDTA, and
      pyrophosphate, J. Cell Biol. 62, 717

(21) BEAUFAY, H., (1966), La centrifuation en gradient de densité.
      Applications) l'étude des organites subcellulaires, Thesis,
      Louvain

(22) LEIGHTON, F., POOLE, B., BEAUFAY, H., BAUDHUIN, P., COFFEY,
      J.W., FOWLER, S., and DE DUVE, C., (1968), The large-scale
      separation of peroxisomes, mitochondria, and lysosomes from
      the livers of rats injected with Triton WR-1339. Improved
      isolation procedures, automated analysis, biochemical and
      morphological properties of fractions, J. Cell Biol. 37, 482

(23) WATTIAUX, R., WATTIAUX-DE CONINCK, S., and RONVEAUX-DUPAL,
      M.F., (1971), Deterioration of rat-liver mitochondria during
      centrifugation in a sucrose gradient, Eur. J. Biochem. 22,
      31

(24) BEAUFAY, H., and BERTHET, J., (1963), Medium composition and
      equilibrium density of subcellular particles from rat liver,
      Biochem. Soc. Symp. 23, 66

(25) WEIBEL, E.R., STÄUBLI, W., GNÄGI, H.R. and HESS, F.A., (1969)
      Correlated morphometric and biochemical studies on the liver
      cell. I. Morphometric model, stereologic methods, and normal
      morphometric data for rat liver, J. Cell Biol. 42, 68

(26) BAUDHUIN, P., EVRARD, P., and BERTHET, J., (1967), Electron
      microscopic examination of subcellular fractions. I. The
      preparation of representative samples from suspension of
      particles. J. Cell Biol. 32,181

(27) BEAUFAY, H., (1969), Methods for the isolation of lysosomes,
      in "Lysosomes in biology and pathology", Vol. 2 (J.T. Dingle
      and H.B. Fell, eds.), 515, North Holland Publishing Co.,
      Amsterdam

(28) AMAR-COSTESEC, A., BEAUFAY, H., FEYTMANS, E., THINES-SEMPOUX,
      D. and BERTHET, J., (1969), Subfractionation of rat liver
      microsomes, in "Microsomes and drug oxidations" (J.R.
      Gillette, A.H. Conney, G.J. Cosmides, R.W. Estabrook, J.R.
      Fouts, and G.J. Mannering, eds.) 41, Academic Press, New
      York

(29) WIBO, M., AMAR-COSTESEC, A., BERTHET, J., and BEAUFAY, H.,
      (1971), Electron microscope examination of subcellular
      fractions, III. Quantitative analysis of the microsomal
      fraction isolated from rat liver, J. Cell Biol. 51, 52

(30) EVANS, W.H., (1970), Fractionation of liver plasma membranes
      prepared by zonal centrifugation, Biochem. J. 116, 833

(31) THINES-SEMPOUX, D., (1972), A comparison between the lyso-
      somal and the plasma membrane, in "Lysosomes in biology
      and pathology", Vol. 3. (J.T. Dingle, ed.) p 278, North-
      Holland Publishing Co., Amsterdam

(32) BERRY, M.N., and FRIEND, D.S. (1969), High-yield preparation
      of isolated rat liver parenchymal cells. A biochemical and
      fine structural study, J. Cell Biol. 43, 506

BINDING OF LIGANDS TO RECEPTORS : THEORY

J.M. Boeynaems
J.E. Dumont

Institut de Recherche Interdisciplinaire (IRIBHN)
Free University of Brussels, School of Medicine,
1000 Brussels, Belgium

Contents

INTRODUCTION

The interaction between ligands and specific binding structures is a general problem which is encountered at different levels in the field of cyclic nucleotide metabolism and action. Some examples of ligands which interact with specific receptor sites in order to modify the activity of adenylate cyclase and other structures modulating cyclic nucleotide concentrations are listed in Table I; cyclic nucleotides exert most of their effects by interacting with specific receptor proteins : the protein kinases in eukaryotes [1] or the cAMP receptor protein in bacteria (CRP) [2].

The general concepts reviewed below have a broad field of application but in the present article we will emphasize their application to membrane hormone receptors.

The concept of hormone receptor contains two distinct but complementary aspects : the receptor binds the hormone and its binding
process gives rise to the hormone primary effect. The molecular
structure and the conformation of the receptor are such that it
should specifically recognize a given hormone, to the exclusion of
others, and that there will be sufficient affinity to allow hormone
binding. Besides this binding component (or "regulatory" unit),
there is another structure more or less physico-chemically independent, which modifies its activity and so expresses the hormone
primary effect, subsequent to the initial binding process.

Several structures exist which specifically bind a hormone but
are not directly involved in the production of its effects : to
distinguish these from the true receptors (3) (Table II), the term
"acceptor" has recently been proposed.

Some cytological, physical and chemical properties of hormone
receptors are listed in Table III.

TABLE I. List of Ligands involved in Cyclic Nucleotide Metabolism and Action	
Hormones :	catecholamines, polypeptides, glycoproteins..
Toxins :	cholera....
Local hormones :	prostaglandins....
Ions and metabolites:	Ca^{++}, glucose....
"Modulators" :	GTP, adenosine, prostaglandins....
Cyclic nucleotides :	cAMP, cGMP

TABLE II.   Hormone "Acceptors"

1. *Inactivating enzymes*

    e.g. - liver plasma membranes for glucagon (4) and insulin (5)

        - kidney plasma membranes for calcitonin (6)

2. *Catabolic enzymes*

    e.g. Catechol-o-methyl transferase (7)

3. *Transport proteins*

    e.g. - albumin, transcortin, TBG, ...

        - catecholamine reuptake

4. *Storing structures*

    e.g. neurophysines, catecholamine granules

5. *Receptor precursors*

    e.g. liver golgi apparatus for insulin (9)

6. *Others ?*

TABLE III.   General Properties of Hormone Receptors

SUBCELLULAR LOCATION	PHYSICAL STATE	CHEMICAL STRUCTURE
PLASMA MEMBRANE: Polypeptides Glycoproteins Catecholamines	Particulate or	Protein or
CYTOSOL: Steroids	Soluble	Lipoprotein or
LYSOSOMES: Steroids ?	or	Glycoprotein or
MITOCHONDRION: Polypeptides ? Thyroid hormones ?	Solubilized	Glycolipid
NUCLEUS: Steroids Thyroid hormones		

EXPERIMENTAL APPROACH TO THE HORMONE-RECEPTOR INTERACTION

Today, the classical method of characterizing hormone receptors
is to measure the binding of labelled analogues of the hormones to
preparations of the receptors. However, at each of its steps, this
methodology can lead to a variety of artefactual results, as illustrated in Table IV. Physical methods, such as circular dichroism
spectroscopy (10, 11), allow the detection of the conformational
changes which are produced by the hormone-receptor interactions and
could thus be used to quantitatively characterize them. These
methods would not be subject to many of the disadvantages listed
in Table IV.

TABLE IV.   Artefacts in Measuring Labelled Hormones binding to
            their receptors

1. *Labelled analogue:*

    - different behaviour from the native one (e.g. after
      iodination)

    - specific radioactivity insufficient to detect scarce
      receptors

2. *Receptor preparation:*

    loss or unmarking of binding sites during tissue homogeni-
    zation or cell fractionation

3. *Incubation*

    - inactivation of the labelled hormone

    - binding to acceptors

    - degradation of the receptors

    - modification of the receptors : temperature, ionic strength,
      pH, Ca^{++}, nucleotides, ...

4. *Separation of bound from free hormone*

    - saturable binding to glass or millipore filters

    - incomplete recovery of bound hormone in centrifugation
      pellet or on millipore filter

    - dissociation of bound hormone during washing

The most crucial problem when measuring hormone binding is to evaluate its relevance to the true receptors, since hormones bind not only to their receptors but also to a variety of "acceptors" (Table II). In fact, since there are two complementary aspects in the concept of receptor, hormone binding and generation of the hormone primary effect, there are two different and complementary experimental approaches to their study : the measurement of hormone binding and the measurement of a hormone primary effect. The progress in the field of cyclic nucleotide research allows measurement of one primary effect apparently common to many hormones, namely adenylate cyclase activation (12, 13). Both approaches have to be combined : if binding alone is studied, it is impossible to discriminate between receptors and acceptors, whereas if only adenylate cyclase activation is measured, it is not possible to distinguish the process of hormone-receptor binding from the subsequent molecular events involved in the generation of the hormonal effect. The controversy over the catecholamine β receptor illustrates well the pitfalls of the classical methodology of binding (Table V) (7, 8, 14). However, in spite of its limitations and potential source of error, the measurement of binding of labelled hormones, when performed with appropriate caution, has been demonstrated to give useful information, provided the data are correctly interpreted (Table VI).

MOLECULAR MODELS OF RECEPTORS

It is of course possible to imagine a virtually infinite number of more or less complicated models describing receptor and hormone interactions, but only simple and realistic models will be considered here (Table VII). They can be classified according to different criteria : the mechanism of coupling between regulatory and effector units, the existence of cooperative interactions between regulatory units and the eventual heterogeneity of these units (existence of "isoreceptors" by analogy with isoenzymes). Regulatory and effector units can be tightly coupled in the absence and the presence of ligand (non-dissociable receptor); tightly coupled in the absence of ligand, they can dissociate from each other in its presence (dissociable receptor) or, on the contrary, they can be independent in the absence of ligand but interact with each other after binding of the ligand to the regulatory unit (two-step model). The meaning of these three different concepts of receptors can be appreciated in the light of the current models of biomembranes (15). The trilaminar membrane model would seem appropriate to the first two models of receptors : the regulatory unit would be integrated in the outer protein layer and the effector unit in the inner layer; signals could be transmitted from the former to the latter directly through protein interaction or by the phospholipids of the central

TABLE V.   The Catecholamine Binding Controversy

1. *LEFKOWITZ ET AL. (1973)*

   - binding of $^3_1$H nor-epinephrine to heart microsomes
   - correlated with β adrenergic effect and adenylate cyclase
     activation
       (agonist specificity
       (affinity
   - different from neural storage vesicles

       (lack of inhibition by reserpine
       (absence of ATP requirement

   = β adrenergic receptor

2. *CUATRECASAS ET AL. (1974)*

   - binding of $^3_1$H nor-epinephrine to fat cells and heart micro-
     somes

   - not correlated with β adrenergic effect

       (lack of stereospecificity (for (-) N,E,)
       (displacement by non-catecholamine catechols
       (non-displacement by non-catechol agonist (soterenol)

   = catechol-o-methyl transferase (COMT)

       (common inhibition by sulfhydryl blocker
       (common stimulation by S-adenosyl methionine

3. *LEFKOWITZ (1974)*

   - binding of $^3_1$H nor-epinephrine to heart microsomes and other
     tissues

   - different from COMT

       (subcellular distribution
       (affinity
       (substrate specificity
       (lack of COMT activity in purified binding protein

   = ??

N.B. Specific radioactivity : (0,01 CI/μM for $^3_1$H nor-epinephrine
                               (1.0 CI/μM for $^{125}_1$I insulin

   ⟶ Non-detection of the scarce β receptors

part of the membrane (34). The tight coupling between both units
fits well with the pseudo-cristalline rigidity of this membrane.
Thermodynamic considerations and experimental data have led to the
fluid and mosaic model of membranes : there is an alternance of
lipids and proteins some of which extend over the whole thickness
of the membrane, and all these molecules diffuse freely in the
membrane plane (15, 52) (Figure 1). The dissociation model is
thought to apply to cyclic AMP dependent protein kinases (16), but
it could also describe the molecular organization of some hormone
responsive adenylate cyclase systems (17-20).

The concept of cooperativity was originally introduced to
describe oxygen binding to hemoproteins, but has been extensively
applied in enzymology (21-26). Extending the concept to hormone
receptors, they would appear to be polymeric molecules in which
the binding of one ligand molecule to a subunit would induce a
conformational change by which the affinity for the ligand of the
neighbouring unoccupied subunits is either increased (positive
cooperativity) or decreased (negative cooperativity).

TABLE VI.	Measurement of Labelled Hormone Binding to Receptors and Acceptors	
PURPOSES :	1.	Choice of a molecular model which adequately accounts for the data
	2.	Estimation of the model's kinetic and equilibrium parameters
	3.	Calculation of thermodynamic constants (ΔG, ΔH, ΔS)
DATA :	1.	Saturation of the receptors (or acceptors) with labelled hormone (at equilibrium)
	2.	Displacement of labelled hormone by cold hormone
	3.	Dilution of the binding component
	4.	Kinetics of association
	5.	Kinetics of dissociation (− chemical dilution (− isotopic dilution (addition of cold hormone) (− combination of chemical and isotopic dilution
	6.	Use of (− agonists (− antagonists
	7.	Effect of temperature (Arrhenius plot)
ANALYSIS :	1.	Graphical representations
	2.	Curve fitting

TABLE VII. Models of Receptor Design

Binding sites homogeneity, no cooperativity	$RE + H \underset{Kd}{\rightleftharpoons} RHE \qquad RE + H \underset{Kd}{\rightleftharpoons} RH + E$	1. $R + H \underset{Kd_1}{\rightleftharpoons} RH$ 2. $RH + E \underset{Kd_2}{\rightleftharpoons} RHE$
Binding sites heterogeneity, no cooperativity	$RE + H \underset{Kd}{\rightleftharpoons} RHE \qquad RE + H \underset{Kd}{\rightleftharpoons} RH + E$ $R'E + H \underset{Kd'}{\rightleftharpoons} R'HE \qquad R'E + H \underset{Kd'}{\rightleftharpoons} R'H + E$	1. $R + H \underset{Kd_1}{\rightleftharpoons} RH$ $R' + H \underset{K'd_1}{\rightleftharpoons} R'H$ 2. $RH + E \underset{Kd_2}{\rightleftharpoons} RHE$ $R'H + E \underset{K'd_2}{\rightleftharpoons} R'HE$
Positive cooperativity	$Kc>1$ $R_2E + H \underset{Kd}{\rightleftharpoons} R_2HE \qquad R_2E_2 + H \underset{Kd}{\rightleftharpoons} R_2HE + E$ $R_2HE + H \underset{Kd/Kc}{\rightleftharpoons} R_2H_2E \qquad R_2HE + H \underset{Kd/Kc}{\rightleftharpoons} R_2H_2 + E$	$Kc>1$ 1. $R_2 + H \underset{Kd_1}{\rightleftharpoons} R_2H$ $R_2H + H \underset{Kd_1/Kc}{\rightleftharpoons} R_2H_2$ 2. $R_2H_2 + E \underset{Kd_2}{\rightleftharpoons} R_2H_2E$
Negative cooperativity	$Kc<1$	$Kc<1$

Legend   R,R' : *Regulatory units*
         E   : *Effector unit*
         Kd,Kd': *Equilibrium dissociation constants*
         Kc : *Cooperativity constant*

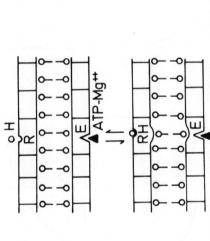
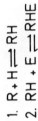
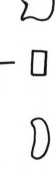

FIGURE 1. *Comparison between the trilaminar and the fluid and mosaic models of plasma membrane.*

R : *regulatory unit; H : hormone (or other ligand); E : effector unit (i.e. adenylate cyclase)*

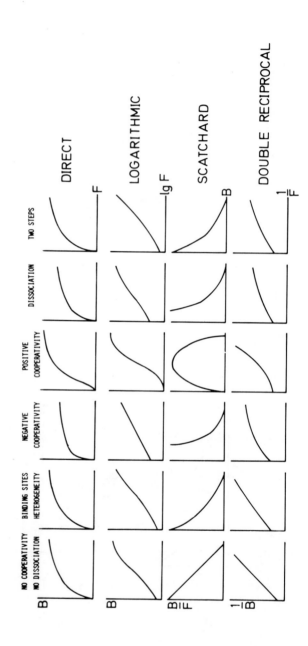

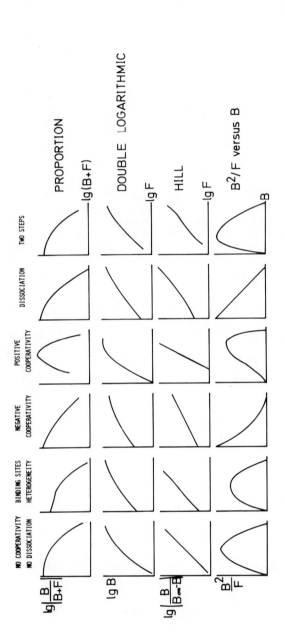

FIGURE 2. Several graphical representations have been simulated for different models of receptors or acceptors.

B : bound hormone concentration; F : free hormone concentration;

$B\infty$ or $(R)_T$: total concentration of binding sites

The parameters characterizing each model are given in Table X and the equations in Table VII, except for cooperativity which was plotted according to the empirical equation of Hill:

$$B = \frac{F^{nH}}{K + F^{nH}}$$

GRAPHICAL REPRESENTATIONS OF SATURATION EXPERIMENTS

The easiest way to analyze saturation experiments is to plot the data in different coordinate systems. The number of possible graphical representations is virtually unlimited : some of them have been listed in Table VIII (27-33). These graphs have a double usefulness : according to their shape, it is possible to choose an adequate model of ligand-receptor interaction, and graphical extrapolation allows then to estimate the model's parameters (Figure 2). The plot most widely used in the field of hormone binding studies is the Scatchard graph : in the case of one class of non-dissociable, tightly coupled and non-cooperative receptors, it is a straight line, with a slope equal to $-1/K_D$ (K_D is the equilibrium dissociation constant) and an abscissa at the origin equal to $(R)_T$ (total concentration of binding sites); when there are two classes of such receptors, it is a hyperbola (Figure 3).

TABLE VIII.   Graphical Representations for Binding Data

NAMES	ORDINATE	ABSCISSA	YEAR OF INTRODUCTION
1.Direct plot, adsorption isotherm	B	F	
2.Logarithmic plot, Bjerrum's formation function, titration curve	B	$\lg F$	1941
3.Double-reciprocal plot, Lineweaver-Burk	$1/B$	$1/F$	1934
4.Half-reciprocal plot, Scott	F/B	F	1956
5.Scatchard, Eadie, Hofstee	B/F	B	1949
6.Hill plot	$\lg \dfrac{B}{(R)t-B}$	$\lg F$	1910
7.Proportion graph, Baulieu and Raynaud	$\lg \dfrac{B}{B+F}$	$\lg (B+F)$	1970
8.Thompson and Klotz	$\lg B$	$\lg F$	1971
9.Boeynaems and Swillens	B^2/F	B	1974

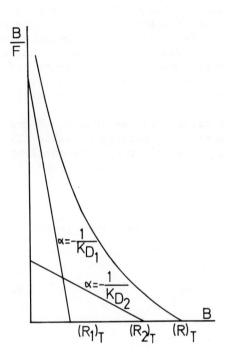

FIGURE 3. Scatchard graph : two classes of independent binding sites. The curve is a hyperbola with two asymptots which characterize the interaction between ligand and each set of sites separately.

$(R_1)T$, $(R_2)T$: total concentration of binding sites

K_{D1}, K_{D2} : equilibrium dissociation constants.

The meaning of a hyperbolic upward concave Scatchard graph, which is often taken as evidence for the existence of multiple receptors with different affinities is in fact ambiguous. It can easily be demonstrated that binding site heterogeneity and negative cooperativity are described by similar equations : both can lead to indistinguishable upward concave hyperbolic Scatchard graphs (25). Moreover, the dissociation model is also characterised by a hyperbolic Scatchard plot, and this is also true, at least for some particular values of the parameters, in the case of a two-step receptor (Figure 4). The B^2/F versus B graph allows one to determine the existence of a dissociable receptor but does not permit discrimination between negative cooperativity and the two-step mechanism. Because of such ambiguities, interpretation of graphical representations clearly requires great caution.

Some empirical values such as (H)0.5, nH and R_H are often used to characterize saturation experiments (Table IX). It is generally believed that (H)0.5 is equal to K_D (the equilibrium dissociation

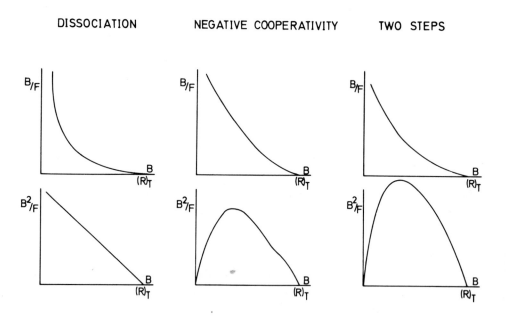

FIGURE 4. Comparison between the Scatchard and the B^2/F versus B representations for three different models of binding. Equations characterizing each model are given in Table VII.

constant of the hormone-receptor interaction). This is not always true, for instance, in the case of a dissociable receptor, $(H)0.5 = \dfrac{K_D \cdot (R)_T}{2}$ and K_D is dimensionless (33). R_H is supposed to be equal to 81, in the absence of cooperativity, less than 81 if there is positive cooperativity and more than 81 for negative cooperativity; in the same conditions, nH would be equal, greater or less than 1, respectively. Table X shows that, both for a dissociable and a two-step receptor, R_H and nH have values typical of negative cooperativity.

METHODOLOGIC ERRORS AND GRAPHICAL REPRESENTATIONS

Several methodologic errors (Table IV) can distort graphical representations and eventually lead to false conclusions. If bound and free hormone are separated before equilibrium of binding has been reached, Scatchard graphs will exhibit an upward convexity, suggestive of positive cooperativity (Figure 5).The same effect will be observed if, during the incubation with binding components, the hormone is inactivated by a zero order process (50) whereas, if the inactivation follows a 1st order kinetics, the shape of the Scatchard graph will not be modified but the apparent affinity will be artefactually lowered (51) (Figure 6).

TABLE IX. Empirical Values used to Characterize Saturation or Concentration-Action Curves

$(H)_{0.5}$ (half saturation concentration)

        Definition : Hormone concentration for which :
                       (half the binding sites are occupied
                       (a half-maximal effect is produced

        Meaning : Supposed index of affinity

$R_H = \dfrac{H_{0.9}}{H_{0.1}}$ *Definition* : Ratio between the hormone concentration for which respectively 90 % and 10 % of the binding sites are occupied

        Meaning : Supposed index of cooperativity

nH (Hill's coefficient)

        Definition : Slope of the Hill's plot

        Meaning : Supposed index of cooperativity

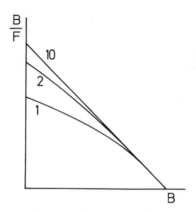

<u>FIGURE 5</u>. *One set of non-dissociable and non-cooperative binding sites : separation of B and F performed after various incubation times. Scatchard plot. F : free hormone concentration; f : fractional occupancy of the binding sites.*

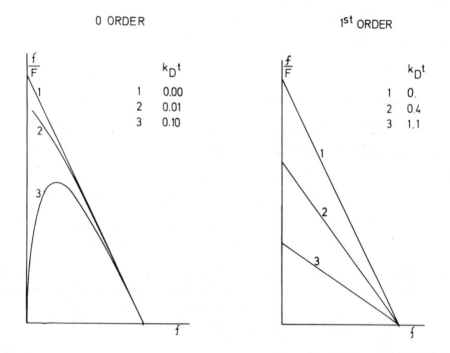

<u>FIGURE 6</u>. *Hormone inactivation by the receptor-containing preparation : comparison between 0 and 1st order kinetics of inactivation. Scatchard plot. Zero order : k_D = nM x min^{-1}; 1st order : k_D = min^{-1}; k_D : inactivation constant; t : time.*

TABLE X

MODEL	n_H	$R_H = \dfrac{(H)0.9}{(H)0.1}$
No cooperativity No dissociation	1	81
Binding sites heterogeneity $(R_1)t = 0.1 \quad Kd_1 = 0.1$ $(R_2)t = 0.9 \quad Kd_2 = 1.0$	0.92	116
Positive cooperativity (Hill)	2	9
Negative cooperativity (Hill)	0.50	6,561
Dissociation $(R)_t = 1 \qquad Kd = 1$	0.61	729
Two steps $(R)_t = 1 \qquad Kd_1 = 1$ $(E)_t = 0.3 \quad Kd_2 = 0.1$	0.81	184

LEGEND :   nH: Hill's index
           (H)0.9: Ligand concentration for which 90 % of the
                      binding sites are occupied
           (H)0.1: Idem 10 %

Characteristic parameters for the different models which are illustrated in Figure 2 and defined in Table   VII.

    The binding can also be measured during the dissociation process, for instance, when free and bound hormone are separated by millipore filtration. In this case, the incubation medium containing both forms of the hormone is eluted on the filter which is then washed with hormone-free buffer. If this washing procedure is too long, some of the bound hormone can dissociate at this time. Let us suppose that there are two sets of receptor sites, one with high affinity and slow dissociation and the other with low affinity and rapid dissociation. If the duration of the washing process increases, the contribution of this second set of sites decreases so that the binding sites appear falsely homogeneous (Figure 7). This consequence may seem unimportant as only the low affinity site will be missed. However, very high affinity sites could also be lost if their kinetic association and dissociation constants were high.

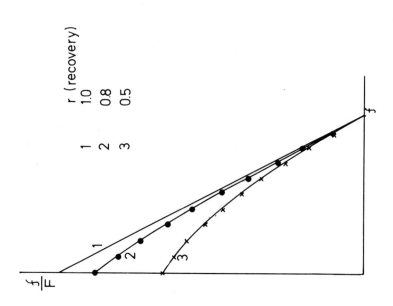
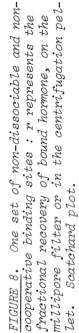

FIGURE 8. One set of non-dissociable and non-cooperative binding sites : r represents the fractional recovery of bound hormone, on the millipore filter or in the centrifugation pellet. Scatchard plot.

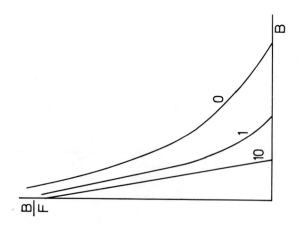

FIGURE 7. Two sets of non-dissociable and non-cooperative binding sites (one with high affinity and slow dissociation, one with low affinity and rapid dissociation) : effect of increasing the duration of washing. Scatchard plot.

TABLE XI : Examples of Recently Proposed Models of Hormone-Receptor Interaction

A. TIGHTLY COUPLED RECEPTORS

1. Homogeneity	Insulin	Fat cells	Kono & Barham	1971
			Cuatrecasas	1971
	HGH	Lymphocyte	Lesniak et al.	1974
	LH	Ovary	Lee & Ryan	1973
	TSH	Thyroid	Verrier et al.	1974
2. Heterogeneity	ACTH	Adrenal	Lefkowitz et al.	1971
	TSH	Thyroid	Manley et al.	1972
	Insulin	Fat cells	Hammond et al.	1972
	Insulin	Liver	Kahn et al.	1974
	Glucagon	Liver	Shlatz & Marinetti	1972
3. Negative cooperativity	Insulin	Lymphocyte	De Meyts et al.	1973
4. Positive cooperativity	TSH	Thyroid	Haye & Jacquemin	1971
	Glucagon	Liver	Rodbell et al.	1974
	Vasopressin	Kidney	Roy et al.	1974
5. Negative & positive cooperativity	Oxytocin	Bladder	Roy et al.	1973
	TSH	Thyroid	Pochet et al.	1974

B. DISSOCIABLE RECEPTOR | Glucagon | Heart | Levey et al. | 1974 |

C. TWO-STEP RECEPTOR

If only a fraction of the total bound hormone is retained on the millipore filter or trapped in a centrifugation pellet, the Scatchard graph is once again distorted : from its upward convexity, a false conclusion of positive cooperativity could be drawn (Figure 8). So, three different types of artefacts (non-quantitative recovery of bound hormone, non-equilibrium conditions, zero order inactivation of hormone) lead to an upward convex Scatchard graph : this peculiar shape is thus not pathognomonic of positive cooperativity.

CONCLUSION

Several models of the molecular organization of hormone receptors have been proposed (Table XI) (35-49). These models differ according to the tissue or the hormone, the authors or the date. In 1970, molecular heterogeneity appeared to be a general rule for membrane hormone receptors. In 1973, this was no longer up to date : cooperativity was proposed as a universal mechanism. Perhaps 1975 will see the fashion of the two-step receptor !

The fundamental question to be asked is : do all the membrane receptors follow the same design, irrespective of hormone or tissue ? In this case, the discrepancies found in the literature would be explained by erroneous methodology and interpretation of results. What might such a universal model, applicable to all hormone receptors, be : cooperativity, dissociation or two-step ? The question is at present unanswered. Conversely, the reported differences could correspond to a reality : glucagon receptors could be positively cooperative in the liver and dissociable in the heart, whereas liver insulin receptors would be negatively cooperative One is then entitled to wonder what is the meaning of the non-universality of hormone receptors design.

REFERENCES

(1) CORBIN, J.D. (1975) in "Regulation of Function and Growth of Eukaryotic Cells by Intracellular Cyclic Nucleotides", ed. J.E. Dumont, B. Brown, N. Marshall, NATO Course, Wépion, 1974 Plenum Publishing Corp., New York

(2) DE CROMBRUGGHE, B., CHEN, B., ANDERSON, W., NISSLEY, S.P., GOTTESMAN, M., PERLMAN, R., PASTAN, I (1971), Nature New Biology, 231, 139

(3) BIRNBAUMER, L., POHL, S.L., KAUMANN, A.J. (1974) in "Advances in Cyclic Nucleotide Research", ed. P. Greengard, G.A. Robison, Raven Press, New York, 4

(4) POHL, S.L., KRANS, H.M.J., BIRNBAUMER, L., RODBELL, M. (1972) J. Biol. Chem., 247, 2295

(5) FREYCHET, P., KAHN, R., ROTH, J., NEVILLE, D.M. (1972) J. Biol. Chem., 247, 3953

(6) MARX, S.J., FEDAK, S.A., AURBACH, G.D. (1972) J. Biol. Chem. 247, 6913

(7) CUATRECASAS, P., TELL, G.P.E., SICA, V., PARIKH, I., CHANG, K.J. (1974), Nature, 257, 92

(8) LEFKOWTIZ, R.J., SHARP, G.W.G., HABER, E (1973) J. Biol. Chem. 248, 342

(9) BERGERON, J.J.M., EVANS, W.H., GESCHWIND, I.I. (1973), J. Cell Biol., 59, 771

(10) SONENBERG, M. (1971), Proceed. Natl. Acad. Sci. US, 68, 1051

(11) SCHNEIDER, A.B., EDELHOCH, H. (1972) J. Biol. Chem., 247, 4986

(12) BIRNBAUMER, L. (1973), Biochim. Biophys. Acta, 300, 129

(13) PERKINS, J.P. (1973) in "Advances in Cyclic Nucleotide Research", ed. P. Greengard, G.A. Robison, Raven Press, New York, 3

(14) LEFKOWITZ, R.J. (1974) Biochem. Biophys. Res. Comm., 58, 1110

(15) SINGER, S.J., NICOLSON, G.L., (1972) Science, 175, 720

(16) BROSTROM, C.O., CORBIN, J.D., KING, C.A., KREBS, F.G. (1971) Proceed. Natl. Acad. Sci. US, 68, 2444

(17) PERKINS, J.P. MOORE, M.H. (1971), J. Biol. Chem., 246, 62

(18) BITENSKY, M.W., GORMAN, R.E., MILLER, W.H. (1972) Science, 175, 1363

(19) KREINER, P.W., KEVINS, J.J. BITENSKY, M.W. (1973) Proceed. Natl. Acad. Sci. US, 70, 1785

(20) LEVEY, G.S., FLETCHER, M.A., KLEIN, I., RUIZ, E., SCHENK, A. (1974) J. Biol. Chem., 249, 2665

(21) MONOD, J., WYMAN, J., CHANGEUX, J.P. (1965), J. Mol. Biol., 12, 88

(22) KOSHLAND, D.E., NEMETHY, G., FILMER, D. (1966) Biochemistry, 5, 365

(23) BRIEHL, R.W. (1963) J. Biol. Chem., 238, 2361

(24) CHANGEUX, J.P., THIERY, J., TUNG, Y., KITTEL, C. (1967) Proceed. Natl. Acad. Sci. US, 57, 335

(25) LEVITZKI, A., KOSHLAND, D.E., (1968) Proceed. Natl. Acad. Sci. US, 62, 1121

(26) HERZFELD, J., STANLEY, H.E. (1974), J. Mol. Biol., 82, 231

(27) DERANLEAU, D.A. (1969), J. Am. Chem. Soc., 91, 4044

(28) HILL, A.V., (1910), J. Physiol., 40, 190

(29) SCATCHARD, G. (1949), Ann. N.Y. Acad. Sci., 51, 660

(30) LINEWEAVER, H., BURK, D. (1934), J. Am. Chem. Soc., 56, 658

(31) BAULIEU, E.E., RAYNAUD, J.P. (1970), Eur. J. Biochem. 13, 293

(32) THOMPSON, C.J., KLOTZ, I.M. (1971), Arch. Biochem. Biophys., 147, 178

(33) SWILLENS, S., VAN CAUTER, E., DUMONT, J.E. (1974), Biochim. Biophys. Acta, 364, 250

(34) RODBELL, M., BIRNBAUMER, L., POHL, S.L. (1969) in "The Role of Adenyl Cyclase and Cyclic 3',5'-AMP in Biological Systems", ed. T.W. Rall, M. Rodbell, P. Condliffe. N.I.H., Bethesda, 59

(35) VERRIER, B., FAYET, G., LISSITZKY, S. (1974), Europ. J. Biochem. 42, 355

(36) KONO, T., BARHAM, F.W. (1971), J. Biol. Chem., 246, 6210

(37) KAHN, C.R., FREYCHET, P., ROTH, J., NEVILLE, D.M. (1974) J. Biol. Chem., 249, 2249

(38) DE MEYTS, P., ROTH, J., NEVILLE, D.M., GAVIN, J.R., LESNIAK, M.A. (1973), Biochem. Biophys. Res. Comm., 55, 154

(39) RODBELL, M., LIN, M.C., SALOMON, Y., (1974), J. Biol. Chem. 249, 59

(40) ROY, C. (1975) in "Regulation of Function and Growth of Eukaryotic Cells by Intracellular Cyclic Nucleotides", ed. J.E. Dumont, B. Brown, N. Marshall, NATO Course, Wépion, 1974, Plenum Publishing Corp.

(41) CUATRECASAS, P. (1971), Proceed. Natl. Acad. Sci. US, 68, 1264

(42) LEFKOWITZ, R.J., ROTH, J., PASTAN, I (1972), Ann. N.Y. Acad. Sci., 195

(43) ROY, C., BOCKAERT, J., RAJERISON, R., JARD, S. (1973) FEBS Letters, 30, 329

(44) LESNIAK, M.A., GORDEN, P., ROTH, J., GAVIN, J.R. (1974) J. Biol. Chem., 249, 1661

(45) SHLATZ, L., MARINETTI, G.V. (1972), Science, 176, 175

(46) HAMMOND, J.M., JARETT, L., MARIZ, I.K., DAUGHADAY, W.H. (1972) Biochem. Biophys. Res. Comm. 49, 1122

(47) POCHET, R., BOEYNAEMS, J.M., DUMONT, J.E. (1974), Biochem. Biophys. Res. Comm., 58, 446

(48) HAYE, B., JACQUEMIN, C. (1971) FEBS Letters, 18, 47

(49) MANLEY, S.W., BOURKE, J.R. HAWKER, R.W. (1972) J. Endocrin., 55, 555

(50) LEE, C.Y., RYAN, R.J. (1973) Biochemistry, 12, 4609

(51) DESBUQUOIS, B., KRUG, F., CUATRECASAS, P. (1974) Biochim. Biophys. Acta, 343, 101

(52) CUATRECASAS, P. (1974), Ann. Rev. Biochem., 43, 169

ON THE MODES OF REGULATION OF INTRACELLULAR CYCLIC AMP:
DESENSITIZATION OF ADENYLYL CYCLASES TO HORMONAL STIMULATION
AND COMPARTMENTALIZATION OF CYCLIC AMP

L. Birnbaumer, J. Bockaert, M. Hunzicker-Dunn,
V. Pliška, and A. Glattfelder

Department of Physiology, Northwestern University Medical
School, Chicago, Illinois; Department of Molecular Medicine, Mayo Medical School, Rochester, Minnesota; Institut
für Molekularbiologie and Biophysik and Institut für Mess-
and Regeltechnik, ETH, Zürich, Switzerland

CONTENTS

1. INTRODUCTION

Intracellular levels of cyclic AMP are generally considered to
be the result of the complex interplay between formation of cyclic
AMP by adenylyl cyclase and removal of cyclic, either through hydrolysis by phosphodiesterase (PDE) or extrusion from the cell by active
or passive transport across the plasma membrane. In addition cyclic
AMP levels may also be determined by unequal distribution throughout
the cell. Of the systems involved in the regulation of intracellular
cyclic AMP levels, other articles in this book deal with the regulation of adenylyl cyclases by stimulatory and inhibitory hormones
and by nucleotides and nucleosides with regulation of PDE activities both in rapid and reversible manners as well as in slow and
possibly protein synthesis dependent manners; and with regulation

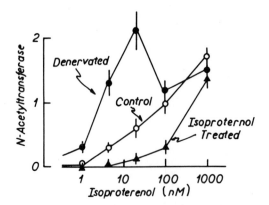

Fig. 1.   Effect of in vivo denervation or isoproterenol treatment on the subsequent sensitivity of explanted rat pineal glands to
in vitro isoproterenol. The synthesis of serotonin N-acetyltransferase vs the concentration of in vitro isoproterenol is shown. Adapted
from Deguchi and Axelrod (1).

of exit rates of cyclic AMP as seen in some cell lines after virus
transformation. This chapter will deal with two other regulatory
mechanisms: 1) hormone-induced desensitization of adenylyl cyclases,
for which good experimental evidence is already available, and 2)
feedback regulated compartmentalization of cyclic AMP, whose existence is still somewhat speculative.

2. REGULATION OF CYCLIC AMP LEVELS BY DESENSITIZATION OF ADENYLYL
CYCLASE TO HORMONAL STIMULATION.

     Experiments with intact animals, tissue slices, or isolated
cells frequently have demonstrated that elevations of cyclic AMP
levels induced by stimulating hormones are followed by a rapid return to basal or close to basal levels, even in the presence of
active hormone. In many systems this return is accompanied by a
loss or diminution of hormone action. For example, Deguchi and
Axelrod (1), exploring the sensitivity to catecholamines of pineal
glands explanted from animals previously exposed to increased or decreased sympathetic stimulation of their glands, found that cyclic
AMP accumulation in response to isoproterenol as well as the resulting induction of serotonin N-acetyltransferase is altered by these
treatments (Figs. 1 and 2). Treatments leading to low or no sympathetic stimulation (denervation or reserpine) resulted in increased cyclic AMP accumulation in response to isoproterenol and in
an increase of the sensitivity to isoproterenol action, i.e. in a
lowering of the concentration of isoproterenol needed to obtain

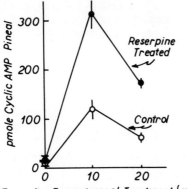

Fig. 2.   Effect of treatment of rats with reserpine on the
capacity of explanted pineal glands to respond to in vitro exposure
to isoproterenol with increased cyclic AMP accumulation.   Adapted
from Deguchi and Axelrod (1).

Table 1
Hormone-specific desensitization of hormonal
stimulation in macrophages of guinea pigs.

Addition to Cells (2 hours)	Adenylyl Cyclase Activity due to		
	PGE_1	Epinephrine	NaF
None	77	63	126
PGE_1	14	52	125
Epinephrine	59	8	122

Adapted from Remold-O'Donnell (2).

half-maximal induction of the N-acetyltransferase activity.   On the
other hand, treatments leading to increased sympathetic stimulation
of the gland (such as constant darkness or injection of isoproterenol) resulted in the opposite effect, i.e. in an increase of the
concentration needed to obtain a half-maximal induction of the
enzyme.   These results suggest that pre-exposure of adenylyl cyclase
systems to their stimulant may result in a loss of responsiveness.
Indeed pre-exposure of cells to specific adenylyl cyclase stimulating agents has resulted in loss of responsiveness of the system
to the stimulating hormones in several other systems as well.
Remold-O'Donnell (2) studied the effect of exposing isolated guinea
pig macrophages to catecholamines and prostaglandins on the response
of the adenylyl cyclase system.   As shown in Table I, adapted from
the report of Remold-O'Donnell, treatment of the cells with either
a catecholamine or a prostaglandin resulted in desensitization of
the adenylyl cyclase system to their own response with little or

no cross-over effect. This clearly indicated that macrophages have
a stimulant-specific process that results in a selective inhibition
of the responsiveness of adenylyl cyclase and raised the question
as to what the mechanism might be by which the desensitization is
induced. We investigated this question by studying the mechanism
by which luteinizing hormone (LH) and human chorionic gonadotrophin
(hCG) exert some of their actions on Graafian follicles of various
species.

Table II
Effect of LH and PGE_1 on cyclic AMP synthesis in
cultured Graafian follicles of rat ovaries

Addition to Culture (18 hours)	Labelled cyclic AMP formed (20') in the presence of		
		LH	PGE_1
None	90	3320	3920
LH	730	830	3220

Adapted from Lamprecht et al. (3).

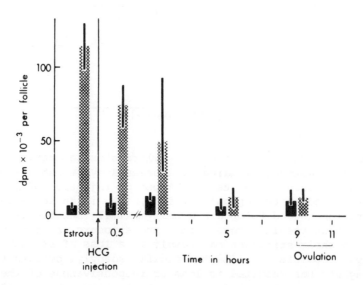

Fig. 3 Effect of in vivo administration of an ovulatory dose of
hCG to estrous rabbits on the capacity of their Graafian follicles
to respond at varying times after hCG to in vitro LH exposure with
an increased accumulation of labelled cyclic AMP obtained in the
absence and the presence of in vitro LH, respectively. (From
Marsh et al., 5.)

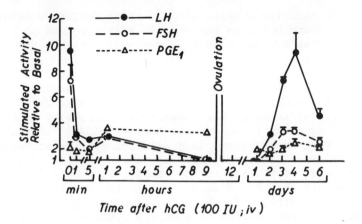

Fig. 4 Effect of in vivo administration of an ovulatory dose of hCG to estrous rabbits on the responsiveness to LH of the adenylyl cyclase system of their Graafian follicles and resulting corpora lutea (CL) formed after ovulation. Estrous rabbits (New Zealand White, 3.5 to 4.5 Kg) were given 100 IU, iv, of hCG (Ayerst) and sacrificed by cervical dislocation at the times indicated on the figures. Their ovaries were removed and immediately cooled to 0° in iced KRB. Estrous and pre-ovulatory Graafian follicles as well as CL resulting from the hCG injection were dissected, kept in iced KRB until homogenization and homogenized (Dounce) in 10 volumes of medium containing 27% (w/w) sucrose, 1.0 mM EDTA and 10 mM Tris-HCl, pH 7.5. The homogenate was filtered through #12 silk screen, diluted with an equal volume of homogenizing medium and assayed for basal and hormonally responsive adenylyl cyclase activities. Adenylyl cyclase incubations were for 10 min. at 37° in medium containing 3.0 mM ATP labelled in the α position with ^{32}P (pH 7.0), 5.0 mM $MgCl_2$, 1.0 mM EDTA, 1.0 mM cyclic AMP, 20 mM creatine phosphate (pH 7.0), 0.2 mg per ml of creatine kinase, 25 mM Tris-HCl pH 7.0, homogenate protein, and when present 10 µg per ml of LH (NIH-LH-B8), FSH (NIB-FSH-Pl) or PGE_1 (Upjohn). The one min. point was obtained by injecting the rabbit followed by immediate cervical dislocation and removal of the ovary. Incubation of estrous follicles dissected in the above described manner with 20 IU per ml of hCG at 22° for 30 min. did not induce any loss of responsiveness of their adenylyl cyclase to either LH or FSH. The 0 min point was obtained with Graafian follicles dissected from ovaries of estros rabbits (no injections). Adenylyl cyclase activities were determined in duplicate incubations. Single points represent one assay in which a minimum of 1 rabbits were used. Mean + SEM is shown where 2 to 6 such assays were performed. Data are expressed as "Activities relative to basal" and were obtained by dividing the activities obtained in the presence of hormonal stimulus by the respective activity obtained in their absence.

   Two laboratories working with Graafian follicles reported, in
1973, that LH and hCG also induced, in what appeared to be the
adenylyl cyclase system, a loss of responsiveness to themselves.
Thus, Lamprecht et al. (3) reported that excised rat graafian follicles when exposed during 18 hr. to LH, loose their capacity to
accumulate follicular cAMP in response to newly added LH, while not
loosing the capacity to do the same in response to PGE_2 (Table II).
Marsh et al. (4) reported that Graafian follicles of estrous rabbits
loose their capacity to accumulate labeled cAMP if the rabbits are
pretreated with an ovulatory (and adenylyl cyclase stimulating) dose
of hCG (Fig. 3). Since this loss of cAMP accumulating capacity after
ovulatory doses of hCG is, in the rabbit, accompanied by a loss of
steroidogenesis (5), the desensitization to LH stimulation was
likely due to a direct effect on the adenylyl cyclase of the follicles. Direct determination of adenylyl cyclase activity in homogenates of rabbit Graafian follicles in our laboratory confirmed
this assumption (Fig. 4 and 5). Note that loss of response (Fig. 4)
is real and not due to an increase of basal activity by bound hCG
(Fig. 5).

   In contrast to other desensitizing processes described in the
literature, the one operative in Graafian follicles leads to loss
of responsiveness very rapidly. This characteristic led us to investigate whether desensitization is obtainable in broken cell preparation. Experiments reported elsewhere had suggested that de-

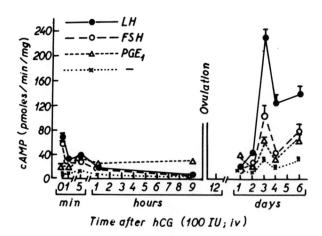

Fig. 5. Same as Fig. 4 but data expressed as absolute activities.
Note that the fall in responsiveness seen in the previous figure
is not due to elevation of the baseline basal activity.

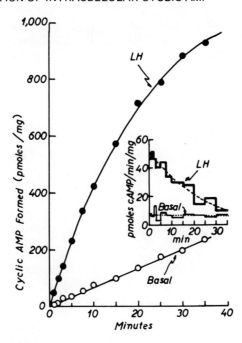

Fig. 6. Non-linearity of LH-stimulated adenylyl cyclase activity
in membranes from pig Graafian follicles. The reaction mixture contained 1.5 mM [α-^{32}P] ATP, 5.0 mM MgCl$_2$, 1.0 mM EDTA, 1.0 mM EGTA,
1.0 mM cyclic AMP, 20 mM creatine phosphate (pH 7.0), 0.2 mg per ml
of creatine kinase, 25 mM Bis-Tris-propane-HCl buffer, pH 7.0, 15μg
membrane protein and, when present 10 μg per ml LH (NIH-LH-B9).
Points represent individual incubations in the absence (0) or presence (0) of LH. Incubations were carried out for the indicated time
at 30°. Inset: Time course of loss of LH-stimulated adenylyl cyclase activity. Same data as in main figure but expressed as rates.
Note that the rate of cyclic AMP accumulation between 30 and 35 min.
was nearly the same in the presence of hormone as in its absence.
Details of the preparation of the membrane particles from pig Graafian
follicles are described by us elsewhere in this book. In other experiments we found that 1. levels of ATP were maintained throughout
the incubation regardless of presence of LH, and 2. that LH addition
to basal at 30 min. results in stimulation with characteristics similar to those seen where LH is added at time zero.

sensitization occurs not only in Graafian follicles of the rat and
the rabbit, but also of the pig, and we therefore prepared membrane
particles from mature (see Channing [6]) Graafian follicles of pigs.
Sufficient quantities can be prepared from pigs to carry out detailed studies of the properties of the adenylyl cyclase system. A
study of the time course of cAMP formation by membrane adenylyl

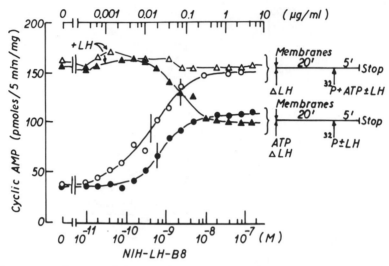

Fig. 7. Dependency of loss of responsiveness to LH on LH concentration and ATP. Graafian follicle membranes were incubated in completed adenylyl cyclase assay medium (see legend to Fig. 6) at 1.25 fold
its final concentration except for the addition of LH, unlabelled ATP
and labeled ATP (5 x 10[6] cpm with sp. act. greater than 5 Ci/mmole)
which were added when indicated. Final volume of first stage of
incubation (20 min. long "desensitization reaction") was 40 ul.
Volume of post-addition was 10 ul. Two sets of determination were
carried out: one without ATP in the desensitization reaction and
the other with 0.625 mM ATP in the desensitization stage of the
incubation. Abscissa, concentration of LH added during the desensitization reaction (shown on the schematic protocol as Δ LH; open
circles, activities of membranes incubated 20 min. in the presence
of varying LH but without ATP and assayed for 5 min. without further
addition of LH; closed circles, activities of membranes incubated
20 min. in the presence of varying LH but without ATP and assayed
for 5 min. with further addition of 10 μg/ml of LH; open triangles,
activities of membranes incubated 20 min. in the presence of ATP
and varying concentrations of LH and assayed for 5 min without
further addition of LH; closed triangles, activities of membranes
incubated 20 min. in the presence of ATP and varying concentrations
of LH and assayed for 5 min. with further addition of 10 μg/ml of
LH. Points represent individual incubations; vertical lines mark
concentrations at which the respective half-maximal effects were
obtained. Apparent K_m values of activation for LH (as assayed in
the final 5-min. adenylyl cyclase assay) were 4.6 x 10[-10] M when
the first stage of incubation was carried out in the absence, and
6.2 x 10[-10] M when carried out in the presence of ATP (the difference is not significant); half maximal desensitization was obtained
with 2.5 x 10[-9] M LH in the desensitization reaction (this 4- to
5-fold difference being highly (p < 0.001) significant). For rest
of details, see legend to Fig. 6.

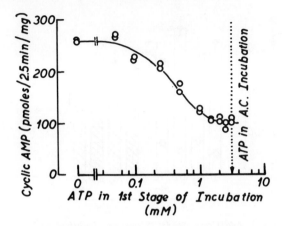

Fig. 8. Dependency of LH-mediated desensitization on ATP concentration. A first (desensitization) stage of incubation was carried out as above at 30° for 20 min. and in the presence of 10 μg per ml of LH and the indicated concentrations of ATP. After 20 min. the second 5 min. stage of incubation was started by addition of 10 ul of medium containing labeled ATP (5 x 10[6] cpm, sp. act. greater than 5 Ci/mmole), 5 μg LH, and varying amounts of unlabeled ATP to give a final concentration of 1.5 mM (marked with a dotted line).

cyclase confirmed that a desensitization mechanism is operative in these membranes. As shown in Fig. 6, adenylyl cyclase activity preceeds linearly under the assay conditions for about 30 to 35 min in the absence but not in the presence of LH. The activity in the presence of LH (6 to 8 times greater than basal at the beginning of the incubation) decays within 35 min. to levels almost identical to basal activity. This loss of stimulated activity was found to be dependent on LH concentration as well as on ATP and not due to metabolism of LH (Fig. 7) since both LH and ATP had to be present during the desensitization stage of the incubation (first 20 min.) and further addition of LH could not overcome the loss of activity. The ATP concentration necessary to obtain half maximal inhibition of LH response is about 0.5 mM (Fig. 8). Loss of responsiveness was found also to require Mg in the incubation (Fig. 9), but was independent of cAMP since the effect could be elicited either in the presence of 1 mM cAMP or when cAMP was substituted by theophylline (Fig. 10). GTP, on the other hand, could not be used in place of ATP (Fig. 11), neither could AMP-PNP, the non-phosphorylating analogue of ATP (Fig. 12). We consistently obtained some loss of LH response when membranes were incubated with ATP-Mg alone (see Fig.

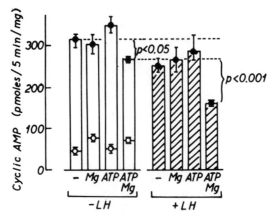

Fig. 9. Dependence of desensitization process on ATP, Mg and LH.
The basic protocol was the same as described in the legend to Fig.
7. Additions of the first stage of incubation (basic medium lack-
ed ATP, $MgCl_2$ and LH) are shown below the respective bars. When
present in the first stage of incubation, ATP was 0.625 mM, $MgCl_2$
(Mg on figure) was 6.25 mM and LH (NIH-LH-B8) was 12.5 µg per ml.
After 20 min. at 30° the second stage of incubation (adenylyl cyclase
assay) was initiated by addition of 10 µl of labeled ATP (5 x 10^6
cpm, sp, act. greater than 5 Ci/mmole) containing the ATP and $MgCl_2$
necessary to complete the adenylyl cyclase assay (final ATP: 0.5 mM
and final $MgCl_2$ added: 5.0 mM) without (o) and with (•) 0.5 µg LH.
o, no LH in first incubation, no LH in second incubation (basal
activities); •, either no LH (open bars) or 12.5 µg per ml of LH
(hatched bars) in first incubation, additional 10 µg per ml LH in
second incubation. Points are means ± range of triplicate determinations (open bars) and of sextuplicate determinations (hatched
bars). Significance of difference was calculated by Students' test.

9 and 10). The reason for this became clear when the dependency of
the desensitizing process on Mg was investigated. As shown in Fig.
13, LH is not an absolute requirement for loss of LH action. Treatment of membrane particles with sufficiently high concentrations
of Mg also resulted in loss of LH responsiveness, the effect of
LH being that of shifting towards lower values the concentration of
Mg required for effectively desensitizing the system to LH stimulation, i.e. that of LH sensitizing the adenylyl cyclase to an ATP and
Mg dependent process whose action leads to a breakdown (uncoupling)
of the receptor-adenylyl cyclase interaction. In other experiments
we established that at 10 µg/ml neither FSH nor PGE_1 (that stimulates pig Graafian follicle adenylyl cyclase 30% as effectively as

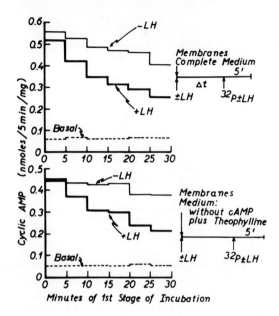

Fig. 10. Lack of an effect of substituting theophylline for cyclic
AMP in the reaction medium on the LH-stimulated desensitization
of the adenylyl cyclase system to respond to LH. The basic protocol is described on the figure. ---, first stage of incubation
carried out in the absence of LH, no LH in the second stage of incubation; continuous lines, LHpresent in the second stage; ____ , no
LH in first stage of incubation, 10 ug per ml LH in second stage of
incubation (control);====, LH present in both stages of incubation.
Note that presence of LH during the first stage of incubation stimulates loss of LH sensitivity regardles of whether the reaction is
carried out in the presence of cAMP (1.0 mM) or theophylline (10 mM).
Rest of incubations were the same as described in the legends to Figs.
6,7, and 9.

LH) induced desensitization to LH, indicating that the effect of
LH is specific and therefore mediated by an LH receptor.

The ineffectivenses of AMP-PNP in supporting the desensitization reaction strongly suggests that desensitization is mediated by
a phosphorylation reaction.

Which of the elements of adenylyl cyclase is phosphorylated
and how does desensitization or uncoupling come about is not yet
known. Roth and collaborators, after careful studies of insulin-
dependent regulation of the concentration of insulin binding sites
on target cells, suggested that certain hormone resistant states
may be associated with loss of hormone receptors (7,8). Thus, one

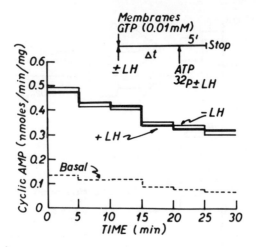

Fig. 11. Lack of LH-stimulated loss of sensitivity to LH when the reactions are carried out in the presence of GTP (10^{-5}M). The loss of LH-stimulated activity during the first stage of incubation in the absence of LH is parallel to the loss of basal activity and is due to the fact that in the presence of GTP the adenylyl cyclase system is less stable to incubation at 30° than in its absence. Rest of incubation conditions were the same as described in the legends to Fig. 6,7, and 9.

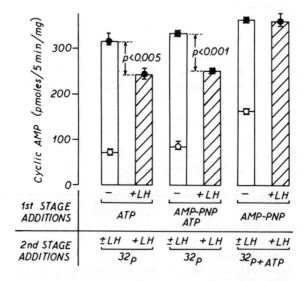

Fig. 12. Lack of capacity of AMP-PNP to support LH stimulated de-sensitization of pig Graafian follicle adenylyl cyclase to LH. The desensitization reaction (20 min, 30°) carried out in the pre-

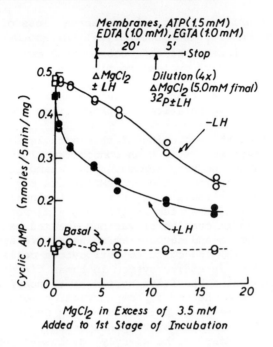

Fig. 13. Dependence of the desensitization process on Mg, lack of need for LH and stimulating effect of LH. The basic protocol is described in the figure. To that effect membrane particles were incubated in the absence (o) or presence (o) of LH (10 µg per ml) for 20 min at 30° in 25 µl of medium containing all adenylyl cyclase reagents and the indicated concentrations of ATP, EDTA, EGTA, and MgCl$_2$ (the last shown as concentration in excess of 3.5 mM on the abscissa). The reaction medium was then diluted with 75 µl of adenylyl cyclase assay reagents containing the same concentrations of ATP, EDTA, EGTA (totalling 3.5 mM) but varying concentrations of MgCl$_2$ to give a constant final concentration during the 5 min. adenylyl cyclase assay of 5.0 mM (total added, i.e. 1.5 mM in excess of 3.5 mM). ____, 10 µg per ml of LH added to the second stage of incubation; ----, no LH added to the second stage of incubation.

---

sence of either ATP (1.25 mM), AMP-PNP (1.25 mM) or both. Rest of conditions are described on the figure and in the legend to Fig. 9. Note that AMP-PNP does not interfere with the LH-stimulated desensitization and that therefore the lack of desensitization seen with AMP-PNP alone is due to its inability to support the desensitization process and not due to a combination of a possible capacity to support the desensitization reaction and a strong inhibitory effect on this same process. Activities were calculated on the basis of labeled ATP converted to cyclic AMP; no corrections were made for AMP-PNP addition.

mechanism of desensitization may be an actual loss of active receptors upon hormone-induced phosphorylation; another may be alteration, via phosphorylation, of the phospholipid environment surrounding the receptor-adenylyl cyclase complex, known to be an important
factor determining optimal receptor-catalytic unit coupling (9,10).
Clearly further investigation is needed to establish the molecular
site(s) affected by the putative phosphorylating process.

As mentioned at the beginning of this article, desensitization
of the adenylyl cyclase system with concomitant loss or diminution
of hormone action may be very common. Thus examples where the
transient nature of the increase of cAMP levels may be due to desensitization of the stimulated system in rat pineal, the catecho-
lamine- and PG-sensitive system in guinea pig macrophages and the
LH-sensitive system in ovaries of various species mentioned above
but also the histamine-and catecholamine-sensitive system in rabbit
cerebellar slices (11) and cultured astrocytoma cells (12), the
catecholamine and PG sensitive system in human fibroblasts (13), and
perhaps the epinephrine-sensitive system of thymocytes (14). It will
be interesting to see whether a phosphorylation mechanism similar
to the one above in membrane particles of pig Graafian follicles is
involved also in the changes of responsiveness of other systems.
These systems may or may not be adenylyl cyclase-dependent, such
as the increased sensitivity of adrenals to ACTH seen after hypophysectomy or morphine tolerance seen in the myenteric plexus of
guinea pig ileum after chronic morphine treatment. Interestingly,
in the latter system (15), morphine tolerance (that expresses itself in a loss of sensitivity of the inhibitory action of morphine
on electrically stimulated plexus activity) is accompanied by subsensitivity to inhibitory catecholamines and supersensitivity to
the excitatory neurotransmitter serotonin.

3. REGULATION OF CYCLIC AMP LEVELS BY COMPARTMENTALIZATION
    OF CYCLIC AMP

While in all of the above mentioned examples of stimulation of
the adenylyl cyclase system led to both a transient increase in cyclic AMP and a diminution (subsensitivity) or loss (desensitization)
of hormone action, there are other systems in which a decline of intracellular cyclic AMP levels is not accompanied by loss of hormone-
and cyclic AMP-dependent effects. In fact, there is often good evidence that cyclic AMP levels decline inspite of continued and stimulated adenylyl cyclase activity. Thus in some cell cultures (16,17)
the accumulation of intracellular cyclic AMP is transient, even
though extrusion (excretion, transport) into the medium continues
almost linearly, suggesting that the adenylyl cyclase activity is not
being shut off by a desensitizing mechanism. The best studied system where both variations of total intracellular cAMP levels and
of the cyclic-dependent ensuing physiologic response to hormonal
stimulation have been extensively described is the rat adipocite.

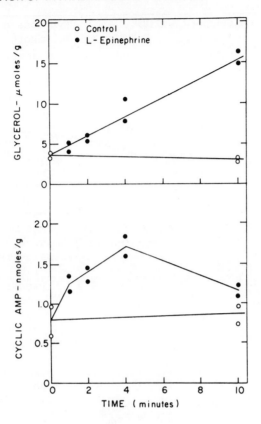

Fig. 14. Time course of epinephrine induced changes of cyclic AMP levels in isolated fat cells and of epinephrine effect on glycerol release. Concentration of epinephrine used (1.1 μM) was saturating with respect to glycerol release. From Manganiello, Murad and Vaughan (20).

This system exhibits the following features, among others, from reports by Butcher and collaborators (18), Kuo and DeRenzo (19), Manganiello et al. (20) and Ho and Sutherland (21), as well as from a more recent paper by Schimmel (22).

    i) Hormonal stimulation leads to transient increases of cyclic AMP levels (18-21).

    ii) Hormonal stimulation leads to continued cellular response (lipolysis) at both maximally and submaximally stimulating concentrations of hormone (19, 20, 22, 23 and Fig. 14 and 15).

    iii) The decline of cyclic AMP levels following hormonal stimulation is associated with a state of refractoriness to stimulation

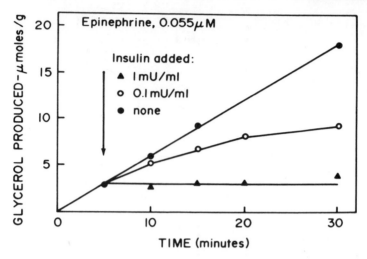

Fig. 15. Time course of epinephrine stimulated glycerol release
from isolated fat cells and effect of insulin. The concentration
of epinephrine used in this experiment is not saturating. From
Vaughan (23).

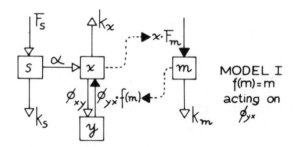

Fig. 16. Diagramatic representation of a model for regulation of
cyclic AMP levels by cyclic AMP dependent feedback modulation of
equilibrium between two cyclic AMP pools of which only one is both
responsible for biologic action of cyclic AMP and susceptible to
hydrolysis by phosphodiesterase.

by either further addition of the same stimulating hormone or of
another adenylyl cyclase stimulating hormone (20, 21, 22).

    iv) Lipolysis is continuously dependent on hormone addition,
since addition of propranolol to epinephrine-stimulated fat cells
results in immediate cessation of lipolysis that can be re-stimu-

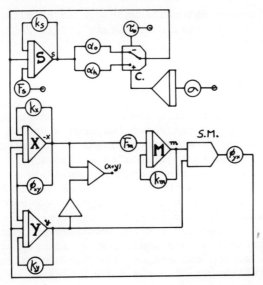

Fig. 17. Setups diagram of PACE TR-10 Analogue Computer with Servomultiplier attachment (S.M.) used to stimulate the model shown in Fig. 16.

lated by addition of another lipolytic hormone such as ACTH (20).

v) Re-stimulation with ACTH of lipolysis in epinephrine-stimu-lated, propranolol-inhibited fat cells at a time when cAMP levels have already declined, is not accompanied by re-stimulation of cAMP levels, i.e. refractoriness to stimulate cyclic AMP levels is not associated with refractoriness to stimulate lipolysis (20)

vi) Partial inhibition of PDE activity with theophylline in the absence of added hormonal stimulus leads to lipolysis without signi-ficant changes in basal cyclic AMP levels (18,19).

vii) Accumulation of cyclic AMP in response to hormonal stimu-lation in the presence of theophylline is potentiated (higher levels are attained) and extended in time (the decline is slower, depending very much on the degree of PDE inhibition achieved and whether fat pads or isolated cells are tested), when compared to that seen in the absence of theophylline (18,21).

viii) After hormonal stimulation, fat cells secrete into the incubation medium a substance, which we shall call modulator, that accumulates slowly with a time course closely related to the decline in cyclic levels and whose addition to fresh cells will inhibit their cyclic accumulating response, i.e., make them refractory to respond to hormonal stimulation by increasing cyclic AMP levels (20,21).

ix)   Incubation of fat cells with cyclic results in both appearance of the cyclic AMP refractory state and in secretion of the
modulator substance.

In view of the fact that the well known cyclic AMP-dependent
lipolytic response did not vary in these experiments in parallel
with the variation of total intracellular cyclic AMP, we explored
some years ago (24, 25), with the aid of an analogue computer, the
possibility that all of the above features might be explained (or
fitted) with a model in which cyclic AMP is distributed in one or
more compartments and is regulated by a feedback loop involving a
modulator substance.   In the search for an explanation for the biphasic cyclic AMP response with maintenance of hormone action we had
first explored a model with a single cyclic AMP compartment and test-
ted the effects of ATP supply or PDE activity; but were unable to
obtain satisfactory results.   After assuming the existence of two
cyclic AMP compartments, one small fed by adenylyl cyclase, susceptible to PDE action and responsible for biological action, and
the other in equilibrium with the first, not fed by adenylyl cyclase,
biologically inert and much larger (we assumed the equilibrium
position favoring the large compartment in a ratio between 10:1
and 100:1), with the equilibrium position regulated by a modulator
substance whose level (synthesis) is under the control of cyclic
AMP in the small compartment, we were able to simulate all of the
then known features of the fat cell system.   This model, which also
includes an ATP compartment, is depicted in the diagram of Fig. 16.
Its mathematical formulation is as follows:

$$d\delta/dt = F_\delta - (\alpha + k_\delta)\ \delta$$

$$dx/dt = \delta\alpha + y\phi_{yx}\delta(m) - x(\phi_{xy} + k_x)$$

$$dy/dt = x\phi_{xy} - y\phi_{yx}\delta(m)$$

$$dm/dt = xF_m - mk_m$$

$$\delta(m) = m$$

where: δ: concentration of ATP (substrate); x: concentration of
cAMP in the small, active compartment; y: concentration of cyclic
AMP in the large, inactive compartment; and m: modulator substance
whose rate of synthesis is dependent on x according to xF_m (this
being a key element in a non-linear feedback mechanism that modulates
the flow of mass between the two cyclic AMP compartments).   Calling
compartments that contain δ, x, y and m as S, X, Y and M, then:
F_δ and F_m zero order rate constants governing the inflow of mass into
S and M respectively; and k_δ, k_x and k_m: first order rate constants
governing the outflow of mass from compartments S, K and M respectively.   A biochemical analogue to k_x is PDE activity or ex-

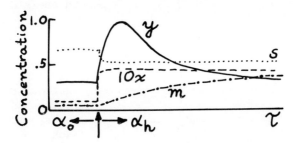

Fig. 18. Simulated time courses of the changes in levels of cyclic AMP in small biologically active compartment (x, represented 10 times expanded), of cyclic AMP in the large biologically inactive compartment (y), of substrate (s), and of modulator substance (m) before and after a 10-fold increase of the parameter α that corresponds to adenylyl cyclase activity (shift from (α_0 to α_h). The following set of constants (machine units) were used: $F_s=0.2$, $k_s=0.4$ $F_m=0.2$, $\Phi_{xy}=0.03$, $\Phi_{yx}=0.01$, $\alpha_0 = 0.005$ and $\alpha_h=0.05$.

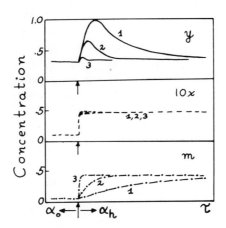

Fig. 19. Effect of rate of turnover of modulator substance m on the simulated time courses of x (shown as $10x$), y and m. Calculations were carried out using the constants described in the legend to Fig. 18 except for F_m and k_m which were varied. Curve 1: $F_m=0.2$ and $k_m=0.02$ (same as in Fig. 18); curve 2. $F_m=1.0$ and $k_m=0.1$ and curve 3: $F_m=5.0$ and $k_m=0.5$. Note that only the absolute values of F_m and k_m were varied while the ratio F_m/k_m was kept constant.

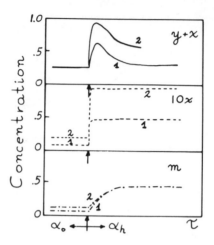

<u>Fig. 20.</u> Effect of 50% decrease of parameter corresponding to phos-
phodiesterase activity on the simulated time courses of x (shown
as $10x$), y and m. Calculations were carried out using the same
constants described in the legend to Fig. 19 for curves 2 except
for k_x which was varied. <u>Curve 1</u>: k_x=0.5 (same as curve 2 in Fig.
19); and <u>curve 2</u>: k_x=0.25.

trusion of cyclic AMP from the cell; that to k_s is ATPase activity
acting on ATP in compartment S. The first order rate constant representing adenylyl cyclase activity is α; Φ_{xy} and Φ_{yx} are first order
rate constants governing the flow of mass from compartment X to Y
and Y to X, respectively. Note that in the above set of equations
the flow of cyclic AMP from Y to X is dependent on the concentration
of modulator according to $\Phi_{yx}\delta(m)$, where $\delta(m)$ has been set to equal
m, thus completing the feedback loop initiated when the rate of formation of m was set to depend on x according to xF_m.

A calculation, carried out with an AEI PACE TR-10 Analogue
Computer (see Fig. 17 for program scheme), showing the variation of
concentration of all components involved after adenylyl cyclase
stimulation (shift from α_0 to α_h) is represented above in Fig. 18.
As can be seen the time course of the hormone induced change in Y
exhibits a maximum followed by decay to levels only slightly higher
than initial. Y follows closely total cyclic AMP ($x + y$), for $y\gg x$.
Notice also that hormonal stimulation leads to a sustained increase
of cAMP in X, the small compartment assumed in the model to be responsible for biological action. Finally, the rate at which modulator increases in M when cyclic AMP levels increase in X merits
comment. In our calculation m increases slowly in accordance with

the observations of Ho and Sutherland (21). Modification of rate
constants of m turnover (F_m and k_m) in such a way that m increases
rapidly in response to cAMP in X, resulted in almost complete obliteration of the biphasic response in Y (Fig. 19) and made it clear
that, if the model is indeed a reflection of what happens in the intact cell, then the slow character of the appearance of modulator
seen by Ho and Sutherland is actually a requisite for both the
appearance of cyclic AMP increases and the slow decline that follows.
Fig. 20 shows that the model is also consistent with the finding
that partial inhibition of PDE activity leads not only to increased
height (potentiation) of cyclic AMP peak detected after hormonal
stimulation of adenylyl cyclase, but also to hormone-like action
(increase of cyclic AMP in X) before hormonal stimulation (compare curves 1 and 2).

It is our belief that mathematical models are only useful if,
in addition to simulating or mimicking what is known of the real
system and providing plausible explanation for some features of
the system (which might previously not have been evident), they
also provide information that can be used to design new experiments,
thus contributing to experimental testing and the, eventual biochemical elucidation of the mechanisms involved. These requisites may
have been fulfilled here. Thus, most of the fat cell features (regarding cyclic AMP and cyclic AMP regulated responses) can be
mimicked with this relatively simple model. In fact, the calculation
presented above were performed during the months of September through
November of 1971, before we knew of the results of Ho and Sutherland
(21), i.e. before we knew of the slow rate of appearance of the
modulator substance and before we knew that synthesis of this substance can be stimulated by exogeneously added cyclic AMP. However
to this date, there is no clear evidence that cyclic AMP is indeed
compartmentalized. Some of our original reasons for assuming compartmentalization included not-only that we needed it in our calculations and that the hormone induced cyclic AMP-dependent lipolytic
effect is persistent in time, but also that resting levels of cyclic
AMP are high and do not result in hormone-like action as expected
from the then known affinity of the cyclic AMP-dependent protein
kinases. Clearly, with the more recent elucidation of the molecular
mechanism by which cyclic AMP activated the catalitic unit of protein kinases and with the realization that intracellular concentrations of protein kinase are of the same order of magnitude as total
intracellular levels of cyclic AMP, i.e. between 10^{-7} and 10^{-6}M,
the last of the above arguments may no longer hold. On the other
hand, the recent description by Rosen's group (26) that the cyclic
AMP binding component of the holoenzyme can exist in a phosphorylated
as well as a non-phosphorylated state and their finding that the
dephospho form appears to dissociate slower from the catalytic
unit, may offer a molecular basis for the regulatory subunit acting
as a cyclic AMP sink. Cyclic AMP bound to the regulatory unit was
shown by Brostrom et al. (27) not to be susceptible to PDE action.

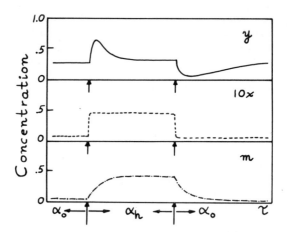

Fig. 21. Effects of removal of hormonal stimulus (down shift from $\alpha_h \rightarrow \alpha_o$) on the simulated time course of x (shown as $10x$), y and m. Calculations were carried out using the same constants described in the legend to Fig. 19 for curve 2.

In addition to "predicting", as it were, the slow time course of accumulation of the modulator substance and its inducibility by cyclic AMP, the model presented above also predicts that the rate of removal is slow. As a consequence, removal of the hormonal stimulus after the hormone stimulated steady state has been reached (i.e. after total cyclic AMP levels have declined) should result, as shown in Fig. 21, in the appearance of a transient decrease of cyclic AMP levels below control. It will be interesting to see whether this prediction is correct or not. A result such as the one depicted in Fig. 21 would suggest that further consideration should be given to the idea that cyclic AMP levels are regulated by a cyclic AMP dependent modulation of the equilibrium between two cyclic AMP pools, only one of which is both responsible for biological action and susceptible to PDE hydrolysis.

In summary, stimulated levels of cyclic AMP may decline via desensitization of adenylyl cyclase (a process that is hormone, specific), via complex-feedback regulation of cyclic AMP compartmentalization, via cyclic extrusion or via cyclic AMP-dependent increases in the levels of PDE. Two or more of these modes of regulation may coexist in a single cell and it may not always be obvious which of them is responsible for or predominating in the phenomenon we are looking at (cf. 13 and 28). Clearly, transient increases in cyclic AMP levels seem to be common phenomena. The in-

triguing question that follows is why do cellular systems have such
sophisticated homeostatic mechanisms that prevent them from being
exposed to high cyclic AMP levels for more than a minimum length
of time.

4. NOMENCLATURE USED

The term adenylyl rather than the original adenyl or the more
often used adenylate has been used throughout this article. We
prefer this name because it more accurately relates to the reaction
catalyzed by the enzyme, i.e. the intramolecular transfer of the 5'-
adenylyl group to its 3' position, and because it accurately describes the substrates of the reaction: 5'-adenylyl pyrophosphate
(ATP) and 5'-adenylyl imidodiphosphate (AMP-PNP). AMP, on adenylate
is therefore automatically excluded as substrate.

5. ABBREVIATIONS USED

AMP-PNP, 5'-adenylyl imidodiphosphate; cAMP, cyclic AMP; CL,
corpus luteum; EGTA, ethylene glycol bis (beta-aminoethyl ether)-
N, N'-tetraacetic acid; FSH, follicle stimulating hormone; hCG,
human chorionic gonadotropin; LH, luteinizing hormone; PDE, cyclic
nucleotide phosphodiesterase; PG, prostaglandin.

6. ACKNOWLEDGEMENTS AND PRESENT ADDRESSES

We wish to express our appreciation for the excellent technical
assistance of Mr. Po-Chang Yang who carried out many of the experiments reported above. Dr. J. Bockaert was a receipient of an International Fellowship (No. FO5 TW 2035, 1973-1974) from the Fogarty
International Center for the Advanced Study in the Health Sciences,
U.S. Public Health Service. This research was supported in part by
Grant HD-06513 from the United States Public Health Services. Present Addresses: L.B.: Department of Cell Biology, Baylor College of
Medicine, Houston, Texas 77025, U.S.A.; J.B.: Laboratorie de Physiologie Cellulaire, College de France, Paris, France; M.H.-D.: Depart-
ment of Biochemistry, Northwestern University Medical School, Chicago,
Illinois, U.S.A.; V.P.: Institut fur Molecularbiologie and Bio-
physik, ETH-Hönggerberg, 8049 Zürich, Switzerland; and A.G.:
Institut für Mess-und Regeltechnik, ETH, 8006, Zürich, Switzerland.

7. REFERENCES

1.   Deguchi, T. and Axelrod, J. (1973). Proc. Nat. Acad. Sci. U.S.
     70, 2411.

2.   Remold-O'Donnell, E. (1974) J. Biol. Chem. 249, 3615.
3.   Lamprecht, S.A., Zor, U., Tsafriri, A. and Lindner, H.R.   (1973)
      J. Endocr. 57, 217.
4.   Marsh, J.M., Mills, T.M. and LeMaire, W.J. (1973) Biochim. Bio-
      phys. Acta 304, 197.
5.   Hilliard, J. and Eaton, L.W. (1971) Endocrinology 89, 522.
6.   Channing, C.P. and Kammerman, S. (1973) Endocrinology 92 531.
7.   Kahn, C.R., Neville, D.M., Jr., and Roth, J. (1973) J. Biol.
      Chem. 248, 244.
8.   Roth, J. (1975) Res. Progr. Horm. Res. 31 (in press).
9.   Pohl, S.L., Krans, H.M.J., Kozyreff, V., Birnbaumer, L. and
      Rodbell, M. (1971) J. Biol. Chem. 246, 4447.
10.   Puchwein, G., Pfeuffer, T. and Helmreich, E.J.M. (1974) J. Biol.
      Chem. 249, 3232.
11.   Kakiuchi, S. and Rall, T.W. (1968) Mol. Pharmacol. 4,367.
12.   Browning, E.T., Schwartz, J.P. and Breckenridge, B. McL. (1974)
      Mol. Pharmacol. 10, 162.
13.   Franklin, T.J. and Foster, S.J. (1973) Nature New Biol. 246,
      146.
14.   Makman, M.H. (1971) Proc. Nat. Acad. Sci. U.S. 68, 885.
15.   Schulz, R., Cartwright, C. and Goldstein, A. (1974) Nature 251,
      329.
16.   Kelley, L.A. and Butcher, R.W. (1974) J. Biol. Chem. 3098.
17.   Moyle, W.R., Kong, Y. Ch. and Ramachrandran, J. (1973) J. Biol.
      Chem. 248, 2409.
18.   Butcher, R.W., Baird, C.E. and Sutherland, E.W. (1968) J. Biol.
      Chem. 243, 1705.
19.   Kuo, J.F. and DeRenzo, E.C. (1969) J. Biol. Chem. 244, 2252.
20.   Manganiello, V.C., Murad, F. and Vaughan, M. (1971) J. Biol.
      Chem. 246, 2195.
21.   Ho, R.J. and Sutherland, E.W. (1971) J. Biol. Chem. 246, 6822.
22.   Schimmel, R.J. (1974) Endocrinology 94, 1372.
23.   Vaughan, M. (1972) in "Insulin Action" (Fritz, I.B., ed.), Aca-
      demic Press, New York, pp. 297.
24.   Birnbaumer, L., Glattfelder, A. and Pliška, V. (1972) Excerpta
      Medica Int. Congr. Ser. No. 256, A393.
25.   Pliška, V., Glattfelder, A. and Birnbaumer, L. (1972) Experientia
      28, 750.
26.   Erlichman, J., Rosenfeld, R. and Rosen, O.M. (1974) J. Biol.
      Chem. 249, 5000.
27.   Brostrom, C.O., Corbin, J.D., King, C.A. and Krebs, E.G. (1971)
      Proc. Nat. Acad. Sci. U.S. 68, 2444.
28.   Franklin, T.J. and Foster, S.J. (1973) Nature New Biol. 246,
      119.

THE INTERACTION OF GLUCAGON WITH ISOLATED PLASMA MEMBRANES OF RAT LIVERS: THE RELEVANCY OF MEASURING BINDING SITES

H. Michiel J. Krans

Department of Endocrinology and Metabolism
University Hospital
Leiden, The Netherlands

Contents

Introduction
Transfer of hormonal message
Iodination of hormones
Measurement of binding
Relation between binding and adenylate cyclase
Binding sites and adenylate cyclase are different entities
Effects of guanyl nucleotides on binding
How reliable is the measurement of binding as indication of the
 first step in translation of the hormonal message?
Degradation of glucagon by its target organ
The functional meaning of receptor sites
Summary

INTRODUCTION

In this presentation I shall review both the older and newer data concerning the binding of glucagon to liver membranes. Special attention will be given to the significance of the binding in relation to physiological responses which can be measured biochemically. Most of the work reported here was done by Rodbell and coworkers[1].

---

[1] The ideas, the mutual interest in experiments and the stimulating discussions of the group consisting of M. Rodbell, L. Birnbaumer, S.L. Pohl and V. Kozyreff are responsible for the reported results.

Glucagon is a peptide molecule of 20 aminoacids, produced in the α-cells of the islands of Langerhans. Binding of glucagon was studied in a subcellular fraction from liver cells, enriched in plasma membranes. The liver responds <u>in vivo</u> to glucagon with stimulation of glycogenolysis and gluconeogenesis. These actions are accompanied by a rise in cyclic AMP content of the liver (1, 2). This is one of the classical examples of cyclic AMP acting as mediator for the action of hormones.

The membranes were prepared according to a modification of the procedure of Neville (3, 4). This preparation consists mainly of membrane sheets usually arranged in pairs, joined by various kinds of cell junctions and some vesicles. With this procedure liver membranes can be prepared in reasonable amounts, and if they are preserved in liquid nitrogen, the properties are unchanged for a long time.

TRANSFER OF HORMONAL MESSAGE

There are good reasons to assume that many peptide hormones affect intracellular processes in the target organ without entering the cell. However, the original experiments of Cuatrecases in which he demonstrated that insulin, coupled to large sepharose particles which could not penetrate through the cell membrane, had effects on fat cells identical to free insulin in solution (5) have been subjected to criticism. For both insulin (6, 7) and growth hormone (8) it has been reported that hormone leaks from the particles and that free hormone accounts for the total biological activity (7). The coupling to sepharose in the presence of albumin may also lead to the formation of hormone-guanidine-albumin complexes, which tend to have a greater hormonal activity than the hormone itself (9). This phenomenon of super activity of hormone may be due to greater resistance of the complex to hormone inactivating processes, which are seen in many biological systems (10).

If peptide hormones do not penetrate the cell membrane the message originated by the hormone must be transferred through the cell. The first step in hormone action will be recognition on the outer surface of the cell. The specific site, which recognizes the hormones is called the receptor. Such a receptor for a poly-peptide hormone is then quite distinct from the steroid receptor, which appears to be a cytoplasmic or nuclear protein, which specifically binds steroid hormones.

For reasons of clarity I will use the term receptor for sites which have a dual function : i.e. binding of hormone to the re-

ceptor elicits a second action. A discussion on the binding of
glucagon is of limited value unless data on physiological responses
are considered.

A membrane bound adenylate cyclase which can be stimulated by
glucagon is present in liver membranes (4, 11). This can be used
for measuring the relation between binding and the metabolic response.

Adenylate cyclase systems in mammalian cells can be activated
by a variety of hormones (12). Robison et al. (13) suggested that
adenylate cyclase was a complex organized system, which contained
regulatory and catalytic sites. Later studies revealed that at
least two distinct components could be distinguished : a recognition
site and a catalytic component (or adenylate cyclase enzyme).

In the model (Figure 1) proposed by Rodbell et al. (14, 15,
16) three parts are distinguished : 1° the receptor, located on
the outer side of the membrane, recognizes the hormone; 2° the
transducer transfers the message, and 3° the effector or ampli-
fier, located on the inner side of the membrane, induces the
changes in metabolism. For many hormones the effector is the
enzyme adenylate cyclase stimulating the formation of cyclic AMP.
This model only serves as a working hypothesis, and furthermore it
does not take into account recent propositions concerning the
structure of the membranes such as the fluid mosaic model (17).

IODINATION OF HORMONES

Supposing that in membranes, free receptors for a specific
hormone are present, addition of a hormone (e.g. glucagon), results
in binding of the hormone. Since only low amounts of hormone
would be bound, the use of labelled hormone is necessary for the
study of binding. For small peptide hormones it is possible to
substitute ^{14}C or ^{3}H for radioactive labelling. For molecules such
as insulin or glucagon too many ^{14}C or ^{3}H atoms have to be substituted to obtain sufficiently high specific activity. About 10,000
atoms of ^{14}C or 100 atoms ^{3}H are required to provide the same
number of counts as can be obtained with 1 atom of ^{125}I.

For iodination of glucagon we must use radioactive iodine.
Iodine is substituted into tyrosine (ortho positions) and to a
lesser degree histidine. The site of the iodination is dependent
on the micro-environment of the tyrosine in the hormone molecule.
Tyrosine on the outside of the peptide molecule is more easily
accessible than tyrosine which is buried inside the molecule.
There is also a general tendency for monoiodotyrosine to be more

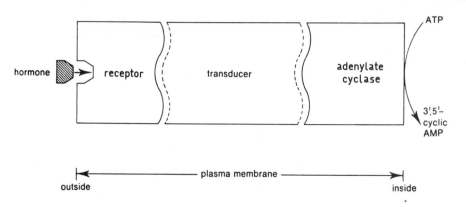

FIGURE 1. *Schmatic representation of the 3 functionally different parts in the membrane (see text).*

rapidly substituted with a second I atom than the initial iodination of tyrosine. (18). It therefore is important to iodinate with low amounts of iodine with high specific activity and to use ratio's of less than one atom of I per molecule of hormone during the iodination.

    To establish whether incorporation of iodine into the tyrosine of the hormone alters the biological activity of glucagon, monoiodoglucagon was prepared from [127]I with a trace amount of ^{125}I added, to monitor the separation of the iodinated and the non-iodinated product. Iodination, using the I_2 method (19), particularly at pH less than neutrality leads to less oxidation and cleavage of peptides than other methods using stronger oxidants. After preparative acrylamide electrophoresis (20) two peaks of labelled hormone were found (Figure 2), which both demonstrated full biological activity. The identity of the two peaks is not clear. One peak may be desamidoglucagon. For an exact description of the method, see reference 20. As shown in Figure 3, monoiodoglucagon showed stimulation of adenylate cyclase identical to the native hormone. These results were obtained when 1 µmol/3.5 mg glucagon was iodinated.

When this method was used for nanograms of hormone it did not yield high specific activity ^{125}I-glucagon. Therefore other methods were necessary. The two methods most frequently used for iodination of hormones are the chloramine-T method (21), and more recently the lactoperoxidase method (22). In both methods oxidizing agents are used to substitute iodine in the hormone. To minimize the damaging effects of oxidizing agents the amounts of chloramine-T have to be kept as low as possible (23).

In the lactoperoxidase method, the danger of partial denaturation of the hormone by the strong oxidizing action of chloramine-T is diminished. Lactoperoxidase oxidizes iodide to iodine and acts also as an iodinase in the iodination of tyrosine. The reaction is pH dependent with an optimal pH of 5.6 (24).

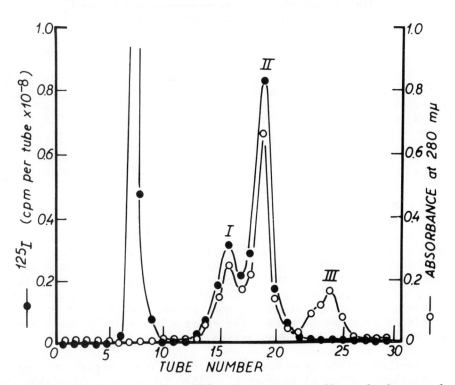

FIGURE 2.   Separation of iodinated from non-iodinated glucagon by preparative gel electrophoresis. The first peak is free iodine, peak III non-iodinated glucagon and peaks I and II are both iodinated, biologically active glucagon. See (20).

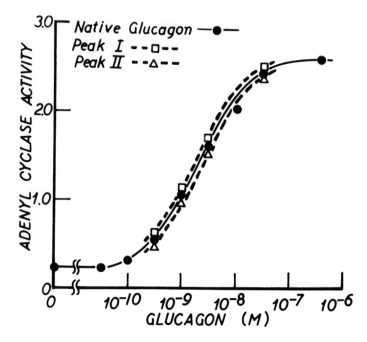

FIGURE 3. *Identical stimulation of adenylate cyclase (expressed in pmoles cyclic AMP/10 min/mg membrane protein) by native glucagon and monoiodoglucagon, prepared by the I_2 method (peaks I and II). See (20).*

Hydrogen peroxide is added as substrate for the oxidation. Hormones and particularly glycoprotein hormones are susceptible to inactivation by hydrogen peroxide (25) and therefore the amount added should be kept to the minimal amount required for the activation of lactoperoxidase. Prolonged incubation times (20-40 minutes), low amounts of enzyme and periodic addition of small amounts of hydrogen peroxide (for example every 10 minutes) has been found to minimize inactivation (24).

Another method used for iodination is the constant current electrolysis method of Rosa et al. (26) in which no oxidizing agents are needed. Iodination is performed by electrolysis of a solution of $K^{131}I$ in the presence of the hormone to be labelled

and the degree of iodination achieved can be varied with the
electrolytic current. If diluted solutions of I are used, a low
degree of iodination can be attained. Notwithstanding its
theoretical simplicity this method is not often used.

We iodinated glucagon using the chloramine-T method (21).
To minimize the chance that more than one atom of I was introduced
into a molecule of glucagon, the ratio I/hormone was kept <1 (10,
20). 10 µl 10^{-4} M solution of glucagon (1 nmole) in 0.6 M sodium
phosphate buffer pH 7.4 were added to 1.0 nmole $Na^{125}I$ (carrier
free) in 5-10 µl 0,1 N NaOH. 10 µl chloramine-T (3.5 ng/ml in
sodium phosphate buffer pH 7.4) were added, rapidly mixed with a
vortex mixer and within 5 sec 50 µl sodium metabisulfite 2 mg/ml
were added and mixed rapidly. 150 µl of 1 % albumin in 10 mM
sodium phosphate buffer pH 7.6 were added immediately and the mixture was applied to a 0.4 ml column of cellulose in a Pasteur
pipet. The column was washed with 1 ml of 1 % albumin prior to
use. After successive elutions with 2 ml of 1 % albumin in 10 %
phosphate buffer and 2 ml water, the active ^{125}I-glucagon was
eluted with 0.1 ml 50 % ethanol in 10 mM Tris-HCl pH 7.6. The
biological activity of ^{125}I-glucagon prepared in this way was
measured by comparing its ability to stimulate adenylate cyclase
activity in liver cell membranes to the stimulation by various
concentrations of unlabelled glucagon.

                        MEASUREMENT OF BINDING

After incubating membranes with labelled glucagon for a given
time the degree of binding can be determined. The bound hormone
must be separated from the free hormone in a system designed to
prevent changes in the proportion of free versus bound, e.g.
centrifugation through hormone free buffers (7, 20), filtration
through membrane filters with (27) or without (28) washing,
repeated centrifugation (29), centrifugation through a layer of
oil (30), Sephadex filtration (31), absorption to insoluble
material (32). For a complete review of these methods see Table
IV in reference (33).

Binding of labelled glucagon was assayed with the following
method (20). Liver membranes (20-50 µg) were incubated in medium
containing 2.5 % albumin, 20 mM Tris HCl pH 7.6, ^{125}I-glucagon and
sometimes 1 mM EDTA in a final volume of 125 µl. Duplicates of
50 µl were layered over 300 µl 2.5 % albumin in 20 mM Tris HCl pH
7.6 in plastic micro test tubes. The tubes were centrifuged in a
Beckman microfuge in a cold room (4°) for 5 minutes. The supernatant fluid was aspirated; the pellet was washed by adding 0.3
ml of a 10 % solution of sucrose without disturbing the pellet,
centrifugation and aspirating the fluid. The tip of the microfuge
tube was cut off with a razor blade just above the pellet. The

tip was counted in a well type scintilation counter. All results were corrected for glucagon bound to the plastic tubes in the absence of membranes.

Incubation of liver membranes with glucagon shows that maximal binding is attained within 15 minutes (Figure 4). Binding of glucagon to liver membranes has also been measured using oxoid membrane filters for separation (28), giving similar results to those using the method described above.

Receptor sites for a given hormone are considered to be specific for that hormone if other hormones do not interfere with the binding of that hormone. Simultaneous incubation of membranes with labelled glucagon and other hormones such as insulin or secretin, or fragments of the glucagon molecule (the peptide 1-21 or 22-29) which do not have biological activity, do not effect binding of the labelled glucagon to membranes (Figure 5). Labelled glucagon is only displaced by the addition of unlabelled native glucagon.

Such specificity of binding is not confined to glucagon, but has been described for many other systems where binding of hormones has been studied. Caution is advised in the design of experiments since many peptide hormones have been shown to bind to a range of inert materials. It is essential that binding should be related to other actions, such as stimulation of adenylate cyclase; however, we should not forget that other effects of hormones besides the activation of adenylate cyclase may yet be demonstrated.

RELATION BETWEEN BINDING AND ADENYLATE CYCLASE

In liver membranes dose-concentration curves of glucagon binding and adenylate cyclase activation by glucagon are essentially identical (Figure 6). The number of binding sites has been estimated at 2.5 pmoles/ml protein (16). At $4 \times 10^{-9}M$ glucagon 50 % of the binding sites are occupied (20) and the activation of adenylate cyclase is half maximal (4). However, under somewhat different assay conditions, Rodbell et al. reported a K_m for adenylate cyclase activation of about $2,5 \times 10^{-10}M$ (34). The parallelism between binding and adenylate cyclase stimulation is an indication that binding is related to stimulation of the catalytic component. Reversible binding to specific receptor sites in the target cells with equilibrium constants that appear to be related to dose response curves has been demonstrated for ACTH (31), glucagon (20), lysine vasopressin (35), arginine vasopressin and oxytocin (36) and for binding and physiological responses for the β-adrenergic receptor of the heart (37, 38). However, critical comparisons of the kinetics of binding and activation of adenylate cyclase are lacking in some of the systems studied.

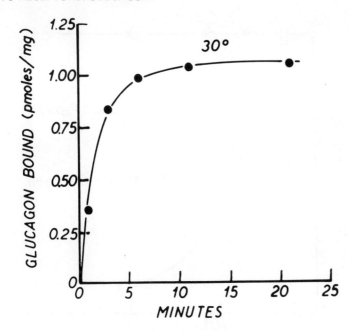

FIGURE 4. Binding of glucagon (3 x 10^{-9} M) reaches its maximum after 10-15 minutes.

It should be noted that,whereas activation of adenylate cyclase is found to be immediate,a steady state for binding is established only after 10 minutes. At steady state,an equilibrium is envisaged to exist between hormone and receptor according to the reversible bimolecular reaction :

$$H + R \rightleftharpoons HR$$

It would be expected that if a great excess of cold glucagon was added to membranes incubated with labelled glucagon, labelled glucagon would be exchanged with the unlabelled hormone and the amount of the radioactive label in the membrane pellet would be expected to be reduced to zero. However, following the addition of a 1000 times excess of cold glucagon to the incubation medium,15 minutes after the addition of a small amount of labelled glucagon, i.e. after a steady state of binding has been established, the

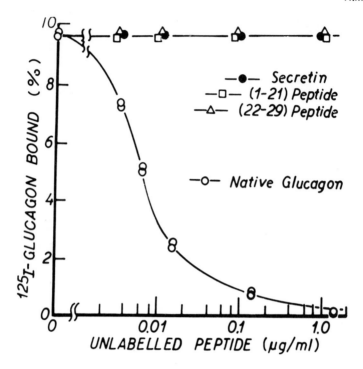

FIGURE 5. *Simultaneous incubation of glucagon with secretin or the biologically inactive glucagon peptide fragments 1-21 or 22-29 does not affect the binding of labelled glucagon. Glucagon bound is expressed as percentage of the total amount of glucagon added to the incubation medium. See (20).*

amount of radioactivity in the pellet was reduced at the most by only 50 % (Figure 7). If, however, excess cold glucagon was added only 1 minute after the start of the incubation with labelled glucagon, the bound activity was then found to be reduced to nearly zero (33). The implication of this finding will be discussed later.

Binding sites and adenylate cyclase are different entities. Membrane function can be modified in specific ways. For example, treatment with detergents such as Lubrol X 100, urea, phospholipase A or trypsin can be shown to affect both binding of hormones and subsequent adenylate cyclase activiation. Increasing concentrations

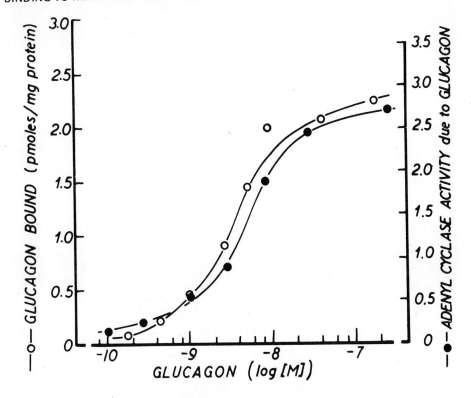

FIGURE 6. *Relation between binding and adenylate cyclase stimulation by glucagon. See (20).*

of urea in the incubation medium (Figure 8) was found to inhibit binding and adenylate cyclase in a parallel way (20).

The effects of enzymatic treatment of cells or membranes have been investigated in other systems. Cuatrecasas (39) reported that phospholipase revealed binding sites for insulin in fat cells, whereas Kono (40) has shown that trypsin may lower the number of insulin receptors, although after removal of trypsin new receptors regenerated spontaneously if the cells were kept under the appropriate conditions.

Phospholipids form an integral part of membrane structure (41). Careful investigation of the effect of phospholipase on liver membranes (Figure 9) revealed that a low enzyme concentration

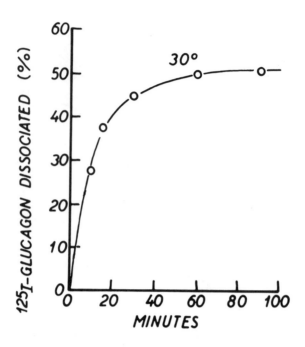

FIGURE 7. _Dissociation of labelled glucagon from the membranes by addition of a thousand-fold excess of cold glucagon to the incubation medium._

lowered the binding of glucagon, but increased the stimulation (both hormonal and fluoride) of adenylate cyclase. However, this may be explained by the observation that phospholipase A gives rise to products which can act as potent surfactants. Conversely, phospholipase C treatment was found to result in a greater loss of adenylate cyclase stimulation than binding. The acidic phospholipids have been shown to be particularly important for the binding of glucagon and the subsequent activation of adenylate cyclase (42). The studies of Levey et al. (43) demonstrated that phospholipids, especially phosphatidylserine, could restore glucagon sensitivity of isolated adenylate cyclase from cat hearts. Although after isolation, adenylate cyclase had lost sensitivity to the hormone, it had retained responsiveness to fluoride.

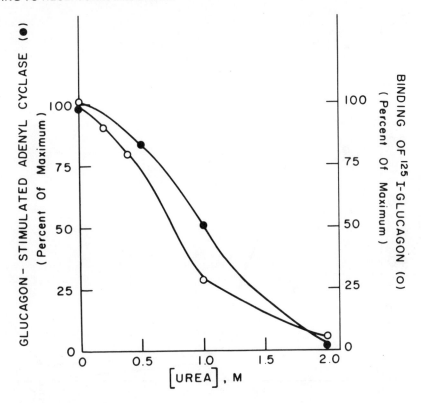

FIGURE 8. *Parallel loss of binding and adenylate cyclase stimulation by adding increasing concentrations of urea to the incubation medium See (20).*

Similarly it has been shown that phospholipids can partially restore binding and glucagon sensitivity of adenylate cyclase in
liver membranes (41).

Such effects of phospholipases may be interpreted as evidence
that the receptor and the adenylate cyclase catalytic subunit are
different entities. Further evidence for this assumption can be
derived from the following findings :

1° Glucagon, lacking its N-terminal amino-acid histidine (des-his-
glucagon) has lost its biological activity, but it competes effectively with glucagon for binding sites, albeit with ten times lower
affinity (Figure 10). Des-his-glucagon has proved to be an important tool in the study of the glucagon receptor (44).

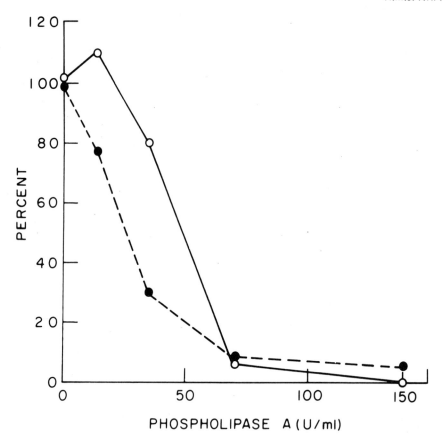

<u>FIGURE 9</u>. *Effect of treatment of membranes with increasing con-
centrations phospholipase A on binding o––––––––o and adenylate
cyclase stimulation by glucagon o–––––––o. See (20).*

2° Preincubation of membranes at 37° with 0.5 M perchlorate
results in a loss of binding and adenylate cyclase stimulation
(45). The response to fluoride is also lost. Pre-treatment at
0° inhibits the adenylate cyclase reaction as indicated by a loss
of sensitivity to both fluoride and hormone, but binding of glucagon and the characteristics of binding such as the time course
of binding, the exchange of unlabelled glucagon and the effects
of nucleotides etc. are found to be unchanged (Figures 11, 12).
It seems that the adenylate cyclase enzyme structure is more
susceptible to perchlorate treatment than the receptor, and can be
modified independently in this manner.

3° Addition of guanosine phosphates, especially GTP[2] and GDP[2]
influences binding (46) and adenylate cyclase stimulation (47).

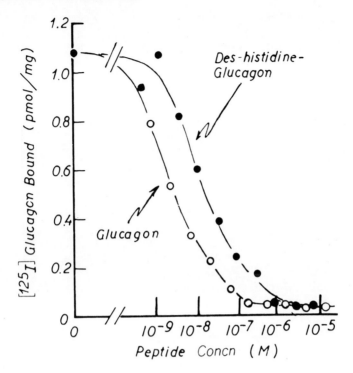

<u>FIGURE 10</u>. *Effect of addition of des-his-glucagon or unlabelled glucagon on the binding of 1.5 x 10^{-9} M ^{125}I-glucagon. See (44).*

EFFECT OF GUANYL NUCLEOTIDES ON BINDING

The first observation that GTP can affect hormone action was unexpected. While comparing binding and adenylate cyclase activation we realized that although the binding studies were performed in a simple incubation medium of Tris-buffer and albumin (20), the medium employed for the study of stimulation of adenylate cyclase contained a number of additions such as ATP[2], an ATP regenerating system and $MgCl_2$ (see (17) for complete details). Incubation of

---

[2] abbreviations : GTP = Guanosine triphosphate
                   GDP = Guanosine diphosphate
                   ATP = Adenosine triphosphate

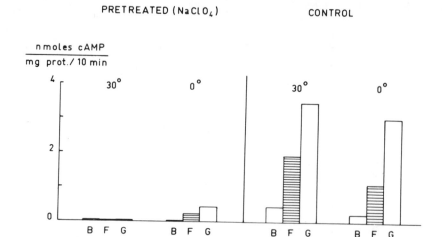

FIGURE 11.   Pretreatment of membranes with NaClO₄ 0.5 M for 30 minutes at both 30° and 0° abolishes basal (B), fluoride stimulated (F) and glucagon stimulated (G) adenylate cyclase activity. See text.

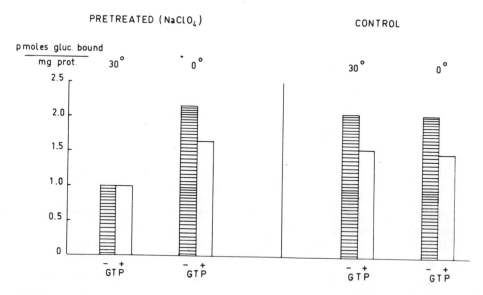

FIGURE 12.   Pretreatment of membranes with NaClO₄ at 0° as in Figure 11 does not affect binding. Addition of GTP 10⁻⁶ M (+) has the same effect as in untreated membranes. See text.

membranes in the latter medium was found to result in a 50 %
decrease in the amount of glucagon bound at equilibrium.

Omitting the different additions systematically showed that
ATP (3 mM) was responsible for the lowering of binding. Addition
of different nucleotides demonstrated that the effect of ATP was
shown to a greater extent by GTP (and GDP) (Table I) and GTP was
the more potent by a factor of 10^3 (Figure 13). GMP or cyclic GMP
were found to have no effect. The lowering of the binding was not
reflected by inhibition or decreased responsiveness of adenylate
cyclase. Addition of GTP was even found to stimulate the adenylate
cyclase of liver membranes or membranes of islet cell tumors (48,
49). The effects of GTP on adenylate cyclase will be discussed
in detail in the appropriate article in this volume by Birnbaumer.

TABLE I

ADDITIONS	BINDING OF GLUCAGON	BOUND ^{125}I-GLUCAGON DISSOCIATED
	pmole/mg protein	%
None	1.15 $\pm$ 0.03	49 $\pm$ 2
CTP	0.75 $\pm$ 0.04	65 $\pm$ 3
UTP	0.71 $\pm$ 0.04	75 $\pm$ 4
ATP	0.59 $\pm$ 0.02	75 $\pm$ 4
GTP	0.43 $\pm$ 0.02	100 $\pm$ 1

Effects of addition of different nucleotides (3 mM final concentration) on binding of glucagon (3 x 10^{-9} M) and on displacement
of bound ^{125}I- glucagon by a great excess (10^{-6} M) cold glucagon.
See (46).

CTP = cytosine triphosphate
UTP = uridine triphosphate

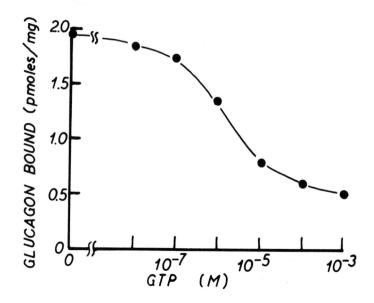

<u>FIGURE 13</u>.   *Effect of GTP on binding of glucagon.   See (46).*

HOW RELIABLE IS THE MEASUREMENT OF BINDING AS AN INDICATION OF THE FIRST STEP IN TRANSLATION OF THE HORMONAL MESSAGE ?

What generates the message sent to the enzyme ? Does the interaction of the hormone with the receptor trigger the signal, or does the occupation of the receptor induce a conformational change in the membrane leading to an activation of adenylate cyclase ? In the latter situation the hormone would have to be released to terminate the message.

Earlier, the observation that bound hormone does not appear to be completely exchanged with the unbound hormone, was discussed. Addition of a hundred-fold surplus of unlabelled glucagon to membranes, loaded with labelled glucagon, showed that not more than

30-40 % of the labelled amount bound was released in 30 minutes
(20). It was also a time dependent process, indicating that the
process of binding and of release was slow. However, addition of
GTP was found to accelerate the exchange, and moreover, instead of
the 40 % reduction in the amount bound following the addition of
an excess of unlabelled glucagon, the labelled glucagon was now
found to be totally exchanged (Table I). It must be emphasized
that what is generally referred to as "binding" is essentially a
measurement of a steady state stimulation established within 10-15
minutes incubation period.

Birnbaumer et al. (50) investigated whether preceding incubations affected the adenylate cyclase reaction. It appeared that
changes in concentrations of glucagon in the incubation medium were
immediately reflected in changes in adenylate cyclase stimulation.
No difference in adenylate cyclase stimulation was seen if the
binding sites were occupied by glucagon prior to incubation for
adenylate cyclase activity or if glucagon was added to the membranes
only at the start of the adenylate cyclase incubation.

They also demonstrated the absence of a lag time in the adenylate cyclase response (Figure 14). If membranes are incubated in
the absence of hormone only a basal production of cyclic AMP is
measured. Addition of 4×10^{-9} M glucagon stimulates cyclic AMP
formation immediately. Des-his-glucagon however, is known to
occupy the binding sites (44), but it does not stimulate adenylate
cyclase. Addition of excess Des-his-glucagon (10^{-6} M) reduces
adenylate cyclase activity to basal within 15 seconds. Subsequent
addition of an excess of glucagon (1×10^{-5} M) restimulates the
adenylate cyclase within 15 seconds. However, the addition of
excess Des-his-glucagon in the presence of ATP 5 minutes after the
addition of glucagon showed that the exchange for Des-his-glucagon
was time dependent and that Des-his-glucagon did not displace the
total bound glucagon as much as native glucagon (Figure 15). The
slow change in binding was not reflected in the changes in adenylate
cyclase stimulation. Thus this was evidence that not all the binding sites might be necessary for glucagon activation of adenylate
cyclase.

Rodbell et al. (34) demonstrated recently that if membranes
were incubated with a very low concentration of glucagon
(7×10^{-11} M), using AMP-PNP[3] as a substrate for adenylate cyclase,
a time lag of about 4 minutes appeared before stimulation of adenylate cyclase was observed. Pre-incubation of the membranes with
glucagon in low concentrations, or addition of GTP (0.1 μM)
abolished this lag time. GTP in the absence of glucagon had no
effect. They concluded that GTP had a permissive effect for the
system and that GTP changed the activation state of adenylate

---

[3] AMP-PNP (= App(NH)p) = 5-adenyl-imido-phosphate

3´5´cAMP FORMED (PMOLES)

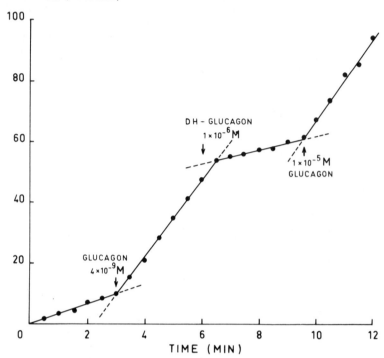

FIGURE 14. *Rapid reaction of adenylate cyclase to changes in the medium. The arrows indicate when additions were added into the medium. See (50).*

cyclase. GTP was also found to stimulate the release of bound glucagon. They found a hyperbolic relationship between the amount of glucagon bound and the maximal activity of adenylate cyclase, concluding that all the specific binding sites for glucagon represented receptors which were linked functionally and structurally to the adenylate cyclase system.

DEGRADATION OF GLUCAGON BY ITS TARGET ORGAN

Another compelling question in the study of the relationship between glucagon and binding sites is the fate of glucagon during the binding and after its release from the binding sites. Is the hormone inactivated by the binding process or are other factors involved ? If the incubation medium,is tested after membranes have been incubated in the medium a fall in biologically active

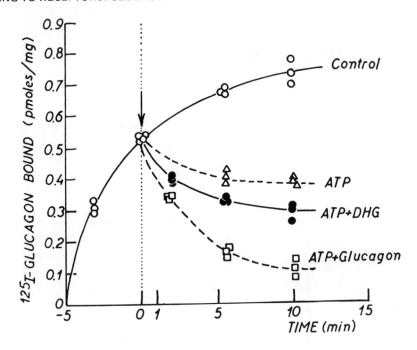

<u>FIGURE 15</u>. Effect of Des-his-glucagon and glucagon on the exchange
of bound glucagon in the presence of ATP. Membranes were preincubated with 2 x 10⁻⁹ M ¹²⁵I-glucagon for 5 minutes, than at zero
time (arrow)   ATP (3.2 mM), ATP + Des-his-glucagon (3 x 10⁻⁶ M) or
ATP + glucagon (3 x 10⁻⁶ M) was added.
An immediate exchange of the bound labelled glucagon was not
observed; after 15 minutes a considerable amount of labelled
glucagon remained bound. See (28).

glucagon is seen (10). This fall was greater than could be
accounted for by the amount of glucagon bound by the membrane.
Almost 50 % of the hormone appeared to be inactivated within a few
minutes of incubation and the inactivation was specific for glucagon. Addition of high concentrations of hormones such as ACTH
or insulin only slightly inhibited the inactivation. Only boiling
the membranes abolished the inactivation. The inactivation was
also inhibited or abolished by pretreatment of the membranes with
agents such as detergents, phospholipase A, trypsin or urea, which
interfere both with binding and activation of adenylate cyclase
(Figure 16). There appears to be parallelism between loss of

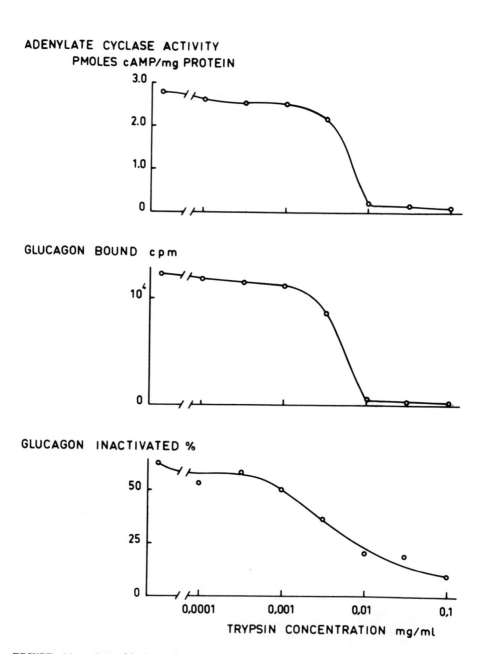

<u>FIGURE 16</u>. *Parallel reduction of adenylate cyclase activation, glucagon binding and glucagon inactivation by treatment with increasing concentrations of trypsin. See (41).*

adenylate cyclase activation, binding and inactivation of the hormone. The following factors suggest that the inactivation sites are not identical to the regulatory sites:

1° Bound glucagon could be removed from the membranes with 2 M urea. This glucagon retained its biological activity and was found to bind in a manner indistinguishable from native glucagon (20).

2° Des-his-glucagon, at concentrations equal to or higher than those required for inhibition of glucagon binding and action, only partially inhibited glucagon inactivation (10).

3° No effect of GTP on the inactivation is seen (10).

THE FUNCTIONAL MEANING OF THE RECEPTOR SITE

After a review of the data on binding we have not resolved the basic question as to the nature of the receptor. Other pertinent questions may be asked, such as is hormone binding a measure of hormone receptor activity ? Is there one class of receptors ? Are there superfluous (spare) receptors ? Do we have to distinguish between acceptors and receptors ? Birnbaumer (33) confines the term acceptor to receptors which lack a dual function in that they do not elicit a secondary response or, in more precise terms, that the secondary response cannot be observed.

For a number of systems two classes of receptors for the same hormone have been described. One class consists of low capacity, high affinity sites with a K_d close to the concentration of hormone present in biological systems and the other high capacity low affinity sites, which even at very high hormone concentration, are not totally occupied. This has been described for a number of hormones such as ACTH (31) and insulin (51). However, we could not find an indication of the existence of two classes of sites for the binding of glucagon to liver membranes (28).

The following arguments derived from our findings are important when considering the function of receptors in general:

1° The number of binding sites determined depends on the incubation medium. Addition of nucleotides change the apparent number of binding sites (20), but no direct effect of nucleotides on activation of adenylate cyclase is seen. Even if in the presence of GTP virtually no binding has been detected, adenylate cyclase can be stimulated by glucagon.

2° The activation of adenylate cyclase is immediate, whereas maximum binding is attained only after 5 or 10 minutes (20, 50). In other systems (37) equilibrium times of 180 minutes have been described. This may indicate that more sites are available than necessary for hormone action. Unfortunately the effects of binding occurring in the first instants are impossible to observe with methods available, and therefore it is at present impossible to determine the nature of binding in the first few seconds.

The question as to what triggers the hormonal response is also unresolved. Patton (52) distinguished two possible mechanisms to relate binding and action, the occupancy theory and the rate theory. Both theories state that hormone receptor interaction follows the law of mass action and that this is the rate limiting step for hormone action. In the occupancy theory the number of occupied sites determines the hormone effect, but in the rate theory the hormone response is proportional to the number of hormone receptor interactions per unit of time. Experimental evidence for the rate theory has not been presented for any system to date.

Birnbaumer and Pohl (27) have tried to construct a curve for glucagon binding according to the formula :

$$H^* \xleftarrow{\quad K_3 \quad} H + R \underset{K_2}{\overset{K_1}{\rightleftharpoons}} HR$$

(H = Hormone, R = Receptor, H^* = inactivated Hormone, K_1 and K_2 are the rate constants of association and dissociation and K_3 is the rate constant of inactivation.)

The curve obtained did not fit with any of Patton's theoretical curves.

The kinetics of binding, the observed response (e.g. the stimulation of adenylate cyclase) and the inactivation of the hormone have to be taken into account in experiments designed to relate binding with other effects.

3° At low hormone concentration (10^{-11} M) the activation of adenylate cyclase by glucagon showed a lag time of 3-4 minutes (34). At this concentration of glucagon addition of GTP accelerated the activation and the lag time disappeared (34). This shows that GTP stimulates the activation of adenylate cyclase and facilitates the transfer of message to the membranes. This is used as evidence to support the theory that GTP causes the receptor to assume a more active state. With present knowledge it is not possible to state that GTP is obligatory for the action of glucagon, but strong evidence exists that this may be so.

4° The apparent number of receptors exceeds the necessary sites for activation of adenylate cyclase, i.e. not everything that appears to bind a hormone is necessarily a receptor.

The "superfluous" or "spare" sites cannot be distinguished from the physiological binding sites with kinetic, electron microscopic or other methods. These sites should be designated simply as reserve receptors. Even under conditions where binding was not maximal and adenylate cyclase was not fully stimulated, a discrepancy between binding of glucagon and adenylate cyclase stimulation was seen (50). The function of these extra sites is an intriguing question, but at present we can only speculate over the answer. They may be evidence of binding sites related to functions which are not mediated by cyclic AMP, part of an inactivating system, storage sites, or even unoccupied sites, which are uncovered after occupancy of neighbouring receptor sites.

Figure 17 is an attempt to summarize the ideas and experimental results discussed in this paper. Receptors (R) may be connected with the adenylate cyclase effector (E), or with effectors for other actions, which cannot be measured. It may be that a receptor has connections with different types of effectors. Some binding sites (R^1) may not immediately be connected with effectors, but these cannot be distinguished from R. The danger of most models is that they may sustain the assumption that receptors are pre-existing structures within a rigidly structured membrane. However, the concept of fluid membrane structure (17) implies the possibility that the availability of receptors is subject to dynamic variation and that it is useless to look for a fixed number of receptors.

The answers to many questions have to await more insight into the structure of the receptor. We know that phospholipids are of paramount importance for the whole system, but we do not know if receptors are biochemical separate entities, or discreet modifications of the basic membrane structure. Receptor isolation has been reported (53), but has made little contribution to the insight into the structure of the receptor. The crucial experiment of recombining the receptor with the basic system to see if activity can be restored has not been successfully carried out. However, the findings of Levey et al. (43) concerning the restoration of the glucagon receptor with phospholipids looks promising. We have to investigate meticulously relationships between different determinants to get more clarity concerning the function of receptors. With our present knowledge it is even difficult to interpret results indicating differences in a number of receptor sites in obese and nonobese animals and man or the possibility of diseases due to modification of receptors (54).

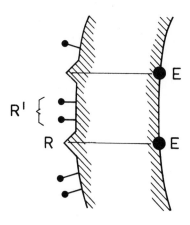

FIGURE 17. Tentative scheme indicating the manner by which receptors may be related to effector elements. See text.

SUMMARY

    To summarize our information concerning the binding of glu-
cagon to liver membranes :

1° Glucagon binds to isolated liver plasma membranes with a maximum of 2.5 pmoles bound per mg protein.

2° The binding is specific for glucagon.

3° Both the binding and the release of bound glucagon are relatively slow processes whereas the activation of adenylate cyclase is
immediate and linear.

4° GTP lowers the maximal number of apparent binding sites but
accelerates the response of the catalytic system.

5° Glucagon is inactivated on separate sites. These sites are
connected but not identical to the active binding sites.

6° Only one class of binding sites is found.

7° Not all the apparent binding sites are necessary for glucagon
action.

8° Actions at the catalytic site do not affect interaction of the binding sites.

9° The number of apparent occupied sites does not determine the potency of the hormone stimulation.

REFERENCES

(1) EXTON, J.H., ROBISON, G.A., SUTHERLAND, E.W. and PARK, C.R. (1971) J. Biol. Chem 246, 6166

(2) JOHNSON, M.E.M., DAS, N.M., BUTCHER, F.R. and FAIN, J.N. (1972) J. Biol. Chem. 247, 3229

(3) NEVILLE, D.M. (1968) Biochim. Biophys. Acta 154, 540

(4) POHL, S.L., BIRNBAUMER, L. and RODBELL, M. (1971) J. Biol. Chem. 246, 1849

(5) CUATRECASAS, P. (1969) Proc. Nat. Acad. Sci. (Wash.) 63, 450

(6) DAVIDSON, M.B., VAN HERLE, A.K. and GERSCHENSON, L.E. (1973) Endocrinology 92, 1442

(7) KOLB, H.J., RENNER, R., HEPP, K.D., WEISS, L. and WIELAND, O.H. (1975) Proc. Nat. Acad. Sci. USA (Wash.), 72, 248

(8) SCHWARTZ, J., NUTTING, D.F., GOODMAN, H.M., KOSTYO, J.L. and FELLOWS, R.E. (1973) Endocrinology 92, 535

(9) WILCHEK, M., OKA, T. and TOPPER, Y.J. (1975) Proc. Nat. Acad. Sci. (Wash.) 72, 1055

(10) POHL, S.L., KRANS, H.M.J., BIRNBAUMER, L. and RODBELL, M. (1972) J. biol. Chem. 247, 2295

(11) BIRNBAUMER, L., POHL, S.L., RODBELL, M. (1971) J. bio. Chem., 246, 1857

(12) ROBISON, G.A., BUTCHER, R.W. and SUTHERLAND, E.W. (1971) Cyclic AMP, Academic Press New York and London

(13) ROBISON, G.A., BUTCHER, R.W. and SUTHERLAND, E.W. (1967) Ann. N.Y. Acad. Sci. 139, 703

(14) RODBELL, M., BIRNBAUMER, L., POHL, S.L. and KRANS, H.M.J. (1970) Acta Diabet. lat. 7 (suppl. 1), 9

(15) BIRNBAUMER, L., POHL, S.L., KRANS, H.M.J. and RODBELL, M.
      (1970) Adv. in Bioch. Psychopharmac. 3, 185, Raven Press,
      New York

(16) RODBELL, M., BIRNBAUMER, L., POHL, S.L. and KRANS, H.M.J.
      (1971) in: Structure Activity Relationships of Protein
      and Polypeptide Hormones, p. 199 (Margoulies, M. and
      Greenwood, F.C., eds.), Excerpta Medica, Amsterdam

(17) SINGER, S.J. and NICOLSON, G.L. (1972) Science 715, 720

(18) RUDINGER, C.F. (1971) in: Radioimmunoassay Methods (Kirkham,
      K.E. and Hunter, W.M., eds.) p. 104, Churchill Livingstone,
      Edinburgh and London

(19) JUNEK, H., KIRK, K.L. and COHEN, L.A. (1969) Biochemistry 8,
      1844

(20) RODBELL, M., KRANS, H.M.J., POHL, S.L. and BIRNBAUMER, L.
      (1971), J. biol. Chem. 246, 1861

(21) HUNTER, W.M. and GREENWOOD,F.C. (1962) Nature 194, 495

(22) THORELL, J.I. and JOHANSON, B.G. (1971) Biochim. Biophys.
      Acta 251, 363

(23) FREYCHET, P., ROTH, J. and NEVILLE, D.M. Jr. (1971) Biochem.
      Biophys. Res. Comm. 43, 400

(24) MIYACHI, Y., VAITUKAITES, J.L., NIESCHLAG, E. and LIPSETT,
      M.B. (1972) J. clin. Endocr. 34, 23

(25) REICHERT, L.E. Jr. (1961) Endocrinology 69, 398

(26) ROSA, U., MASSAGLIA, A., PENNISI, F., CORZANI, J. and ROSSI,
      C.A. (1967) Biochem. J. 103, 407

(27) CUATRECASAS, P. (1971) J. biol. Chem. 246, 6522

(28) BIRNBAUMER, L. and POHL, S.L. (1973) J. biol. Chem. 248,
      2056

(29) DEKRETSER, D.M., CATT, K.J. and PAULSEN, C.A. (1971)
      Endocrinology 80, 332

(30) GLIEMANN, J., ØSTERLIND, K., VINTEN, J. and GAMMELTOFT, S.
      (1972) Biochim. Biophys. Acta 286, 1

(31) LEFKOWITZ, R.J., ROTH, J., PRICER, W. and PASTAN, I (1970)
      Proc. Nat. Acad. Sci. (Wash.), 65, 745

(32) LEFKOWITZ, R.J., ROTH, J. and PASTAN, I (1970) Nature 228,
      864

(33) BIRNBAUMER, L., POHL, S.L. and KAUMANN, A.J. (1974) Adv. in
      Cyclic Nucleotid. Res. 4, 239

(34) RODBELL, M., LIN, M.C. and SALOMON, Y. (1974), J. biol. Chem.
      249, 59

(35) BOCKAERT, J., ROY, C., RAJERISON, R. and JARD, S. (1973)
      J. biol. Chem. 248, 5922

(36) BIRNBAUMER, L. and YANG, P.C. (1974) J. biol. Chem. 249,
      7848

(37) LEFKOWITZ, R.J., O'HARA, D.S. and WORSKOW, J. (1973) Nature
      New Biology 244, 79

(38) KAUMANN, A.J. and BIRNBAUMER, L., (1974) J. biol. Chem. 249,
      7874

(39) CUATRECASAS, P. (1971) J. biol. Chem. 246, 6532

(40) KONO, T. and BARHAM, F.W. (1971) J. biol. Chem. 246, 6210

(41) POHL, S.L., KRANS, H.M.J., KOZYREFF, V., BIRNBAUMER, L. and
      RODBELL, M. (1971) J. biol. Chem. 246, 4447

(42) RUBALCAVA, B. and RODBELL, M. (1973) J. biol. Chem. 248, 3831

(43) LEVEY, G.S., FLETCHER, M.A., KLEIN, J., RUIZ, E. and SCHENK,
      A. (1974) J. biol. Chem. 249, 2665

(44) RODBELL, M. BIRNBAUMER, L., POHL, S.L. and SUNDBY, F. (1971)
      Proc. nat. Acad. Sci. (Wash.) 68, 909

(45) KRANS, H.M.J., BIRNBAUMER, L., POHL, S.L. and RODBELL, M.
      (1972), Eur. J. clin. Invest. 2, 202

(46) RODBELL, M., KRANS, H.M.J., ROHL, S.L. and BIRNBAUMER, L.
      (1971) J. biol. Chem. 246, 1872

(47) RODBELL, M. BIRNBAUMER, L., POHL, S.L. and KRANS, H.M.J.
      (1971) J. biol. Chem. 246, 1877

(48) RODBELL, M. (1973) Fed. Proc. 32, 1854

(49) GOLDFINE, J.D., ROTH, J. and BIRNBAUMER, L. (1972) J. biol.
      Chem. 247, 1211

(50) BIRNBAUMER, L., POHL, S.L., RODBELL, M. and SUNDBY, F.
      (1972) J. biol. Chem. 247, 2038

(51) FREYCHET, P., ROTH, J. and NEVILLE D.M. Jr. (1971) Proc.
      Nat. Acad. Sci. (Wash.) 68, 1833

(52) PATTON, W.M. (1961) Proc. Roy. Soc. London B 154, 21

(53) QUATRECASAS, P. (1971) Proc. Nat. Acad. Sci. (Wash.) 68,
      1264

(54) KAHN, C.R., NEVILLE, D.M. Jr. and ROTH, J. (1973) J. biol.
      Chem. 248, 244

HORMONE BINDING TO RECEPTORS : VASOPRESSIN

Christian Roy
Serge Jard
Tomislav Barth[1]
Rabary Rajerison
Joël Bockaert

Laboratoire de Physiologie Cellulaire
Collège de France
F-75231 Paris 05 (France)

(1) Present address : Institute of Organic Chemistry
    and Biochemistry, Czechoslovak Academy of Sciences
    16610 Prague 6 (Czechoslovakia)

Contents

INTRODUCTION

It is now clearly established that the primary action of anti-diuretic hormone on the mammalian kidney consists in the activation of a membrane-bound adenylate cyclase present in the tubular cells from the responding parts of the nephron (1, 2). Membrane fractions prepared from the kidney medullary portion contain a vasopressin-sensitive adenylate cyclase (3 - 8); they exhibit the expected high sensitivity to the hormone and marked stereospecificity towards the natural neurohypophysial peptides and artificial structural analogues (7, 9 - 11). These acellular preparations thus appear to be a convenient biological material for a tentative

97

characterization of the hormonal receptors involved in the response
of the mammalian kidney to vasopressin. The purpose of the present
paper is to discuss some of the methodological and technical problems encountered during the course of recent studies by this group,
on the pig kidney lysine-vasopressin receptor (4, 9 - 12).

METHODOLOGICAL AND TECHNICAL CONSIDERATIONS

A hormonal receptor is defined by its ability : 1° - to
specifically bind the hormonal molecule (a reversible dose-dependent
binding must be demonstrable in the range of physiological hormone
concentrations); 2° - to trigger the sequence of events leading to
a regulatory response of the target cells. The criteria which are
usually retained for the characterization of a hormonal receptor
are based on the demonstration of several correlations between
binding and response with respect to time and dose dependency,
structural requirements for binding and response, cellular and
zoological specificity, effects of various treatments both chemical
and physiological, ontogenic development, etc. A correct interpretation of such binding-response relationship implies that
adequate responses could be given to the main following questions :
is the response a function of receptor occupancy, turnover rate of
the bound hormone or of any other characteristics of the hormone-
receptor interaction ? - What is the nature of the coupling function
(quantitative relationship between hormone-receptor interaction and
response) ? - Is the entire population of receptors involved in the
response (coupled versus uncoupled receptors). Are there several
kinds of binding sites, and is it possible to easily discriminate
between them ?

For the experimental characterization of a hormonal receptor
coupled to adenylate cyclase, the main following prerequisites
must be fulfilled : the procedure used for the membrane preparation
must preserve the stability of the adenylate cyclase activity and
its responsiveness to hormonal stimulation. The membranes must be
free of enzymes inactivating the hormonal molecule. Finally the
radioactive hormone used for binding studies must possess high
specific radioactivity and biological potency.

Previous experiments indicated that gentle homogeneization of
pig or rat kidney medullary tissue preserves adenylate cyclase
responsiveness to neurohypophysial peptides together with high
sensitivity and stereospecificity towards natural hormones and a
large series of structural analogues (4, 11). Extensive washing
of the low speed sediment (600 x g) from the tissue homogenate in
an hypotonic medium containing 10 mM Tris-HCl pH 8, 3.3 mM $MgCl_2$
and 1 mM EDTA, led to an enzyme preparation free from enzymic
activities inactivating the hormone or its structural analogues

and from most of the components responsible for non specific
absorption of the labelled hormone (non specific binding is
defined as the component of total binding which cannot be inhibited
by a large excess of unlabelled hormone). Tritium labelling of
the tyrosyl residue in the lysine-vasopressin molecule (13)
followed by purification on a neurophysin-sepharose column led to
a radiochemically pure and highly labelled (5 - 12 Ci/mM) hormonal
preparation. The biological potency of the {^{3}H}-LVP used was
identical to that of the native hormone on usual biological tests
including pig and rat kidney adenylate cyclase activation. The
latter observation is of primary importance since as will be discussed below the quantitative relationship between receptor
occupancy and adenylate cyclase activation depends on the structure
of the active peptide tested.

BINDING OF LYSINE-VASOPRESSIN TO PIG KIDNEY PLASMA MEMBRANES

The binding of {^{3}H}-LVP to pig kidney plasma membranes is a
time dependent process. As indicated by Figure 1 an equilibrium
was reached within 7 to 10 minutes when incubating membranes at
30°C in the presence of 10^{-8} M free hormone. Vasopressin binding
was reversible when decreasing the hormonal concentration in the
incubation medium to a very low value. The binding time course
was highly temperature and hormone concentration dependent. The
time needed to reach the equilibrium value was decreased when
increasing the temperature or the concentration of hormone in the
incubation medium. These two observations suggest that the rate
limiting step for the formation of the hormone-membrane complex is
the interaction itself rather than some physical process such as
diffusion and/or uptake of the hormone by closed membrane vesicles.
Both the association and dissociation curves can be adequately
described by a mono exponential process (Figure 1) as expected
from a reversible binding of the hormone to a homogeneous population of receptor sites. The rate constants for the hormone-
receptor complex formation and dissociation

$$(k_1 = 1.5 \times 10^{+7} M^{-1}min^{-1}, \quad k_{-1} = 0.03 \ min^{-1})$$

can be deduced from the semi logarithmic plots given in Figure 1.
The values obtained are in good agreement with those deduced from
the determination of the association time course at two different
hormone concentrations in the incubation medium, as well as with
the apparent Km value for hormone binding (see Figure 2). A dose
dependent specific binding is observable in a 10^{-9} to 10^{-7} M concentration range. The maximal binding capacity is close to 1.0 pM/
mg protein and the concentration leading to half the maximal
binding (apparent Km) is 2×10^{-8} M. Lysine-vasopressin binding
is slightly cooperative (Hill coefficient : n = 1.5). The satur-
ability of lysine-vasopressin binding to pig kidney membranes is

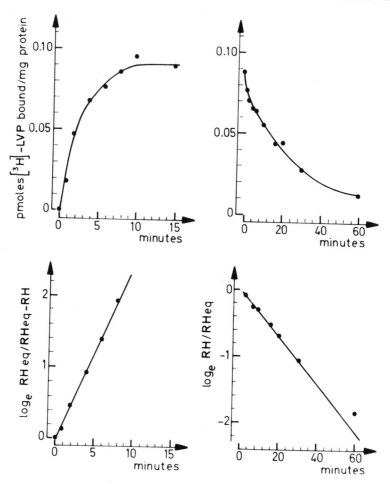

FIGURE 1.   Time course of association and dissociation of {³H}
vasopressin with renal plasma membrane receptors.

   A pig kidney membrane fraction (0.31 mg protein) was incubated
in a final volume of 100 μl with 10⁻⁸ M {³H} vasopressin and the
binding was measured as a function of time at 30°C(association
curve : left part).   The incubation medium contained 100 mM Tris-
HCl, pH 8;   1 mM MgCl₂;   0.25 mM ATP and 1 mM cyclic AMP. At the
end of the incubation period, assay medium was diluted with 2 ml
of a medium identical to the assay mixture and filtered immediately
(association process) on Millipore filter EAWP 0.45 μm.   Filters
were then washed by three times 10 ml of a solution containing
0.1 % bovine serum albumine, 10 mM Tris-HCl, pH 8 and 1 mM MgCl₂
kept at 4°.   To test the reversibility of binding, the enzyme was
first incubated at 30°C for 15 minutes in the presence of {³H}

                                                  (continued)

Figure 1 (continued)

vasopressin (10^{-8} M). The hormonal concentration was then lowered to 5 x 10^{-10} M by dilution with the incubation medium without hormone. Residual binding was measured as a function of time after dilution. The semilogarithmic plots of the association and dissociation curves are shown in the lower part of the figure (From Bockaert et al.) (4).

further illustrated by the competition experiment depicted in Figure 3. A dose dependent inhibition of {^{3}H}-LVP (10^{-8} M) binding is obtained when adding increasing amounts of unlabelled LVP to the incubation medium. Such competition experiments can be used to estimate the apparent affinity of any unlabelled peptide for the lysine-vasopressin receptor (see legend to Figure 3). Incidently, it can be noted that there is a fairly good agreement between the Km values for vasopressin binding deduced either from the {^{3}H}-LVP binding curve (Figure 3, left graph) or from the competition curve. This is a further confirmation that the {^{3}H}-LVP used is a good radioactive marker of the natural hormone.

From the above described binding studies it can be concluded that membrane fractions prepared from pig kidney medulla contained a limited number of binding sites for lysine-vasopressin. Binding is reversible; there is no indication of a large heterogeneity in the population of sites as regards their affinity for the hormone. The dissociation curve was adequately described by a mono exponential process and the Hill coefficient for the concentration binding curve at equilibrium, was higher than unity. In the explored concentration range only one category of binding sites is detectable. The observed rate constants for the hormone-membrane complex formation allow precise time-course studies and validate the use of a millipore filter technique for the separation of bound from free hormone.

CORRELATIONS BETWEEN HORMONE BINDING AND ADENYLATE CYCLASE ACTIVATION

For all the experiments to be described below, both hormone binding and adenylate cyclase activation were measured on the same enzyme preparation and under identical experimental conditions.

As indicated by Figure 4, lysine-vasopressin binding and adenylate cyclase activation followed similar time-courses after addition of a submaximal amount of hormone to the incubation medium. This observation can be taken as evidence that the response is a function of receptor occupancy rather than a function of the fre-

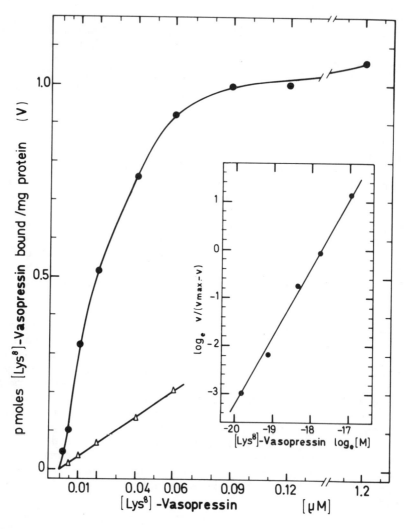

<u>FIGURE 2</u>. *Effect of hormonal concentration on {³H}-vasopressin*
binding to pig kidney membranes.
Lysine-vasopressin specific binding on membranes (0.185 mg) was
measured after 20 minutes incubation at 30°C in the presence of
increasing amounts of hormone. For hormonal concentrations of up
to 6 x 10⁻⁸ M only {³H} vasopressin was used. For higher con-
centrations, the labelled hormone was diluted with appropriate
amounts of unlabelled peptide. The lower curve (Δ) describes the
development of non-specific binding when the labelled peptide con-
centration within the incubation medium is increased. The Hill
transformation of binding curve is given in the inside panel
(n = 1.52 ± 0.11). (From Roy et al. (12)).

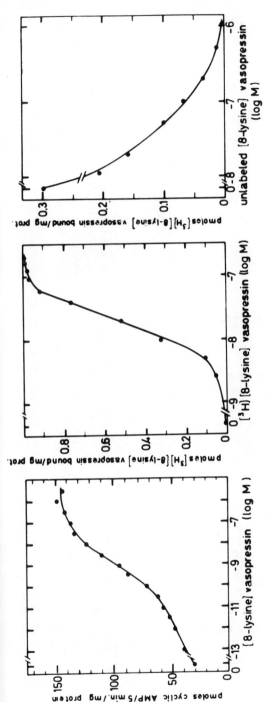

FIGURE 3. Effect of lysine-vasopressin on pig kidney adenylate cyclase : enzyme activation and hormone binding.

Both adenylate cyclase activation (left panel) and binding (middle panel) were measured under identical experimental conditions (see 12) in the presence of the indicated amounts of lysine-vasopressin.

The right part of the figure shows the effect of increasing concentrations of unlabelled vaso-pressin on the binding of a constant amount of {3H}-vasopressin (10⁻⁸M). Maximal inhibition of radioactivity binding observed in the presence of unlabelled peptide added was considered as a non specific component and subtracted from each experimental value.
The concentration of unlabelled peptide giving 50 % inhibition of the {3H} lysine vasopressin specific binding was 3.6 x 10⁻⁸ M. This value is close to the value equal to 1.5 x apparent Km, which can be calculated by assuming that the unlabelled peptide behaves like a pure compe-titive inhibitor of the {3H} lysine vasopressin and by taking into account that {3H} lysine-vasopressin concentration used is equal to 10⁻⁸M, i.e. 0.5 x apparent Km. From Roy et al. (12).

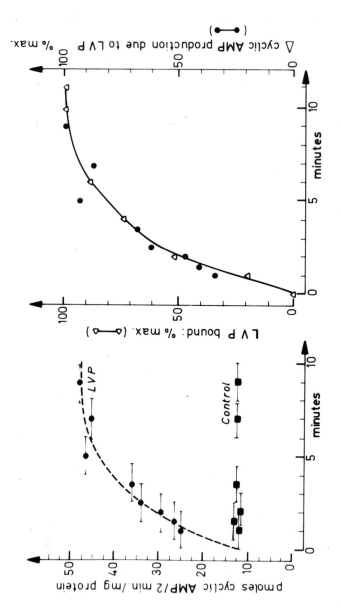

FIGURE 4. Time course of adenylate cyclase activation by lysine-vasopressin.
Left panel : Adenylate cyclase activity was measured during successive 2-minute periods as a function of time after adding vasopressin $10^{-8}M$ to the incubation medium. Samples without hormone were used as a control. The enzyme activation (increase in activity above control value) was calculated. The experimental values were used to construct the curve given in the right panel.
Right panel: Comparison of the time courses for $[^3H]$-vasopressin $(10^{-8}M)$ binding ($\triangle$) and adenylate cyclase activation ($\bullet$). From Bockaert et al.

quency of hormone-receptor interactions (rate theory). The fre-
quency of hormone-receptor interaction is given by : k_1 {H}{R};
(k_1 association rate constant, {H} and {R} = concentrations of
free hormone and unoccupied receptor respectively). It is maximal
at zero time when {R} is equal to the total amount of receptor
present and then progressively decreases towards an equilibrium
value. The time required to obtain a steady state adenylate
cyclase activation depends on the hormonal concentration tested.
Using supramaximal vasopressin concentrations, it was verified that
enzyme activation reached its equilibrium value almost instantaneously. From the above conclusions, it is obvious that the determination of adenylate cyclase activity by the amount of cyclic AMP
formed during a short period of time following the addition of
hormone to the incubation medium can lead to underestimate the
enzyme activation especially when low hormonal concentrations are
used. When looking for correlations between binding and response
it is thus necessary to measure both these two parameters under
equilibrium conditions. Comparison of the dose dependencies for
LVP binding and enzyme activation at equilibrium (Figure 5) indicated that the hormone concentration needed to saturate the membrane binding sites is identical to that leading to a maximal
enzyme activation. However the binding and activation curves are
not superimposable. A large adenylate cyclase activation was
observable in a concentration range for which a very small fraction
of the receptor sites are occupied by the hormone. As illustrated
by Figure 5, these observations could be accounted for by the
existence of a non linear coupling between receptor occupancy and
adenylate activation. However, to test this hypothesis, it is
necessary to exclude the possibility that the detected binding
sites are not the physiological receptors involved in adenylate
activation. In such a situation one can reasonably expect the
structural requirements for the attachment of the hormonal molecules to the physiological receptors to be different from the
structural requirements for the attachment to the detected binding
sites. Recent studies (9, 10) using a series of 32 lysine-vasopressin and oxytocin structural analogues failed to reveal such
differences. Each analogue was tested for its ability to activate
the adenylate cyclase and to inhibit the binding of {^{3}H}-LVP.
Without exception, all the analogues which were able to interact
with the adenylate cyclase as full or partial agonists were also
able to inhibit {^{3}H}-LVP binding (a typical experiment is illustrated by Figure 6). The maximal inhibition obtained was identical to that induced by the unlabelled vasopressin itself indicating that the entire population of vasopressin binding sites is
accessible to these analogues. Furthermore, the concentration of
peptide needed to obtain the saturation of the membrane binding
sites corresponded fairly well to that eliciting maximal enzyme
activation (Figure 7). This type of correlation was extended (10)
to a group of peptides which behaved as competitive inhibitors of

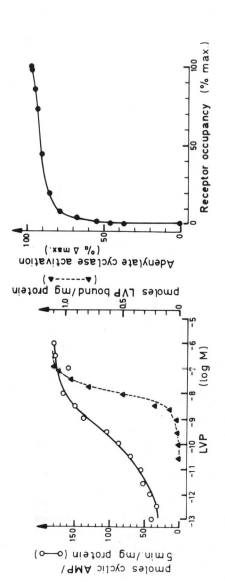

FIGURE 5. Receptor occupancy-adenylate cyclase activation relationship.
Left panel : The dose dependent adenylate cyclase activation and vasopressin binding were
determined under equilibrium conditions and on the same enzyme preparation (pig kidney adenylate cyclase).
Right panel : For each of the LVP concentrations used the percent saturation of the receptor
was calculated as well as the percent enzyme activation. The enzyme activation was plotted
as a function of receptor occupancy. From Jard et al. (14).

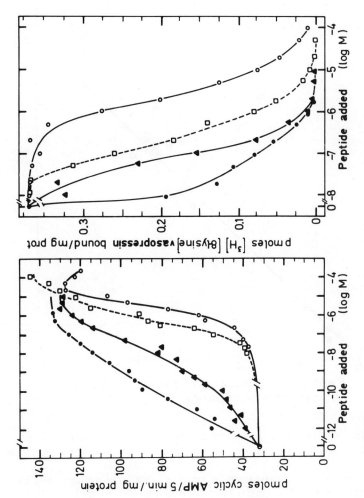

FIGURE 6. Specificity of hormone binding and adenylate cyclase activation.
The following peptides lysine-vasopressin (●), arginine-vasopressin (▲), deamino-{D-Arg⁸}
vasopressin (O-O) and deamino-6-carba-{Arg⁸} vasopressin (□-□) were tested for their
ability to activate the pig kidney adenylate cyclase (left panel) and to inhibit {³H}-vaso
pressin (10⁻⁸ M) binding (right panel). From Roy et al. (9)

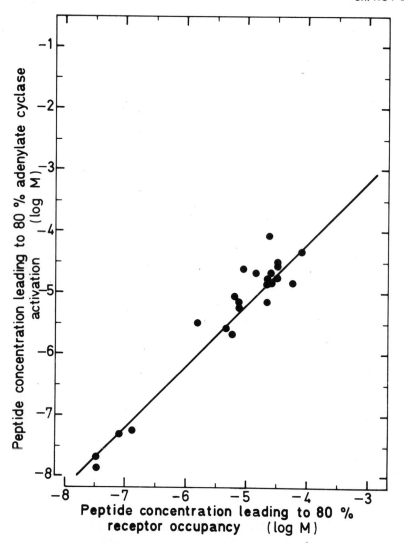

FIGURE 7. *Relation between peptide concentrations needed to satu-*
ration of vasopressin binding sites and maximal adenylate cyclase
activation.
Each point on the graph corresponds to a given structural analogue
of lysine-vasopressin (for details see Roy et al. (10)). For each
analogue the peptide concentration needed to obtain 80 % of maximal
adenylate activation was deduced from the corresponding dose-response
curve and plotted as a function of the peptide concentration leading
to a 80 % saturation of the receptor sites. The latter value was
deduced from competition experiments similar to those in Figure 6.
From Jard et al. (14).

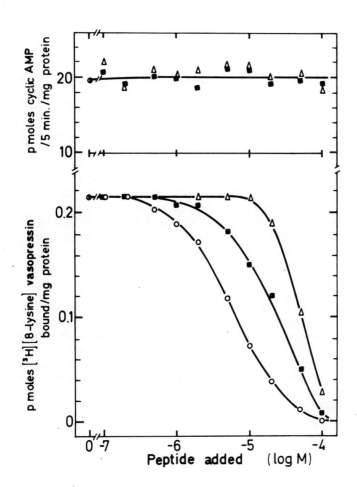

FIGURE 8.   Effects of two competitive inhibitors of lysine-vasopressin on {³H}-vasopressin binding to pig kidney membranes.
Upper part : Increasing amounts of pivaloyl-methyloxytocin (■)
and carbamoyl-methyloxytocin (Δ) were tested for their action on
adenylate cyclase.
Lower part : The abilities of these two peptides to compete with
{³H} {Lys⁸}-vasopressin binding (10⁻⁸ M) were tested. Oxytocin
(o) was used as a reference in this experiment. From Roy et al.
(10).

lysine-vasopressin both for the attachment to the binding sites
and enzyme activation (Figure 8). The apparent Km deduced from
binding studies was very close to the apparent Ki for the inhibition of adenylate cyclase activation. Such striking similarities
between the structural requirements for binding and action
strongly suggest that the detected binding sites are the physiological vasopressin receptors involved in adenylate cyclase
activation and, as a consequence, that the quantitative relationship between receptor occupancy and enzyme activation (the coupling
function) is a non linear one. It was further shown that the
coupling function depends on the structure of the active peptide
used (9, 10). Among the series of structural analogues tested an
almost continuous transition can be observed from analogues of
usually low affinity for which the coupling function is almost
linear to the natural antidiuretic hormones lysine and arginine-
vasopressins exhibiting a marked non linear coupling.

The activation-receptor occupancy relationship for lysine-
vasopressin was also affected by the chemical composition of the
incubation medium especially by its magnesium content. The initial
slope of the coupling function is significantly decreased at low
Mg^{2+} concentration (1 mM) as compared to that at high Mg^{2+} (16 mM).

The existence of a non linear coupling is suggestive of an
indirect activation process, the receptor and the adenylate cyclase
being distinct molecular entities coupled through the intermediary
of the membrane structure. It was recently demonstrated that the
vasopressin receptor and adenylate cyclase activity could be
extracted in soluble and active forms from the membrane structure
by the use of the non ionic detergent Triton X 100. The sensitivity
of the adenylate cyclase activation by vasopressin was lost after
membrane solubilization (12).

Acknowledgments

The experimental work reported in this paper was supported by
the "Centre National de la Recherche Scientifique" : RCP grant 220
and by the "Délégation générale à la recherche Scientique et Technique" : grant N° 73-3-1206.

REFERENCES

(1) BROWN, E., CLARKE, D.L., ROUX, V., and SHERMAN, G.H. (1963)
     J. Biol. Chem. 238, PC 852

(2) GRANTHAM, J.J. and BURG, M.B. (1966) Amer. J. Physiol. 211,
     255

(3) ANDERSON, W.A. Jr. and BROWN, E. (1963) Biochim. Biophys.
     Acta, 67, 674

(4) BOCKAERT, J., ROY, C., RAJERISON, R. and JARD, S. (1973)
     J. Biol. Chem. 248, 5922

(5) CAMPBELL, B.J., WOODWARD, G. and BORBERG, V. (1972) J. Biol.
     Chem. 247, 6167

(6) CHASE, L.R. and AURBACH, G.D. (1968) Science 159, 545

(7) DOUSA, T., HECHTER, O., SCHWARTZ, I.L. and WALTER, R. (1971)
     Proc. Nat. Acad. Sci. 68, 1693

(8) MARUMO, F. and EDELMAN, I. (1971) J. Clin. Invest. 50, 1613

(9) ROY, C., BARTH, T. and JARD, S. (1975) J. Biol. Chem. 250,
     3149

(10) ROY, C., BARTH, T. and JARD, S. (1975) J. Biol. Chem. 250,
     3157

(11) RAJERISON, R., MARCHETTI, J. ROY, C., BOCKAERT, J. and JARD,
     S. (1974) J. Biol. Chem. 249, 6390

(12) ROY, C., RAJERISON, R., BOCKAERT, J. and JARD, S. (1975).
     J. Biol. Chem. (in press)

(13) PRADELLES, P., MORGAT, J.L., FROMAGEOT, P., CAMIER, M.,
     BONNE, D., COHEN, P., BOCKAERT, J. and JARD, S. (1972)
     F.E.B.S. Letters 26, 189

(14) JARD, S., ROY, C., BARTH, T., RAJERISON, R. and BOCKAERT, J.
     (1975) Advances in Cyclic Nucleotides Research, Raven Press
     N.Y., Vol. 5, 31

EFFECTS OF CHOLERAGEN AND FLUORIDE ON ADENYLATE CYCLASE

Martha Vaughan

Laboratory of Cellular Metabolism
National Heart and Lung Institute
National Institutes of Health
Bethesda, Maryland 20014, USA

CONTENTS

A role for adenylate cyclase and cyclic AMP in the mediation of effects of a number of hormones on specific target cells has been extensively documented. There are, on the other hand, no known physiological counterparts to the effects of choleragen and of fluoride. These agents are capable of increasing adenylate cyclase activity in a variety of tissues. It may be inferred, therefore, that they act through components of the adenylate cyclase complex that are shared by many types of cells.

ACTIVATION OF ADENYLATE CYCLASE BY CHOLERAGEN

Choleragen is an exotoxin produced by Vibrio cholerae. It is a protein of molecular weight 84,000, composed of two different subunits with several intrachain disulfide bridges but no free sulfhydryl groups (1,2). Purified choleragen (1) has been found to activate adenylate cyclase in intestine, fat cells, liver, thyroid, platelets, leukocytes, cultured adrenal tumor and melanoma cells (3-12). It appears that all of the biological effects of the toxin may be secondary to adenylate cyclase activation.

113

The action of cholera toxin was initially studied in vivo by introducing it into ligated loops of small intestine in dogs or rabbits and measuring the resultant accumulation of fluid. The effect of the toxin was remarkable in that it became evident only after a delay of 15-30 min (13). In addition, the continued presence of choleragen was not required. Exposure of the intestine to choleragen for only a few minutes followed by washing produced, after the usual lag period, accelerated fluid secretion that persisted for many hours (14). In fact, the effects of even brief exposure to choleragen seem to be essentially irreversible.

Cuatrecasas extensively studied the binding of ^{125}I-choleragen to liver membranes and fat cells (15-18). At 24° or at 37°, binding of the ^{125}I-choleragen was essentially complete in 5 min (15). Specific binding to fat cells (15) and effects on lipolysis were proportional to choleragen concentration over similar ranges. The dissociation constant for the formation of the initial choleragen-receptor complex was of the order of 0.5 nM (15). With continuing incubation at temperatures above 24°, however, dissociation of the ^{125}I-choleragen became progressively slower and less extensive (17). These observations correlate with the demonstration that after a brief period of exposure the continued presence of choleragen was unnecessary for the production of functional effects on intestine (14), adrenal (11), or fat cells (7,17).

Specific antiserum added to the toxin before exposure of the tissue will prevent its effects (19). With adrenal cells, antiserum was largely effective even when added 15 min after choleragen (11), but in leukocytes (10) the capacity to reverse choleragen effects with antiserum was lost more rapidly.

Gangliosides found in plasma membranes can bind choleragen and prevent its biological effects (20). This is specifically a property of the monosialoganglioside, G_{M1} (15,16,21-25). After choleragen is bound to the cell, however, it is not readily removed (16) nor are its biological effects prevented (11) by added gangliosides. There is evidence that ganglioside G_{M1} may be the choleragen "receptor" or a part of it (15,16,26), and it has been reported (16) that new functional choleragen receptors can be generated by incubation of fat cells with ganglioside G_{M1}.

In addition to choleragen, Finkelstein and Lo Spalluto (1) purified from the growth medium of the Vibrio cholerae a protein, evidently a portion of choleragen, which they termed "choleragenoid" (27). It is immunologically identical with choleragen but has a molecular weight of 58,000 and does not produce choleragen-like effects on intestine (1) or fat cells (19). After incubation with choleragenoid, fat cells exhibit no lipolytic response to choleragen. When added after 15 min, however, choleragenoid does not prevent the lipolytic effect of choleragen (18). From studies of binding of ^{125}I-choleragenoid and the effects of unlabeled choleragenoid on choleragen binding Cuatrecasas (18) concluded that both probably interact in a similar manner with the same receptors on the cell surface, although the subsequent alterations in the complex that lead to activation of adenylate cyclase with choleragen do not occur when the receptor is occupied by choleragenoid. It has been suggested that choleragenoid is the portion of the choleragen molecule that is responsible for the initial binding to the ganglioside receptor (18,26,28).

The changes that occur in the cells following the initial binding of choleragen and result after 15 to 60 min in activation of adenylate cyclase are largely unknown. They are temperature dependent (17) but evidently do not require continuing synthesis of RNA or protein (10,17).

The striking aspects of the effects of choleragen on adenylate cyclase, the slowness with which activation occurs after the relative rapid initial binding of the toxin, and the apparent irreversibility of the toxin-activated state are in obvious contrast to the rapid onset and reversal of hormonal activation. Data concerning the hormonal responsiveness of the choleragen-activated adenylate cyclase are somewhat conflicting. O'Keefe and Cuatrecasas (12) found that, at the time the adenylate cyclase of melanoma cells was maximally active after exposure of the cells to choleragen, no increase in activity was demonstrable when melano-cyte-stimulating hormone was added to the assay system. Chen et al. (29) reported that the elevated adenylate cyclase activity of the intestinal mucosa from patients with cholera could be further stimulated with prostaglandin E_1. Gorman and Bitensky (8) found that choleragen activated hepatic adenylate cyclase to the same level as that produced by epinephrine acting on adenylate cyclase from normal liver and the toxin-activated cyclase was not responsive to epinephrine, although its responsiveness to glucagon was unimpaired.

We have consistently found that a maximally effective concentration of isoproterenol stimulates the fat cell adenylate cyclase to the same extent in preparations already activated with choleragen as it does in those from control cells, and the concentration dependency of the isoproterenol response is unaltered by choleragen. Whether this means that the catalytic units of the adenylate cyclase that are susceptible to activation by choleragen are different from those that are under hormonal control remains to be determined. Quantitative interpretation of effects of hormones on adenylate cyclase in broken cell preparations is complicated by the fact that in many cases the maximal stimulation that can be demonstrated is apparently much less than that which occurs in the intact cell, and the concentrations of hormones required to produce activation of cyclase are considerably greater than those that are effective in the intact tissue. The suggestion that choleragen may in some way stabilize the adenylate cyclase and its hormonal responsiveness (30) could account for the observations of Hewlett et al. (7) that epinephrine had a greater effect on the choleragen-activated fat cell cyclase than it did on the enzyme from control cells. In any case, the relationship between the effects of choleragen and those of hormones on adenylate cyclase remains unclear.

EFFECTS OF FLUORIDE ON ADENYLATE CYCLASE

Activation of Adenylate Cyclase by Fluoride

In early studies, Rall and Sutherland (31) found that adenylate cyclase activity in liver homogenates was increased by fluoride. It is now well known that fluoride enhances the activity of adenylate cyclase from most mammalian tissues, and it has often been stated, erroneously, that the activity observed in the presence of fluoride represents "total" adenylate cyclase. Fluoride activation of adenylate cyclase has been studied chiefly by adding it to the assay system. It has, however, been reported that incubation of adenylate cyclase preparations from rat parotid (32), brain (33), or liver (34) with fluoride resulted in activation that was not reversed when the fluoride concentration was lowered by dilution, by washing, or by dialysis of the enzyme before assay. Perkins and Moore (33) described in some detail this apparently irreversible activation of the brain cyclase and noted that it was dependent on temperature and fluoride concentration. In the following discussion, some characteristics of the effects of fluoride added to the assay system are compared with those produced when the fat cell adenylate cyclase is incubated with fluoride and then assayed in its effective absence.[1]

---

[1] In the experiments of Manganiello and Vaughan (36) referred to here, all incubations and adenylate cyclase assays were carried out at 30°. The assay system (pH 8.0) contained 6.6 mM $MgCl_2$, 3.3 mM ATP (with an ATP regenerating system) and 0.8 mM cyclic AMP. Basal activity and that assayed in the presence of fluoride was essentially independent of ATP concentration (with Mg^{++} always in excess) between 1.5 and 10 mM. Incubation of adenylate cyclase preparations (with or without fluoride) was carried out in a medium containing Tris buffer, pH 7.4, and 2.5 mM $MgCl_2$.

Stimulation of fat cell adenylate cyclase activity by fluoride in the assay system occurs very rapidly, often with no discernible delay (31,35) and accumulation of cyclic AMP usually proceeds at a constant rate for 20 min or more. In our studies (36), as previously reported (37), plots of adenylate cyclase activity vs concentration of fluoride in the assay system were sigmoidal and no effects were observed with <0.5 mM fluoride. Stimulation was half maximal with about 2 mM sodium fluoride, maximal with 3 mM, and tended to diminish with concentrations above 8 mM (36). Reversal of stimulation with concentrations of fluoride greater than optimal (35,37,38) has been attributed to a decrease in the Mg^{++} ion concentration (37,38) but may also be due to inhibition of adenylate cyclase by fluoride (see below).

When cyclase preparations were incubated with fluoride (followed by dilution so that the concentrations of fluoride introduced into the assay were negligible in terms of effects on adenylate cyclase activity), the activity apparently increased rapidly during the first 5 min and much more slowly thereafter (36). The "initial rate" of activation and the extent of activation after 20 min were dependent on fluoride concentration. Activation under these conditions could be demonstrated with concentrations of fluoride lower than those required to produce stimulation in the assay. Preparations previously incubated with fluoride produced cyclic AMP at a constant rate in the assay for at least 20 min (36). This is consistent with the earlier observations (32-34) that after incubation with fluoride activation was not reversed by prolonged washing or dialysis.

In the assay system, 1.5 mM sodium pyrophosphate, which had little effect on basal adenylate cyclase, essentially abolished fluoride stimulation of adenylate cyclase (39). Although 1.5 mM pyrophosphate, when present initially, effectively prevented fluoride activation and when added after 2.5 min rapidly reversed it, pyrophosphate added after 5 min had a smaller effect. After 10 min fluoride activation was reversed less than 40% by the addition of pyrophosphate (36). The adenylate cyclase activated by preincubation for 20 min with 5 mM fluoride was inhibited only slightly by 1.5 mM pyrophosphate in the assay system (36). When added with fluoride to the cyclase during incubation before assay, however, 1.5 mM pyrophosphate markedly decreased activation and 6 mM essentially completely prevented it. After incubation of the enzyme with fluoride for 5 min, the addition of pyrophosphate effectively abolished further activation, but there was no decline in activity with continued incubation for 15 min (36). It appears that the adtivation produced by fluoride, whether during prior incubation or in the assay system, is initially largely preventable or reversible with pyrophosphate but relatively rapidly becomes irreversible.

It seems probable that the capacity to reverse fluoride activation by dilution is likewise diminished during incubation of the cyclase, thus accounting for the apparent "time course of fluoride activation" when the enzyme is incubated with fluoride for various periods and then assayed in its absence. All of the available evidence is consistent with the view that, when the enzyme is initially exposed to fluoride (at 30°), whether in the assay system or simply in buffer at pH 7.4, the adenylate cyclase is rapidly activated to a level dependent on the concentration of fluoride. Within the first few minutes, the activation is largely reversible either by the addition of pyrophosphate or by removal of fluoride, but with continuing incubation at 30°, the fluoride-activated enzyme becomes no longer susceptible to inactivation by these means.

Whereas the capacity to reverse the fluoride-activated state appears to be rapidly lost, the responsiveness of the enzyme to fluoride stimulation was maintained for at least 20 min under the assay conditions (although it diminished rapidly during incubation in Tris buffer, pH 7.4) (36). The effect of the assay medium in this case appeared to be one of stabilizing the capacity of the enzyme to respond to fluoride. In both media the stabilities of basal enzyme activity and of the enzyme already activated by fluoride were similar, and in both media the reversibility of fluoride activation was rapidly lost (36). All of these observations are consonant with the hypothesis that activation of the cyclase by fluoride and its reversal are enzyme-dependent processes (35). In this view, incubation of the cyclase preparations at 30° could cause inactivation of these converting enzymes and/or depletion of the necessary cofactors, although other explanations are equally possible with the limited information available at present. Based on studies of a different type, Najjar and co-workers (40,41) have recently suggested that fluoride activation of adenylate cyclase may be enzymatically controlled.

One would like to be able to compare the characteristics of the cyclase activated by incubation with fluoride before assay with those of the cyclase activated by assay in the presence of fluoride, but interpretation of such experiments is complicated by the fact that fluoride present in the assay can inhibit the cyclase activated in several different ways (see below). It seems most probable, however, that fluoride activation of adenylate cyclase is the same process whether it occurs in the assay system or is achieved by incubation of the enzyme with fluoride.

Fluoride stimulation of adenylate cyclase differs in many ways from that caused by peptide hormones or catecholamines. Birnbaumer et al. (37) compared effects of fluoride on the fat cell cyclase with those of ACTH. In particular, they noted that the apparent K_m for fluoride activation was significantly increased

when the assay temperature was decreased from 37° to 30°. It was
also shown that the magnitude of activation by 10 mM fluoride was
distinctly greater at 37° than it was at 30°, whereas the effect
of ACTH increased little between 30 and 37°. Harwood and Rodbell
(38) further showed that activation by fluoride was minimal in
assays at temperatures below 25°, although hormonal stimulation
was demonstrable even at 10°. It has been repeatedly found in
studies of adenylate cyclase from several sources that activity in
the presence of a hormone plus fluoride is equivalent to that
observed with fluoride alone. (This is discussed further in relationship to the inhibitory effects of fluoride.) On the other
hand, after activation of the fat cell cyclase by preincubation
with fluoride, the addition of isoproterenol in the assay system
(without fluoride) caused a further increase in activity, although
the increment was only a fraction of that produced by isoproterenol
with the enzyme not exposed to fluoride (36). One can only conclude
that the relationship between fluoride activation and hormonal
activation of adenylate cyclase remains to be defined as does the
mechanism of action of fluoride which may or may not involve
enzymatic modification of the cyclase complex.

Inhibition of Adenylate Cyclase by Fluoride

Harwood and Rodbell (38) showed that under conditions in which
hormonal stimulation of fat cell adenylate cyclase was greater than
that produced by fluoride, specifically at assay temperatures of
30° or below, fluoride in concentrations as low as 1 mM caused
inhibition of hormonal stimulation. As discussed below, fluoride
also inhibits the choleragen-stimulated adenylate cyclase and the
enzyme activated by preincubation with fluoride.

In our studies (36), the activity of the fat cell adenylate
cyclase was greater in the presence of 100 μM isoproterenol than
it was in the presence of 5.3 mM fluoride. (These concentrations
of the respective agents in the assay caused maximal stimulation
of adenylate activity.) When fluoride was present with isoproterenol, the rate of cyclic AMP accumulation was decreased to the
level of that observed with fluoride alone, and when fluoride was
added after 3 min or 7 min to assays containing isoproterenol,
the new lower rate was established with no discernible delay,
demonstrating the rapidity with which fluoride inhibition occurs
(36).

In the presence of 100 μM isoproterenol, 0.5 mM fluoride significantly decreased cyclase activity; with 5 mM fluoride activity
was equal to that observed with fluoride alone and was independent
of isoproterenol concentration (36), as previously reported (38).
Thus, it might appear that at this concentration fluoride completely

prevents hormonal stimulation of the enzyme, and the activity observed is due entirely to fluoride (38), the resultant of its stimulatory and inhibitory effects. It has not been possible, however, to determine experimentally whether this interpretation is, in fact, correct.

As previously mentioned, stimulation of fat cell cyclase by fluoride was essentially completely prevented with 1.5 mM sodium pyrophosphate. This concentration of pyrophosphate had little effect on activity in the presence of isoproterenol or isoproterenol plus 5.3 mM fluoride; i.e., pyrophosphate in a concentration that prevented activation by fluoride did not interfere with its inhibitory effect (36). In these circumstances (with fluoride, isoproterenol and pyrophosphate present) it was apparent that the effect of isoproterenol was not completely inhibited by fluoride, since the addition of propranol to block isoproterenol stimulation of cyclase returned activity to the basal level (36).

Birnbaumer et al. (37) originally reported that adenylate cyclase activity assayed in the basal state or in the presence of fluoride was enhanced by Mn^{++} ion. We found that 3.3 mM $MnCl_2$ roughly doubled both basal activity and the increment produced by fluoride while activity in the presence of isoproterenol was unaffected. With 3.3 mM $MnCl_2$ the activity in the presence of isoproterenol plus fluoride tended to be slightly higher than that produced by isoproterenol alone and was equivalent to that observed with fluoride alone, suggesting that perhaps Mn^{++} interferes with the inhibitory effects of fluoride. When $MnCl_2$ was added to the assay at various times in the presence of fluoride, there was an immediate increase in the rate of cyclic AMP formation (36). If the effect of manganese is viewed as one of preventing fluoride inhibition, it would appear that the inhibitory effects of fluoride are rapidly reversible as well as immediate in onset.

The choleragen activated adenylate cyclase from fat cells was inhibited by fluoride in a concentration-dependent manner essentially identical to that observed for the isoproterenol-stimulated enzyme (36). As was the case with isoproterenol, regardless of the degree of activation produced by the toxin, when assayed in the presence of 5.3 mM fluoride, the activity was equal to that of the cyclase from control cells assayed with the same concentration of fluoride (36). Although 3.3 mM $MnCl_2$ had little effect on the basal activity of the enzyme from the toxin-treated cells, it, in descriptive terms, reversed the inhibitory effect of fluoride as it did in the presence of isoproterenol and permitted demonstration of fluoride stimulation of the toxin-treated enzyme (36).

The fat cell adenylate cyclase activated by prior incubation with 5 mM fluoride was also inhibited by fluoride added to the assay system over a concentration range very similar to that found for fluoride inhibition of isoproterenol activation (36).   Inhibition of the fluoride-activated enzyme by fluoride was apparently prevented by $MnCl_2$, which also somewhat increased the activity of the fluoride-activated enzyme.   The latter observation could mean that even after dilution the cyclase activated by prior incubation with fluoride remains slightly inhibited by fluoride.

In summary, fluoride can inhibit the fat cell adenylate cyclase, whether it is activated by hormones, by choleragen, or by fluoride itself. Fluoride inhibition is essentially immediate in onset, and, if one looks upon the effect of Mn^{++} as one of preventing fluoride inhibition, it may be rapidly reversible.   It can be demonstrated under conditions in which fluoride activation of the cyclase is not observed, e.g., at temperatures below 25° (38) or in the presence of pyrophosphate (36).   If, as suggested by Harwood and Rodbell (38), fluoride inhibits hormonal stimulation at some point on the pathway between the formation of hormone-receptor complex and augmentation of adenylate cyclase activity, then it may be necessary to postulate another mechanism by which fluoride inhibits the enzyme activated by toxin or by fluoride.   Insofar as we have studied them, however, the characteristics of the inhibitory effects of fluoride appear to be similar, whether the cyclase is activated by choleragen, isoproterenol, or fluoride itself.

Although, at present, information concerning the inhibitory effects of fluoride is related specifically to the fat cell adenylate cyclase, it seems likely that just as the capacities to be activated by fluoride and by choleragen are apparently general properties of many mammalian cyclases, so is susceptibility to fluoride inhibition.   Thus, as we learn more about all of these processes, we may gain a better understanding of some of the basic mechanisms through which adenylate cyclase activity is controlled in all tissues.

REFERENCES

1. Finkelstein, R. A., and Lo Spalluto, J. J.   (1970) J. Infect. Dis. 121: 563.

2. Lo Spalluto, J. J., and Finkelstein, R. A. (1972) Biochim. Biophys. Acta 257: 158.

3. Kimberg, D. V., Field, M., Johnson, J., Henderson, A., and Gershon, E. (1971) J. Clin. Invest. 50: 1218.

4. Sharp, G. W. G., and Hynie, S. (1971) Nature 229: 266.

5. Sharp, G. W. G., Hynie, S., Lipson, L. C., and Parkinson, D. K. (1971) Trans. Ass. Am. Phys. 84: 200.

6. Evans, D. J., Jr., Chen, L. C., Curlin, G. T., and Evans, E. G. (1972) Nature New Biol. 236: 137.

7. Hewlett, E. L., Guerrant, R. L., Evans, D. J. Jr., and Greenough, W. B. (1974) Nature 249: 371.

8. Gorman, R. E., and Bitensky, M. W. (1972) Nature 235: 439.

9. Zieve, P. D., Pierce, N. F., and Greenough, W. B. (1971) Johns Hopkins Med. J. 129: 299.

10. Bourne, H. R., Lehner, R. I., Lichtenstein, L. M., Weissman, G., and Zurier, R. (1973) J. Clin. Invest. 52: 698.

11. Wolff, J., Temple, R., and Cook, G. H. (1973) Proc. Nat. Acad. Sci. U.S.A. 70: 2741.

12. O'Keefe, E., and Cuatrecasas, P. (1974) Proc. Nat. Acad. Sci. U.S.A. 71: 2500.

13. Finkelstein, R.A. (1969) Tex. Rep. Biol. Med. 27: 181.

14. Pierce, N. F., Greenough, W.B., and Carpenter, C.C. (1971) Bacteriol. Rev. 35: 1.

15. Cuatrecasas, P. (1973) Biochemistry 12: 3547.

16. Cuatrecasas, P. (1973) Biochemistry 12: 3558.

17. Cuatrecasas, P. (1973) Biochemistry 12: 3567.

18.   Cuatrecasas, P. (1973) Biochemistry 12: 3577.

19.   Vaughan, M., Pierce, N.F., and Greenough, W. B. (1970) Nature 226: 658.

20.   van Heyningen, W.E., Carpenter, C. C., Pierce, N. F., and Greenough, W. B. (1971) J. Infect. Dis. 124: 415.

21.   van Heyningen, W. E. (1973) Naunyn-Schmiedebergs Arch. exp. Path. Pharmak. 276: 289.

22.   King, C. A., and van Heyningen, W. E. (1973) J. Infect. Dis. 127: 639.

23.   Holmgren, J., Lönnroth, I., and Svennerholm, L. (1973) Scand. J. Infect. Dis. 5: 77.

24.   Holmgren, J., Lönnroth, I., and Svennerholm, L. (1973) Infect. Immunol. 8: 208.

25.   Davis, J., Tyrrell, D. A. J., Ramsdew, B. W., Louis, I. N., and Milne, R. G. (1973) Exp. Mol. Pathol. 18: 1.

26.   van Heyningen, W. E. (1974) Nature 249: 415.

27.   Finkelstein, R. A., Peterson, J. W., and Lo Spalluto, J. J. (1971) J. Immunol. 106: 868.

28.   van Heyningen, S. (1974) Science 183: 656.

29.   Chen, L. C., Rohde, J. E., and Sharp, G. W. G. (1972) J. Clin. Invest. 51: 731.

30.   Beckman, B., Flores, J., Witkun, P. A., and Sharp, G. W. G. (1974) J. Clin. Invest. 53: 1202.

31.   Rall, T. W., and Sutherland, E. W. (1958) J. Biol. Chem. 232: 1065.

32.   Schramm, M., and Naim, E. (1970) J. Biol. Chem. 245: 3225.

33.   Perkins, J. B., and Moore, M. M. (1971) J. Biol. Chem. 246: 62.

34.   Birnbaumer, L., Pohl, S. L., Rodbell, M., and Sundby, F. (1972) J. Biol. Chem. 247: 2038.

35.   Vaughan, M., and Murad, F. (1969) Biochem. 8: 3092.

36. Manganiello, V. C., and Vaughan, M. Unpublished observations.

37. Birnbaumer, L., Pohl, S. L., and Rodbell, M. (1969) J. Biol. Chem. 244: 3468.

38. Harwood, J. P., and Rodbell, M. (1973) J. Biol. Chem. 248: 4901

39. Birnbaumer, L., Pohl, S. L., and Rodbell, M. (1971) J. Biol. Chem. 246: 1857.

40. Constantopoulos, A., and Najjar, V. A. (1973) Biochem. Biophys. Res. Commun. 53: 794.

41. Layne, P., Constantopoulos, A., Judge, J. F. X., Rauner, R. and Najjar, V. A. (1973) Biochem. Biophys. Res. Commun. 53: 800.

STIMULATION OF ADENYLATE CYCLASE IN THE THYROID

N.J. Marshall

Department of Nuclear Medicine
The Middlesex Hospital Medical School
Thorn Institute of Clinical Science
Mortimer Street
London W1N 8AA (United Kingdom)

Contents

INTRODUCTION

In 1962 Klainer et al. (1) reported the presence of an adenylate cyclase in the thyroid, responsive to the pituitary hormone, TSH[1]. Since then, research has mainly been directed towards determining the relevance of cyclic AMP as a regulator

---

[1] *ABBREVIATIONS:*   TSH = *thyroid stimulating hormone*
                       TSIg = *thyroid stimulating immunoglobulins*
                       PG = *prostaglandin*

of the thyroid follicular cell, particularly in response to TSH.
However, during the course of this work, many other compounds
have been tested as potential stimulators of adenylate cyclase
in the thyroid. In this paper, evidence that thyroidal adenylate
cyclase can be activated by compounds as diverse as immunoglobulins, prostaglandins and catecholamines as well as TSH will
be discussed. It is, as yet, too soon to debate the physiological
significance of these responses and discussion is directed towards
characterisation of the response to each different group of
agonists, and consideration of the influence this might bear on
our ultimate concept of the hormone-receptor/membrane adenylate
cyclase system(s) operative in the thyroid.

TSH STIMULATION OF ADENYLATE CYCLASE IN THE THYROID

The evidence that TSH activation of thyroid follicular
cell metabolism is mediated by intracellular cyclic AMP was
comprehensively reviewed by Schell-Frederick and Dumont (2) and
Dumont (3). It was concluded that the several criteria necessary
to establish the role of cyclic AMP as the second messenger to
the trophic hormone were partially fulfilled for most responsive
metabolic processes, the clearest exception being TSH stimulation
of phospholipid metabolism. The copious literature cited will
not be reviewed in this presentation, but more recent reports
describing (i) TSH activation of adenylate cyclase in membrane
preparations, (ii) the modification of this process and (iii) TSH
binding to thyroid tissue and its relationship to adenylate
cyclase activation will be discussed.

Stimulation of Plasma-Membrane Associated Adenylate Cyclase by TSH

Yamashita and Field (4) and Wolff and Jones (5) reported
TSH activation of adenylate cyclase in plasma membrane-enriched
subcellular fractions from the bovine thyroid. Wolff and Jones
carefully appraised tissue disruption conditions, since the
responsiveness of the final preparation to TSH appeared sensitive
to physical stresses applied during homogenisation, and finally
detailed a procedure yielding responsive membranes. The adenylate
cyclase copurified (80 to 150 fold) with a number of enzymes considered to be plasma-membrane markers and out of a number of poly-

peptide hormones tested was found to respond solely to TSH and
human chorionic thyrotrophin. However, both these membranes and
those described in several subsequent investigations, have proved
fairly insensitive to TSH. For example, whereas levels of TSH
in sera from euthyroid subjects rarely exceed 8-10µU/ml, Wolff
and Jones report that concentrations of at least 1 mU/ml of bovine
TSH were necessary to activate adenylate cyclase in plasma membranes from the bovine thyroid; the incubation conditions were
those found to be optimal for stimulation (5mM MG^{++}, 2.5 mM ATP,
10 mM theophylline, an ATP regenerating system and 25 mM Tris-HCl
buffer, ph 7.5). However, Pochet et al. (6) have reported more
sensitive membrane preparations from horse thyroid (half-maximal
stimulation was observed at 1.2 mU bovine TSH/ml). Whether this
was due to species differences or the different preparative procedure employed (7) is not certain. Curiously, Wolff and Jones
observed that even with doses as high as 500 mU TSH/ml stimulation of adenylate cyclase continued to increase with no indication of a plateau in response. Subsequent experience in the
author's laboratory, using techniques identical to Wolff and
Jones, have shown this characteristic as well as the sensitivity
to TSH, to vary from one preparation to another (see Figure 1),
and saturable systems have been described by other laboratories
(6,8,9,10).

The accumulation of cyclic AMP in response to incubation
of membranes with TSH appears relatively stable, with little
evidence of decline during incubation periods of at least 30
minutes. Persistence of stimulation after washing thyroid tissue,
previously exposed to TSH, with hormone-free medium (11,12,13) and
direct investigation for TSH inactivation during incubation with
thyroid slices (14), suggests that the hormone is not actively
degraded during the incubation period. In this respect TSH
acting on the thyroid contrasts with other systems such as glucagon or insulin acting on the liver (15,16).

Modification of TSH Stimulation of Adenylate Cyclase

As with other hormone-receptor/adenylate cyclase systems
the molecular events which occur in the membrane are far from
understood. One way of investigating this problem further is to
test the effects of compounds which might be predicted to perturb
the system in a characteristic manner and hence allow one to
deduce the involvement of a specific component. In the following

subsections, the effects of (a) ionic environment, (b) nucleotide triphosphates and (c) agents which might be expected to disturb membrane structure will be discussed. Inhibition of TSH stimulation with prostaglandin antagonists is considered elsewhere (Section III, and the paper in this volume by Jacquemin).

a. Ionic Environment

        In studies using isolated membranes from the thyroid both TSH binding (discussed later) and stimulation of adenylate cyclase was sensitive to ionic environment. During the course of detailed investigations, Wolff and coworkers (5,17) reported that K^+ slightly increased the response of adenylate cyclase to TSH, but Ca^{++} and Li^+, and to a lesser extent Na^+ were inhibitory. These findings were largely in agreement with those reported by Burke (18,19) from studies using sheep thyroid homogenates. However, as would be expected, parallel effects were not necessarily observed in cellular systems. For example Williams (20) observed inhibition of TSH stimulation of cyclic AMP accumulation in mouse thyroid lobes upon reduction of Na^+ or increase of Ca^{++}, but Li^+ was without effect. Kendall-Taylor (21), however, reported that Li^+ (20mM) almost completely abolished TSH stimulation of ^3H-adenosine incorporation into cyclic AMP in mouse thyroid lobes. Yamashita et al. (22) and van Sande and Dumont (23) detected no modification of basal or TSH stimulated cyclic AMP levels in dog thyroid slices after replacement of most Na^+ by K^+, although omission of Ca^{++} and the addition of EGTA appeared to somewhat reduce TSH stimulation. As discussed elsewhere in this volume (see Dumont et al.) changing intracellular levels of Ca^{++} were found to only slightly effect TSH stimulation of cyclic AMP accumulation in dog thyroid slices, compared with other metabolic parameters such as glucose carbon-1-oxidation.

        Van Sande and coworkers (23,24) have demonstrated that iodide inhibited TSH stimulation of cyclic AMP formation in tissue slices from thyroids of many different species. Our observation that high levels of iodide did not inhibit TSH stimulation of adenylate cyclase in membrane preparations from the bovine thyroid (unpublished) is compatible with their conclusions that inhibition resulted from the formation of an intracellular iodine containing compound. In neither of the above systems was iodide stimulation of basal adenylate cyclase observed, but Burke (25) has reported stimulation of adenylate cyclase in the sheep thyroid by NaI (10^{-5} to 10^{-3} M), although NaI also proved inhibitory to TSH and PGE stimulation.

b. Nucleoside Triphosphates

Wolff and Hope-Cook (26) investigated the effects of purine nucleotides on the response of adenylate cyclase to TSH in membrane preparations from the bovine thyroid. Various nucleotides were found to enhance the response, but ITP proved the most potent. A time-lag in the onset of ITP-modulated enhancement of cyclic AMP production in response to TSH was observed. Verrier et al. (9) reported that GTP enhanced TSH stimulation of adenylate cyclase in membranes prepared from the pig thyroid, but Sato et al. (27) reported little effect of GTP on TSH stimulation in human thyroid plasma membranes, especially in comparison with its marked potentiation of PGE_2 stimulation, using identical conditions.

Interestingly, it has been demonstrated that ITP, when present at concentrations ranging from $10\mu M$ to $1mM$, changed the Scatchard plot of the relation between TSH concentration and adenylate cyclase activation from a hyperbole to a curve exhibiting a maximum with downward concavity. This was interpreted as being due to change from negative to positive cooperativity (6,28). Boeynaems et al. (28) reported that in the horse thyroid ITP increased basal and TSH stimulated adenylate cyclase activity, and TSH stimulation was therefore not necessarily increased by the nucleotide. This also appears to be true for GTP modification of adenylate cyclase activity in membranes prepared from the hyperplastic guinea pig thyroid (8).

5'-guanylylimidodiphosphate was reported to be a potent activator of adenylate cyclase in bovine thyroid membranes, and this stimulation was further enhanced by TSH (29).

c. Agents potentially disruptive to membrane structure

In the thyroid, as in many other systems examined, (30-33), phospholipids appear to play an essential role in hormonal stimulation of adenylate cyclase (34). Yamashita et al. (35) reported that treatment of thyroid slices with phospholipase C inhibited TSH elevation of cyclic AMP levels. Subsequently, Yamashita and Field (36) demonstrated the effect using pre-treaded plasma membranes, confirming the suggestion that membrane lipids are important for TSH stimulation of adenylate cyclase. The phenomenon was reversible, since response to TSH was partially restored if phospholipids, in particular phosphatidyl choline, were added to the membranes after phospholipase A treatment. Although in this study no attempt was made to localise the site of specific requirements for phospholipids, Haye and Jacquemin (37) reported that binding of labelled TSH to thyroid tissue was

partially inhibited after pretreatment with phospholipase C,
suggesting involvement at the receptor site. More recently,
Bashford et al. (38) have reported a sharp increase in TSH
binding to thyroid plasma membranes at incubation temperatures
about 30°, which was coincident with a marked change in temperature dependence of the motional characteristics of 3 membrane-
bound fluorescent probes. This indicated that lipid mobility
may be an important factor for TSH binding.

        Further evidence for phospholipid components in the TSH
receptor/adenylate cyclase system may be derived from observations
of inhibition by "membrane-active" agents; at least some of
these probably act by distorting phospholipid organisation within
membrane structure. Wolff and Jones (5,39) demonstrated that
phenothiazines such as chlorpromazine, detergents, in particular
cetyl pyridinium chloride, basic compounds such as cobramine B
and polylysine, polyenes such as filipin and the ionophores
valinomycin, gramicidin or monensin A, inhibited TSH stimulation
of adenylate cyclase in membrane preparations from the bovine
thyroid without reducing basal activity. These agents did not
effect fluoride stimulation at concentrations inhibitory to TSH
activation, but some enhanced fluoride stimulation at higher
concentrations. We have shown (40) that TSH stimulation of
adenylate cyclase in membrane preparations is also sensitive to
propranolol. Since D and L propranolol were equipotent,
inhibiting in a non-competitive manner, and inhibition was also
observed with quinidine, but not practolol, the results were
interpreted to indicate inhibition due to the "local-anaesthetic"
activity of these compounds. The high concentrations of propranolol required to produce inhibition (10^{-4} to 10^{-3} M) were
consistent with this conclusion; it is noteworthy that propranolol has been shown to be effective over this concentration
range in systems ranging from TSH stimulation of release of
radioiodine from intact mouse thyroid lobes (41), activation of
glucose oxidation in bovine thyroid slices (42), augmentation of
adenylate cyclase activity, ^{3}H cyclic AMP formation and cyclic AMP
levels in dog thyroid slices (35), as well as adenylate cyclase
in plasma membranes, although this drug has also been shown to
act on components of the follicular cell other than the receptor-
adenylate cyclase system (41,43,44,45). It is also possible that
α-adrenergic antagonists can modify membrane structure in an
analagous manner, since these were found to inhibit TSH stimulation of adenylate cyclase in membrane preparations when present
at relatively high concentrations (46). When three α-antagonists,
thymoxamine, phenoxybenzamine, and phentolamine were investigated
over concentrations ranging from 10^{-7} to 5×10^{-3} M, potentiation
of TSH stimulation was observed prior to inhibition; such
diphasic modification of the response of adenylate cyclase has
also been observed with "membrane active" agents, such as

chlorpromazine (39) and propranolol (40, 47).

The diversity of compounds inhibiting TSH activation of adenylate cyclase together with lack of stereospecificity suggests that the inhibition cannot be due to interaction with the TSH receptor. It is likely, particularly in view of the diphasic modification often observed, that the inhibition is another example of the membrane-stabilisation/destabilisation phenomenon. Seeman (48) reviewing the action of many "membrane-active" compounds on widely differing cellular and subcellular systems, noted that membrane stabilisation occurred at concentrations of the order of $10^{-6}M$, and breakdown of membrane structure (destabilisation) at higher concentrations ($10^{-3}M$). It is of course interesting that basal adenylate cyclase activity generally appeared to be uninfluenced by such changes induced in membrane structure, and this emphasizes the independence of the TSH receptor and the catalytic subunit.

TSH Binding and its Relation to Stimulation of Adenylate Cyclase

In 1966 Pastan et al. (11) reported that TSH interacted with a receptor located at a site on the thyroid follicular cell which was accessible to anti-TSH antibody and trypsin. This interaction appeared to be a necessary prerequisite for stimulation of glucose-1-^{14}C oxidation. However, they were unable to detect binding of labelled TSH to specific receptor sites, probably due to the methodology used, but recently, several groups have described binding of TSH to thyroid tissue. Table 1 lists some of the studies reported.

As is apparent from Table 1 TSH binding has been described in many different thyroid tissue preparations, and as discussed critically by Field (60), the range of values for receptor affinity may reflect both this variable and the widely different experimental conditions used. Several attempts have been made to correlate binding with stimulation of adenylate cyclase activity (8-10,57), in some cases demonstrating that the dose-response curve for stimulation of the enzyme closely corresponded to that for saturation of hormone binding, analogous to the relationship described between glucagon and liver plasma-membrane adenylate cyclase (see paper by Krans in this volume).

Wolff et al. (53) reported correlation between the relative potencies of TSH and its α and β subunits in displacing TSH bound to bovine membranes and adenylate cyclase activation. Further comparison between TSH, its subunits, and luteinising hormone and its β-subunit, lead to the conclusion that the β-

Table 1. Studies on TSH binding to thyroid tissue

	Ref.	Thyroid tissue preparation used for binding	Affinity* constant
Schell-Frederick and Dumont (1970)	2	Isolated bovine cells	————
Haye and Jacquemin (1971)	37	Porcine and ovine slices	————
Manley et al. (1972)	49	Slices from hyper-plastic guinea-pig thyroid	$3.8 \times 10^8 M^{-1}$
Mehdi et al. (1973)	50	Bovine thyroid membranes	————
Amir et al. (1973)	10	Bovine thyroid membranes	$2.0 \times 10^7 M^{-1}$
Lissitzky et al. (1973)	51	Cultured, isolated porcine cells	$1.0 \times 10^9 M^{-1}$
Verrier et al. (1974)	9	Cultured, isolated porcine cells. Membranes prepared from above cells	$1.9 \times 10^9 M^{-1}$ $0.6 \times 10^9 M^{-1}$
Goldfine et al. (1974)	52	Bovine thyroid membranes	————
Wolff et al. (1974)	53	Bovine thyroid membranes	————
Moore and Wolff (1974)	54	Bovine thyroid membranes	2.2 to 3.1 x $10^8 M^{-1}$
Manley et al. (1974)	8	Membranes from hyperplastic guinea-pig thyroid	$2 \times 10^9 M^{-1}$
Smith and Hall (1974)	55	Guinea-pig thyroid membranes	$2.6 \times 10^{10} M^{-1}$
Smith and Hall (1974)	56	Human thyroid membranes	$2.7 \times 10^9 M^{-1}$
Kotani et al. (1975)	57	Bovine thyroid membranes	$1.1 \times 10^8 M^{-1}$

Table 1.   Studies on TSH binding to thyroid tissue (continued)

	Ref.	Thyroid tissue preparation used for binding	Affinity* constant
Mehdi and Nussey (1975)	58	Human thyroid membranes	——
Bashford et al. (1975)	38	Human thyroid membranes 25°C Human thyroid membranes 37°C	$8 \times 10^9 M^{-1}$ $4.7 \times 10^9 M^{-1}$
Marshall et al. (1975)	59	Human thyroid membranes. Human thyroid membranes $(+10^{-3}M$ propranolol$)$	$3.5 \times 10^9 M^{-1}$ $8.0 \times 10^9 M^{-1}$

*A single value does not indicate linear Scatchard plot,   but the value of the highest affinity observed.

subunit of TSH was the prime component for stimulation of biological activity, but the α-subunit, whilst exhibiting the minimum intrinsic activity, caused marked enhancement of both binding
and activation by the β-subunit in intact TSH.

In a recent report, Kotani et al. (57) confirmed GTP
potentiation of TSH stimulation of adenylate cyclase in bovine
thyroid membranes, and reported that as with other systems (61-
64) this appeared to be associated with a reduction of hormone
binding. In contrast however, Manley et al. (8), using membranes
isolated from hyperplastic guinea-pig thyroids, and Moore and
Wolff (54) using bovine thyroid membranes reported that bound TSH
was not displaced by concentrations of ITP and GTP which enhanced
adenylate cyclase activity. The reason for this discrepancy is
not at present apparent.

In a detailed study on the effect on TSH binding of agents shown to modify TSH stimulation of adenylate cyclase, no simple correlation could be demonstrated (54). For example, whereas Ca^{++}, Na^+, and Li^+ affected enzyme activity and binding in parallel, K^+ and Mg^{++} enhanced adenylate cyclase activity but decreased binding, but chlorpromazine, ITP, GTP, cetyl pyridinium chloride, gramicidin S and valinomycin altered adenylate cyclase but not binding, whilst phospholipase A and filipin inhibited enzyme activity, but enhanced binding. To the latter group we would add compounds with "quinidine-like local-anaesthetic activity" such as propranolol (Table 1).

Thus, although studies of the binding of TSH to thyroid tissue preparations have reported correlation with activation of adenylate cyclase in many respects, the finding of agents which modify these functions independently emphasizes their discreet nature and suggests that the relationship between them is complex.

IMMUNOGLOBULIN STIMULATION OF ADENYLATE CYCLASE IN THE THYROID

In 1956 Adams and Purves (65) interpreted the results of a guinea-pig bioassay for TSH in an astute manner to demonstrate the presence of a component present in thyrotoxic sera, distinguishable from TSH, which stimulated the guinea-pig thyroid. This component, since shown to be an immunoglobulin G (66–68) was soon reported to mimic many of the actions of TSH, both in vivo and in vitro, and has been implicated in the aetiology of thyrotoxicosis (69, 70). Due to the increased time-period required to elicit a maximum response to this immunoglobulin G (12 hours compared with 3 hours for TSH in a McKenzie bioassay (71)) and the slow decay rate once maximum response had been achieved, the stimulating antibodies were referred to as Long-Acting-Thyroid-Stimulators (LATS); however, recent work has revealed the inadequancy of such terminology (72) and for the purpose of this article they will be referred to as thyroid stimulating immunoglobulins (TSIg).

It is now established that an early site of action of TSIg on thyroid follicular cells is activation of adenylate cyclase. In the following discussion, present knowledge concerning the mode of immunoglobulin stimulation of adenylate cyclase in thyroid tissue will be summarised.

Studies with non-Human Thyroid Tissue

TSIg stimulation of adenylate cyclase has now been studied in tissue preparations from a variety of species. In 1968 Gilman and Rall (73) reported that a human globulin preparation containing thyroid stimulatory activity, as judged by a mouse bioassay, did not increase the cyclic AMP content of bovine thyroid slices during 10 to 60 minute incubations, either in the presence or absence of theophylline (1mM). However, failure to elicit a response may have been due to species specificity of the immunoglobulins (74). This might also explain the variation of potency of immunoglobulins from different thyrotoxic sera, when tested on plasma-membrane factions from the bovine thyroid (5,26). However, in 1970 Levey and Pastan (75) reported that immunoglobulins from three hyperthyroid sera compared with euthyroid controls, stimulated adenylate cyclase activity in bovine and canine thyroid homogenates. At the same time, Kaneko et al. (76) demonstrated increased adenylate cyclase activity in dog thyroid slices, which showed a delay in onset compared with TSH and correlated with a delay in stimulation of glucose oxidation. Incubation with TSH (1mU/ml) resulted in a significant increase in cyclic AMP accumulation in the slices after only 3 minutes, whereas a parallel experiment with the immunoglobulin showed a significant increase only after 30 minutes. The TSIg had no demonstrable effect on phosphodiesterase activity. Kendall-Taylor (77) reported stimulation of adenylate cyclase activity in intact mouse thyroid glands by a purified IgG from a thyrotoxic patient, and again, the response was slow compared with that to TSH, (the maximum being reached after 90 minutes, compared with a 20-minute period for a slightly less potent dose of TSH). A delayed response to TSIg using a similar in vitro system was also reported by Zakarija and McKenzie (78). However, it would be unwise to conclude that this delay in activation of adenylate cyclase explains the prolonged response of in vivo systems to TSIg, since studies with other in vitro systems have reported no such time lag (79,80). In this context, it will be interesting to determine whether the kinetics of the adenylate cyclase response to the Fab portion of the immunoglobulin is the same as that to TSH, since this fragment has been reported to produce a short-acting response similar to TSH, in the McKenzie bioassay (81) and also displace TSH bound to human thyroid membranes (74). Molecular dissection of the immunoglobulin into H and L chains (82,83) and comparison of the kinetics of response to individual and recombined chains could similarly yield valuable information concerning molecular events associated with immunoglobulin activation of adenylate cyclase.

Wolff and Hope-Cook (26) reported stimulation of adenylate cyclase in bovine thyroid membranes by sera and immunoglobulins from thyrotoxic patients and ITP and GTP were found to enhance the response.

Yamashita and Field (84) have compared TSH stimulation of adenylate cyclase in bovine thyroid membranes with that induced by immunoglobulins known to stimulate the mouse thyroid. The immunoglobulin stimulation was dose-dependent and saturable, but the maximum response achieved was less than that produced by TSH. Moreover, incubation of the membranes with the immunoglobulins at 0° for 30 minutes reduced the response to TSH. Clearly, to cause such inhibition, the immunoglobulin could be acting either by inhibiting TSH binding, or TSH activation of adenylate cyclase, or both processes. Since the inhibition appeared to be non-competitive, Yamashita and Field concluded that the inhibition was not due to competitive inhibition of TSH binding and that the inhibition may have been a consequence of a more generalised modification of membrane structure by the immunoglobulin. However, it is also possible that competitive inhibition of binding may occur together with non-specific inhibition of subsequent acti-vation of adenylate cyclase.

Fayet et al. (85) reported that LATS positive serum would displace TSH bound to isolated porcine thyroid cells, and Manley et al. (86) reported that immunoglobulins from thyrotoxic sera displaced TSH bound to membranes prepared from hyperplastic guinea-pig thyroids. This confirmed an earlier suggestion that the binding protein, identified as a 4S protein (87) might be a component of the cell membrane (88). A similar finding was reported by Smith and Hall (55) using thyroids from normal guinea pigs. Comparing the responses to immunoglobulins from euthyroid and thyrotoxic serum and the latter preabsorbed with human thyroid membranes Manley et al. (86) correlated displacement with acti-vation of adenylate cyclase. Detailed study of the displacement of labelled TSH by the immunoglobulins showed:

i)   the extent of displacement of TSH was dependent on the con-
     centration of immunoglobulins;

ii) displacement of TSH by immunoglobulins appeared to be due to
     a reduction in the number of available binding sites and not
     a reduction in affinity of the receptors for the hormone;

iii) simultaneous combination of the immunoglobulins and TSH to
     the same receptor could not be detected in experiments
     subjecting solubilised receptor preparations to gel-filtration
     chromatography.

These results were considered to be consistent with the concept that the immunoglobulin bound to the TSH receptor, sub-sequently activating adenylate cyclase.

Studies with Human Thyroid Tissue

Screening of thyrotoxic sera by a mouse bioassay has always revealed a significant proportion (40-60%) in which TSIg could not be detected. At present, this field is subject to considerable reappraisal in the light of results from experiments whichstress the importance of human specific antibodies (70) – probably those often detected in a so-called LATS-protector assay. This controversy will not be discussed in this presentation, but is mentioned to emphasize the clinical relevance of investigating TSIg interaction with human thyroid tissue. In 1973, Kendall-Taylor (89) reported stimulation of adenylate cyclase in human thyroid slices by immunoglobulins from thyrotoxic sera, and this has subsequently been confirmed by Onaya et al. (90). More recently, attempts have been made to correlate immunoglobulin displacement of TSH bound to membrane preparations from the human thyroid, and potency as activators of adenylate cyclase, with thyrotoxicosis (55,56,74,91-94). Although the results are equivocal, examples can be cited of immunoglobulins from thyrotoxic sera which both displace TSH bound to human thyroid tissue and stimulate adenylate cyclase. The ability to displace TSH from human thyroid membrane preparations appears to be associated with the Fab part of the immunoglobulin molecule, i.e. the fragment reported to cause a short-acting (TSH-like) response in the McKenzie bioassay (74,81).

In studies of the interaction between immunoglobulins and human thyroid tissue insufficient experimental control of the many inherent variable parameters probably accounts for the discrepancies reported. It must be remembered that each preparation of pathologically occurring immunoglobulins is heterogenous, and it is not inconceivable that the two phenomena of TSH displacement and stimulation of adenylate cyclase might be affected by different molecular species (84,94). Furthermore, the human thyroid tissue used in these studies is often only available because of its abnormality, and careful controls should be applied before final interpretation of results. However, detailed investigation of this problem generally concluded that the TSH adenylate cyclase system of thyroids from thyrotoxic subjects did not differ from controls (95,96), although Takasu et al. (97) reported that the latter was more sensitive to TSH and that the resulting stimulation was particularly sensitive to low doses of thyroid hormones. However, basal and TSH responsive adenylate cyclase activities of non-functioning thyroid nodules have been reported to be greater than in adjacent normal tissue (98-100).

Thus the results reported to date concerning the nature of the interaction between immunoglobulins, TSH and the receptor-

adenylate cyclase system in the thyroid, suggest that the immunoglobulins bind to TSH receptors and stimulate adenylate cyclase in
a manner analagous to the hormone. However, it will be important
to ascertain whether once bound to the receptor, activation of
adenylate cyclase is obligatory for all immunoglobulins. Although
the receptor site is thought to be intimately associated with
adenylate cyclase, the receptor binding reaction and enzyme activation are likely to be discrete processes; on this basis it
might be anticipated that antibodies which bind to the receptor,
but which do not activate adenylate cyclase will be reported, and
that these may correlate with certain hypothyroid conditions.

The mechanism whereby an immunoglobulin might bind to a
receptor specific for a pituitary polypeptide hormone, and activate adenylate cyclase is as yet little understood. However, it
is hoped that the above discussion illustrates the challenge TSIg
presents to those seeking a unifying concept of hormone receptor-
adenylate cyclase systems.

PROSTAGLANDIN STIMULATION OF ADENYLATE CYCLASE
IN THE THYROID

Prostaglandin stimulation of adenylate cyclase activity
in thyroids of several different species has frequently been
demonstrated (for a review see (101)). The greatest response,
both in terms of least effective dose, and magnitude of maximal
stimulation has generally been obtained with PGE_1 and PGE_2, and
the effects of the former have been investigated particularly
closely.

PGE_1 stimulation of adenylate cyclase in the thyroid
differs from that due to TSH. For example, whereas the dose
response curve to TSH varies for different membrane preparations
from the bovine thyroid, that to PGE_1, as well as catecholamines
and fluoride, is relatively consistent (Figure 1). Also the
maximal effect due to PGE_1 is usually less than that achieved with
TSH (102,103), and the prostaglandin receptor/adenylate cyclase
system appears to be more labile to tissue disruption than that
for TSH (5,40).

Wolff and Hope-Cook (26) reported that in the presence of
1 mM ATP, addition of purine nucleotides increased responsiveness
of adenylate cyclase in bovine thyroid membranes to PGE_1. However,
whereas ITP (20 μM) was the most effective for TSH, GTP (20 μM)
proved more effective for PGE_1 and this suggests that the two
agonists stimulated adenylate cyclase via independent pathways.

Sato et al. (27) reported that GTP and GDP markedly increased PGE_2 stimulation of adenylate cyclase in membranes prepared from human thyroids.

PGE_1 binding to membrane preparations from the bovine thyroid has been studied (104). A receptor affinity of $2.6 \times 10^8 M^{-1}$ was reported in the presence of 5mM Ca^{++} at pH 7.0, and bound PGE_1 was displaced by PGE_2, $PGF_1\alpha$, arachidonic acid and 7-oxa-13-prostynoic acid (the latter to less than 15% of control value). Moreover, binding was inhibited by purine nucleotides, and the order of potency correlated with effects on stimulation of adenylate cyclase. Such characteristics were thought consistent with a physiological binding site for PGE_1. TSH displaced labelled PGE_1, but only at high concentrations (600 mU/ml caused displacement to 50% of control value), and since displacement was observed in the presence of other polyeptide hormones, including insulin, ACTH and HCG, as well as ribonuclease, at comparable protein concentrations, it was concluded that this was due to non-specific effects. Coupled with the finding that PGE_1 does not displace TSH bound to bovine thyroid membranes (54,57) this suggests that PGE_1 and TSH do not share a common receptor binding site.

It might be hoped that studies investigating stimulation of adenylate cyclase with combined maximal and submaximal doses of PGE_1 and TSH, would indicate whether separate receptor systems were bound to a common adenylate cyclase subunit. However, at present conflicting results prevent decisive conclusions.

Burke and coworkers, examining many parameters of response of the thyroid to TSH, including activation of adenylate cyclase, reported inhibition by PGE_1 (105,106). Following the observation that TSH increased endogeneous prostaglandin synthesis in the thyroid they proposed a negative feedback system for prostaglandin modulation of TSH stimulation (107). However, the concept of negative feedback is complicated by the finding that prostaglandin inhibitors such as 7-oxa-13-prostynoic acid, polyphloretin phosphate or SC 19220 inhibit, rather than enhance TSH stimulation (105,106). In contrast, Mashiter et al. (102), reported additivity between maximal PGE_1 and sub-maximal TSH, but not for maximal PGE_1 added to maximal TSH in dog thyroid slices. This finding has been confirmed by Spaulding and Burrow (103), when studying both increases in cyclic AMP concentration and protein kinase activation in calf thyroid slices. However, Wolff and Hope-Cook (26) reported additivity between maximal doses of PGE and TSH acting on bovine thyroid plasma membranes.

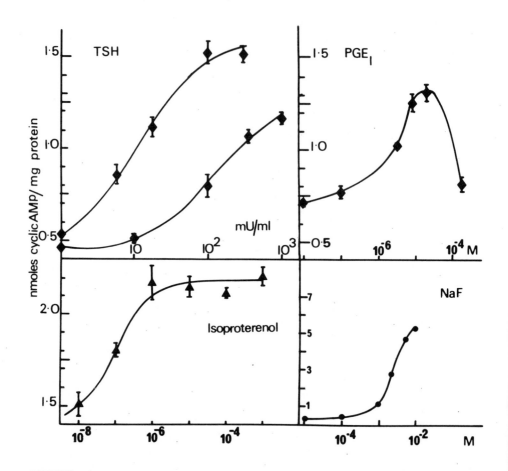

FIGURE   1

Response of adenylate cyclase in bovine thyroid plasma membranes
to TSH, PGE₁, isoproterenol and NaF. Representative dose-response
curves are shown, different membrane preparations being used for
each curve. Adenylate cyclase determinations were in quadruplica-
te each being assayed for cyclic AMP in duplicate, and the results
were expressed as mean ± S.E.M. Taken from results accrued by
Sigrid von Borcke, Harold Meinhold and the author.

The possibility that prostaglandins may play an intermediary role, promoting rather than inhibiting TSH stimulation of adenylate cyclase activity has also been suggested and is discussed in detail by Jacquemin (this volume). This hypothesis largely stems from the observation of inhibition of TSH stimulation with prostaglandin inhibitors. However, a prostaglandin synthesis inhibitor, indomethacin, has at best been found to only partially inhibit TSH stimulation of cyclic AMP formation when present at concentrations which completely inhibited TSH stimulation of prostaglandin synthesis in the pig thyroid (108,109). Moreover, this compound neither effected TSH activation of protein kinase in the calf thyroid (103) nor TSH stimulation of adenylate cyclase activity in plasma membranes from the bovine thyroid (110). Furthermore, although another prostaglandin antagonist, polyphloretin phosphate, inhibited TSH stimulation of adenylate cyclase activity in mouse thyroid lobes, it enhanced prostaglandin stimulation (111); similar results have been obtained in the author's laboratory, using plasma membrane preparations from the bovine thyroid (unpublished). So far the clearest picture has been obtained with the prostaglandin antagonist 7-oxa-13-prostynoic acid, which consistently inhibited TSH stimulation in all systems studied (105), but seems to act at a step subsequent to the binding process since it did not displace TSH bound to beef thyroid plasma membranes significantly (54).

Thus although it is well established that prostaglandins bind to membrane associated receptors of the thyroid and stimulate adenylate cyclase activity, the exact nature of any relationship between these phenomena and TSH stimulation is obscure. Furthermore, as demonstrated by Field and coworkers (112,113), when investigating the in vitro response of adenylate cyclase to several prostaglandins, it cannot be assumed that stimulation of this enzyme, in particular by $PGF_1\alpha$ is associated with increased intracellular cyclic AMP concentrations or C-1-glucose oxidation.

CATECHOLAMINE STIMULATION OF ADENYLATE CYCLASE IN THE THYROID

The question of whether catecholamines stimulate thyroid function, and the corollary that thyroid metabolism may be under some form of adrenergic control has been argued for considerable time - for a recent review of this topic see (114). In this paper, relatively recent evidence that catecholamines activate thyroid adenylate cyclase and the relevance of this to stimulation of other metabolic functions, in particular iodide metabolism, will be briefly discussed.

Melander (115) reported stimulation of release of iodine from thyroids of T4-suppressed and hypophysectomised mice, following the injection of several biogenic amines including isoproterenol, adrenaline and noradrenalin. Since the stimulation due to isoproterenol and adrenalin was potentiated by theophylline, it was suggested that cyclic AMP may mediate the effect. Pretreatment of the mice with α-adrenergic antagonists inhibited stimulation due to adrenalin and noradrenalin, but not that due to isoproterenol. However, isoproterenol stimulation was inhibited by l- but not d-propranolol, and it was concluded that this agonist acted on a β-adrenergic receptor linked to adenylate cyclase. Thus the mouse thyroid offers another example of a β-adrenergic receptor linked to adenylate cyclase,which, as discussed by Robison et al. (116) has been observed in many other tissues.

Utilising dispersed but viable cells from the calf thyroid, Maayan and Ingbar (117) reported that catecholamines stimulated uptake and organification of ^{127}I, the order of potency being isoproterenol > adrenalin > noradrenalin. However, adrenalin stimulation was not potentiated by theophylline, and was sensitive to inhibition by phentolamine, but not propranolol. In subsequent work (118,119), it was reported that adrenalin and adrenochrome stimulated adenylate cyclase activity of isolated calf thyroid cells, and that adrenalin also increased incorporation of ^{14}C-labelled mixed amino acids into proteins, ^{3}H-uridine into RNA and oxidation of D-glucose-1-^{14}C to ^{14}CO$_2$. The latter effect was inhibited by both phentolamine and propranolol. Melander et al. (120) reported that isproterenol stimulation of iodide organification, but not uptake, was inhibited by phentolamine, but not propranolol. Thus it was suggested that stimulation of iodide metabolism in isolated bovine thyroid cells by adrenalin may be mediated by α-adrenergic receptors and that cyclic AMP did not mediate the response. However, as discussed below, in several systems in which cyclic AMP accumulation and adenylate cyclase activation have been studied in the bovine thyroid, results indicate the presence of β-adrenergic receptors.

Gilman and Rall (73) reported adrenalin stimulation of cyclic AMP accumulation in bovine thyroid slices. The system was saturable, with a half-maximal response to adrenalin at $3X10^{-6}$M, and the response was more rapid than that to TSH. Since adrenalin stimulation proved sensitive to the β-adrenergic antagonist dichloro-isoproterenol, but less so to phenoxybenzamine, they concluded mediation by a β-adrenergic receptor. More recently, Spaulding and Burrow (47,121) described stimulation of both cyclic AMP levels and protein kinase activity by l-isoproterenol acting on calf thyroid slices. They report a somewhat more sensitive system with half-maximal stimulation at $7X10^{-8}$M, concentrations as low as 10^{-8}M significantly increasing protein kinase activity. Stereospecific blockade by l-propranolol (6×10^{-6}M) of both adenylate cyclase activation and stimulation of protein kinase activity by isoproterenol (6×10^{-7}M) was observed. In this study phentolamine (10^{-4}M) failed to inhibit isoproterenol stimulation, and combined maximal doses of isoproterenol and TSH resulted in levels of cyclic AMP that were not significantly greater than those with TSH alone.

Given the observation that adrenalin stimulated cyclic AMP formation in dispersed bovine thyroid cells and tissue slices, we investigated the possibility that catecholamines might activate adenylate cyclase in plasma-membrane preparations from the bovine thyroid. Using the preparative procedure described by Wolff and Jones (5), we observed stimulation by dl-isoproterenol, l-adrenalin and l-noradrenalin (122). The system was saturable, half-maximal stimulation being achieved with concentrations of the order of 10^{-7}M isoproterenol and the magnitude of the response was generally less than that to TSH (Figure 1). As discussed previously for prostaglandin stimulation, some membrane preparations proved sensitive to TSH but not catecholamines or prostaglandins; this may account for the previous report by Wolff and Jones (5) that catecholamines did not stimulate adenylate cyclase in membrane preparations from the bovine thyroid.

Both as judged by the criteria of the relative potency of agonists (isoproterenol > adrenalin > noradrenalin), and the stereospecific, competitive inhibition of isoproterenol stimulation by l-propranolol, we concluded that stimulation was via a β-adrenergic receptor linked to adenylate cyclase. Inhibition of isoproterenol stimulation was also observed with phentolamine, but the relatively high doses necessary suggested a non-adrenergic mechanism, possibly related to that causing inhibition of TSH stimulation (46).

Although analysis of the response of the bovine thyroid to catecholamines has not been as detailed as that for the response of rat liver, the results discussed above suggest an apparent paradox for the thyroid similar to that observed for rat liver (see paper in this volume by Exton). Thus, whereas β-adrenergic receptors appear to be present in the bovine thyroid, and as has been found in many other tissues (116) are linked to adenylate cyclase, other studies reveal that catecholamine stimulation of parameters such as iodide metabolism are sensitive to α-adrenergic antagonists. Clearly, much work remains to be done with the thyroid; for example, relative potencies of the adrenergic agonists as stimulators of intracellular cyclic AMP accumulation, iodide metabolism and glucose oxidation should be closely investigated, and in particular, the potency of α-agonists

such as phenylephrine determined, together with an examination of
the possibility that heterogeneous cell-populations in the experimental tissue contribute to the results. However, it appears
likely that the dual-model concept suggested by Exton et al. for
the rat liver may also apply to the bovine thyroid such that a
physiological catecholamine might stimulate thyroid function both
via a cyclic AMP mediated pathway, and one linked to an α-
adrenergic receptor.

     Thus results from recent research into stimulation of the
bovine thyroid by catecholamines tempt one to question the obligatory nature of the role of cyclic AMP in stimulating many
metabolic functions in the follicular cell.

STIMULATION OF ADENYLATE CYCLASE IN THE THYROID BY (i) FLUORIDE (ii) BACTERIAL PRODUCTS AND (iii) BIOGENIC AMINES

     Space permits only brief mention of other stimulators of
adenylate cyclase in the thyroid, which have been described, but
not investigated as closely as those detailed above.

i. As in many other systems, fluoride has been shown to stimulate thyroidal adenylate cyclase in broken cell preparations. In
general, the response is greater than that seen with TSH, and
occurs over a relatively restricted concentration range (Figure
1). Integrity of membrane structure does not appear to be as
critical for fluoride stimulation, and it is considered to act
on the catalytic subunit directly. For example, concentrations
of agents (e.g. phospholipase C, chlorpromazine, propranolol)
which inhihit TSH stimulation, cause insignificant change in
the response to fluoride (36,39,40,123). However, solubilization
of membranes with Lubrol PX was found to result in inhibition of
fluoride stimulation, and unlike TSH, the response was not restored by the addition of phosphatidylcholine (36). An as yet
unexplained finding is the observation that fluoride stimulated
guanylate cyclase, but not adenylate cyclase in bovine thyroid
slices (124). In contrast to TSH and PGE_1 stimulation of adenylate cyclase, fluoride stimulation has been reported to be
inhibited by ITP and GTP (26,27).

ii. Mashiter et al. have studied cholera enterotoxin stimulation
of adenylate cyclase in slices of canine thyroid (125). Perhaps
the most striking characteristic (discussed in greater detail
elsewhere in this volume - see Vaughan) was the delay (25 minutes)
before the onset of stimulation. However, when the tissue was
"pulsed" with only a 5-minute exposure to the toxin, washed, and
then incubated in toxin free medium, persistent stimulation was

observed, indicating rapid binding of the enterotoxin. One
possible explanation of the time lag could be that after rapid
binding the toxin must be converted to another form before
activating adenylate cyclase. It is also possible that the activation occurred only after mediation by an intermediate
reaction within the cell, explaining the failure of the toxin to
activate adenylate cyclase in tissue homogenates. Mashiter et
al. (125) also reported a small degree of activation of canine
thyroid slices by Escherichia coli enterotoxin, with an even
greater delay prior to the onset of activation (120 minutes).
However, unlike cholera enterotoxin, the latter appeared to
stimulate some metabolic processes such as ^{14}C-glucose oxidation
without mediation by cyclic AMP. Stimulation of many metabolic
functions of the thyroid have also been reported following the
addition of specific fractions derived from the growth medium
of Chlostridium perfringens (126).

iii. Finally, mention should be made of the potential of biogenic
amines, other than the catecholamines, as stimulators of adenylate
cyclase in the thyroid. In particular a recent report by Sato et
al. (127) described stimulation of adenylate cyclase in membrane
preparations from the human thyroid by histamine and serotonin.

CONCLUSION

This paper has discussed recent evidence that adenylate
cyclase in thyroids of different species responds to stimulators
ranging from a pituitary polypeptide hormone, immunoglobulins,
prostaglandins, catecholamines and biogenic amines, inorganic
ions and products from the growth medium of microorganisms. At
present we can do little more than list the characteristics of
the responses, and only comment with reservations on questions
concerning the relevance of a given stimulation to thyroid
physiology or pathology. Perhaps the most immediate question,
however, which relates both to thyroid physiology and more
generally to our ideas concerning hormone-receptor/adenylate
cyclase systems, is that of the interelationships between the
systems producing the activation of adenylate cyclase. During
the above discussion it was clear that the response to the individual groups of agonists was distinguished by features
peculiar to each, but that it was not possible to conclude that
the responses were therefore mediated by separate receptors or
catalytic units. Current opinion favours the idea that whereas
thyroid stimulating antibodies interact directly with the
receptor for TSH, prostaglandins, catecholamines, and biogenic
amines such as histamine, stimulate via different receptor
systems. Investigations in progress at present will hopefully
decide whether such a system, perhaps envisaged as a fluid
mosaic of receptors with different specificities associated in

an unknown manner with adenylate cyclase applies. At present, the general two-step fluidity hypothesis involving lateral diffusion of a hormone-receptor complex within the plane of the membrane, and interaction of this with adenylate cyclase can still serve as a useful working hypothesis for the thyroid membrane as well as other systems (128). The dynamic nature of receptor systems was recently emphasised in a study of choleratoxin induced redistribution of ganglioside GM1 in lymphocyte membranes (129)

Thus it is hoped that further detailed characterisation of the activation of adenylate cyclase in the thyroid will enable a composite model to be established, relating the receptor-adenylate cyclase systems in operation to each other. One future approach, yet to be fully exploited, could be to use tumour cell lines responsive to only some of the stimulators mentioned above, as described by Macchia et al. (130).

Although TSH stimulation of adenylate cyclase has been particularly closely investigated, any final model for this hormone-receptor/adenylate system will be influenced by the results of studies with other stimulators. For example, the concept of the mechanism of action of TSH will have to allow for similar stimulation by species specific immunoglobulins, and in spite of evidence for receptors specific for prostaglandins, the action of TSH does not appear to be totally independent of these fatty acids. Moreover, study of catecholamine stimulation of iodine metabolism indicates that cyclic AMP may mediate only one control system of this essential metabolic parameter. Thus, although we are as yet far from perceiving the final model, it is hoped that this discussion has illustrated how characterisation of stimulation by one agonist can cause reappraisal of conclusions concerning the mechanism of action of apparently unrelated agonists.

ACKNOWLEDGEMENT

The author wishes to thank Professor Deborah Doniach and Drs. Barry Brown and Gordon Malan for helpful discussion during the preparation of this paper.

REFERENCES

(1) KLAINER, L.M., CHI, Y.M., FRIEDBERG, S.L., RALL, T.W., and
     SUTHERLAND, E.W. (1962), J. Biol. Chem. 237, 1239

(2) SCHELL-FREDERICK, E., and DUMONT, J.E. (1970) in Biochemical
     Actions of Hormones, ed. G. Litwack, Academic Press, New
     York and London, 415

(3) DUMONT, J.E. (1971), Vitam. Horm. 29, 287

(4) YAMASHITA, K. and FIELD, J.B. (1970) Biochim. Biophys. Res.
     Comm. 40, 171

(5) WOLFF J., and JONES, A.B. (1971) J. Biol. Chem. 246, 3939

(6) POCHET, R., BOEYNAEMS, J.M. and DUMONT, J.E. (1974) Biochem.
     Biophys. Res. Comm. 58, 446

(7) BRUNETTE, D.M., and TILL, J.E. (1971) J. Mem. Biol. 5, 215

(8) MANLEY, S.W., BOURKE, J.R. and HAWKER, R.W. (1974) J.
     Endocrinol. 61, 419

(9) VERRIER, B., FAYET, G. and LISSITZKY, S. (1974) Eur. J.
     Biochem. 42, 355

(10) AMIR, S.M., CARRAWAY, T.F., KOHN, L.D., and WINAND, R.J.
     (1973) J. Biol. Chem. 248, 4092

(11) PASTAN, I., ROTH, J., and MACCHIA, V. (1966) Proc. Natl.
     Acad. Sci. U.S. 56, 1802

(12) MALAN, P.G., STRANG, J. and TONG, W. (1974) Endocrinology
     96, 397

(13) DERUBERTIS, F.R., CHAYOTH, R., ZOR, U. and FIELD, J.B.
     (1975) Endocrinology 96, 1579

(14) BOEYNAEMS, J.M., GOLDSTEIN-GOLAIRE, J. and DUMONT, J.E.
     (1973) Endocrinology 93, 1227

(15) POHL, S.L., KRANS, M.J., BIRNBAUMER, L., and RODBELL, M.
     (1972) J. Biol. Chem. 247, 2295

(16) FREYCHET, P., KAHN, R., ROTH, J., NEVILLE, D.M. Jr. (1972)
     J. Biol. Chem. 247, 3953

(17) WOLFF, J., BERENS, S.C. and JONES, A.B. (1970) Biochem. Biophys. Res. Comm. 39, 77

(18) BURKE, G. (1970) Biochem. Biophys. Acta 220, 30

(19) BURKE, G. (1970) Endocrinology, 86, 353

(20) WILLIAMS, J.A. (1972) Endocrinology, 91, 1411

(21) KENDALL-TAYLOR, P. (1972) J. Endocrinology, 54, 137

(22) YAMASHITA, K., BLOOM, G. and FIELD, J.B. (1971) Metabolism 20, 943

(23) VAN SANDE, J., and DUMONT, J.E. (1973) Biochim. Biophys. Acta, 313, 320

(24) VAN SANDE, J., GRENIER, G., WILHEMS, G. and DUMONT, J.E. (1975) Endocrinology, 96, 781

(25) BURKE, G. (1970) J. Clin. Endocrinol. Metab., 30, 76

(26) WOLFF, J. and HOPE-COOK, G. (1973) J. Biol. Chem., 248, 350

(27) SATO, S., YAMADA, T., FURIHATA, R. and MAKIUCHI, M. (1974) Biochim. Biophys. Acta, 332, 166

(28) BOEYNAEMS, J.M., VAN SANDE, J., POCHET, R., and DUMONT J.E. (1974) Mol. Cell Endocrinol. 1, 139

(29) LONDOS, C., SALOMON, Y., LIN, M.C., HARWOOD, J.P., SCHRAMM, M., WOLFF, J. and RODBELL, M. (1974) Proc. Nat. Acad. Sci. USA, 71, 3087

(30) POHL, S.L., KRANS, H.M., KOZYREFF, V., BIRNBAUMER, L. and RODBELL, M. (1971) J. Biol. Chem. 246, 4447

(31) CUATRECASAS, P. (1971) J. Biol. Chem., 246, 6532

(32) LEVEY, G.S. (1971) Biochem. Biophys. Res. Com., 43, 108

(33) LEVEY, G.S. (1971) J. Biol. Chem., 246, 7405

(34) MACCHIA, V., TAMBURRINI, O., and PASTAN, I. (1970) Endocrinology, 86, 787

(35) YAMASHITA, K., BLOOM, G., RAINARD, B., ZOR, U. and FIELD, J.B. (1970) Metabolism, 19, 1109

(36) YAMASHITA, K., and FIELD, J.B. (1973) Biochim. Biophys.
     Acta, 304, 686

(37) HAYE, B., and JACQUEMIN, C.R. (1971) FEBS Letters 18, 47

(38) BASHFORD, C.L., HARRISON, S.L., RADDA, G., and MEHDI, Q.
     (1975) Biochem. J., 146, 473

(39) WOLFF, J. and JONES, A.B. (1970) Proc. Natl. Acad. Sci. US
     65, 454

(40) MARSHALL, N.J., VON BORCKE, S. and MALAN, P.G. (1975)
     Endocrinology, 96, 1513

(41) KENDALL-TAYLOR, P. and MUNRO, D.S. (1970) Clin. Sci., 39,
     781

(42) LEVEY, G.S., ROTH, J. and PASTAN, I. (1969) Endocrinology,
     84, 1009

(43) ZOR, U., BLOOM, G., LOWE, I.P. and FIELD, J.B. (1969)
     Endocrinology, 84, 1082

(44) ONAYA, T. and SOLOMON, D.H. (1969) Endocrinology, 85, 1010

(45) BURKE, G. (1969) Metabolism, 18, 961

(46) MARSHALL, N.J., VON BORCKE, S., SHARDLOW,S., and MALAN, P.G.
     Proc. of IXth FEBS Meeting, Budapest, 1974, 129

(47) SPAULDING, S.W. and BURROW, G.N. (1974) Nature 254, 347

(48) SEAMAN, P.M. (1966) Int. Rev. Neurobiol., 9, 145

(49) MANLEY, S.W., BOURKE, S.R. and HAWKER, R.W. (1972)
     J. Endocrinol., 55, 555

(50) MEHDI, S.Q., NUSSEY, S.S., GIBBONS, C.P. and EL KABIR, D.J.
     (1973) Biochem. Soc. Trans. 1, 1005

(51) LISSITZKY, S., FAYET, G., VERRIER, B., HENNEN, G., JAQUET,
     P. (1973) FEBS Letters, 29, 20

(52) GOLDFINE, I.D., AMIR, S.M., PETERSEN, A.W., and INGBAR, S.H.,
     (1974) Endocrinology, 95, 1228

(53) WOLFF, J., WINAND, R.J. and KOHN, L.D. (1974) Proc. Natl.
     Acad. Sci. USA, 71, 3460

(54) MOORE, W.V. and WOLFF, J. (1974) J. Biol. Chem., 249, 6255

(55) SMITH, B.R. and HALL, R. (1974) FEBS Letters, 42, 301

(56) SMITH, B.R. and HALL, R. (1974) The Lancet,(ii), 427

(57) KOTANI, M., KARIYA, T. and FIELD, J.B. (1975) Metabolism, 24, 959

(58) MEHDI, S.Q., and NUSSEY, S.S. (1975) Biochem. J., 145, 105

(59) MARSHALL, N.J., FLORIN-CHRISTENSON, A., and VON BORCKE, S. (submitted for publication)

(60) FIELD, J.B. (1975), Metabolism, 24, 381

(61) RODBELL, M., BIRNBAUMER, L., POHL, S.L. and KRANS, M.J. (1971), J. Biol. Chem., 246, 1877

(62) KRISHNA, G., HARWOOD, J.P., BARBER, A.J. and JAMIESON, G.A. (1972), J. Biol. Chem., 247, 2253

(63) BILEZIKIAN, J.P. and AURBACH, G.D. (1974), J. Biol. Chem., 249, 157

(64) RODBELL, M., KRANS, H.M.J., POHL, S.L. and BIRNBAUMER, L. (1971) J. Biol. Chem., 246, 1872

(65) ADAMS, D.D. and PURVES, H.D. (1956) Proc. Univ. Otago, med. sch., 34, 11

(66) ADAMS, D.D. and KENNEDY, T.H. (1962) Proc. Univ. Otago, med. sch., 40, 6

(67) McKENZIE, J.M. (1962), J. Biol. Chem., 237, 3571

(68) COHEN, S. and PORTER, R.R. (1964) Adv. in Immunol., 4, 287

(69) McKENZIE, J.M. (1968) Physiol. Rev., 48, 252

(70) KENDALL-TAYLOR, R. (1975) Clinics in Endocrinology and Metabolism, 4, 319

(71) McKENZIE, J.M. (1958) Endocrinology, 63, 372

(72) ADAMS, D.D., DIRMIKIS, S., DONIACH, D., EL KABIR, D.J., HALL, R., IBBERTSON, H.K., IRVINE, W.J., KENDALL-TAYLOR, P., MANLEY, S.W., MEHDI, S.Q., MUNRO, D.S., PURVES, H.D., SMITH, B.R. and STEWART, R.H. (1975) Lancet (i), 1201

(73) GILMAN, A.G. and RALL, T.W. (1968), J. Biol. Chem., 243, 5867

(74) HALL, R., SMITH, B.R. and MUKHTAR, E.D. (1975) Clin. Endocrinol., 4, 213

(75) LEVEY, G.S. and PASTAN, I. (1970), Life Sciences, 67

(76) KANEKO, T., ZOR, U. and FIELD, J.B. (1970), Metabolism, 19, 430

(77) KENDALL-TAYLOR, P. (1972), J. Endocrinol., 52, 533

(78) ZAKARIJA, M. and McKENZIE, J.M. (1973) Metabolism, 22, 1185

(79) ENSOR, J., KENDALL-TAYLOR, P., MUNRO, D.S. and SMITH, B.R. (1971), J. Endocrinol., 49, 487

(80) SHISHIBA, Y., SOLOMON, D.H., and DAVIDSON, W.D. (1970) Endocrinology, 86, 183

(81) DORRINGTON, K.J., CARNEIRO, L. and MUNRO, D.S. (1966), Biochem. J., 98, 858

(82) MEEK, J.C., JONES, A.E., LEWIS, U.J. and VANDERLAAN, W.P., (1964) Proc. Natl. Acad. Sci. USA, 52, 342

(83) SMITH, B.R., DORRINGTON, K.J., and MUNRO, D.S. (1969) Biochem. Biophys. Acta, 192, 277

(84) YAMASHITA, K. and FIELD, J.B. (1972), J. Clin. Invest., 51, 463

(85) FAYET, G., VERRIER, B., GIRAUD, A., LISSITZKY, S., PINCHERA, A., ROMALDINI, J.H. and FENZI, G. (1973), FEBS Letters, 32, 299.

(86) MANLEY, S.W., BOURKE, J.R., and HAWKER, R.W. (1974), Endocrinology, 61, 437

(87) SMITH, B.R. (1971) Endocrinology, 46, 45

(88) BEALL, G.N., DONIACH, D., ROITT, I., and EL-KABIR, D.J. (1969) J. Lab. Clin. Med., 73, 988

(89) KENDALL-TAYLOR, P. (1973), Br. Med. J., 3, 72

(90) ONAYA, T., KOTANI, M., TAKSHI, Y. and OCHI, Y. (1973) J. Clin. Endocrinol. Metab., 36, 859

(91) MUKHTAR, E.D., SMITH, B.R., PYLE, G.A., HALL, R. and VICE, P.
     (1975), Lancet (i), 713

(92) SMITH, B.R. and MUKHTAR, E.D. (1975) Seventh International
     Thyroid Conference, Boston, Abstract 139

(93) SCHLEUSENER, H., KOTULLA, P., KRUCK, I. and GEISSLER, D.
     (1975) Seventh International Thyroid Conference, Boston,
     Abstract 140

(94) Orgiazzi, J. Williams, D.E., Chopra, I.J. and Solomon, D.H.
     (1975) Seventh International Thyroid Conference, Boston,
     Abstract 138

(95) FIELD, J.B., LARSEN, P.R., YAMASHITA, K., CHAYORTH, R.,
     (1974) J. Clin. Endocrinol. Metab., 39, 942

(96) ORGIAZZI, J., CHOPRA, I.J., WILLIAMS, D.E. and SOLOMON, D.H.
     (1975) J. Clin. Endocrinol. Metab., 40, 248

(97) TAKASU, N., SATO, S., TSUKUI, T., YAMADA, T., FURIHATA, R.
     and MAKIUCHI, M. (1974) J. Clin. Endocrinol. Metab., 39,
     772.

(98) DE RUBERTIS, F., YAMASHITA, K., DEKKER, A., LARSEN, P.R.
     and FIELD, J.B. (1972), J. Clin. Invest., 51, 1109

(99) LARSEN, P.R., YAMASHITA, K., DEKKER, A., and FIELD, J.B.
     (1973) J. Clin. Endocrinol. Metab., 36, 1009

(100) FIELD, J.B., LARSEN, P.R., YAMASHITA, K., MASHITER, K., and
      DEKKER, A. (1973) J. Clin. Invest., 52, 2404

(101) MASHITER, K. and FIELD, J.B. (1974) The Prostaglandins, 2,
      49

(102) MASHITER, K., MASHITER, G.D. and FIELD, J.B. (1974)
      Endocrinology, 94, 370

(103) SPAULDING, S.W. and BURROW, G.N. (1975) Endocrinology, 96,
      1018

(104) MOORE, W.V. and WOLFF, J. (1973) J. Biol. Chem., 248, 5705

(105) SATO, S., SZABO, M., KOWALSKI, K. and BURKE, G. (1972)
      Endocrinology, 90, 343

(106) BURKE, G. (1974) Endocrinology, 94, 91

(107) BURKE, G., CHANG, L. and SZABO, M. (1973) Science N.Y., 180, 872

(108) HAYE, B., CHAMPION, S. and JACQUEMIN, C. (1973) FEBS Letters 30, 253

(109) CHAMPION, S., HAYE, B., and JACQUEMIN, C. (1974) FEBS Letters 46, 289

(110) WOLFF, J. and MOORE, W.V. (1973) Biochem. Biophys. Res. Comm. 51, 34

(111) MELANDER, A., SUNDLER, F. and INGBAR, S.H. (1973) Endocrinology, 92, 1269

(112) FIELD, J.B., DEKKER, A., ZOR, U. and KANEKO, T. (1971) Ann. N.Y. Acad. Sci., 180, 278

(113) ZOR, U., KANEKO, T., LOWE, I.P., BLOOM, G., and FIELD, J.B. (1969) J. Biol. Chem., 244, 5189

(114) MELANDER, A., ERICSON, L.E., and SUNDLER, F. (1974) Life Sciences (Minireview) 14, 237

(115) MELANDER, A., (1971) Acta Endocrinologica Kbh, 66, 151

(116) ROBISON, G.A., BUTCHER, R.W. and SUTHERLAND, E.W. (1971) Cyclic AMP, Academic Press, NY

(117) MAAYAN, M.L. and INGBAR, S.H. (1968) Science N.Y., 162, 124

(118) MAAYAN, M.L. and INGBAR, S.H. (1970) Endocrinology, 87, 588

(119) MAAYAN, M.L., SHAPIRO, R. and INGBAR, S.H. (1973) Endocrinology, 92, 912

(120) MELANDER, A., SUNDLER, F., and WESTGREN, U., (1973) Endocrinology, 93, 193

(121) SPAULDING, S.W. and BURROW, G.N. (1975) Seventh International Thyroid Conference, Boston, Abstract 11

(122) MARSHALL, N.J., VON BORCKE, S., and MALAN, P.G. (1975) Endocrinology, 96, 1520

(123) BURKE, G. (1970) Endocrinology, 86, 346

(124) YAMASHITA, K. and FIELD, J.B. (1972) J. Biol. Chem., 247, 7062

(125) MASHITER, K., MASHITER, G.D., HAUGER, R.L. and FIELD, J.B. (1973) Endocrinology, 92, 541

(126) MACCHIA, V., BATES, R.W. and PASTAN, I. (1967) J. Biol. Chem. 242, 3726

(127) SATO, A., HASHIZUME, K. and ONAYA, T. (1975) Seventh International Thyroid Conference, Boston, Abstract 10

(128) CUATRECASAS, P. (1974) Ann. Rev. Biochem., 43, 169

(129) REVESZ, T. and GREAVES, M. (1975) Nature, 257, 103

(130) MACCHIA, V., MELDOLESI, M.F. and CHIARELLO, M. (1972) Endocrinology, 90, 1483

GUANYLATE CYCLASE

David L. Garbers, Ted D. Chrisman,
and Joel G. Hardman

Department of Physiology
Vanderbilt University School of Medicine
Nashville, Tennessee 37232

Contents

The abbreviations used are as follows: guanosine 3',5'-monophosphate, cyclic GMP; adenosine 3',5'-monophosphate, cyclic AMP; inosine 3',5'-monophosphate, cyclic IMP; 2'-deoxyguanosine 3',5'-monophosphate, cyclic dGMP.

INTRODUCTION

The natural occurrence of cyclic GMP was first reported in 1963 by Ashman *et al*. (2) who isolated the nucleotide from rat urine. In 1969 Goldberg *et al*. (32) and Ishikawa *et al*. (50) detected cyclic GMP in tissues from mammals and lower phyla. In the same year, three laboratories published reports of an enzyme, guanylate cyclase, that catalyzed the formation of cyclic GMP from GTP in cell-free systems (47, 50, 84, 99). Since then, a number of properties of guanylate cyclase have been extensively studied. This is a review of these properties and of some methodologic considerations based on our own work and on published literature.

METHODS OF ASSAY

Isotopic

A number of assays for guanylate cyclase involve the formation of radioactive cyclic GMP from radioactive GTP. These assays employ (^{14}C)GTP (84), (^{3}H)GTP (14, 45, 72), or (^{32}P)GTP (97, 99, 101). Advantages and disadvantages of the three isotopes have been discussed by Schultz (82). The main problems with isotopic assays are maintenance of low assay blanks, adequate purification of the radioactive cyclic GMP formed, and the relatively high cost.

Careful attention to the construction of an adequate assay blank cannot be overemphasized, especially with preparations of low activity. In some cases, a high assay blank results from the failure to adequately purify the labelled cyclic GMP. A blank problem also can result from a contaminant in the radioactive GTP that copurifies with cyclic GMP. In the latter case, purification of the labelled substrate on various ion-exchange resins or on other systems prior to assay, may alleviate the problem. However, with some batches of (^{3}H)GTP, we have found that prior purification does not effectively reduce an assay blank caused by an unidentified radioactive contaminant that seems to form in the GTP preparation with storage. A sometimes less obvious source of a blank problem is the potential non-enzymatic formation of cyclic GMP from GTP during the assay incubation or as a result of the method of terminating the incubation (55).

Purification of radioactive cyclic GMP has been accomplished by the use of aluminium oxide columns (72, 97, 101), QAE-Sephadex columns (83, 86), polyethyleneimine-cellulose columns or thin layer plates (10, 14, 83, 84), Dowex-50 columns (47, 50, 83), high pressure ion-exchange columns (11), and Dowex-1 formate columns (33). Often, a single chromatographic step does not yield adequate purification of cyclic GMP. Salt (e.g. $ZnCO_3$, but not $BaSO_4$)

coprecipitation of other guanine nucleotides can be useful in conjunction with column chromatography (14).

  With any source of guanylate cyclase, it is mandatory to verify
the identity and purity of the radioactive product being measured
regardless of the assay method used. Demonstrations of constancy
of specific activity after repurification with another system and
conversion to radioactive 5'-GMP by purified cyclic nucleotide
phosphodiesterase are relatively straightforward to carry out, but
are all too often not done. Even apparently minor changes in assay
conditions may require careful reconfirmation of the identity of the
radioactive product being measured. This requirement is well
exemplified by the recent report that the inclusion of glycerol and
other alcohols in an adenylate cyclase assay mixture resulted in
the formation of a novel nucleotide that migrated with cyclic AMP
in several chromatographic systems (78).

                              Non-Isotopic

  Guanylate cyclase activity also can be determined with non-
radioactive GTP as substrate. The cyclic GMP formed can be measured in principle by one of several assays that detect the nucleotide in picomole and subpicomole amounts. These assays include
immunoassay (92), enzymatic cyclic (33), enzymatic conversion to
radioactive GDP (86), protein binding (20, 71, 73), and activation
of cyclic GMP-dependent protein kinases (63). Most if not all of
these assays provide more sensitivity than do assays that employ
radioactive substrate, but they can be less precise and more
laborious.

                            Assay Conditions

  No single set of conditions can be said to be optimal for all
guanylate cyclase assays; the best system for one tissue or cell
type may not be the best or even an adequate system for other
tissues. Careful attention to certain factors may, however, avoid
unnecessary delays in the development of a satisfactory assay
system. The most important fact that must be kept in mind is that,
as with other enzymes, meaningful assays of the activity of guanylate cyclase - as opposed to the qualitative demonstration of its
presence - require conditions under which the accumulation of
cyclic GMP is proportional to the amount of enzyme present and is
linear with the time of incubation.

  Buffers should not be chosen solely on the basis of their pK_a
values, particularly for studies involving metal effects. Certain
buffers, for instance, may be strong metal binding agents (91), and

this can complicate the interpretation of kinetic data involving metals. Glycylglycine, often used as a buffer, has log binding constants for Mg^{2+} and Mn^{2+} of 1.1 and 1.7, respectively (36). Although metal binding by tris (hydroxymethyl)aminomethane (Tris) is negligible (36), binding constants for metals with nucleoside triphosphates are considerably lower in Tris than in other types of buffers (74), probably because of the formation of Tris-nucleotide complexes. We routinely use triethanolamine as a buffer, but other substances that are weak metal binding agents and that have pK_a values between 7 and 8 are also available (36).

The pH of the assay is often selected at or near the pH optimum of the enzyme, which is between 7.5 and 8.0 (see later section). When kinetic studies are contemplated, there are advantages in maintaining the assay pH near 8.0, because GTP exists primarily as GTP^{4-} at higher pH values, and $HGTP^{3-}$ can be neglected (74). Thus, since binding constants for various divalent metals with GTP^{4-} are very high (74, 91), it is generally possible to consider the free metal concentration to be the total metal in excess of GTP (17). Results from kinetic studies can be misleading when calculations are based on total metal concentrations rather than on metal in excess of GTP. When GTP is the variable substrate, excess and not total metal must be kept constant, otherwise more than one variable must be considered.

When guanylate cyclase activity is being measured in very crude protein mixtures, loss of GTP due to enzymes other than guanylate cyclase is a major problem, especially when reaction velocities are to be determined at GTP concentrations that are less than saturating. GTP-regenerating systems can be used (e.g. 7, 100), but they may create more problems than they solve. Phosphoenolpyruvate inhibits guanylate cyclase (47), and the creatine phosphate-creatine phosphokinase system can, under some conditions, increase the activity of the enzyme from sea urchin sperm independently of GTP regeneration and, under other conditions, can apparently inhibit the enzyme (41). Moreover, dependence on a substrate-regenerating system for the maintenance of linear reaction velocities creates the necessity to constantly check potential modifiers of guanylate cyclase for effects on the regenerating system.

With particulate guanylate cyclase preparations from both sea urchin sperm and rat lung, sodium azide inhibits GTPase sufficiently to allow linear cyclic GMP accumulation at low GTP concentrations (14, 26). An example of the effect of azide on rat lung guanylate cyclase is shown in Figure 1. Under these conditions, azide has no effect on enzyme activity at early time points, when the reaction velocity is essentially linear, but at later time points, when the reaction velocity decreases in its

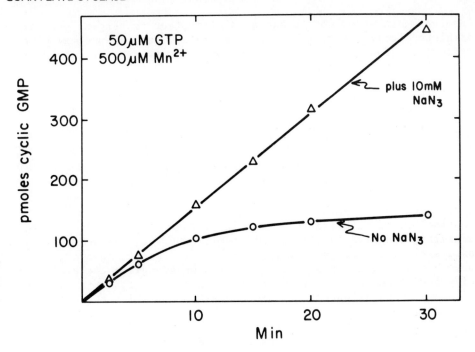

Figure 1. The effect of sodium azide on the rate of cyclic GMP formation by a Triton-dispersed particulate guanylate cyclase preparation from rat lung. Aliquots (containing 45 µg protein) were incubated with the GTP, Mn^{2+} or sodium azide concentrations indicated in the Figure. Incubations were conducted as described in reference (14).

absence, azide maintains a constant reaction rate. This effect correlates with an inhibition by azide of inorganic phosphate release from GTP. The use of azide may present complications though; at GTP concentrations below 5 µM, azide can inhibit slightly the soluble guanylate cyclase activity from rat lung (15), and it can increase the activity of at least some preparations of adenylate cyclase under conditions where ATP levels are stable (51).

Since guanylate cyclase appears to contain critical SH groups (see section General Properties - Apparent Importance of Sulfhydryl Groups for Guanylate Cyclase), another consideration involves whether or not to add a thiol-protecting reagent such as dithiothreitol. As will be discussed later, such agents may have different effects on guanylate cyclase activity depending on assay conditions and on the source of the enzyme. Potential binding or change in oxidation state of metals by a thiol reagent conceivably could lead to complications. However, with sea urchin sperm and rat lung guanylate cyclases, we have observed no kinetic differences with respect to metal or to GTP when assays were carried out or without 1 to 2 mM dithiothreitol.

Another very important consideration regarding assay conditions is the prevention of or correction for cyclic GMP degradation by phosphodiesterases that are present in virtually all currently used preparations of guanylate cyclase. We have routinely used methylxanthines as inhibitors of phosphodiesterase activity, and high levels of cold cyclic GMP also may be useful in assays with radioactive GTP (97, 100). At present, however, possible direct effects of these agents on guanylate cyclase activity cannot be completely ruled out. In any event, it is mandatory with any preparation to estimate the extent to which the cyclic GMP formed is lost by the action of phosphodiesterase during the incubation. Otherwise, the apparent guanylate cyclase activity may be meaningless as an estimate of the actual activity.

Finally - and perhaps anticlimactically - it should be pointed out that assaying guanylate cyclase (or, for that matter, other potentially regulatable enzymes) under optimal conditions, may not always be desirable. While perhaps best for studies involving distribution, purification and partial characterization, optimal conditions may obscure potential regulatory mechanisms. The biochemical literature contains many examples of enzymes (e.g. one form of cyclic nucleotide phosphodiesterase (81) that exhibit allosteric behavior and other regulatory potential only or most clearly under conditions of suboptimal pH or substrate or cofactor concentrations.

DISTRIBUTION

Distribution among Tissues and Phyla

Guanylate cyclase has been detected in all mammalian tissues examined with the exception of whole blood (99) and sperm (39, 43). The richest sources of guanylate cyclase are the spermatozoa of various invertebrates including sea urchin sperm, clam, scallop, tube worm, and abalone (39, 40, 42), where the activities are several hundred-fold greater than activities in any mammalian tissue yet studied. Of the various mammalian tissues or cell types studied, retina (38) and platelets (8, 9) contain the highest guanylate cyclase activity. Rat lung and small intestine also have relatively high guanylate cyclase activity, while skeletal muscle, fat and thymus have much lower activities (47, 50, 58, 72, 84, 99).

Subcellular Distribution

Early studies of mammalian guanylate cyclase indicated that its activity in most tissues was found primarily in the supernatant fraction of homogenates (7, 47, 84, 99). In the light of these early studies, mammalian guanylate cyclase was considered to be a primarily soluble enzyme, a feature that clearly distinguished it from adenylate cyclase. In contrast to most tissues, however, rat small intestine (50) and sea urchin sperm (39, 42) were shown to contain mainly or entirely particulate guanylate cyclase activity. Triton X-100, a non-ionic detergent, markedly increased the activity of these particulate guanylate cyclases and solubilized or dispersed them.

When mammalian tissues that were initially thought to contain primarily or entirely soluble guanylate cyclase activity were re-examined in the presence of detergent (14, 45, 46, 56), the apparent distribution of the enzyme between soluble and particulate fractions was markedly altered. The presence of detergent revealed substantial activity in particulate fractions that was not expressed in the absence of detergent. Thus, most mammalian tissues contain guanylate cyclase activity associated in varying relative amounts with both soluble and particulate fractions. The soluble and particulate activities appear to differ in several respects, which are discussed in detail in the following section.

The subcellular location of all the particulate form of guanylate cyclase is not yet defined, but at least some of it appears to be on the plasma membrane. Schultz *et al.*(87) demonstrated guanylate cyclase activity associated with partially purified plasma membranes from rat kidney. Particulate guanylate cyclase activity in rat brain seems to be associated with synaptosomal plasma membranes (37). Using sea urchin sperm, Gray and Drummond (40, 41) have been able to assign most of the guanylate cyclase to the plasma membrane of the sperm tail. In collaborative studies with Dr. Sidney Fleischer in the Department of Molecular Biology at Vanderbilt, we have recently demonstrated that highly purified plasma membranes from rat liver contain guanylate cyclase with a specific activity approaching that of the activity in the cytosol.

GENERAL PROPERTIES

Nucleotide Substrate Specificity

Soluble Enzyme. Initial studies on soluble guanylate cyclase showed that GTP was a substrate for cyclic GMP formation, whereas GMP and GDP were not (47, 50, 84, 99). Highly phosphorylated guanosine derivatives, e.g. guanosine tetraphosphate, have not been tested as substrates. Guanylate cyclase located in soluble fractions of mammalian tissues does not detectably use ATP as an alternate substrate to form cyclic AMP or cyclic GMP (47, 84, 99).

More recently, ITP and dGTP have been shown to be used as substrates by a partially purified guanylate cyclase preparation from rat lung to yield cyclic IMP and cyclic dGMP, respectively (24, 31). The relative rates of cyclic GMP, cyclic dGMP and cyclic IMP formation by the preparation from rat lung under V_{max} conditions are 1.0, 1.7 and 0.1, respectively. Evidence that guanylate cyclase is responsible for both cyclic IMP and cyclic dGMP formation is tentative, and is primarily based on competitive inhibition of guanylate cyclase by dGTP, competitive inhibition of deoxyguanylate cyclase by GTP, and similar gel filtration profiles of inosinate, guanylate and deoxyguanylate cyclase activities (24, 31). We have detected no cyclic dGMP formation from dGMP, but we have detected its formation from dGDP at 0.5 % of its rate of formation from dGTP (28), which could be due to contamination of the dGDP with dGTP.

Particulate Enzyme. In addition to GTP, ITP and dGTP also seem to be used as substrates *in vitro* by the particulate guanylate cyclase from sea urchin sperm (24, 31). The relative rates of cyclic GMP, cyclic dGMP and cyclic IMP formation from saturating concentrations of GTP, dGTP and ITP were different from those found with the soluble enzyme from rat lung being 1.0, 0.5 and 0.08, respectively. Preincubation of sea urchin sperm particles with trypsin altered in a very similar manner guanylate, inosinate and deoxyguanylate cyclase activities, and various metals and metal-nucleotide combinations protected the three cyclase activities to comparable degrees against trypsin. Inosinate, deoxyguanylate and guanylate cyclase activities were also inactivated by heat at similar rates. Although particulate adenylate and guanylate cyclases appear to be separate and distinct proteins (see discussed in the following section : Similarities in some Properties of Adenylate and Guanylate Cyclases), the possibility remains open that adenylate cyclase and the particulate form of guanylate cyclase are capable of forming at very low rates cyclic GMP and cyclic AMP, respectively, from the corresponding triphosphates.

Pyrophosphate Formation

With soluble guanylate cyclases from rat lung and liver, the enzyme reaction seems to be analogous to that of adenylate cyclase (48, 79, 95). When α-(^{32}P)GTP is used as a substrate, the specific activity of the resulting cyclic (^{32}P) GMP is essentially the same as that of the (^{32}P)GTP (45). When β, γ -(^{32}P)GTP is used, however, no significant radioactivity is recovered in cyclic GMP.

Recently pyrophosphate formation has been demonstrated with a partially purified soluble guanylate cyclase preparation from rat lung (25). Pyrophosphate and cyclic GMP were formed in virtual 1:1 ratios under a variety of conditions. Enzyme activities cata-lyzing the formation of the two substances were stimulated to the same extent by Ca^{2+}, inhibited to the same extent by other nucleo-tides and eluted in the same fractions from columns of Bio-Gel A·5m and DEAE-Sephadex.

pH Optimum

A pH optimum between 7.5 and 8.0 (in the presence of Mn^{2+}) has been determined for soluble guanylate cyclases from lung (47, 99), liver (47), and brain (72), and for the particulate enzyme from sea urchin sperm (39, 40).

Apparent Importance of Sulfhydryl Groups for Guanylate Cyclase

Activity. Heavy metals (e.g. Zn^{2+}, Hg^{2+}, Cd^{2+}) inhibit soluble guanylate cyclase from lung (47, 99) and platelets (9), and sulf-hydryl group-protecting agents such as dithiothreitol protect against the metal inhibition. p-Chloromercuriphenyl sulfonate in-activates the soluble liver enzyme (98), and p-hydroxymercuribenzoate inactivates the particulate enzyme from sea urchin sperm (27). N-ethylmaleimide inactivates the soluble enzymes from rat (15) and human lung (54) and the particulate enzymes from rat lung (15) and sea urchin sperm (27). Dithiothreitol or similar agents again protect against such inactivation. Some batches of commercial dialysis tubing contain a material that inactivates guanylate cyclase unless dithiothreitol is present (47) or unless the tubing is rigorously treated (14).

An increase in activity of soluble guanylate cyclases in crude extracts of human platelets (8) and rat lung (14) occurs with incubation of the preparations. This increase in activity is pre-vented by thiol group-protecting agents. Thus, both reduced and oxidized sulfhydryl groups may be involved in the maintenance of optimal guanylate cyclase activity, although other interpretations of these findings are possible.

Metal Ion Requirements and Kinetics

Soluble Enzyme. With all soluble guanylate cyclases studied, Mn^{2+} has been found to be the preferred metal for optimal activity (e.g. 3, 7, 12, 14, 65, 84, 97, 99). With activity from rat lung, substituting Mg^{2+} or Ca^{2+} for Mn^{2+} reduces the activity to 10 to 20 % of that observed with Mn^{2+} (12, 14, 47, 99). Epidermal guanylate cyclase is about 15 % as active with Ca^{2+} or Fe^{2+} as with Mn^{2+} (65). Guanylate cyclase from platelets is only 5 % as active with Ca^{2+} as with Mn^{2+}, but it is 65 % as active with Mg^{2+} and 35 % as active with Fe^{2+} as with Mn^{2+} (9).

In initial studies on lung guanylate cyclase, Mn^{2+} in excess of GTP was found to be required for optimal activity (47, 99), but the nature of the requirement for excess metal was not defined. A requirement for excess Mn^{2+} could mean (a) that there is a metal site on guanylate cyclase, (b) that free GTP is a potent inhibitor of the enzyme, or (c) that a combination of these possibilities exists.

A free metal binding site appears to be present on rat lung soluble guanylate cyclase (12, 14). Reciprocal plots as a function of excess Mn^{2+} at various fixed levels of MnGTP show downward concavity (Figure 2). When similar data are plotted as a function of MnGTP, however, reciprocal plots are linear and intersecting; this suggests that a Mn^{2+} binding site exists on guanylate cyclase and that free GTP is not a potent enzyme inhibitor (30). The explanation for the downward concavity of the Mn^{2+} reciprocal plots (Figure 2) is not known, but multiple enzymes or multiple Mn^{2+} binding sites on one enzyme are possible explanations. The dissociation constant for Mn^{2+}, estimated from the intersection of the extrapolated slopes nearest the left vertical axis, is about 0.5 mM. Although Mn^{2+} in excess of the GTP concentration is generally required for maximum activity, the metal becomes inhibitory at higher concentrations (14, 65, 72).

The kinetic behaviour of the rat lung soluble guanylate has also been studied using Mg^{2+} or Ca^{2+} (14). The reciprocal plots, unlike those with Mn^{2+} are linear, and the apparent Michaelis constants are 0.1 mM for Mg^{2+} and 0.4 mM for Ca^{2+}.

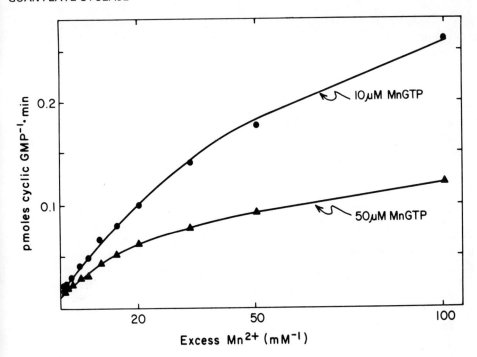

Figure 2.   _Reciprocal plots of cyclic GMP formation as a function of excess_ Mn^{2+} _with a soluble guanylate cyclase preparation from rat lung. The incubation mixture contained 30 μg protein and either 10 μM MnGTP or 50 μM MnGTP; excess_ Mn^{2+} _was varied over the indicated range (0.01 to 1.0 mM). Assays were conducted as described in reference (14)._

Particulate Enzyme. The effects of metals on particulate guanylate cyclases may depend in part on whether the particulate enzyme is assayed in the presence or absence of detergent. To date only one particulate enzyme, that from sea urchin sperm, has been studied extensively in both the absence and presence of a detergent (26, 29). The behaviour of this enzyme may be useful in predicting some properties of particulate guanylate cyclases from mammalian tissues, which often have been studied only in the presence of a detergent. The properties of the particulate enzymes from sea urchin sperm and rat lung are indeed very similar with regard to metal effects when both enzymes are studied in the presence of detergent.

Guanylate cyclase activities in particulate fractions from rat lung (12, 14) and sea urchin sperm (26, 29, 39, 44) require Mn^{2+} as a metal co-factor. When Ca^{2+} or Mg^{2+} is substituted for Mn^{2+}, rat lung and sea urchin sperm enzyme activities are less than 1 % of those measured with Mn^{2+} (12, 14, 26, 29, 39). When Fe^{2+} is substituted for Mn^{2+}, sea urchin sperm guanylate cyclase activity is about 10 % of that observed with Mn^{2+} (26).

With suboptimal concentrations of MnGTP, Mn^{2+} in excess of GTP is required for optimal activity of the particulate enzyme (12, 14, 26, 29, 39, 44). At high concentrations of Mn^{2+}, more pronounced inhibition is observed with the particulate than with the soluble enzyme (12, 14, 26, 39, 41, 44, 56, 57). The concentration at which Mn^{2+} in excess of GTP inhibits seems to depend on whether or not detergent is present (26). Reciprocal plots as a function of excess Mn^{2+} at fixed MnGTP concentrations are shown in Figure 3 for the sea urchin sperm guanylate cyclase. When no Triton X-100 was present (left panel), Mn^{2+} failed to inhibit the enzyme at concentrations up to 2 mM, but when Triton was present (right panel), inhibition was clearly evident at excess Mn^{2+} concentrations above 1 mM.

Reciprocal plots as a function of excess Mn^{2+} at fixed concentrations of MnGTP are linear for the particulate enzymes from rat lung (Figure 4) (12, 14) and sea urchin sperm (26, 29). The plots intersect at a common point to the left of the vertical axis, which again suggests that free GTP is not a potent inhibitor of guanylate cyclase (30). The estimated dissociation constant for Mn^{2+} is 0.20 mM for the rat lung enzyme (Figure 4) in the presence of Triton and 0.32 mM for the sea urchin sperm enzyme in the absence of Triton (29).

An unusual feature of the kinetic behaviour of both the lung and sea urchin sperm particulate enzymes is that the Michaelis constant for Mn^{2+} approaches zero as MnGTP becomes saturating (Figure 4). This type of behaviour, which has been observed with other metal-activated enzymes (17, 18, 66, 69, 70) can be explained by assuming that (a) Mn^{2+} must bind to guanylate cyclase before MnGTP can bind, but that (b) after MnGTP binds, Mn^{2+} need not leave the enzyme at the end of a catalytic cycle (17). Thus, at saturating MnGTP, Mn^{2+} is required in only stoichiometric amounts with enzyme; since the enzyme concentration is low, the requirement for excess Mn^{2+} seems to disappear.

That sea urchin sperm guanylate cyclase can bind free metals has been confirmed by studies showing that metals protect the

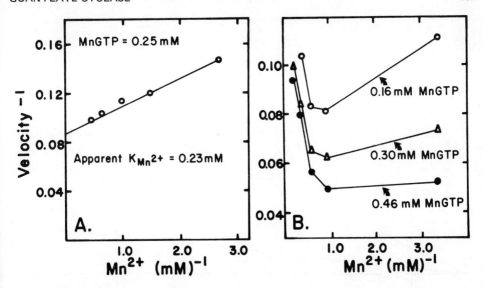

Figure 3. _Reciprocal plots of sea urchin sperm particulate guany-_
late cyclase activity as a function of Mn^{2+}. _Reciprocal velocities_
are plotted as a function of reciprocal free Mn^{2+} concentrations
at the indicated fixed MnGTP concentrations. _Enzyme activity was_
estimated in the absence (A) and presence (B) of 1 % Triton X-100.
Velocities are nanomoles of cyclic GMP formed 10 min^{-1}·80 µg pro-
tein $^{-1}$. _Reproduced from reference (26)._

enzyme against heat denaturation (27). Sea urchin sperm guanylate
cyclase is inactivated by preincubation at 37°, but the addition
of various metals protects the enzyme against thermal inactivation.
The ability of Mn^{2+} to protect the enzyme is shown in Figure 5.
From this type of data, enzyme-metal dissociation constants can be
calculated. The dissociation constant calculated for Mn^{2+} (0.12
mM) agrees reasonably well with the kinetic constant of 0.32 mM
determined by other means (29), suggesting that estimates of
binding constants in both types of experiments reflect binding at
the same site.

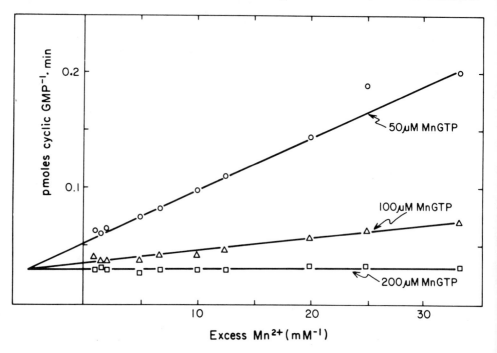

Figure 4. *Reciprocal plots of cyclic GMP formation as a function of excess Mn²⁺ with a Triton-dispersed particulate guanylate cyclase preparation from rat lung. The incubation mixture contained 45 μg protein and varying concentrations of excess Mn²⁺ (0.03 to 1.0 mM) at the indicated MnGTP concentrations. Reproduced from reference (14).*

Metal-GTP Kinetics

<u>Soluble Enzyme.</u> All available kinetic data are consistent with the assumption that guanylate cyclase uses as substrate the metal nucleotide complex. In all studies on soluble guanylate cyclases, reciprocal plots as functions of MnGTP have been linear (7, 12, 14, 72, 87, 98, 99). Apparent Michaelis constants for MnGTP for the bovine lung, rat lung, human lung, guinea pig heart, rat liver, rat kidney, rat heart and rat brain guanylate cyclases have been reported to be 0.3 mM (99), 0.05 mM (61), 0.2 mM (54), 0.14 mM (64), 0.04 mM (97), 0.4 mM (7), 0.07 (57), and 0.23 mM (72), respectively. The apparent Michaelis constant for MgGTP for the rat lung enzyme is about 0.1 mM and that for CaGTP is about 10 μM (14).

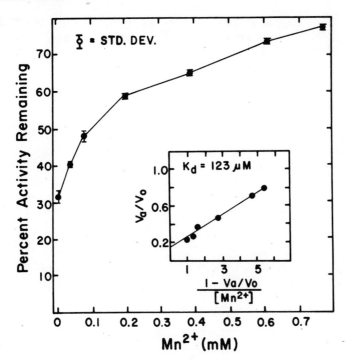

Figure 5. Protection of sea urchin sperm particulate guanylate cyclase against heat inactivation by Mn^{2+}. Preincubation mixtures contained 50 mM triethanolamine buffer at pH 7.8, 0.5 mM dithiothreitol, 80 μg protein, and the Mn^{2+} concentrations shown in the figure in a final volume of 0.48 ml. After preincubation for 20 minutes at 37°, an aliquot was assayed for remaining guanylate cyclase activity. Control preincubations were carried out at 0.2° with all Mn^{2+} concentrations (27). The estimated K_d (inset) was 123 μM. Va and Vo on the inset are inactivation rates in the presence and absence of Mn^{2+}. Reproduced from reference (27).

A true Michaelis constant for MnGTP (estimated at saturating Mn^{2+}) has been determined only for the rat lung enzyme (14). This was found to be 5 to 10 μM, and the dissociation constant for MnGTP was estimated to be about 12 μM. Since the kinetic patterns exhibited by the particulate enzyme are not linear as a function of reciprocal MnGTP (see below), it is important to point out that the linear kinetic patterns of the soluble enzyme are not altered by the addition of detergent (14).

Particulate Enzyme. Reciprocal plots as functions of MnGTP have
been reported to be linear (16, 38) or concave upward (12, 14, 26,
29, 58). An example of reciprocal plots that are concave upward
(indicating positive cooperative behaviour) is shown in Figure 6
for the Triton-dispersed particulate enzyme from rat lung. The
Hill plot (inset, Figure 6) is linear with a slope of 1.6; this
indicates that at least two MnGTP molecules bind to the enzyme.
The MnGTP concentration at which the velocity equals one-half of
$V_{max}(S_{0.5})$ is 70 µM. Similar concave patterns have been seen with
the Triton-dispersed enzyme from sea urchin sperm (26), with a
Hill plot slope of about 1.5 and an $S_{0.5}$ value of about 0.13 mM.
In the absence of Triton, the sea urchin sperm enzyme still displays apparent positive cooperative behaviour, with no appreciable
change in the Hill plot slope or in the $S_{0.5}$ value (26).

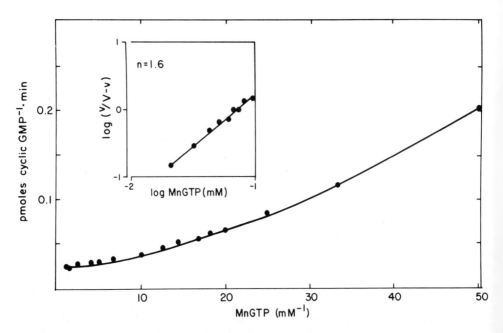

FIGURE 6. *Reciprocal plot of cyclic GMP formation as a function of*
MnGTP concentration with a Triton-dispersed particulate guanylate
cyclase preparation from rat lung. The incubation mixture contained
45 µg protein, the indicated amounts of MnGTP and 0.75 mM excess
Mn^{2+}. Inset : Hill plot taken from the data. Reproduced from
reference 14.

Effects of Ca^{2+} and Other Divalent Cations in Combination with Mn^{2+}

Soluble Enzyme. Under certain conditions, the addition of Ca^{2+} in the presence of Mn^{2+} can result in an increased rate of cyclic GMP formation (7, 13, 14, 45, 46, 72, 76). The response of the soluble enzyme from rat lung to the addition of 3 mM Ca^{2+} over a range of Mn^{2+} concentrations is shown in Figure 7. The apparent stimulation of enzyme activity due to Ca^{2+} is most noticeable when total GTP is in excess of total Mn^{2+}. As Mn^{2+} concentrations are increased, the apparent stimulation by Ca^{2+} diminishes.

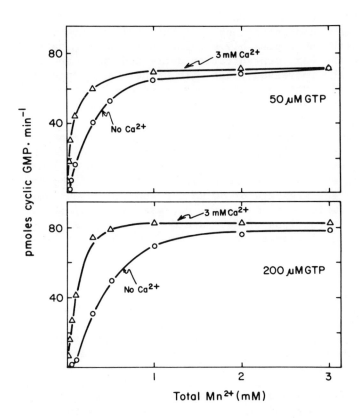

FIGURE 7. Effects of Ca^{2+} on a soluble guanylate cyclase preparation from rat lung as a function of total Mn^{2+} concentration. Ca^{2+} (final concentration of 3mM) was added to the incubation mixture in the presence of the indicated amounts of Mn^{2+} at either 50 µM GTP (upper panel) or at 200 µM GTP (lower panel). Assay conditions were as described in reference 14, from which the figure is reproduced.

As pointed out previously, when Ca^{2+} is substituted completely for Mn^{2+}, soluble guanylate cyclase activity from rat lung is reduced to 10 to 20 % of that observed in the presence of Mn^{2+}. The apparent weak ability of CaGTP (in the presence of excess Ca^{2+} to serve as a substrate compared to MnGTP could be a reflection of Ca^{2+} substituting very poorly for Mn^{2+} at a metal cofactor site on the enzyme. Thus, CaGTP might be an effective substrate in the presence of a small amount of Mn^{2+}. When a small amount of Mn^{2+} (10 µM) is added in the presence of varying amounts of Ca^{2+} under the conditions given in Figure 8, a marked increase in the rate of cyclic GMP formation is seen (upper panel). The lower panel of Figure 8 shows the calculated concentrations of free Mn^{2+}, CaGTP and MnGTP when Mn^{2+}, Ca^{2+}, and GTP are present in the incubation mixture simultaneously. Calculations were based on stability constants of 25,000 M^{-1} for CaGTP and 353,000 M^{-1} for MnGTP (26). At the lower Ca^{2+} concentrations, the Mn^{2+}-related increase in rate occurred with MnGTP possibly serving as the predominant substrate. Increasing the Ca^{2+} concentration decreased MnGTP and increased Mn^{2+}: thus the increased rates with higher Ca^{2+} concentrations in the presence of Mn^{2+} appear to have been due to free Mn^{2+} promoting more effective use of CaGTP as a substrate (14).

When Mg^{2+} was substituted for Ca^{2+} under the conditions of Figure 8, the addition of 10 µM Mn^{2+} had no demonstrable effect on enzyme activity (14). Furthermore, the addition of 3 mM Ba^{2+}, Sr^{2+} or Mg^{2+} did not increase the apparent activity of the soluble preparation in the presence of 50 µM GTP and 100 µM Mn^{2+} (14), conditions under which Ca^{2+} markedly increases activity (Figure 8). Thus, the interactions of Ca^{2+} and Mn^{2+} with the soluble form of guanylate cyclase appear to be unique compared to those of other divalent cations.

Particulate Enzyme. In the presence of Mn^{2+}, the effects of Ca^{2+} on particulate enzymes from lung (13, 14), heart (56, 57, 58) and sea urchin sperm (26, 44) can be either inhibitory or stimulatory, depending on conditions. With sea urchin sperm guanylate cyclase, Ca^+ can stimulate the enzyme in the absence of detergent, but in the presence of detergent, Ca^{2+} stimulation is essentially lost and inhibition becomes predominant (26). The effects of Ca^{2+} on sea urchin sperm guanylate cyclase have also been studied as a function of temperature (44). Ca^{2+} seems to act only as an inhibitor at temperatures less than 25°, whereas it can stimulate enzyme activity at higher temperatures. With detergent-dispersed guanylate cyclases from both heart and lung, Ca^{2+} seems to act predominantly as an inhibitor (14, 56, 57, 58).

In the absence of detergent, Ca^{2+}, Ba^{2+}, Sr^{2+} and Mg^{2+} were all capable of increasing the activity of the sea urchin sperm enzyme when Mn^{2+} and GTP were equimolar (26). This increase in

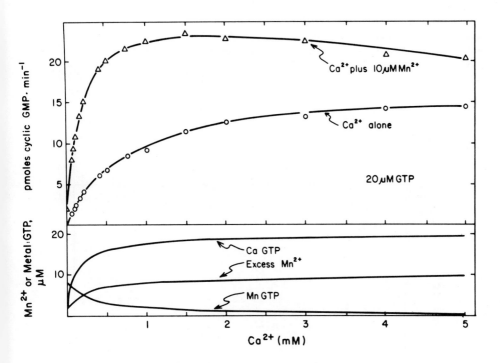

Figure 8. *Effects of low Mn^{2+} concentration on the rate of cyclic GMP formation by a soluble guanylate cyclase preparation from rat lung in the presence of 20 µM GTP and varying amounts of Ca^{2+}.*

Upper panel : Results of addition of 10 µM Mn^{2+} to the incubation mixture containing varying amounts of Ca^{2+} (0 to 5 mM).

Lower panel : Calculated concentrations of excess Mn^{2+}. MnGTP and CaGTP when Ca^{2+}, 10 µM Mn^{2+} and 20 µM GTP were present simultaneously in the incubation medium (see text). Reproduced from reference (14).

activity could be at least partially accounted for by simply an
increase in free Mn^{2+} concentration caused by the complexing of
GTP with the other metal. However, even at relatively low GTP
concentrations (15 μM) and with Mn^{2+} concentrations well in excess
of GTP, Ca^{2+}, Sr^{2+} and Ba^{2+} still significantly increased cyclic
GMP production (Figure 9). As the total GTP concentration was increased, the degree of stimulation in the presence of Ca^{2+} or Sr^{2+}
decreased (Figure 10), despite maintenance of a fixed total concentration of Ca^{2+} or Sr^{2+} and a fixed concentration of free Mn^{2+},
suggesting that the relative concentrations of CaGTP or SrGTP and
MnGTP were determining factors in the observed response (26). The
concave upward reciprocal plots normally observed in the presence
of MnGTP (see previous section) were changed to linear patterns in
the presence of SrGTP or CaGTP.

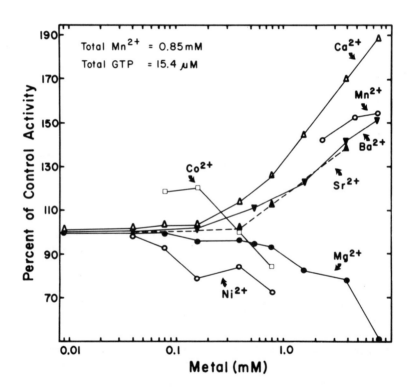

FIGURE 9. *The effect of various metals on particulate guanylate*
cyclase activity from sea urchin sperm when the GTP concentration
is low and the Mn^{2+} concentration is in excess of GTP. The activity
with no added metal other than Mn^{2+} was 0.3 nanomoles cyclic GMP
formed min^{-1} mg $protein^{-1}$ at 30°. Reproduced from reference 26.

These results suggest that particulate guanylate cyclase from at least one source, sea urchin sperm, contains multiple nucleotide binding sites and that stimulation of cyclic GMP formation by Ca^{2+}, Sr^{2+} and perhaps other metals may reflect interaction of a metal GTP complex with the enzyme as either an effector, substrate or both.

Further evidence in support of this conclusion comes from studies of the abilities of metal-nucleotides to protect sea urchin sperm guanylate cyclase against inactivation by heat and by N-ethylmaleimide (27). Both CaGTP and MnGTP, but not GTP, protected the enzyme against thermal denaturation. Neither CaGTP nor MnGTP protected maximally, however, unless the metal concentration exceeded that of GTP. At fixed free Mn^{2+} or Ca^{2+} concentrations, protection curves appeared to be sigmoidal, suggesting multiple binding sites. MnATP also protected against heat inactivation, but CaATP was virtually ineffective. When inactivation by N-ethylmaleimide was studied, the enzyme was found to be effectively protected by CaGTP and MnATP but only slightly if at all by MnGTP. The CaGTP protection curves against N-ethylmaleimide were hyperbolic instead of sigmoidal, suggesting that an N-ethylmaleimide-reactive amino acid occurs at but one of the CaGTP binding sites.

Effects of Nucleotides Other than GTP

Soluble Enzyme. Nucleoside tri- and diphosphates inhibit soluble guanylate cyclases (47, 50, 97, 99). Thompson et al. (97) determined a K_i for ATP (apparently a competitive inhibitor) of 11 µM for the rat liver enzyme. dGTP has been shown to competitively inhibit the rat lung enzyme, with a K_i of 10 µM (24, 31).

Particulate Enzyme. The sea urchin sperm enzyme has been extensively studied with respect to the effects of other nucleotides on its activity (29). At high MnGTP levels (greater than 0.1 mM), nucleoside tri- and diphosphates inhibit, but at low MnGTP (20 µM or less) some of these nucleotides are capable of activating the enzyme (Figure 11). Activation by nucleotides of a positively cooperative enzyme is not unexpected (59). At a MnGTP concentration of 7 µM, MnADP, MndATP, MndGTP and MnATP all activated at low concentrations (the MnATP data are not shown). At concentrations of 50 to 100 µM, the triphosphates began to inhibit the reaction, whereas MnADP continued to activate up to about 200 µM. In the presence of 1 mM ADP, neither MnATP nor MndGTP activated the enzyme. These data, along with the kinetic data previously discussed, suggest that the nucleotides bind to a regulatory site before binding to the catalytic site. The activation of guanylate cyclase at low concentrations of MnGTP by the other nucleotides could be due to their binding to a

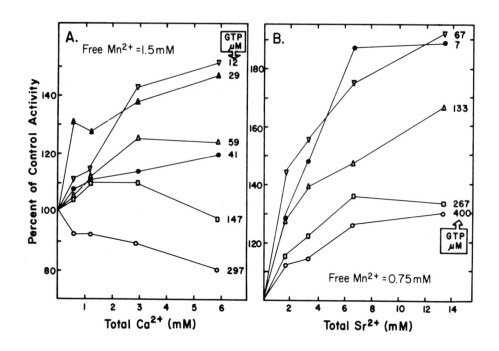

FIGURE 10. The effects of Ca^{2+} and Sr^{2+} on particulate guanylate cyclase activity from sea urchin sperm as a function of the GTP concentration.

A. Total GTP concentrations were fixed and total Ca^{2+} concentrations varied as shown in the figure. Total Mn^{2+} concentrations were adjusted to maintain the free Mn^{2+} concentration at about 1.5 mM. Activities with no Ca^{2+} added ranged from 30 picomoles of cyclic GMP formed min^{-1} mg protein $^{-1}$ at 12 μM GTP to 1270 at 294μM GTP.

B. Total GTP concentrations were fixed and total Sr^{2+} concentrations varied as shown in the figure. Total Mn^{2+} concentrations were adjusted to maintain the free Mn^{2+} concentration at about 0.75 mM. Activities with no Sr^{2+} added ranged from 0.12 nanomole of cyclic GMP formed min^{-1} mg protein $^{-1}$ at 12 μM GTP to 11.4 at 400 μM GTP. Reproduced from reference 26.

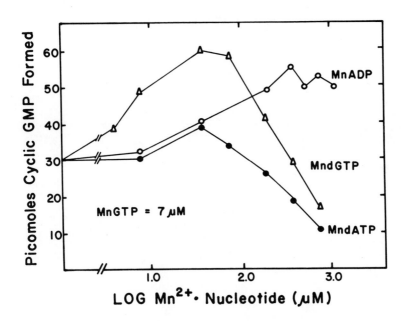

FIGURE 11. _Activation of sea urchin sperm particulate guanylate_
cyclase by MndGTP, MndATP, or MnADP. MnGTP and free Mn^{2+} con-
centration were 7 μM and 1.6 mM, respectively. The ordinate
represents the pmoles of cyclic GMP formed 12 min^{-1} 80 μg of
protein^{-1}. Reproduced from reference 29.

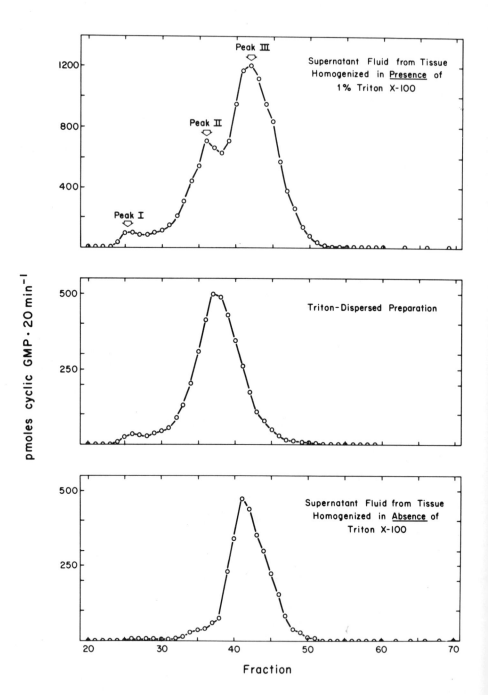

FIGURE 12. Gel filtration of particulate and soluble guanylate
cyclases from rat lung. Reproduced from reference 14.
Upper panel: 2 g of rat lung were homogenized in 8 ml of a solution
containing 50 mM triethanolamine, pH 7.0, 1 mM dithiothreitol and
1% Triton X-100. The homogenate was centrifuged at 32,000 x g
(40 min), and 4 ml of the supernatant fluid were added to a 2.5 x
35 cm column of Bio-Gel A·5m equilibrated in the same medium used
for homogenization. The 2.6-ml fractions were collected and 0.1
ml of each fraction was assayed for guanylate cyclase activity in
the presence of 1 mM $MnCl_2$ and 0.1 mM GTP. The final concentration
of Triton X-100 was 0.2% in the incubation mixture.
Middle panel: Rat lung was homogenized in 9 volumes of medium,
centrifuged and the pellet was washed in the medium three times and
resuspended to one-sixth of the volume of the original homogenate
in medium containing 1% Triton X-100. After centrifugation, the
pellet was discarded and 4 ml of the supernatant fluid were
applied to the same column and assayed as described above.
Lower panel: 1 g of rat lung was homogenised in 9 ml of a solution
containing 50 mM triethanolamine, pH 7.0, and 1 mM dithiothreitol,
and the homogenate was centrifuged at 32,000 x g (40 min). The
supernatant fluid was brought to 1 % Triton X-100, and 4 ml of the
mixture were applied to the Bio-Gel A·5m column and assayed as
described above.

regulatory site which MnGTP can also bind to, but does not saturate at low concentrations. The inhibition seen at higher concentrations of the other nucleotides could be explained by their competing with MnGTP at the catalytic site. Since MnADP did not inhibit at higher concentrations, it may not compete effectively at the catalytic site. Higher concentrations of MnGTP (0.1 mM and above) probably saturate the regulatory site. Inhibition by the other nucleotides at these MnGTP concentrations could, then, result from competition at both catalytic and regulatory sites. Thus, depending on the intracellular concentration of GTP, other nucleotides in the cell could possibly function as either activators or inhibitors of sea urchin sperm and perhaps other particulate guanylate cyclases.

Behaviour of Soluble and Particulate Enzymes on Gel-filtration

Columns. Kimura and Murad (56, 57, 58) and Chrisman et al. (12, 14) have shown differences in the behaviour of particulate and soluble guanylate cyclases on gel-filtration columns. The behaviour of rat lung particulate and soluble guanylate cyclases on Bio-Gel A 5m columns is shown in Figure 12. When the 32,000 x g (40 minutes) supernatant fluid prepared by homogenization of the tissue in the presence of Triton was applied to the column (which was also equilibrated with detergent), three peaks of activity were eluted (Peaks I, II and III, upper panel). Only peak I (void volume) and the larger peak II were seen when the detergent-dispersed particulate enzyme was applied to the same column (middle panel). The lower panel shows that a single peak of activity (corresponding to peak III of the upper panel) was eluted when supernatant fluid prepared by homogenization of tissue in the absence of detergent was added to the column in the presence of detergent. Approximate apparent molecular weights based on gel filtration elution profiles are 450,000 and 800,000 for soluble and particulate forms, respectively. The extent of aggregation and the possible influence of adhering macromolecules on these apparent molecular weights are unknown. Kimura and Murad (56, 57, 58) have filtered Triton-treated whole homogenates from rat heart, lung, and liver on Bio-Gel P 300, Sephadex G-200 and Sepharose 4B columns and have similarly concluded that separable peaks, apparently analogous to peaks II and III of Figure 12, represent the particulate and soluble enzymes, respectively.

White et al. (100) have partially purified (445-fold) the soluble guanylate cyclase from bovine lung, using ammonium sulfate, DEAE-cellulose chromatography, ultrafiltration and gel filtration. Two peaks of activity were collected from gel filtration columns. A minor peak was eluted in the void volume and a major peak was retained by the column. The apparent molecular weight of the activity in the major peak was 300,000 (102).

SIMILARITIES IN SOME PROPERTIES OF ADENYLATE
AND GUANYLATE CYCLASES

The initial observations on guanylate cyclase indicated that
this enzyme differed in several respects from adenylate cyclase,
but some of these differences now appear to be more quantitative
than qualitative. It is difficult to make precise and straightforward comparisons of all properties of the two enzymes, since
rarely have both enzymes from the same tissue been systematically
compared in the same laboratory. Aside from substrate specificity
and partial solubility, the responsiveness of the enzymes to various
hormones and neurotransmitters in cell-free systems constitutes the
most conspicuous difference between the two enzymes (see following
section).

The catalytic mechanisms, not surprisingly, appear to be quite
similar if not identical. Both enzymes require divalent cation
(see section on Metal Ion Requirements and Kinetics and (77)); both
use metal nucleotide as substrate (see section on Metal-GTP Kinetics
and (77)); both can use the corresponding 2'-deoxynucleotide as
substrate (see section on Nucleotide Substrate Specificity and (49)).

Initially, the two cyclases appeared to have strikingly different
divalent cation requirements. Guanylate cyclase was shown to be
much more active in the presence of Mn^{2+} than Mg^{2+} (47, 84, 99), and
adenylate cyclase was considered to require Mg^{2+}, although it had
been shown very early to use Mn^{2+} effectively (94). Subsequently,
adenylate cyclase from a variety of tissues has been shown to be
at least as active if not much more active with Mn^{2+} than with Mg^{2+}
(52, 77), and adenylate cyclase activity from at least two sources
is detectable only in the presence of Mn^{2+} (23, 39, 43). Thus, the
divalent cation specificities of the enzymes appear to be more
similar than different, the major difference being that Mg^{2+}
generally substitutes less effectively in the guanylate cyclase
than in the adenylate cyclase reaction. Indeed, differences in
cation requirements seen to be as great among different sources of
one of the cyclases as between the two cyclases.

Kinetically, the enzymes seem to be similar in some respects
and perhaps different in others. Guanylate cyclase has a free
metal site that is necessary for activity (see section on Metal
Ion Requirements and Kinetics). Adenylate cyclase also appears
to require free metal (5, 21), although there is some disagreement
about this point (19). A possible major difference between the two
enzymes is that at least some particulate guanylate cyclases display positive cooperative patterns with respect to MnGTP concentration (see section on Metal-GTP Kinetics), whereas there has been
no report of such behaviour for adenylate cyclase. Both cyclases,
however, do appear to contain multiple nucleotide binding sites.

The stimulation of sea urchin sperm particulate guanylate cyclase by low concentrations of ATP (see Section on Effects of Nucleotides other than GTP) may be analogous to the activation of adenylate cyclase by low concentrations of GTP (80).

The lack of fluoride sensitivity of guanylate cyclase (7, 47, 99) contrasts with the marked sensitivity to activation shown by adenylate cyclase from many sources (77, 94). However, adenylate cyclase from several sources is not activated by fluoride, and fluoride-sensitive adenylate cyclases can be rendered insensitive to the anion under some conditions (23, 39, 43, 52).

Their intracellular locations were at first thought to constitute a major qualitative difference in the two enzymes. In contrast to mammalian adenylate cyclase, well known to be a membrane-bound enzyme, mammalian guanylate cyclase was thought to be confined primarily to the cytosol fraction of most tissues. However, as pointed out in Section on Subcellular Distribution, mammalian guanylate cyclase was later shown to be associated with membrane fractions as well as with soluble fractions of a variety of tissues. Although particulate and soluble guanylate cyclase activities differ in several of their properties, the possibility that soluble activity may represent displaced particulate activity cannot be ruled out.

Thus, adenylate and guanylate cyclases have several superficially similar properties. Whether or not analogous mechanisms are involved in the regulation of adenylate cyclase and the membrane associated form of guanylate cyclase remains to be determined.

EFFECTS OF HORMONES AND NEUROTRANSMITTERS ON
GUANYLATE CYCLASE ACTIVITY IN CELL FREE SYSTEMS

Guanylate cyclase was shown in early experiments to be insensitive to a number of hormones that activate adenylate cyclase in cell-free systems (47, 67, 87). Several hormones, neurotransmitters and other agents are known to increase the content of cyclic GMP in a variety of cell types (34, 35). These agents include acetylcholine and several other substances that do not commonly raise (and may in some cases lower) cyclic AMP levels.

By analogy with the stimulation of adenylate cyclase by agents that increase intracellular cyclic AMP levels, it might be expected that agents that increase intracellular cyclic GMP levels would stimulate or activate guanylate cyclase in cell-free systems. This would not hold, of course, for agents that act on phosphodiesterase. Reported effects or lack of effects of cholinergic and other agents on guanylate cyclase activity in broken cells are listed in Table 1.

TABLE I. Reported effects of hormones, neurotransmitters and other
agents on guanylate cyclase activity in cell-free systems.

AGENT	TISSUE OR CELL	REPORTED EFFECT
acetylcholine and other cholinergic agents	heart (103), gall bladder (1), pancreatic islets (68) adrenal (90), platelet, thyroid (53)	stimulation
"	heart (58, 64), brain (72), epidermis (65), spleen (15), sea urchin sperm (44), liver (15, 97), lung (15, 62, 93)	none
secretin	pancreatic islets (68), pancreas (96), stomach (96), brain (96), liver (96), lung (96), small intestine (96), skeletal muscle (96)	stimulation
"	heart (96), lung (15), liver (15)	none
"	iris (96)	inhibition
pancreozymin	pancreatic islets (68) liver (97)	stimulation none
fibroblast growth factor	fibroblast (89)	stimulation
ACTH	adrenal (67)	none
angiotensin II	adrenal (67)	none
norepinephrine	pancreatic islets (68), lung (61) adrenal (67), epidermis (65)	inhibition none
epinephrine	pancreatic islets (68) heart (47), liver (47)	inhibition none
phenylephrine	liver (15)	none
methoxamine	liver (97)	none

184   D.L. GARBERS, T.D. CHRISMAN, AND J.G. HARDMAN

TABLE I. (continuation)

AGENT	TISSUE OR CELL	REPORTED EFFECT
glucagon	liver (47, 92, 97)	none
serotonin	liver (97)	none
	platelet (53)	inhibition
insulin	liver (47, 97)	none
hydrocortisone	liver (98)	none
histamine	liver (97)	none
parathyroid hormone	kidney (87)	none
thyrocalcitonin	"	none
oxytocin	"	none
vasopressin	"	none

There are obvious discrepancies among reports of effects of some agents on guanylate cyclase activity, the reasons for which are not clear. The reported effects involve a variety of tissues, and it is possible that guanylate cyclases from all tissues do not respond to cholinergic or other agents in the same manner (or at all). There are in addition, however, discrepancies among reports dealing with the effects of an agent on the same tissue, heart for example. There are several possible reasons for the existence of such discrepancies.

First, guanylate cyclase may require for its regulation co-factors or conditions that in some laboratories have been (perhaps unknowingly) included in the incubation mixture but which in other laboratories have not. In virtually all instances where hormone effects have been sought, a limited set of assay conditions have been employed. Conceivably the ability of a hormone or neuro-transmitter to stimulate guanylate cyclase activity in a cell-free system may be strongly dependent on substrate concentration, pH, ionic composition of the medium or other factors. The apparent requirement for GTP in the hormonal stimulation of adenylate cyclase (80) could have an analogy in a requirement for a co-factor, perhaps a nucleotide, for hormonal stimulation of guanylate cyclase.

Second, assay procedures used in some laboratories simply could have been inadequate. Several of the reports referred to in Table 1 are in the form of abstracts, and the reliability of the assay techniques were not documented and thus cannot be evaluated.

Third, the effect of a potential modifier may be restricted to either the soluble or the particulate form of guanylate cyclase. In all probability the factors and mechanisms involved in regulation of the soluble form of guanylate cyclase in a tissue may be quite different from those involved in regulation of the membrane-associated form. The sensitive form of the enzyme may not have been the form that was studied in some cases, and in other cases, especially where whole homogenates were used, the activity of the sensitive form could have been very small relative to that of an insensitive form and thus have been obscured.

Fourth, sensitivity of guanylate cyclase to stimulation by hormones or neurotransmitters may involve a very labile system, the integrity of which could be disrupted by some ordinary homogenization techniques. There are indeed precedents (e.g. 75) for lability of the hormone sensitivity of adenylate cyclase systems to mechanical disruption.

Finally, some hormones or neurotransmitters may act to alter indirectly guanylate cyclase activity in intact cells, perhaps through primary effects on cation distribution or some other process, thus making the search for their direct effects on the enzyme in a cell-free system predestined to failure. In several tissues, a number of agents that raise cyclic GMP levels, including acetylcholine and depolarizing K^+ concentrations, require Ca^{2+} for their effects (22, 85, 88). In at least one tissue, the ductus deferens of the rat, changing the Ca^{2+} concentration in the medium alone brings about marked changes in the tissue content of cyclic GMP (85). These observations prompted the suggestion that elevations in cyclic GMP levels in response to cholinergic and other agents (that are known or thought to alter Ca^{2+} distribution) occur secondarily to elevations in the concentration of Ca^{2+} in the cytoplasm (85). Guanylate cyclase activity is reported to be reduced by exposure of rod outer segments to light (4, 60, 76), which is said to increase the phosphodiesterase activity of these structures (6). Such phenomena also conceivably could be secondarily linked to primary changes in ion fluxes. Although Ca^{2+} can, under certain conditions, be shown to have apparent stimulatory effects on guanylate cyclase activity in cell-free systems (see Section on Effects of Ca^{2+} and Other Divalent Cations in Combination with Mn^{2+}, these effects at present cannot be said to be of physiologic importance in the control of guanylate cyclase activity in intact cells.

Since at least some particulate guanylate cyclases exhibit apparent allosteric kinetic behaviour, one possible means of regulating their activities is by altering the concentration of an allosteric effector. The membrane-associated enzyme from sea urchin sperm seems to have multiple binding sites for nucleotides, and nucleotides other than GTP, including ATP, can either stimulate or inhibit it depending on their concentrations and on the GTP concentration (see previous section). Therefore, the activity of the enzyme could be sensitive to a change in the concentration of ATP, or perhaps another nucleotide, occurring in its immediate vicinity. Such a change might occur in response to primary effects of hormones or neurotransmitters on cation flux or distribution which in turn could alter the activity of a membrane-associated ATPase.

The probability that guanylate cyclase can be indirectly if not directly controlled by hormones, neurotransmitters, and other factors is high. However, clear and confirmed demonstrations of such regulation in simple systems is lacking. Hopefully our understanding of the fundamental properties of the enzyme in both its soluble and particulate forms will soon be extensive enough to allow more than just an empirical approach in studying its regulation.

Acknowledgments

The authors' research cited in this review was supported by NIH grants GM-16811, HL-13996, and AM-07462. Dr. Garbers was a recipient of postdoctoral fellowships from the NIH (1-F02-HD-53268-01) and the American Cancer Society (Pf-861). The excellent assistance of Ms. Marvist Parks and Ms. Janice Suddath is deeply appreciated.

REFERENCES

(1) AMER, M.S., and MCKINNEY, G.R. (1973), The Pharmacologist 15, 157 (Abs)

(2) ASHMAN, D.F., LIPTON, R., MELICOW, M.M. and PRICE, T.D. (1963), Biochem. Diphys. Res. Commun. 11, 330

(3) BARMASCH, M., PISAREV, M.A., and ALTSCHULER, N., (1973), Acta Endocrin. Panam. 4, 19

(4) BENZINGER, R.E., FLETCHER, R.T., and CHADER, G.J. (1974), Science 183, 86

(5) BIRNBAUMER, L., POHL, S.L., and RODBELL, M. (1969), J. Biol. Chem. 244, 3468

(6) BITENSKY, M.W., MIKI, N., MARCUS, F.R., and KEIRNS, J.J.
     (1973), Life Sciences 13, 1451

(7) BÖHME, E. (1970), Eur. J. Biochem. 14, 422

(8) BÖHME, E., and JAKOBS, K.H. (1973), International Research
     Communications System 3, 1

(9) BÖHME, E., JUNG, R., and MECHLER, I. (1974) in "Methods in
     Enzymology" (J.G. Hardman and B.W. O'Malley, Vol Eds) Vol. 38
     199, Academic Press, N.Y.

(10) BÖHME, E., and SCHULTZ, G. (1974) in "Methods in Enzymology"
     (J.G. Hardman and B.W. O'Malley, Vol Eds) Volume 38, 27,
     Academic Press, N.Y.

(11) BROOKER, G. (1972) in "Methods in Molecular Biology" (M.
     Chasin, ed.) Vol. 3, 82, Dekker, New York

(12) CHRISMAN, T.D., GARBERS, D.L., and HARDMAN, J.G. (1974) Fed.
     Proc. 33, 1250 abs.

(13) CHRISMAN, T.D., GARBERS, D.L., and HARDMAN, J.G. (1974)
     Abstract, Second International Conference on Cyclic AMP,
     Vancouver, in "Advances in Cyclic Nucleotide Research"
     (1975) (G.I. Drummond, P. Greengard and G.A. Robison, eds.)
     Vol. 5, 823, Academic Press, New York

(14) CHRISMAN, T.D., GARBERS, D.L., PARKS, M.A., and HARDMAN, J.G.
     (1975) J. Biol. Chem., 250, 374

(15) CHRISMAN, T.D. and HARDMAN, J.D., unpublished observations

(16) CLARK, V.L., and BERNLOHR, R.W. (1972) Biochem. Biophys. Res.
     Commun. 46, 1570

(17) CLELAND, W.W. (1970) in "The Enzymes" (ed. by P.D. Boyer) II,
     1-65, Academic Press, New York

(18) CLELAND, W.W., DANENBERG, K.D., and SCHIMERLIK, M.I. (1972)
     Fed. Proc. 31, 850 abs.

(19) DEHAËN, C. (1974) J. Biol. Chem. 249, 2756

(20) DINNENDAHL, V. (1974) Naunyn-Schimedeberg's Arch. Pharmacol.
     284, 55

(21) DRUMMOND, G. and DUNCAN, L. (1970) J. Biol. Chem. 245, 976

(22) FERRENDELLI, J.A., KINSCHERF, D.A., and CHANG, M.M. (1973)
     Mol. Pharmacol. 9, 445

(23) FLAWIA, M.H. and TORRES, H.N. (1972) J. Biol. Chem. 247, 6873

(24) GARBERS, D.L., CHRISMAN, T.D. and HARDMAN, J.G. (1974) Abstracts, Second Int. Conference on Cyclic AMP, Vancouver, in "Advances in Cyclic Nucleotide Research" (1975), (G.I. Drummond, P. Greengard and G.A. Robison, eds.) Vol. 5, 823, Academic Press, New York.

(25) GARBERS, D.L., CHRISMAN, T.D., SUDDATH, J.L., and HARDMAN, J.D. (1975) Arch. Biochem. Biophys, 166, 135

(26) GARBERS, D.L., DYER, E.L., and HARDMAN, J.G. (1975) J. Biol. Chem. 250, 382

(27) GARBERS, D.L. and HARDMAN, J.G. 1975, J. Biol. Chem. 250, 2482

(28) GARBERS, D.L. and HARDMAN, J.G., unpublished observations

(29) GARBERS, D.L., HARDMAN, J.G. and RUDOLPH, F.B. (1974) Biochemistry, 13, 4166

(30) GARBERS, D.L. and JOHNSON, R.A., manuscript in preparation

(31) GARBERS, D.L., SUDDATH, J.L., and HARDMAN, J.G. (1975) Biochim. Bipphys. Acta, 377, 174

(32) GOLDBERG, N.D., DIETZ, S.B., and O'TOOLE, A.G. (1969) J. Biol. Chem. 244, 4458

(33) GOLDBERG, N.D. and HADDOX, M.K. (1974) in "Methods in Enzymology" (J.G. Hardman and B.W. O'Malley, Vol. Eds.) Vol. 38, 73, Academic Press, N.Y.

(34) GOLDBERG, N.D., HADDOX, M.K., HARTLE, D.K., and HADDEN, J.W. (1973) "Pharmacology and the Future of Man". Proc. 5th International Congress of Pharmacology, San Francisco, Vol. 5, 146, Karger, Basel, Switzerland

(35) GOLDBERG, N.D., O'DEA, R.F., and HADDOX, M.K. (1973) "Advances in Cyclic Nucleotide Research" 3, 155

(36) GOOD, N.E., WINGET, G.D., WINTER, W., CONNOLLY, T.N., IZAWA, S., and SINGH, R.M.M. (1966) Biochemistry 5, 467

(37) GORIDIS, C. and MORGAN, I.G. (1973) FEBS LETTERS 34, 71

(38) GORIDIS, C., VIRMAUX, N., URBAN, P.F., and MANDEL, P. (1973) FEBS LETTERS 30, 163

(39) GRAY, J.P. (1971) "Cyclic AMP and Cyclic GMP in Gametes" Ph.
      D. Dessertation, Vanderbilt University Medical School Library,
      Nashwille, Tennessee

(40) GRAY, J.P. and DRUMMOND, G.I. (1973) Proc. Can. Fed. Biol. Soc.
      16, 79 (abs.)

(41) GRAY, J.P. and DRUMMOND, G.I. (1974) Fed. Proc. 33, 1250 (abs.)

(42) GRAY, J.P., HARDMAN, J.G., BIBRING, T., and SUTHERLAND, E.W.
      (1970) Fed. Proc. 29, 608 (abs.)

(43) GRAY, J.P., HARDMAN, J.G., HAMMER, J.L., HOOS, R.T. and
      SUTHERLAND, E.W. (1971) Fed. Proc. 30, 1267 (abs.)

(44) GRAY, J.P., LUK, D., and DRUMMOND, G.I. (1974) Abstracts,
      Second Int. Conference on Cyclic AMP, Vancouver, "Advances in
      Cyclic Nucleotide Research" (1975) (G.I. Drummond, P. Green-
      gard and G.A. Robison, eds.) Vol. 5, 823, Academic Press,
      New York

(45) HARDMAN, J.G., BEAVO, J.A., GRAY, J.P., CHRISMAN, T.D.,
      PATTERSON, W.D., and SUTHERLAND, E.W. (1971) Ann.N.Y. Acad.
      Sci. 185, 27

(46) HARDMAN, J.G., CHRISMAN, T.D., GRAY, J.P., SUDDATH, J.L., and
      SUTHERLAND, E.W. (1973) "Pharmacology and the Future of Man".
      Proc. 5th International Congress of Pharmacology, San
      Francisco, Vol. 5, 134, Karger, Basel, Switzerland

(47) HARDMAN, J.G. and SUTHERLAND, E.W. (1969) J. Biol. Chem.
      244, 6363

(48) HAYAISHI, O., GREENGARD, P., and COLOWICK, S.P. (1971) J.
      Biol. Chem. 246, 5840

(49) HIRATA, M. and HAYAISHI, O. (1966) Biochem. Biophys. Res.
      Comm. 24, 360

(50) ISHIKAWA, E., ISHIKAWA, S., DAVIS, J.W., and SUTHERLAND, E.W.
      (1969) J. Biol. Chem. 244, 6371

(51) JOHNSON, R.A., and PILKIS, S.J. (1974) Abstracts, Second
      International Conference on Cyclic AMP, Vancouver, in
      "Advances in Cyclic Nucleotide Research" (1975) (G.I.
      Drummond, P. Greengard, and G.A. Robison, eds.) Vol. 5, 808
      Academic Press, New York

(52) JOHNSON, R.A., and SUTHERLAND, E.W. (1973), J. Biol. Chem.
      5114

(53) JUNE, R., MECHLER, I., MOCIKAT, S., and BÖHME, E. (1972)
      Naunyn-Schmiedeberg's Archives of Pharmacology, 294 (Supp.)
      R59

(54) KIM, G., and SILVERSTEIN, E. (1974) Fed. Proc. 33, 1250
      (abs.)

(55) KIMURA, H., and MURAD, F. (1974) J. Biol. Chem. 249, 329

(56) KIMURA, H., and MURAD, F. (1974) Abstracts, Second Inter-
      national Conference on Cyclic AMP, Vancouver, in "Advance
      Cyclic Nucleotide Research" (1975) (G.I. Drummond, P. Green-
      gard and G.A. Robison, ed.) Vol. 5, 822, Academic Press,
      New York

(57) KIMURA, H. and MURAD, F. (1974) Fed. Proc. 33 (Part I), 479

(58) KIMURA, H. and MURAD, F. (1974) J. Biol. Chem. 249, 6910

(59) KOSHLAND, D.E., Jr. (1970) in "The Enzymes" (Boyer, P.D. ed)
      3rd Ed. Vol. 1, 341

(60) KRISHNA, G., KRISHNAN, N., FLETCHER, T., and CHADER, G.
      (1974) Abstracts, Second International Conference on Cyclic
      AMP, Vancouver, in "Advances in Cyclic Nucleotide Research"
      (1975) (G.I. Drummond, P. Greengard and G.A. Robison, eds.)
      Vol. 5, 823

(61) KRISHNAN, N., and KRISHNA, G. (1974) Fed. Proc. 33, 1250
      (abs.)

(62) KRISHNAN, N., and KRISHNA, G. (1974) Abstracts, Second
      International Conference on Cyclic AMP, Vancouver, in
      "Advances in Cyclic Nucleotide Research" (1975) (G.I.
      Drummond, P. Greengard, G.A. Robinson, eds.) Volume 5,
      820, Academic Press, New York

(63) KUO, J.F., LEE, T.P., REYES, P.L., WALTON, K.G., DONNELLY,
      T.G., Jr., and GREENGARD, P. (1972) J. Biol. Chem. 247, 16

(64) LIMBIRD, L.E., and LEFKOWITZ, R.J. (1974) Abstracts, Second
      International Conference on Cyclic AMP, Vancouver, in
      "Advances in Cyclic Nucleotide Research" (1975) (G.I.
      Drummond, P. Greengard and G.A. Robison, eds.) Volume 5, 823
      Academic Press, New York

(65)   MARKS, F., (1973) Biochim. Biophys. Acta 309, 349

(66)   McCLURE, W.R., LARDY, H.A., and KNEIFEL, H.P. (1971) J. Biol.
       Chem. 246, 3569

(67)   McMILLAN, B.H., NEY, R.L., and SCHORR, I. (1971) Endocrinology
       89, 281

(68)   MONTAGUE, W. and HOWELL, S.L. (1974) Abstracts, Second Int.
       Conference on Cyclic AMP, Vancouver, in "Advances in Cyclic
       Nucleotide Research" (1975) (G.I. Drummond, P. Greengard and
       G.A. Robison, eds.) Vol. 5, 822, Academic Press, New York

(69)   MORRISON, J.F., and EBNER, K.E. (1971) J. Biol. Chem. 246,
       3977

(70)   MORRISON, J.F. and EBNER, K.E. (1971) J. Biol. Chem. 246,
       3985

(71)   MURAD, F., MANGANIELLO, V., and VAUGHAN, M. (1971) Proc. Nat.
       Acad. Sci. (USA) 68, 736

(72)   NAKAZAWA, K. and SANO, M. (1974) J. Biol. Chem. 249, 4207

(73)   O'DEA, R.F., BODLEY, J.W., LIN, L., HADDOX, M.K., and GOLD-
       BERG, N.D. (1974) in "Methods in Enzymology" (J.G. Hardman
       and B.W. O'Malley, Vol. Eds.) Vol. 38, 85, Academic Press,
       N.Y.

(74)   O'SULLIVAN, W.J. and PERRIN, D.D. (1964) Biochemistry 3, 18

(75)   ØYE, I. and SUTHERLAND, E.W. (1966) Biochim. Diophys. Acta
       127, 347

(76)   PANNBACKER, R.G. (1973) Science 182, 1138

(77)   PERKINS, J.P. (1973) "Adv. Cyclic Nucleotide Research"
       (P. Greengard and G.A. Robison, eds.) 3, 1

(78)   PETRACK, B., MA, D., and SHEPPY, F. (1974) J. Biol. Chem.
       249, 3661

(79)   RALL, T.W. and SUTHERLAND, E.W. (1962) J. Biol. Chem. 237,
       1228

(80)   RODBELL, M., BIRNBAUMER, L., POHL, S.L., and KRANS, H.M.
       (1971) J. Biol. Chem. 246, 1877

(81)   RUSSELL, T.R., TERASAKI, W., and APPLEMAN, M.M. (1973) J.
       Biol. Chem. 248, 1334

(82) SCHULTZ, G. (1974) in "Methods in Enzymology" (J.G. Hardman
      and B.W. O'Malley, Vol. Eds.) Vol. 38, 115, Academic Press,
      New York

(83) SCHULTZ, G., BÖHME, E., and HARDMAN, J.G. (1974) in "Methods
      in Enzymology" (J.G. Hardman and B.W. O'Malley, Vol. Eds.)
      Vol. 38, 9, Academic Press, New York

(84) SCHULTZ, G., BÖHME, E., and MUNSKE, K. (1969) Life Sciences
      8, 1323

(85) SCHULTZ, G., HARDMAN, J.G., SCHULTZ, K., BAIRD, C.E., and
      SUTHERLAND, E.W. (1973) Proc. Nat. Acad. Sci. (USA) 70, 3889

(86) SCHULTZ, G., HARDMAN, J.G., SCHULTZ, K., DAVIS, J.W., and
      SUTHERLAND, E.W. (1973) Proc. Nat. Acad. Sci. (USA) 70, 1721

(87) SCHULTZ, G., JAKOBS, K.H., BÖHME, E., and SCHULTZ, K. (1972)
      Eur. J. Biochem. 24, 520

(88) SCHULTZ, G., Schultz, K., and HARDMAN, J.G. (1974) Meta-
      bolism, in press

(89) SEIFERT, W., and RUDLAND, P.S. (1974) Abstracts, Second
      Int. Conference on Cyclic AMP, Vancouver, in "Advances in
      Cyclic Nucleotide Research" (1975) (G.I. Drummond, P.
      Greengard and G.A. Robison, eds.) Vol. 5, 822, Academic Press
      New York

(90) SHIMA, S. (1974) Abstracts, Second Int. Conference on Cyclic
      AMP Vancouver, in "Advances in Cyclic Nucleotide Research"
      (1975) (G.I. Drummond, P. Greengard and G.A. Robison, ed.)
      Vol. 5, 823, Academic Press, New York

(91) SILLEN, L.G. and MARTELL, A.E. (1971) "Stability Constants
      of Metal Ion Complexes, "Supplement 1, The Chemical Society,
      Burlington House, London

(92) STEINER, A.L., PAGLIARA, A.S., CHASE, L.R., and KIPNIS, D.M.
      (1972) J. Biol. Chem. 247, 1114

(93) STONER, J., MANGANIELLO, V.C., and VAUGHAN, M. (1974 Mol.
      Pharmacol. 10, 155

(94) SUTHERLAND, E.W., RALL, T.W., and MENON, T. (1962) J. Biol.
      Chem. 237, 1220

(95) TAKAI, K., KURASHINA, Y., SUZUKI, C., OKAMOTO, H., UEKI, A.,
      and HAYAISHI, O. (1971) J. Biol. Chem. 246, 5843

(96)   THOMPSON, W.J., JOHNSON, D.G., LAVIS, V.R., and WILLIAMS,
       R.H. (1974) Endocrinology 94, 276

(97)   THOMPSON, W.J., WILLIAMS, R.H., and LITTLE, S.A. (1973)
       Arch. Biochem. Biophys. 159, 206

(98)   THOMPSON, W.J., WILLIAMS, R.H., and LITTLE, S.A. (1973)
       Biochim. Biophys. Acta 302, 329

(99)   WHITE, A.A. and AURBACH, G.D. (1969) Biochim. Biophys. Acta
       191, 686

(100) WHITE, A.A., NORTHUP, S.J., and ZENSER, T.V. (1972) in
       "Methods in Cyclic Nucleotide Research" (Chasin, M., ed.)
       125, Marcel Dekker, New York

(101) WHITE, A.A., and ZENSER, T.V. (1971) Anal. Biochem. 41, 372

(102) WHITE, A.A., and ZENZER, T.V. (1974) in "Methods in Enzymo-
       logy" (J.G. Hardman and B.W. O'Malley, Vol. Eds.) Vol. 38,
       192, Academic Press, New York

(103) WHITE, L.E., IGNARRO, L.J., and GEORGE, W.J. (1973). The
       Pharmacologist 15, 157 (abs.)

REGULATION OF CYCLIC AMP PHOSPHODIESTERASE ACTIVITY

Martha Vaughan

Laboratory of Cellular Metabolism
National Heart and Lung Institute
National Institutes of Health
Bethesda, Maryland 20014, USA

CONTENTS

Insofar as is known at present, a cell can regulate its content of cyclic AMP in only two ways - by modifying the activity of adenylate cyclase which controls the rate of cyclic AMP formation, and by altering the activity of the phosphodiesterases which convert cyclic AMP to 5'-AMP[1]. Conceivably, control could also be exerted through processes related to extrusion of cyclic AMP from the cells or through enzymes that might catalyze the conversion of cyclic AMP to compounds other than 5'-AMP. There is today, however, no evidence that such mechanisms do play a role in regulation of cyclic AMP concentration in mammalian cells.

---

[1]Abbreviations: 5'-AMP, 5'-adenosine monophosphate; ACTH, adrenocorticotropic hormone; PGE_1, prostaglandin E_1.

Probably, at least in part because cyclic AMP was discovered as the "second messenger" for epinephrine and glucagon in the liver (1), research in the field was focussed for at least 10 years on adenylate cyclase and agents that control its activity. Only in the past few years has there been a growing recognition of the importance of regulation of phosphodiesterase activity and also only recently a general awareness of the complexity of the phosphodiesterase systems for cyclic AMP degradation. In early studies, phosphodiesterase was almost always assayed in supernatant fractions of tissue homogenates with high concentrations of cyclic AMP as substrate. It is now well known that most cells contain phosphodiesterase activities with two (or more) apparent Michaelis constants for cyclic AMP and some of the modifications of phosphodiesterase activity that have been described seem to be confined to a high affinity component of the enzyme, i.e., may be demonstrated only when assays are carried out with low concentrations of cyclic AMP. In addition, in the fat cell as described below, the effects of insulin, dexamethasone and lipolytic hormones on phosphodiesterase activity are evidently localized to a fraction of the enzyme that is particulate.

A wide variety of drugs, ions and nucleotides, as well as specific proteins and other molecules that are normally found in cells, can inhibit or activate phosphodiesterase when added to the assay system. The physiological significance of many of these is unknown but at least certain of them may well play a role in regulation of intracellular phosphodiesterase activity. Several groups have now provided evidence from different types of studies that intracellular phosphodiesterase activity can be influenced by hormones as well as by cyclic AMP itself. In our laboratory and others, the search for ways in which cells might accomplish functional control of cyclic AMP degradation was initiated by measuring phosphodiesterase activity in specific situations in which available data on cyclic AMP metabolism may well have been explicable by alterations in the activity of this enzyme.

The following discussion is concerned with four ways in which phosphodiesterase activity can be altered in intact cells. Two of these that are rapid in onset and readily reversible have been studied in fat cells. The slower more chronic changes in phosphodiesterase activity that evidently depend on protein synthesis have been investigated for the most part in cultured cells.

EFFECT OF INSULIN ON FAT CELL PHOSPHODIESTERASE ACTIVITY

In fat cells, insulin can prevent or reverse the effects of epinephrine (also ACTH[1] and other hormones that activate adenylate

cyclase) on accumulation of cyclic AMP and on lipolysis. These
effects of insulin could presumably result either from a decrease
in adenylate cyclase activity or an increase in phosphodiesterase
activity. The phosphodiesterase activity in homogenates of fat
cells exhibits two Michaelis constants for cyclic AMP (2-7). A
major portion of the high-affinity phosphodiesterase is apparently
particulate whereas most of the high K_m activity is recovered
in the supernatant (4,5). Under some circumstances, it is possible
to obtain particulate fractions that contain little or no low
affinity phosphodiesterase (7).

     After incubation of fat cells with insulin, phosphodiesterase
activity in whole homogenates assayed with low substrate concentrations (but not with high) was increased as initially reported
by Loten and Sneyd (2). The effects of insulin were, however,
much larger when activities in the particulate fractions were
compared (5). No effects of insulin on phosphodiesterase in the
supernatant fractions were demonstrable (5,6), and, in fact, the
total increment in activity produced by insulin was accounted for
by the increment in the 100,000 g pellet fraction (5). In a long
series of experiments, incubation of fat cells with insulin,
1 mU/ml for 10 min, conditions that produce a maximal effect,
increased the activity of this fraction by about 70% (5). Kinetic
studies revealed only an increase in V_m with no change in K_m.
produced by insulin (5,6). The particulate fractions in which
phosphodiesterase activity was increased by insulin were also
enriched in 5'-nucleotidase and adenylate cyclase but no effects
of insulin on the activities of these enzymes were demonstrable (5).

     The activity of the high affinity particulate phosphodiesterase
from control fat cells was increased by low concentrations of
heparin, EGTA, or dithiothreitol and inhibited by deoxycholate (5).
The enzyme from insulin-treated cells responded similarly to these
agents. On the other hand, incubation at 45° for 5 min before
assay decreased the activity of the control enzyme about 50% and
completely abolished the insulin-induced increment so that the
activities of both types of preparations were equal and the residual
activity in both was stable for at least 30 min at 45° (5). If this
treatment distinguishes a heat labile phosphodiesterase that can be
activated by exposure of cells to insulin from a heat stable
phosphodiesterase that cannot, insulin may, in fact, increase the
activity of the former enzyme by 200%.

     In summary, the activity of a particulate, perhaps membrane-
bound, high-affinity phosphodiesterase can be increased in a rapid,
reversible and specific fashion by exposure of intact fat cells
to insulin. This effect could be sufficient to account for the
effects of insulin on fat cell cyclic AMP content and on lipolysis.

EFFECTS OF INTRACELLULAR CYCLIC AMP CONCENTRATION ON FAT
CELL PHOSPHODIESTERASE ACTIVITY

On addition of epinephrine or ACTH to fat cells, the cyclic AMP content rises rapidly, reaching a maximum in 4 to 7 min and then declining (8,9). If the hormone-stimulated rate of cyclic AMP formation remained constant during this period, there would necessarily be some change in the rate of cyclic AMP degradation to account for the transient nature of cyclic AMP accumulation. In fact, the studies of Zinman and Hollenberg (6) as well as those in our laboratory (7) have shown that when the cyclic AMP content of fat cells is increased with epinephrine or ACTH, with theophylline or dibutyryl cyclic AMP, an increase in phosphodiesterase activity can be demonstrated. The increment in activity appears to result from an increase in V_m of a particulate, low K_m phosphodiesterase (6,7).

In our studies (7), a significant increase in particulate phosphodiesterase activity was observed 2 min after the addition of epinephrine, ACTH or theophylline to fat cells. It reached a maximum in 5 min and then declined after 5 or 10 min. When cyclic AMP content and phosphodiesterase activity were assayed in the same experiment, the changes in phosphodiesterase always paralleled the changes in cyclic AMP content and the decline in phosphodiesterase activity tended to lag behind the fall in cyclic AMP.

In maximally effective concentrations, epinephrine or ACTH or both together produced identical changes in fat cell cyclic AMP content with time (9). Likewise the increases in fat cell phosphodiesterase activity produced by epinephrine, ACTH or both together (after 7 min of incubation) were identical (7). When the effect of epinephrine on cyclic AMP was prevented with propranolol, there was no increase in phosphodiesterase activity and when propranolol was added to cells 5 min after epinephrine, both the cyclic AMP content and the phosphodiesterase activity fell to basal levels within 2 min (7). Thus, under several conditions in the presence of epinephrine, ACTH and/or theophylline, the activity of a particulate, high-affinity phosphodiesterase in fat cell could be rapidly altered, always in parallel with, and probably as a consequence of, changes in the concentration of its substrate, cyclic AMP.

As discussed above, insulin also produced a rapid increase in the activity of a low K_m particulate phosphodiesterase in the fat cells. The effect of insulin differed, however, from that of the so-called lipolytic agents in that it was sustained as long as insulin was present and was associated with no change in fat cell cyclic AMP content (7). In addition, the phosphodiesterase activity maximally elevated with theophylline plus ACTH could be further increased by insulin (7). It, therefore, seems clear that, whether insulin and ACTH (for example) alter the activity of the same or different phosphodiesterases, the mechanisms by which they act are different.

EFFECTS OF PROLONGED ELEVATION OF CYCLIC AMP ON PHOSPHODIESTERASE ACTIVITY

In contrast to the transient increase in cyclic AMP content that results in fat cells when a hormone that stimulates adenylate cyclase is added, in cultured mouse fibroblasts (L-cells), after the addition of PGE_1,[1] the cyclic AMP content rises rapidly and then remains at essentially the same maximal level for several hours. By 12 hr, however, it has declined considerably and it cannot be elevated again by addition of fresh PGE_1 (10). This developing refractoriness to PGE_1 could be secondary to increasing phosphodiesterase activity over that period.

As do most mammalian cells, the L-cells contain phosphodiesterase activity with two apparent Michaelis constants for cyclic AMP (10,11). In homogenates of cells incubated with PGE_1 for 24 hr assayed with a relatively low concentration of cyclic AMP as substrate, the phosphodiesterase activity was increased 30 to 100% over that in control cells (10). When assayed at high substrate concentrations, on the other hand, the activity in the PGE_1-treated cells was not increased but tended to be lower than that in control cells, i.e., the activity of a high affinity phosphodiesterase was increased by the incubation of cells with PGE_1 (10). Phosphodiesterase activity was likewise increased in L-929 cells and in 3T3 cells incubated with dibutyryl cyclic AMP (10,11).

In cells in which the cyclic AMP content was maintained at elevated levels by the continued presence of one of these agents, phosphodiesterase activity continued to rise for 48 or more hours (10,11). The increase in activity was prevented with cycloheximide or actinomycin D (10,11) and, on the basis of experiments reported by d'Armiento et al. (11), was probably the result of synthesis of new enzyme rather than synthesis of an activator. Thus it appears that, in fibroblasts, synthesis of a high affinity phosphodiesterase may be controlled by the concentration of its substrate, cyclic AMP.

It seems probable that in many types of cells, cyclic AMP can act as an inducer of phosphodiesterase. Uzunov et al. (12) found that in cloned astrocytoma cells, the activity of a specific component of the phosphodiesterase was increased after incubation for 6 hr with norepinephrine which activates adenylate cyclase in these cells. Isoproterenol as well as dibutyryl cyclic AMP can increase phosphodiesterase activity in lymphoma cells and from studies with this system, Bourne et al. (13) obtained evidence that a cyclic AMP-dependent protein kinase plays a role in the induction of phosphodiesterase synthesis by cyclic AMP.

EFFECTS OF STEROID HORMONES ON PHOSPHODIESTERASE ACTIVITY

In several tissues the effects of hormones that increase adenylate cyclase activity are enhanced by steroid hormones. Effects of this type could result from a steroid induced decrease in phosphodiesterase activity. In HTC hepatoma cells which have been extensively used to study the induction of tyrosine amino-transferase by corticosteroids, epinephrine causes accumulation of cyclic AMP (14). After incubation for 2 days with 1 μM dexamethasone, the cyclic AMP content of the hepatoma cells was increased as was the rise induced by epinephrine (14). Accompanying this apparent increase in sensitivity to epinephrine was a 30 to 40% decrease in phosphodiesterase activity (14). The percentage decrease was the same whether assays were carried out with high or with low concentrations of cyclic AMP as substrate. Thus, although the homogenates of the HTC cells contained phosphodiesterase activity with two K_m's for cyclic AMP, the effect of dexamethasone was not demonstrably localized to one or another form of the enzyme.

The effect of dexamethasone on phosphodiesterase in the hepatoma cells was specific in that it was not mimicked by α-methyl testosterone, a steroid which also fails to induce tyrosine amino-transferase in these cells. In addition, the dexamethasone-induced decrease in phosphodiesterase activity was accompanied by no decrease in phosphatase activity (14). Senft et al. (15) found that phosphodiesterase activity was increased in several tissues in adrenalectomized rats and could be restored to control levels by treating the animals with α-methyl prednisolone. In other studies (5), treatment of intact rats with dexamethasone for 24 to 36 hr caused a decrease in phosphodiesterase activity measured in fat cell homogenates and this effect of dexamethasone was apparently confined to a component of the particulate phosphodiesterase. It is probable that corticosteroids can also decrease phosphodiesterase activity in cultured human fibroblasts (16).

Other types of steroid hormones may also bring about a decrease in phosphodiesterase activity in specific tissues. In toad bladder, for example, where vasopressin activates adenylate cyclase and causes accumulation of cyclic AMP, its effects are dramatically magnified when tissues are incubated with aldosterone for several hours before vasopressin addition (17) and a small but significant decrease in phosphodiesterase activity has been demonstrated under these conditions (18). It should be remembered that in the studies thus far published, the magnitude of the steroid effects on phosphodiesterase may have been grossly underestimated in the sense that when whole homogenate activity is assayed under a given set of conditions, changes in the activity of the specific component of the phosphodiesterase may tend to be masked or minimized.

The mechanism by which the steroid hormones decrease phosphodiesterase activity remains to be elucidated. On the basis of the relatively long time required and the information available concerning other effects of these hormones it seems probable that, as previously stated, "dexamethasone influences the synthesis of a protein that regulates the level of the phosphodiesterase itself or modifies its catalytic activity" (14). In any case, there is considerable evidence that the so-called permissive effects of steroid hormones on cyclic AMP mediated processes in many tissues may be a result of a steroid-induced decrease in phosphodiesterase activity.

In conclusion, there is a growing body of data to support the view that regulation of cyclic AMP degradation is of importance in the physiological control of intracellular cyclic AMP content, whether as a result of acute changes in phosphodiesterase activity, such as those effected by insulin and by cyclic AMP, or consequent to more chronic modulation of phosphodiesterase activity in which it appears that steroid hormones and cyclic AMP itself can play a part. With a better understanding of the phosphodiesterase systems, it now seems probable that they may rival the adenylate cyclases in the complexity of their regulatory properties and the difficulties encountered in attempting to obtain an explanation for these at the molecular level.

REFERENCES

1. Sutherland, E.W. and Rall, T.W. (1958) J. Biol. Chem. 232: 1077.

2. Loten, E.G. and Sneyd, J.G.T. (1970) Biochem. J. 120: 187.

3. Thompson, W.J. and Appleman, M.M. (1971) J. Biol. Chem. 246: 3145.

4. Vaughan, M. (1972) in Insulin Action (Fritz, I.B., ed.) pp 297-318, Academic Press, N.Y.

5. Manganiello, V.C. and Vaughan, M. (1973) J. Biol. Chem. 248: 7164.

6. Zinman, B. and Hollenberg, C.H. (1974) J. Biol. Chem. 249: 2182.

7. Pawlson, L.G., Lovell-Smith, C.J., Manganiello, V.C. and Vaughan, M. (1974) Proc. Nat. Acad. Sci. USA 71: 1639.

8. Butcher, R.W., Baird, C.E. and Sutherland, E.W. (1968) J. Biol. Chem. 243: 1705.

9. Manganiello, V.C., Murad, F. and Vaughan, M. (1971) J. Biol. Chem. 246: 2195.

10. Manganiello, V.C. and Vaughan, M. (1972) Proc. Nat. Acad. Sci. USA 69: 269.

11. d'Armiento, M., Johnson, G.S. and Pastan, I. (1972) Proc. Nat. Acad. Sci. USA 69: 459.

12. Uzunov, P., Shein, H.M. and Weiss, B. (1972) Science 180: 304.

13. Bourne, H.R., Tomkins, G.M. and Dion, S. (1973) Science 181: 952.

14. Manganiello, V.C. and Vaughan, M. (1972) J. Clin. Invest. 51: 2763.

15. Senft, G., Schultz, G., Munske, K. and Hoffman, M. (1968) Diabetologia 4: 330.

16. Manganiello, V.C., Breslow, J. and Vaughan, M. (1972) J. Clin. Invest. 51: 60a.

17. Stoff, J., Handler, J.S. and Orloff, J. (1972) Proc. Nat. Acad. Sci. USA 69: 805

18. Stoff, J.S., Handler, J.S., Preston, A.S. and Orloff, J. (1973) Life Sciences 13: 545.

THEORETICAL SIMULATION OF THE cAMP SYSTEM

S. Swillens
E. Van Cauter
M. Paiva
J.E. Dumont

Institut de Recherche Interdisciplinaire
University of Brussels, School of Medicine
1000 Brussels (Belgium)

Contents

INTRODUCTION

During the last few years, the number and diversity of systems, tissues and experiments in the field of cyclic nucleotides research have become so large that it is now very difficult to integrate the data into a single model. There is therefore an urgent need for a systematic theoretical study of the basic questions of "why" and "how" for each of the main subsystems of the intricate reaction network which operates in the living cell.

Such a theoretical investigation is based upon the use of models which are simply straightforward descriptions of the current ideas. Sometimes as will be shown below, the translation of general concepts into mathematical formulations is already sufficient to elucidate some puzzling results. But generally, a model will be used as a tool to stimulate comparison of theoretical with experimental results.

It has to be emphasized that such models are always approximate since they are based on the present knowledge of the system and must include assumptions when experimental facts are lacking. However, a satisfactory model for a mechanism may be defined as the simplest formulation accounting for all the experimental results. Attempts to fit experimental data will lead to relevant results only if the model includes a minimum number of parameters.

It should be realised that a model is never an end in itself but always a tool which allows subsequent verification of the validity of the description, prediction of some unknown results, and the explanation of some known facts. Finally, crucial experiments may be performed to confirm or invalidate the theoretical results.

In this paper, we present a theoretical investigation of two mechanisms of the cyclic AMP system. The first mechanism is the protein kinase activation by cyclic AMP. The study shows the actual significance of the binding and activation constants and emphasizes the importance of a thorough treatment of the data. In the second part, the consequences of the localisation on the membrane of key enzymes, such as adenylate cyclase and phosphodiesterase, on the cyclic AMP intracellular distribution and metabolism are shown. Quantitative results obtained by numerical simulation illustrate the conclusions.

PROTEIN KINASE AND CYCLIC AMP

The most prevalent protein kinase consists of two subunits : the regulatory subunit R and the catalytic subunit C which is inactive when bound to R. The binding of a molecule of cyclic AMP to the regulatory subunit leads to the release of the catalytic subunit which is then fully active :

$$\text{cyclic AMP} + \text{R-C} \rightleftharpoons \text{RcyclicAMP} + \text{C}$$

The study of such a binding mechanism includes the investigation of the relationship between cyclic AMP concentration and kinase activity which is related to the concentration of free catalytic subunit and investigation of the cyclic AMP binding to the regulatory subunit as a function of the cyclic AMP concentration. In this model, here-referred to as model 2, one molecule of C is released when one molecule of cyclic AMP is bound to R. Therefore, the kinase activation and the cyclic AMP binding are two strictly parallel processes induced by cyclic AMP and, the same theoretical study holds for both (Figure 1).

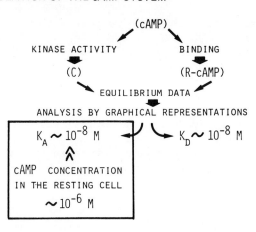

Figure 1. *Theoretical study of kinase activation and cyclic AMP binding*

Initially, before any model was proposed, the activation reaction was studied as an enzymatic reaction. Indeed, the dissociation constant K_D and the half-activation constant K_A, both of them corresponding to the Michaëlis-Menten constant (K_m) of enzymatic reactions were introduced : K_D is the reciprocal of the equilibrium constant and K_A is the total concentration of cyclic AMP needed for half maximal activation of the kinases.

The theory of enzymatic reactions provides graphical representations of equilibrium data (the double reciprocal plot or Lineweaver-Burk plot (1) and the Scatchard or Hofstee plot (2)) which allow the determination of these constants by linear fitting. These representations were used to analyze equilibrium data on cyclic AMP binding and kinase activation. Most studies have led to numerical values of K_D and K_A in the range of 10^{-8} to 10^{-7}M. On the other hand, the cyclic AMP concentration in the resting cell is of about 10^{-6}M.

Since this concentration is much higher than the K_A value, the question of how the cyclic AMP concentration can regulate the kinase activity arises. Three possible answers are:

- cyclic AMP does not regulate kinase activity. The bulk of information on cyclic AMP-protein kinase interaction suggests the contrary;

- a large part of free cyclic AMP is sequestrated so that the
  concentration of cyclic AMP able to bind with kinase is very
  low (3,4). However, the search for such a sequestrating
  structure has been unfruitful until now. Moreover, some studies
  have drawn a good correlation between the total levels of cyclic
    AMP   and degree of kinase activation in intact cells (5,6,7);

- the K_A estimations have no physiological meaning.

        Theoretical considerations developed hereafter demonstrate
the validity of this last answer.

        We have recently shown that the Lineweaver-Burk and
Scatchard representations may not be used when the binding
reaction occurs according to model 2 and therefore the constants
K_D and K_A estimated from such an analysis have no meaning (8). It
is of interest to compare model 2 with the model of enzymatic
reaction :

$$\text{cyclic AMP} + \text{RC} \rightleftharpoons \text{cyclic AMP-RC}$$

which will be here referred to as model 1.

        Model 1 describes the reversible binding of a ligand to a
receptor leading to the formation of an active complex. The
equilibrium constant K_{eq} for the two models are :

$$K_{eq}^{(1)} = \frac{(\text{cAMP-RC})}{(\text{cAMP})\,(\text{RC})} \qquad \text{for model 1}$$

$$K_{eq}^{(2)} = \frac{(\text{RcAMP})\,(\text{C})}{(\text{cAMP})\,(\text{RC})} \qquad \text{for model 2}$$

$K_{eq}^{(1)}$ has the dimension of the reciprocal of a concentration
whereas $K_{eq}^{(2)}$ is dimensionless. Its reciprocal $K_D^{(2)}$ is of
course also dimensionless.

        Binding experiments give equilibrium concentrations of
bound cyclic AMP as a function of the total concentration of cyclic
AMP. If the reaction occurs according to model 1, the Lineweaver-
Burk plot is linear and allows the determination of $K_{eq}^{(1)}$ and of
the total concentration of the receptor $(R-C)_t$ (Figure 2A) whereas
in the case of model 2, the representation is not linear at all
(Figure 2B). However, a few points could be fitted by a straight
line because of the very slight curvature with this method of
plotting. Nevertheless, $K_{eq}^{(2)}$ may not be evaluated as usual
because of the non correspondence between the model and the linear
representation. Moreover, the procedure is clearly misleading
since the equilibrium constant obtained is not dimensionless. The

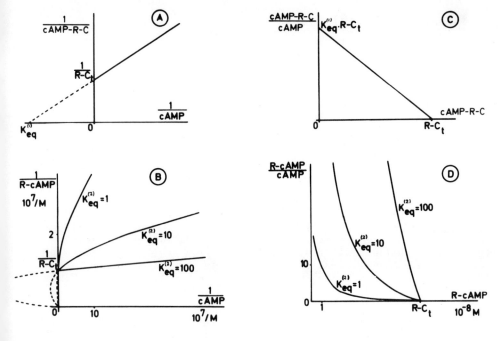

Figure 2. *Theoretical Lineweaver-Burk plots for model 1, (A) and*
model 2, (B) and theoretical Scatchard plots for model 1, (C) and
model 2, (D). R.C$_t$ refers to the total concentration of kinase.
cAMP, R-cAMP and cAMP-R-C refer to equilibrium concentrations.
For model 2, three curves are plotted for the following values of
$K_{eq}^{(2)}$: 1; 10; 100. If these curves were fitted by straight
lines as if the reaction occurred according to model 1, one could
estimate $K_{eq}^{(1)}$: 10^8/M; 2.5×10^8/M; 12×10^8/M. (Reprinted
from Swillens et al. (8)).

same conclusions arise in the case of the Scatchard plot : it is
linear for model 1 (Figure 2C) but not for model 2 (Figure 2D).

Since these methods do not allow the determination of
$K_{eq}^{(2)}$ through linear fittings, we proposed a new representation,
the "B^2/F vs B plot", which is linear in the case of model 2 :
the ratio of the square of bound cyclic AMP to free cyclic AMP
is plotted against bound cyclic AMP (Figure 3). The slope of the
straight line gives the equilibrium constant $K_{eq}^{(2)}$.

Thus, it is of interest that the use of the different
representations can exclude one or both models only by analysing

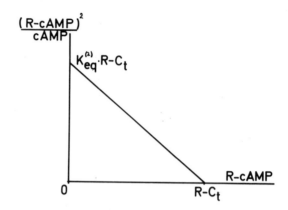

Figure 3.   *Theoretical "B²/F vs B" plot for model 2. R.C_t refers to the total concentration of kinase. R-cAMP and cAMP are the equilibrium concentrations of bound and free cAMP. The slope of the curve is equal to $-K_{eq}^{(2)}$. (Reprinted from Swillens et al. (8)).*

the shape of the experimental curves (Figure 4).   Nevertheless, we must caution that a satisfactory fitting is never a proof of the validity of the assumed model.   Thus, the misuse of theoretical analysis valid only for the enzymatic reactions corresponding to the Michaëlis-Menten model has led to incorrect estimations of $K_{eq}^{(2)}$ in the literature.

The same error has been made concerning the K_A concept. For the enzymatic reaction, the constant K_m corresponds to the concentration of substrate needed for half maximal activation of the enzyme because it is assumed that the enzyme concentration is much lower than the substrate concentration.

For the kinase activation by cyclic AMP, K_A is not a con-stant and this is true for model 1 as well as for model 2.   The actual K_A is higher than or equal to the half total concentration of kinase $(RC)_t$ (Figure 5).   In the case of model 2, we obtain :

$$K_A = \frac{1}{2} (RC)_t \{1 + K_D^{(2)}\} \qquad (1)$$

under the following conditions :

a) the reaction is described by model 2;

b) the total concentrations of regulatory subunits and of cata-lytic subunits are equal;

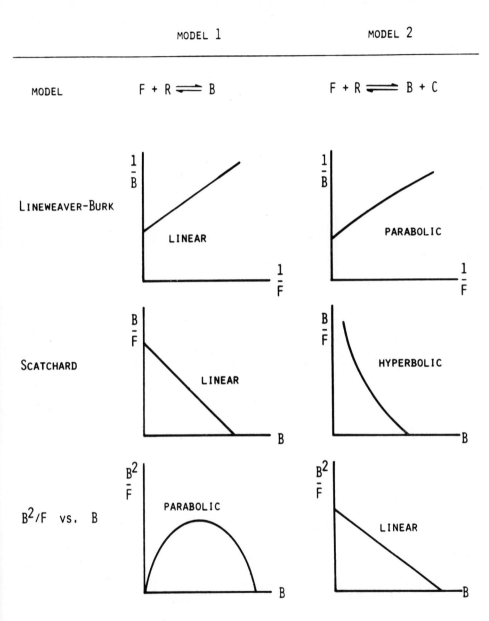

Figure 4. Characteristics of the three theoretical representations for models 1 and 2 (F : free ligand; R : receptor; B : bound ligand; C : active unit)

cAMP BINDING TO PROTEIN KINASE

	Model 1 (USED IN BINDING STUDIES)	Model 2 (DERIVED FROM SEPARATION STUDIES)
MODEL	$cAMP+R\text{-}C \underset{K_-}{\overset{K_+}{\rightleftharpoons}} cAMP\text{-}R\text{-}C$	$cAMP+R\text{-}C \underset{K_-}{\overset{K_+}{\rightleftharpoons}} R\text{-}cAMP+C$
CHARACTERISTICS	UNDISSOCIATED ACTIVE COMPLEX	DISSOCIABLE REGULATORY AND CATALYTIC UNITS
DISSOCIATION CONSTANT $K_D=\dfrac{1}{K_{EQ}}=\dfrac{K_-}{K_+}$	$\sim 10^{-8}$ M	STILL TO BE MEASURED
DIMENSION OF K_{EQ}	RECIPROCAL OF CONCENTRATION	DIMENSIONLESS
ACTIVATION "CONSTANT" K_A	NOT CONSTANT $.5(R\text{-}C)_{TOTAL} + K_D$	NOT CONSTANT $.5(R\text{-}C)_{TOTAL} (1 + K_D)$

Figure 5. Characteristics of model 1 and model 2.

c) the substrate for C does not dissociate the complex RC;

d) the complex RC is inactive;

e) the catalytic subunit C is fully active;

f) the enzymatic reaction catalyzed by C does not displace the equilibrium state, i.e., C is not sequestrated by the substrate.

It can be shown that even if one of these assumptions is false and rejected, the value of K_A lies at least in the range of the total concentration of cyclic AMP binding sites if only the protein kinase activity parallels the cyclic AMP binding (9). An evaluation of the total amount of specific binding sites for cyclic AMP has been performed in dog thyroid cell. The experiment (following the Gilman method) presented in Figure 6 shows the binding of cyclic AMP, i.e. the concentration of occupied sites as a function of the total concentration of cyclic AMP. The binding on both homogenate and supernatant (20000g for 20 minutes) have been investigated. At least up to 100 μM of total cyclic AMP, the binding curves did not exhibit any plateau, i.e. the binding process was not saturated. This suggests that a non-specific binding occurs which may be evaluated by extrapolating the slope of the curve at the highest concentrations of cyclic AMP. This non-specific binding was similar for both preparations used. It probably has no physiological meaning as it may play a role only for very high unphysiological concentrations of cyclic AMP.

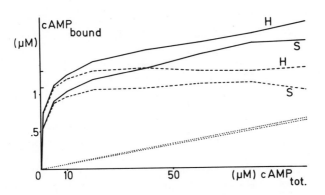

Figure 6. Cyclic AMP binding in dog thyroid homogenate (H) and supernatant (S) by using the Gilman method (————) : experimental results; (....) : non-specific binding; (—————) : specific binding. The concentrations refer to the intracellular volume of a dog thyroid.

This non-specific concentration has thus been deduced from the
experimental results in order to give the specific binding. The
maximal capacity of specific protein binding sites in dog thyroid
cell for cyclic AMP is therefore about 1 μM, i.e. very similar
to basal cyclic AMP concentration.

We can conclude that K_A is also in the range of basal
cyclic AMP concentration and thus the hypothesis of the existence
of sequestrating structure is not necessary. Moreover, if such
a sequestration exists, it cannot be demonstrated by means of the
Gilman method and thus would not consist of protein structure
which would be retained on Millipore filter.

It has to be noted that, as shown by eq (1), K_A is proportional to the total concentration of kinase and thus decreases
when the dilution factor increases. Therefore, a change of the
kinase concentration in the assay would cause a displacement of
the kinase activation curve. Recent experimental work reported
by Beavo and coworkers (10) indeed confirms this theoretical
conclusion.

The hypothesis 7 seems to be of some interest as it is
probably quite irrelevant. Indeed if we suppose that the reaction
transforming a substrate S in a product P is catalysed by the
subunit C of the protein kinase, the system can be described as :

$$cAMP + R\text{-}C \rightleftharpoons R\text{-}cAMP + C$$

$$C + S \underset{k_2}{\overset{k_1}{\rightleftharpoons}} C\text{-}S \overset{k_3}{\longrightarrow} P + C$$

where C-S is the active complex in the Michaëlis-Menten reaction,
Thus, if the binding of C to the substrate S prevents the regulatory subunit R to recognize the specific binding site of C,
the last reaction affects the equilibrium state of cyclic AMP
binding because of the consumption of free catalytic subunit by
the complex C-S. The activity of protein kinase is in this case
equal to k_3 (C-S). Kinetics experiment are usually performed in
the following conditions: - the total concentration of substrate
(casein, histones, phosphorylase kinase, ...) is much higher
than the total concentration of kinase : $(S)_t \gg (R\text{-}C)_t$

- the concentration of substrate is much higher than the
Michaëlis-Menten constant $K_m = \dfrac{k_2 + k_3}{k_1}$, i.e., the enzyme is

functioning at V_{max} : $(S)_t \gg k_m$.

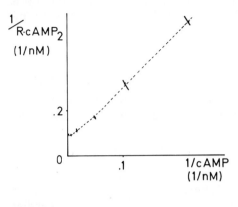

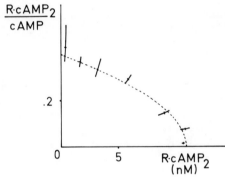

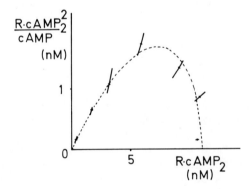

Figure 7. *Fitting of experimental data by model 3 in a Lineweaver-Burk, a Scatchard and a "B^2/F vs B"-plot. Mean and range of triplicates are represented by solid lines*

Under these conditions, the whole available amount of catalytic subunits binds to the substrate S. Thus the binding of cyclic AMP to protein kinase leads to a complete disappearance of either of cyclic AMP or R-C depending on the respective total concentrations of cyclic AMP and R-C. In other words, if $(cAMP_t < (R-C)_t$, the whole amount of cyclic AMP is bound to R and thus $(CS) = (R-C)_t - (R-C)$. On the other hand, if $(cAMP)_t \geqslant (R-C)_t$, the whole amount of C is dissociated from R and bound to S and thus $(C-S) = (R-C)_t$. In this last case, the maximal activity is obtained and is equal to $k_3(R-C)_t$. Therefore half maximal activity is obtained when $(cAMP)_t = \frac{1}{2}(R-C)_t$; i.e.

$K_A = \frac{1}{2}(R-C)_t$. It is noteworthy that K_A does not depend on the dissociation constant of the cyclic AMP binding reaction but only on the total concentration of kinase. Moreover, the value of K_A obtained in such a way has no physiological significance as the conditions of the experiment are not fulfilled in the cell.

Experimental results on the cyclic AMP binding on protein kinase of skeletal muscle have been obtained by Van Sande (to be published) using the Gilman method (11), where bound cyclic AMP concentration is evaluated from the amount of labelled cyclic AMP retained on millipore filters. The results of mathematical treatment and different plottings are quite unexpected. Indeed, the curve in the Scatchard plot has a downward concavity instead of the expected upward one and the "B^2/F vs B"-plot is not linear and shows a maximum.

The only simple model leading to the same type of curves in each of the graphical representation is :

$$2cAMP + RC \rightleftharpoons RcAMP_2 + C$$

Two moles of cyclic AMP would thus be required to activate one mole of holoenzyme. The same conclusion was drawn by Beavo et al. (10) as a result of the determination of the molecular weight of the protein kinase in skeletal muscle. Figure 7 shows how this model fits our experimental data represented by the means and the ranges of triplicates. Each point of a triplicate has a different abscissa because the independent variable of the system is the total concentration of cyclic AMP and not the concentration of bound or free cyclic AMP. This hypothetical model has the property that only one catalytic subunit should be bound to one molecule of regulatory subunit. If it is assumed that the regulatory subunit is a dimeric protein which is able to bind two molecules of cyclic AMP as well as two molecules of catalytic subunit, the graphical representations become quite different and cannot account for our experimental results (Figure 8).

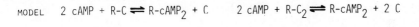

MODEL $2\ cAMP + R\text{-}C \rightleftharpoons R\text{-}cAMP_2 + C$ $2\ cAMP + R\text{-}C_2 \rightleftharpoons R\text{-}cAMP_2 + 2\ C$

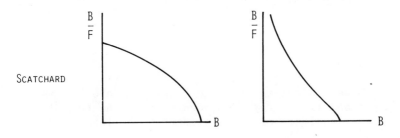

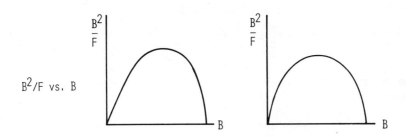

Figure 8.   *Theoretical Scatchard and "B^2/F vs B"-plot for models where two moles of cyclic AMP bind to one mole of holo-enzyme.*
(B : bound cyclic AMP;   F : free cyclic AMP)

However, such results obtained from this type of analysis of the data should always be considered very cautiously. Indeed certain experimental work indicates that under Gilman conditions the millipore filters do not retain all of the kinase and thus the concentration of bound cyclic AMP measured here referred to as RcAMP' only corresponds to a fraction of the actual concentration RcAMP.

$$p = \frac{RcAMP}{RcAMP'} \tag{2}$$

The "loss" of bound cyclic AMP is characterised by the parameter

$$\alpha = \frac{RcAMP - RcAMP'}{RcAMP} \tag{3}$$

It follows from eq (2) and (3) that

$$\alpha \equiv \frac{p - 1}{p} \tag{4}$$

$$0 \leq \alpha \leq 1 \tag{5}$$

$$P \geq 1 \tag{6}$$

When measured values of bound cyclic AMP are systematically underestimated and if the reaction occurs according to model 2, the mathematical analysis of the representations leads to the following conclusions (12) :

a) The "B^2/F vs B" plot becomes hyperbolic and curve intersects the x-axis at the points $x = 0$ and $x = RC'_t$. If x_m refers to the abscissa of the maximum, we have:

$$K_D = \frac{\alpha}{x^2_m} (RC'_t - x_m)^2 \tag{7}$$

b) In the Scatchard representation, the curve intersects the y-axis at the point

$$y_o = \frac{1}{p - 1} \quad \text{and thus}$$

$$\alpha = \frac{1}{1 + y_o} \tag{8}$$

c) The curvature in the Lineweaver-Burk changes as a function of the α value.

If x_m and y_o may be determined with good accuracy, then eq(7) and (8) provide the numerical values of the unknown parameter K_D and α (without performing any fitting).

It is of interest that Lineweaver-Burk and Scatchard plots become linear when

$$\frac{p - 1}{p} = K_D^{(2)}$$

Thus, for a critical value p_c (or α_c) of the parameter p (or α), the observed linearity of these two representations would lead to a rejection of model 2 and acceptance of model 1 even though model 2 applies. The critical values are:

$$p_c = \frac{1}{1 - K_D^{(2)}} \tag{9}$$

and thus $\quad \alpha_c = K_D^{(2)}$ $\hspace{9cm}$ (10)

Figure 9 summarises these conclusions. The values of the parameters were chosen as follows :

$$(R-C)'_t \;=\; 10^{-8}M \text{ and } K_D \;=\; \frac{1}{11}$$

It follows from eq(9) and (10) that $p_c = 1.1$ and $\alpha_c = .091$.

Table 1 summarises the possible shapes of Lineweaver-Burk and Scatchard plots in the case of model 2 for different values of p or α. It is noteworthy that the shapes of these two representations leading to model 1 (linearity) or to the conclusion of a positive cooperativity can appear only if $K_D^{(2)} < 1$ because in this case $\alpha > \alpha_c \equiv K_D^{(2)}$, thus a downward concavity in the Scatchard plot requires that $K_D^{(2)} < 1$.

This artefact could explain the aspect of the plotted experimental data. Figure 10 shows the fitted curve with the following parameter values:

$$\alpha = .56 \quad \text{or p} = 2.25$$

$$K_D^{(2)} = .18$$

$$(R-C)_t = 5.10^{-8}M$$

It seems unlikely that millipore filters could not retain more than 44% of the kinase amount. Therefore, even if the shape of the representations may be explained by this artefact, the numerical analysis of the parameters rejects model 2 despite the improvement in the description of the experimental system.

It is thus suggested that model 2 is not satisfactory but further elaboration on this subject requires more experimental data. Anyway, this example again shows us the need to use available methods corresponding to the considered model. Moreover, it is noteworthy that a positive result giving a good fitting is never a proof of the validity of the model and of its underlying assumptions, especially if Lineweaver-Burk or Hill plots are used. Indeed, these two representations are not suitable methods to analyse the validity of models as they share the common property of not allowing discrimination of hypothetical models. This low sensitivity results from their respective inverse and logarithmic scales which hide the differences in the shapes of plotted curves.

TABLE 1. POSSIBLE ASPECTS OF LINEWEAVER–BURK AND SCATCHARD PLOTS
FOR MODEL 2

The parameter α and p characterise the systematic underestimation of the bound complex. The critical parameters α_c and p_c are defined by eq(9) and (10)

	TYPE OF CONCAVITY IN:		Conclusion "a priori"
	Lineweaver–Burk plot	Scatchard plot	
α(or p) $>$ α_c(or p_c)	upward	downward	positive cooperativity
α(or p) $=$ α_c(or p_c)	no concavity	no concavity	model 1 applies
α(or p) $<$ α_c(or p_c)	downward	upward	negative cooperativity

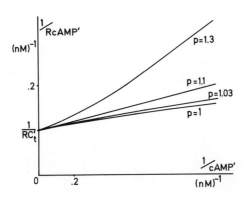

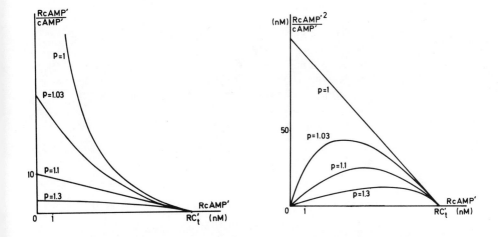

Figure 9. *Lineweaver–Burk, Scatchard and "B²/F vs B" plots for model 2 when the measure of bound cyclic AMP is underestimated. R-cAMP' refers to the measured concentration of bound cAMP. The parameter 'p' characterises the underestimation*

220

S. SWILLENS ET AL.

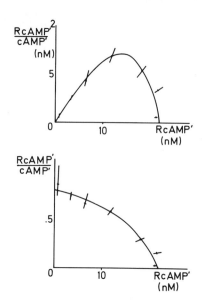

Figure 10. *Fitting of experimental data by model 2 when the measure of bound cyclic AMP is underestimated. Mean and range of triplicates are indicated in the "B²/F vs B" representation (upper plot) and in the Scatchard representation (lower plot). R-cAMP' and cAMP' correspond to the measured values.*

CONSEQUENCES OF THE INTRACELLULAR DISTRIBUTION OF
PHOSPHODIESTERASES

Intracellular cyclic AMP is hydrolyzed by at least two types of phosphodiesterases characterised by different maximal activities and different affinities for the substrate. Moreover, one phosphodiesterase with low activity and high affinity appear to be located at the plasma membrane, whereas the other one appears to be in the cytosol (13,14,15,16). Assuming that the two phosphodiesterases coexist in the same cell and that both exert their action on cyclic AMP, the advantage for any cell of such a dual enzyme system is not obvious. One consequence of this situation may be the amplification of hormonal stimulus and the

minimization of the consumption of ATP needed by cyclic AMP metabolism (17). Moreover, the activity of these two enzymes could be
regulated by different factors.

In most cell types, adenylate cyclase is a membrane bound
enzyme. Intracellular cyclic AMP propagates the hormonal stimulus
in the cell, from the plasma membrane to its sites of action.
The location of these sites depends in part on the cellular
structure and on the physiological function of the tissue. For
instance, it has been reported that the plasma membrane of the
bovine renal collecting duct epithelial cell contains antidiuretic
hormone sensitive adenylate cyclase only at its basal-lateral
(contraluminal) component, whereas the apical (luminal) membrane
contains a cyclic AMP-sensitive phosphorylating system consisting
of a membrane-bound protein kinase and its membrane-bound substrate. This intrinsic protein kinase is not present in the contraluminal membrane (18). The thyroid cell also exhibits a
"polarity" resulting from the structure of the thyroid follicles.
Only the basal part of the plasma membrane is exposed to the stimulating hormone, and therefore, the sites of synthesis of cyclic
AMP are located on the basal membrane. On the other hand, many
effects of the hormonal stimulus take place in the proximity of
the apical membrane. Thus to transmit the hormonal stimulus the
molecules of cyclic AMP must diffuse through the whole cytoplasm.
Even if the cell has a spherical symmetry (i.e. there is no
"polarity"), the molecules of cyclic AMP have first to diffuse
to their sites of action, usually not located at the plasma
membrane.

The activation level of the intracellular system whatever
its location depends on the local concentration of cyclic AMP
thus on the spatial distribution of cyclic AMP. Moreover, the
kinetics of the system are affected by the transport of cyclic
AMP into the cytoplasm. Therefore, it seemed to be of interest
to show how the locations of adenylate cyclase and phosphodiesterase affect the distribution of cyclic AMP and thus
distribution of the activation level of the cyclic AMP dependent
effects (19). A theoretical treatment and a numerical simulation
of this system are presented as follows.

Let us consider a theoretical system which consists of a
synthesis by A and a degradation by P of a component S. These
two reactions and the possible transport of S take place in a
closed homogeneous medium which is chosen cylindrical to simplify
the computations (Figure 11). This cylindrical symmetry does not
affect the conclusion of the study at all.

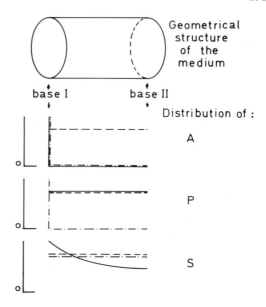

Figure 11. One-dimensional diffusion in a homogeneous medium. Qualitative spatial distribution of a component S synthesized by A and degraded by P.
(—·—·—·—) A and P are located at base I. Therefore S is homogeneously distributed
(————) A and P are soluble. Therefore S is homogeneously distributed
(————) A is located at base I whereas P is homogeneously distributed in the medium. In this case, the concentration of S is lower at base II than the concentration at base I. (Reprinted from Swillens et al. (9))

Case 1

The molecules of A are concentrated at the base I, whereas the molecules of P are distributed homogeneously into the whole medium. Let x be any point of the medium not situated on the base I. At this point, S is degraded by P but is not synthesized because of the lack of A. Thus, there exists a flux of S to this point and consequently a gradient of concentration if transport occurs by diffusion. The concentration of S at base II is lower than at base I.

Case 2

a) If both A and P are located at the base I, S is neither synthesized nor degraded at any inner point x. Since there is no diffusion flow of S in the steady state, the spatial distribution of S is homogeneous.

b) If both A and P are distributed homogeneously in the whole medium, then S is also distributed homogeneously because its synthesis and catabolism occur at the same place.

It clearly appears from this discussion that the gradient of S concentration, e.g. cyclic AMP, depends on the respective location of A, e.g. adenylate cyclase and P, e.g. phospho-diesterases. Whatever the structure of the cell, the distribution of cyclic AMP and consequently the distribution of the level of stimulation are homogeneous when the modulators are located at the same places (case 2 - a), b)). Thus, in the case of cyclic AMP the location of adenylate cyclase and of one phosphodiesterase with high affinity for cyclic AMP at the plasma membrane reduces the gradient of cyclic AMP resulting from the activity of cytosol phosphodiesterase. This fact even if it is not the justification of the location of one phosphodiesterase type, is nevertheless a consequence of this location.

Let us remark that the assumption of an homogeneous medium does not affect the interpretation of the results. Indeed, the cell is a highly structurated medium but this structure acts as a delay factor in the diffusional transport of the molecules. It is taken into account by considering a lower diffusion coefficient for cyclic AMP transport in the thyroid cell affects the kinetics of the system.

Some estimations of the apparent coefficient of diffusion D of molecules as nucleotides in the "cell water" have been made (20,21,22,23) : we can accept the values $10^{-7} cm^2/$ sec and $10^{-6} cm^2/sec$ as limits of possible D. Assuming that the distance between the basal and apical membranes is equal to $10^{-3}cm$, the characteristic diffusion time of a molecule of cyclic AMP in such a cell would lie between .5 sec and 5 sec. Thus a molecule of cyclic AMP can induce its effect at the apical membrane after a few seconds required for its transport between the two membranes. Since the time for the thyroid cell to reach the half-activated state is greater than 1 minute (24), the delay due to the trans-port of cyclic AMP should not appreciably affect the kinetics of activation.

The characteristics of the transmission by cyclic AMP thus ensures a rapid and uniform response of the whole system to the external stimulus. However, the consumption of ATP resulting from the cyclic AMP metabolism whatever the level of stimulation would be is higher if the source and the sink of cyclic AMP were located on the membrane.

Digital simulation of the transmission of the hormonal signal (e.g. cyclic AMP) in the thyroid cell has been performed on a Wang 2200 and CDC 6500 digital computers by using a stochastic method based on a generalisation of the one-dimension random walk (25,26). In this method the chemical reactions take place in a number of discrete channels in each of which the cyclic AMP concentration is assumed homogeneous; the random-walk of molecules between adjacent channels simulates diffusion. Thus diffusion process is considered as a one-dimension process since the thyroid cell has a cylindrical symmetry and we assume no radial concentration gradient. This is a consequence of the great number of receptors in the basal membrane and of the assumption of homogeneous medium.

Numerous data on the elements of the system (Table 2) have been obtained using results from our laboratory on thyroid studies (27) and from observations obtained using the liver (16, 18). The conclusions drawn from this simulation are very general and do not depend on the values used.

Figure 12 shows the influence of the localisation of the phosphodiesterase on the basal membrane. The homogeneity of the cyclic AMP distribution in the steady state may be characterised by the ratio:

$$R = \frac{B - A}{M}$$

where B, A and M are respectively the highest (basal membrane), the lowest (apical membrane) and the mean concentration of cyclic AMP. The relative range R which measured the heterogeneity of cyclic AMP distribution, is given for different cases in Table 3. It appears clearly that the presence of a membrane bound phosphodiesterase greatly minimizes the heterogeneity of cyclic AMP concentration around the mean concentration.

We have considered here the simplest hypothesis that the whole amount of cyclic AMP present in the cell participates in its action, especially in the activation of protein kinase. The concentrations of free cyclic AMP deduced from the stimulation must reflect the level of activation.

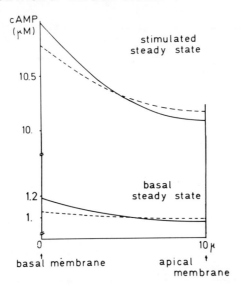

Figure 12. *Theoretical distribution of cyclic AMP in thyroid cell. It is assumed that the distance between the two membranes is equal to 10^{-3}cm and that the coefficient of diffusion D is equal to 10^{-7}cm^2/sec.*
(———) Unrealistic case : two soluble phosphodiesterases
*   Mean cyclic AMP levels : basal : $1.03\ 10^{-6}$M*
*   stimulated : $1.04\ 10^{-5}$M*

(– – –) Realistic case : one membrane bound phosphodiesterase
*   and one soluble phosphodiesterase*
*   Mean cyclic AMP levels : basal : $1.01\ 10^{-6}$M*
*   stimulated : $1.04\ 10^{-5}$M*
(Reprinted from Swillens et al. *(19))*

        The numerical simulation shows that the transport of cyclic AMP does not affect the rate of activation of the cell. Indeed, let δt^+ (δt^-) be the time needed for the transition from the unstimulated (stimulated) steady state to the half activated state for cyclic AMP. Without taking diffusion into account, the time transitions are equal to $\delta t^+ = 59$ sec and $\delta t^- = 45$ sec. If the "diffusion-reaction" coupled system were simulated, the time transitions do not vary significantly (about 1%) with $D = 10^{-7}$cm^2/sec.

TABLE 2. NUMERICAL VALUES OF PARAMETERS USED IN THE THEORETICAL SIMULATION

<u>Adenylate cyclase</u>	— basal activity = $2.8 \ 10^{-6}$M/min
	— stimulation factor by TSH = 4
<u>Phosphodiesterase I</u>	— (soluble enzyme)
	— $K_m = 4.10^{-5}$M
	— $V_m = 3.7 \ 10^{-5}$M/min
<u>Phosphodiesterase II</u>	— (membrane bound enzyme)
	— $K_m = 10^{-6}$M
	— $V_m = 3.7 \ 10^{-6}$M/min

The simulation also shows that for a given level of cyclic AMP concentration at the apex, adenylate cyclase activity is lower when one phosphodiesterase is bound at the basal membrane, i.e., to achieve a definite level of stimulation, is then more economical for the cell even though more cyclic AMP is hydrolyzed at the basal membrane. However, in terms of adenylate cyclase activity (i.e., ATP consumption) required to elicit a given stimulation, these advantages are small (about 1%).

If the enzymatic systems responsible for this synthesis and degradation of a metabolite have the same location in the cell, a more homogeneous distribution of this metabolite is ensured. In the case of the thyroid cyclic AMP system, digital simulation shows that the diffusion process is relatively fast and plays little role in the kinetics of cyclic AMP action in the cell.

CONCLUSION

In this paper, two elements of the cyclic AMP system were theoretically investigated. First, the study of the protein kinase mechanism allowed a comparison of two models of binding. It was emphasized that graphical representations of equilibrium data are valid only when the corresponding model applies. The misuse of these representations can lead to a wrong evaluation of the constants characterising the reaction. It has been shown that the so-called activation constant K_A of the kinase is not a constant since it depends on the total concentration of kinase :

TABLE 3. THEORETICAL SPATIAL DISTRIBUTION OF CYCLIC AMP IN THE THYROID CELL

$R = \dfrac{B - A}{M}$ where B, A and M are respectively the highest, the lowest and the mean concentrations of cyclic AMP

	Basal steady state		*Stimulated steady state*	
	10^{-6}	10^{-7}	10^{-6}	10^{-7}
— Realistic case (membrane bound + soluble phosphodiesterases)				
D (cm^2/sec)	10^{-6}	10^{-7}	10^{-6}	10^{-7}
R	.007	.073	.005	.060
— Unrealistic case (two soluble phosphodiesterases) (given for comparison)				
R	.023	.221	.009	.088

thus, the reported experimental low K_A does not require a hypothesis of compartmentalisation for cyclic AMP in the cell to
explain the regulatory role of the nucleotide. The use of
graphical representations such as Scatchard plot and "B^2/F vs B"
plot also allows one to reject a proposed model and to improve
the description of the system or the interpretation of experimental results.

Secondly, the theoretical simulation of the cyclic AMP
metabolism and diffusion shows that a consequence of the actual
localisation of adenylate cyclase and phosphodiesterases in the
cell is a higher intracellular homogeneity of the cyclic AMP
concentration and of the stimulation level of the cyclic AMP
dependent effects. Moreover, the diffusion of cyclic AMP in the
cell ensures a rapid intracellular transmission of the hormonal
stimulus.

REFERENCES

(1) LINEWEAVER, H., and BURK, D. (1934), J. Amer. Chem. Soc.,
     56, 65

(2) SCATCHARD, G., SCHEINBERG, I.H. and ARMSTRONG, S., (1950),
     J. Amer. Chem. Soc., 72, 535

(3) EXTON, J.H., LEWIS, S.B., HO, R.J., ROBISON, G.A. and
     PARK, C.R., (1971), Ann. N.Y. Acad. Sci., 185, 85

(4) LARNER, J. and VILLAR-PALASI, C., (1971), Curr. Top. Cell
     Reg., 3, 195

(5) DO KHAC, L., HARBON, S. and CLAUSER, H.J. (1973), Eur. J.
     Biochem., 40, 177

(6) MONTAGUE, W. and HOWELL, S.L. (1973), Biochem. J., 134, 321

(7) SODERLING, T.R., CORBIN, J.D., and PARK, C.R. (1973), J.
     Biol. Chem., 248, 1822

(8) SWILLENS, S., VAN CAUTER, E., and DUMONT, J.E. (1974),
     Biochem. Biophys. Acta, 364, 250

(9) SWILLENS, S. and DUMONT, J.E. (submitted for publication)

(10) BEAVO, J.A., BECHTEL, P.J. and KREBS, E.G. (1974), Proceed.
     Natl. Acad. Sci., 71, 3580

(11) GILMAN, A.G. (1970), Proceed. Natl. Acad. Sci. US, 67, 305

(12) SWILLENS, S. and DUMONT, J.E. (1975), Biochem. J., 149, 779

(13) APPLEMAN, M.M., THOMPSON, W.J. and RUSSELL, T.R. (1973)
     Advances in Cyclic Nucleotide Research, 3, 65

(14) MANGANIELLO, V. and VAUGHAN, M. (1973) J. Biol. Chem., 248,
     7164

(15) RUSSEL, T.R. and PASTAN, I (1973), J. Biol. Chem., 248, 5835

(16) RUSSEL, T.R., TERASAKI, W.L. and APPLEMAN, M.M. (1973), J.
     Biol. Chem., 248, 1334

(17) BOEYNAEMS, J.M., VAN SANDE, J., POCHET, R., and DUMONT, J.E.
     (1974) Mol. Cell Endocr., 1, 139

(18) SCHWARTZ, I.L., SHALTZ, L.J., KINNE SAFFRAN, E. and KINNE, R.
     (1974) Proceed. Natl. Acad. Sci. US, 71, 2595

(19) SWILLENS, S., PAIVA, M. and DUMONT, J.E. (1974) FEBS Letters,
     49, 92

(20) DICK, D.A.T. (1959), Exptl. Cell Res., 17, 5

(21) KUSHMERICK, M.J. and PODOLSKY, R.J. (1969), Science, 166,
     1297

(22) HOROWITZ, S.B. and MOORE, L.C. (1974), J. Cell Biol., 60,
     405

(23) FENICHEL, I.R. and HOROWITZ, S.B. (1963) Acta Physiol. Scand.
     60, suppl. 221

(24) VAN SANDE, J. and DUMONT, J.E. (1973) Biochim. Biophys. Acta,
     313, 320

(25) SWILLENS, S. and PAIVA, M., (1975), Simulation, 25, 33

(26) PAIVA, M. and PAIVA-VERETENNICOFF, I, (1972), Bull. Math.
     Biophys., 34, 457

(27) POCHET, R., BOEYNAEMS, J.M. and DUMONT, J.E. (1974), Biochem.
     Biophys. Res. Comm., 58, 446

(28) THOMPSON, J.W., LITTLE, S.A. and WILLIAMS, R.H. (1973),
     Biochemistry, 12, 1889

CONTROL OF METABOLIC PROCESSES BY cAMP-DEPENDENT PROTEIN PHOSPHORYLATION

Jackie D. Corbin, Thomas R. Soderling, Peter H. Sugden, Stanley L. Keely, and Charles R. Park

Department of Physiology, School of Medicine
Vanderbilt University, Nashville, Tennessee   37232

I. INTRODUCTION

Protein phosphorylation and dephosphorylation are catalyzed by protein kinases and phosphoprotein phosphatases according to the following general equation:

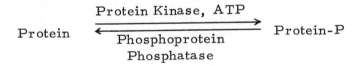

$$\text{Protein} \quad \xrightleftharpoons[\substack{\text{Phosphoprotein} \\ \text{Phosphatase}}]{\text{Protein Kinase, ATP}} \quad \text{Protein-P}$$

In mammalian tissues several types of protein kinases have been identified.   These include casein or phosvitin kinase, phosphory-lase kinase, and pyruvic dehydrogenase kinase (1). Since glycogen synthetase kinase (2, 3), phosphorylase kinase kinase (4), histone kinase (5), and lipase kinase (6, 7) are now believed to be the same protein kinase, and this enzyme is stimulated by or dependent on cAMP for activity, it is referred to as a cAMP-dependent protein kinase.   This enzyme has a widespread occurrence in various tis-sues and species (8) and is believed to be the mediator of many, if not all, of the effects of cAMP in mammalian tissues.   Enzymes which are physiological substrates for the cAMP-dependent protein kinase, e. g. , phosphorylase kinase, exhibit changes in enzymatic activity during phosphorylation or dephosphorylation.   There have been reports of in vitro phosphorylation of several other protein fractions in mammalian tissues catalyzed by cAMP-dependent protein kinases.   Some of the phosphorylatable proteins have been used as substrates for assay of enzyme activity (9). The physiological significance of phosphorylation of these substrates is not clear in all cases, however, because of the broad substrate specificity of this enzyme in vitro. More convincing proof of specificity could be provided if (A) the phosphorylation can be shown to be associated with enzyme activity or other changes; (B) phosphorylation occurs in intact cells and is stimulated by cAMP elevating agents; or (C) the ability of the substrate to be phosphorylated or activated in vitro is affected by hormonal treatment of intact animals or tissues.

A specific inhibitor of cAMP-dependent protein kinase exists in mammalian tissues (10). The physiological role of this small (MW = 26,000), heat-stable protein remains obscure. The protein inhibitor has been an important tool for investigating the protein kinases. In fact, studies using the inhibitor led to the discoveries of cAMP-dependent protein kinase mediation of phosphorylase kinase activation, glycogen synthetase inactivation, and hormone-sensitive lipase activation (3, 4, 6).

The cAMP-dependent protein kinases from several tissues and species have been shown to consist of a regulatory subunit (R), which binds cAMP, and a catalytic subunit (C), which catalyzes protein phosphorylation (11). When bound to C, the R subunit inhibits its catalytic activity. When cAMP binds to the R subunit of the holoenzyme, dissociation of the holoenzyme into its constituent R and C subunits occurs. The free C subunit catalyzes phosphorylation of the substrate proteins. These interactions are illustrated in the following general equation.

$$RC + cAMP \rightleftharpoons R \cdot cAMP + C \qquad [1]$$

It has recently been shown that a form of the protein kinase holoenzyme (RC) from beef heart (12) or from rabbit skeletal muscle (13) is a dimer. These enzymes are activated by cAMP according to equation 2.

$$R_2C_2 + 2\ cAMP \rightleftharpoons R_2 \cdot cAMP_2 + 2\ C \qquad [2]$$

As was discussed in a recent review (14) it is apparent from Eq. 1 or 2 that the degree of activation of the protein kinase by cAMP depends not only on the concentration of cAMP but also on the concentration of the protein kinase holoenzyme. If that is the case, the usual discrepancy between the low values for the apparent K_a of cAMP (10^{-9} to 10^{-7} M) determined using dilute preparations of the enzyme and the actual cellular cAMP level (10^{-7} to 10^{-6}

M) can be explained. The protein kinase concentration in mammalian cells is usually 10^{-7} to 10^{-6} M (14) and might require a relatively high concentration of cAMP for one-half maximum activation. From a similar approach and other theoretical considerations, essentially the same conclusions have been drawn by Swillens et al. (15). It was previously proposed that compartmentalization of cellular cAMP might explain the poor agreement between the cAMP concentration requirement of the isolated kinase and the cell concentration of cAMP (16). Although compartmentalization of cAMP cannot be ruled out, it is not necessary if the above considerations are applied.

A major fringe benefit of the discovery of the cAMP-dependent protein kinase is that since cAMP binds tightly to the R subunit, the holoenzyme can be used to assay the cyclic nucleotide. The binding assay of Gilman (17) is the most widely used of the assays that have been developed. Assays for cAMP utilizing enzyme activity changes have also been reported (18). In retrospect the original assay for cAMP of Sutherland and Rall (19) was based on stimulation of the phosphorylase kinase kinase (protein kinase) by cAMP in liver extracts.

II. HORMONAL EFFECTS ON cAMP-DEPENDENT PROTEIN KINASES IN INTACT TISSUES

The elucidation of both the protein kinase subunit composition and the mechanism of dissociation by cAMP (see Eq. 1 and 2) have made it possible to study the effects of hormones on the enzyme in intact tissues. The detailed methodology for performing such studies in rat adipose tissue was recently developed in our laboratory (20). The essential feature of the procedure involves stabilization of the position of the equilibrium shown in Eq. 1 during homogenization and preparation of the tissue for assay. Using the described procedures this laboratory reported an investigation of the effects of hormones on activation of the adipose tissue protein kinase (21). It was found that hormonal alteration of the tissue cAMP level caused a parallel change in protein kinase activation. Epinephrine-induced elevation of cAMP increased the fraction of the protein kinase present in the active free C subunit form (i.e., the protein kinase activity ratio increased) and insulin reduced the epinephrine effect on both cAMP and protein kinase.

In some instances, hormonal effects on the protein kinase and also on metabolic systems thought to be mediated by cAMP can be observed where no measurable change in the tissue level of cAMP can be detected (22). A possible explanation is that cAMP could be compartmentalized within the cell and that the "active pool" of cAMP is a small component of the total as discussed above. It is also possible that other mechanisms exist for hormonal control of the protein kinase. It should be pointed out that a small change in intracellular cAMP could be sufficient to elicit a large stimulation of protein kinase. This would especially be the case if cAMP has cooperative effects on the enzyme in the cell. The isolated kinase does show cooperativity with respect to cAMP as indicated by a Hill constant greater than one (23).

III. MULTIPLE FORMS OF cAMP DEPENDENT PROTEIN KINASE

Several forms of the cAMP-dependent protein kinase have been found in tissues (1). Although some of the forms could be products of proteolytic degradation or dissociation of subunits (24), it is clear that more than a single form of native protein kinase exists in several tissues (25). At least one form of the kinase from rabbit skeletal muscle (13) and from beef heart (12) have been purified essentially to homogeneity. The molecular weights of these enzymes are 160,000 and 174,000 for the muscle and heart enzymes, respectively. The stoichiometry of the subunit interactions are as depicted in Equation 2. The molecular weight of the R dimer from beef heart is 98,000, and that from rabbit skeletal muscle is 96,000. The C subunit, which probably dissociates from the R subunit as the monomer, has a molecular weight of approximately 40,000 for both the beef heart and rabbit skeletal muscle enzymes. The catalytic subunit is a globular protein but the regulatory subunit exhibits substantial asymmetry (12).

The procedure developed for determination of the state of activation of the protein kinase in intact rat adipose tissue was also applied for studies of immature rat testis (26). The procedure had to be modified, however, for similar studies in rat heart (25). As can be seen in Figure 1 rat heart contains predominantly a different type of cAMP-dependent protein kinase from that in adipose tissue. This type elutes from DEAE-cellulose columns at < 0.1 M NaCl. A second smaller fraction of cAMP-dependent heart enzyme elutes at > 0.1 M NaCl. The peak of activity which does not bind to the column was determined to be the cAMP-independent free C subunit. Only a trace of the total adipose tissue cAMP-dependent protein kinase elutes at < 0.1 M NaCl, the majority eluting in an asymmetric peak at > 0.1 M NaCl. The shoulder of activity in the main peak may correspond with the second peak of cAMP-dependent heart kinase. The rat liver protein kinase is the most complicated since at least three peaks of cAMP-dependent activity are resolved by the procedure. The two main liver peaks may correspond with the two peaks

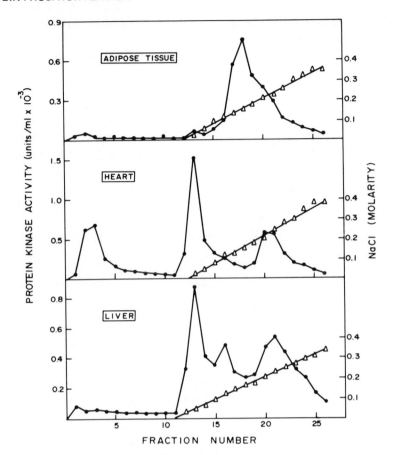

Fig. 1.   DEAE-cellulose chromatography of cAMP-dependent
protein kinase in crude extracts of rat adipose tissue, heart and
liver.   Homogenates of adipose tissue (2 ml/g), heart (4 ml/g)
and liver (4 ml/g) were prepared at 4° in 10 mM potassium phosphate, pH 6. 8, containing 1 mM EDTA and then centrifuged at
20, 000 x g for 45 min.   DEAE-cellulose (DE 11) columns (0. 9 x
4 cm) were equilibrated in the same buffer and 4 ml adipose tissue,
2 ml heart or 2 ml liver supernatant was applied.   The heart extract was always chromatographed as a control for adipose tissue
and liver at the same time on an identical column using the same
gradient flasks.   A tube led from the mixing flask to a Y-connector
which led to each of the two columns.   After washing each column
with ⌐50 mls of the above buffer, a linear gradient (0-0. 4 M) of
NaCl was started.   Each gradient flask contained 100 ml.   A 20 µl
aliquot of each fraction (⌐5ml) was assayed for protein kinase
(●——●) as described earlier (20) using histone as substrate.
Sodium ion (△—△) was measured by a Beckman cationic electrode.

of heart enzyme but there is also an intermediate peak of cAMP-dependent activity present.

The types of protein kinase from several rat tissues were recently studied in our laboratory in relation to the dissociation and reassociation of their corresponding R and C subunits (25). It was found that those enzymes which elute from DEAE-cellulose at < 0.1 M NaCl are more easily dissociated into subunits by treatment with high salt or histone than are those which elute at > 0.1 M NaCl. Furthermore, the dissociated subunits of the former type of kinase reassociate very slowly when compared with the latter type. An example of a dissociation experiment is shown in Table I. It can be seen that a five minute incubation in the presence of histone is sufficient to cause a substantial dissociation of the first peaks of cAMP-dependent protein kinase from rat heart or liver.

Table I. Dissociation of different types of cAMP-dependent protein kinase by histone

Rat Tissue Source	DEAE-Cellulose Protein Kinase Peak	Protein Kinase Activity Ratio	
		Preincubated without histone	Preincubated with histone
Adipose Tissue	1	0.15	0.22
Heart	1	0.07	0.69
	2	0.15	0.19
Liver	1	0.12	0.64
	2	0.18	0.53
	3	0.27	0.29

DEAE-cellulose chromatography of tissue extracts was performed as described in Fig. 1. The peaks of protein kinase from Fig. 1 used for the experiment were as follows: adipose tissue = fraction 18; heart = fraction 13 (peak 1) and fraction 21 (peak 2); liver = fraction 13 (peak 1), fraction 16 (peak 2); and fraction 21 (peak 3). The fractions were dialyzed 5-10 hours against three changes of 10 mM potassium phosphate (pH 6.8) containing 1 mM EDTA. To a 200 μl aliquot was added 10 μl H_2O or 15 mg/ml histone (Sigma Type II-A) for 5 min at 30°. Aliquots (20 μl) were then assayed for protein kinase in the presence and absence of 2 μM cAMP (substrate = histone) and the activity ratio was determined by dividing the activity in the absence to that in the presence of cAMP.

The adipose tissue kinase, the second peak of heart enzyme, and the third peak of liver enzyme are relatively stable to dissociation by histone. The intermediate type of liver kinase is partially dissociated by histone. The protein kinase types thus form a pattern in relation to their elution from DEAE-cellulose: the tighter the binding to DEAE-cellulose, the less dissociable are the protein kinases into R and C subunits.

Up to this point most of our studies have been done using the rat as a source of tissue. It is clear that there is tissue specificity in regard to the type(s) of kinase present. We have also found variations between species of animals. For example, rat and mouse hearts contain predominantly the holoenzyme form which elutes from DEAE-cellulose at < 0.1 M NaCl; whereas, rabbit and human hearts contain about equal amounts of the low and high salt-eluted forms. Beef heart contains almost entirely a form which elutes at > 0.1 M NaCl. Beef liver, in contrast to rat liver (see Fig. 1) contains primarily a form which elutes at > 0.1 M NaCl. As mentioned before, the type(s) of protein kinase present in tissues determines the conditions which are used to homogenize tissues and prepare extracts for assay after hormonal treatment. Before intact tissue studies are carried out it is important, therefore, to consider tissue and species variations in the types of kinase present.

Since the cAMP-dependent protein kinase consists of dissimilar subunits, it was of interest to determine whether the various types of kinase from rat adipose tissue, heart, and liver contain different R subunits, C subunits, or both. Since the R subunit dissociates from C in the presence of cAMP, the chromatographic behavior of each subunit can be studied if the holoenzyme is first incubated with cAMP. The R subunit can be assayed by [^{3}H] cAMP binding and the C subunit by catalytic activity. The free C subunit elutes in the flow-through volume if DEAE-cellulose chromatography of crude extracts of adipose tissue, heart, or liver is carried out following incubation with   1 mM cAMP (data not shown). This might be expected since the C subunit has a higher isoelectric point than the holoenzyme. The cAMP-binding protein profile from adipose tissue (Fig. 2, top panel) exhibits two main peaks of activity. The second peak predominates and probably corresponds to the R subunit composing the main holoenzyme form of adipose tissue shown in Fig. 1. At present the reason for the existence of a significant proportion of the cAMP-binding protein as a minor first peak is not clear. The cAMP-binding protein profile of heart (Fig. 2, middle panel) indicates two main peaks of activity also. The first peak predominates and probably corresponds with the R subunit composing the first peak of holoenzyme shown in Fig. 1. The second peak probably corresponds with

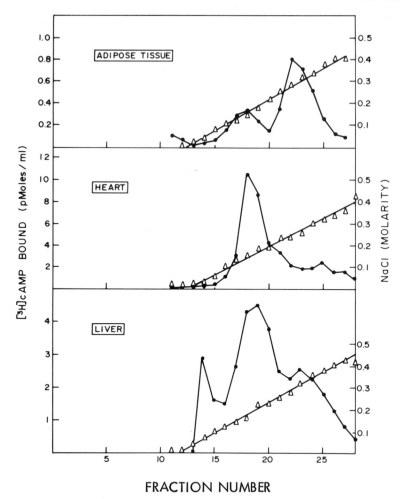

FRACTION NUMBER

Fig. 2. DEAE-cellulose chromatography of cAMP-dependent
protein kinase regulatory subunits of crude extracts of rat adipose
tissue, heart and liver. Cold cAMP was added to a final concentration of 1 mM for 60 min at 0° to supernatant fractions prepared
as described in Fig. 1. Chromatography was also performed as
described in Fig. 1. The cAMP binding protein (●——●) was deter
mined according to the method of Gilman (17) by incubating 100 μl
aliquots of the fractions at 30° with 100 μl of a solution containing
50 mM potassium phosphate (pH 6.8), 1 mM EDTA, 0.5 mg/ml
histone, 2 M NaCl, and 1 μM [^{3}H] cAMP (specific activity = 4.34
CPM per femtomole). The incubation time was 30 min. Sodium
ion (△——△) was determined as described in Fig. 1.

the R subunit of the second peak of holoenzyme of Fig. 1. Since
the first peak of heart R subunit elutes at the same salt concentration as the first peak of adipose tissue R, these R subunits could
be either very similar or identical. It may be recalled (see Fig. 1)
that the main adipose tissue holoenzyme elutes at a slightly lower
salt concentration than does the second peak of heart enzyme. This
appears to be the case also for the main adipose tissue R subunit,
which elutes from the column at a slightly lower salt concentration
than does the second peak of heart R subunit. These R subunits
are therefore not identical. As was the pattern for the liver holoenzyme (Fig. 1), the cAMP-binding protein profile of this tissue
extract is the most complicated as can be seen in Fig. 2 (bottom
panel). The liver profile is the most difficult to interpret, but there
is some resemblance in the salt elution of the second and third
cAMP-binding protein peaks from liver and the two peaks of heart
R subunit. The first peak of liver cAMP-binding protein, which
elutes at < 0.1 M NaCl, is probably not an R subunit. We have
studied extensively a protein from beef liver which elutes at a similar salt concentration. This protein binds adenosine and 5'-AMP
in addition to cAMP.

Although one cannot rule out the possibility that the free R subunits either dissociate into monomers or are hydrolyzed by proteolytic enzymes, it is clear that the profiles of the R subunits tend to
reflect the patterns of the respective holoenzymes on DEAE-cellulose columns, with the exception that the R subunits bind to the
column more tightly than the corresponding holoenzymes. It appears,
therefore that the different types of holoenzymes from rat adipose
tissue, heart and liver contain different types of R subunits. To
date, we have been unable to distinguish different types of C subunits
from these tissues. Since this subunit exhibits a net positive charge
at neutral pH, we have attempted separation of C subunit forms by
cation exchange chromatography. Phosphocellulose column profiles
of C are shown in Fig. 3. Only one peak of activity appears if either
adipose tissue, heart or liver are used as the source. There is no
significant difference in the profiles of the C subunit from these tissues. We have also detected no significant difference in the sedimentation behavior of the C subunits in sucrose density gradients
(data not shown). It would appear that the C subunits of the various
forms of holoenzyme from these three rat tissues are either very
similar or identical. This conclusion would be supported by the
lack of substrate specificity and other properties of the holoenzyme
which relate to catalytic activity (1). Since the holoenzymes contain
different R subunits, it would be more likely to find differences in
regulatory properties of the holoenzymes which relate to the R sub-

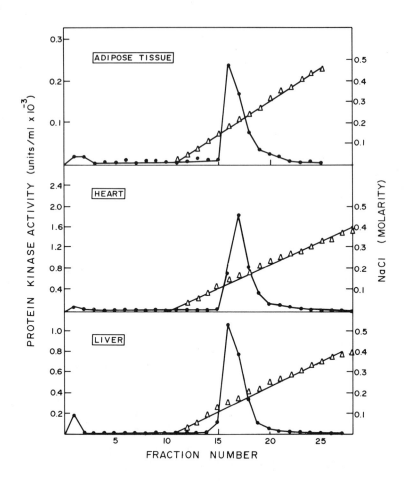

Fig. 3.   Phosphocellulose chromatography of the protein kinase
catalytic subunits of crude extracts of rat adipose tissue, heart
and liver.   Supernatant fractions of tissues were prepared as
described in Fig. 1 in 10 mM sodium phosphate (pH 6.5) containing 1 mM EDTA.   Cold cAMP was added to a final concentration
of 1 mM to 2 ml aliquots of each for 60 min at 0° and the samples
were applied to 0.9 x 4 cm phosphocellulose columns equilibrated
in the same buffer.   Chromatography and assay of protein kinase
(●— ●) were performed as described in Fig. 1 except for the
buffer used and the NaCl gradient (△ — △) was 0-0.5 M NaCl.

unit.   Some possible regulatory modifications of R will be discussed below.

It is also of interest that the forms of the R subunit which
bind to DEAE-cellulose columns more tightly also bind to the C
subunit with higher affinity.   This suggests that the difference in
net charge between the R and C subunits contributes significantly
to formation or stabilization of the RC complex.   This would explain why at neutral pH the form of the R subunit with the higher
net negative charge (binds tightly to DEAE-cellulose) binds more
tightly to a net positively charged C subunit.   It is not meant to
imply that net charge difference is the only attractive force between
R and C; there must also be specific bonds which link these two proteins.

Some of the reasons for the existence of multiple forms of
cAMP-dependent protein kinase can now be summarized.

1.   Isozymic forms.   The two peaks of rat heart enzyme (see
     Fig. 1) may be examples of protein kinase isozymes which
     differ in their R subunit composition.
2.   Subunit dissociation. R_2C_2, R_2C, and RC forms may exist.
3.   Proteolytic digestion.
4.   Phospho- and dephospho-forms (see discussion below).

IV.   EFFECTS OF MgATP

It has been reported that MgATP stimulates the reassociation
of the isolated R and C subunits of a form of protein kinase from
rabbit skeletal muscle (11).   Haddox, et al. have also reported that
MgATP increases the requirement of the protein kinase holoenzyme
for cAMP (27).   These authors demonstrated that MgATP binding
occurs in parallel with the effect of MgATP on the enzyme.   Bechtel
and Beavo found that two moles of MgATP are bound per holoenzyme,
but that no high affinity binding to the isolated R or C subunits occurs
(13).   We reported that concentrations of MgATP as low as 1 μM
prevent the salt or histone-induced dissociation of the first peak of
holoenzyme from rat heart (25).   This effect is observed in the
absence of cAMP.   The data are consistent with the hypothesis that
MgATP elicits a tighter binding of R to C.   Whether this occurs as
a result of MgATP binding to R or C, or by formation of a MgATP
bridge between the two subunits (13) remains to be established.

It is of interest that the MgATP effects discussed above were
all obtained using protein kinases which elute from DEAE-cellulose
columns at < 0.1 M NaCl.   Rosen, et al. reported that a purified
beef heart protein kinase will catalyze autophosphorylation (12).
The phosphate is incorporated into the R subunit of the enzyme and
causes the holoenzyme to become more dissociable by cAMP.   In

our hands the beef heart enzyme elutes from DEAE-cellulose at
> 0.1 M NaCl; therefore, the enzyme is a different type from those
for which MgATP binding studies have been done. In summary,
there appear to be at least three functions served by MgATP: [1]
a phosphate donor for phosphorylation of proteins other than the
kinase; [2] a phosphate donor for autophosphorylation of the R subunit, which produces a more dissociable RC complex and; [3] by
binding to the enzyme MgATP produces a less dissociable RC
complex. Whether or not all of these are separate functions requires further study. It will also be of interest to determine if the
various MgATP effects are regulatory and/or specific for different
isoenzymes of protein kinase.

V. TRANSLOCATION

We have reported (28) that when rat hearts are perfused with
high concentrations of epinephrine and methylxanthine, which nearly
completely activates the protein kinase, the total kinase activity in
the 12,000 x g supernatant fraction is reduced to about 50% of that
in controls. This reduction is probably due to preferential binding
of the free catalytic subunit to the 12,000 x g particulate fraction.
Jungmann, et al. (29) recently reported that elevation of the tissue
cAMP causes the translocation of the ovarian cytoplasmic R · cAMP
complex and C to nuclear acceptor sites. Korenman, et al. (30)
observed the translocation of the uterine cytoplasmic catalytic subunit of protein kinase to the microsomal fraction when cAMP was
elevated. According to Palmer, et al. (31) glucagon stimulation of
perfused rat livers causes an increase in a nuclear-associated
cAMP-independent protein kinase, presumably the catalytic subunit
of protein kinase. It should be pointed out that in the investigations
thus far there is little evidence for specificity of translocation of
the kinase subunits to particulate fractions of tissues. Since the C
protein exhibits a high isoelectric point it might be expected to bind
in a nonspecific manner to proteins or other compounds of opposite
charge. This may be the case in heart tissue since binding of C to
the particulate fraction of heart homogenates is not altered by boili:
or trypsin treatment but can be prevented or reversed by extractior
with 100 mM KCl. Furthermore, the hormone effect could be mim.
icked by adding cAMP to the homogenates. It will be necessary to
establish whether or not translocation is a specific physiological
event in tissues. One must bear in mind also the possibility that a
small fraction of the total C subunit binding to particulate fractions
of heart could be specific. Removal of the high background of the C
subunit bound nonspecifically to particulate fractions could be accor
plished by first treating with low salt media. This would allow for

studies of specific C subunit binding to a substrate or receptor.

VI. PHOSPHOPROTEIN PHOSPHATASES

Although a large volume of information is available concerning protein kinase(s), relatively little is known about the phosphoprotein phosphatase(s). Study of the phosphatases has been complicated by their instability during purification. Recently, study of these enzymes has increased following the suggestion that some effects of insulin may be mediated through them.

One of the most active areas of research on phosphoprotein phosphatases concerns their substrate specificity. As is the case for protein kinase, a single phosphatase might act on glycogen synthetase, phosphorylase kinase, hormone-sensitive lipase, and other enzymes. Zieve and Glinsmann (32) have observed that glycogen synthetase phosphatase and phosphorylase kinase phosphatase co-purify from skeletal muscle. Moreover, the phosphorylated forms of glycogen synthetase and phosphorylase kinase are competitive substrates for this phosphatase. Kato and Bishop (33) have demonstrated that highly purified muscle synthetase phosphatase can also utilize phosphohistone as substrate. Present evidence therefore suggests that a single phosphatase can act on glycogen synthetase, phosphorylase kinase, and histone.

There is confusion as to whether this same phosphatase also dephosphorylates phosphorylase, a protein which is not a substrate for the protein kinase. Riley, et al. (34), Villar-Palasi (35), and Kato and Bishop (32) have reported that phosphorylase is not a substrate for the skeletal muscle phosphatase which catalyzes dephosphorylation of either glycogen synthetase or phosphorylase kinase. On the other hand, Nakai and Thomas (36) have presented evidence suggesting that phosphorylase is a substrate for the heart phosphatase. Homogeneous liver phosphorylase phosphatase can also dephosphorylate glycogen synthetase (37).

It is apparent that much more work is required to resolve these questions of substrate specificity. These studies are complicated by the fact that several of the substrates contain both "specific" and "nonspecific" phosphorylation sites. "Nonspecific" phosphates are those that are not associated with changes in the enzyme activity. This situation has been well documented with phosphorylase kinase (38), and glycogen synthetase (39).

Many of the metabolic processes involving protein phosphorylation-dephosphorylation are under hormonal regulation. One of the actions of insulin in many tissues is to promote conversion of glycogen synthetase from the D form to the more active I form. As is evident from equation 3 a net increase in synthetase I could result from either

$$\text{Synthetase I} \xrightleftharpoons[\text{Phosphoprotein Phosphatase}]{\begin{array}{c}\text{protein kinase}\\ \text{cAMP, Mg}^{++}\text{, ATP}\end{array}} \text{Synthetase D} \qquad [3]$$

inactivation of protein kinase or from activation of the phosphatase. Inactivation of protein kinase by insulin has been demonstrated under certain conditions as discussed earlier. Activation of phosphoprotein phosphatase in liver by insulin has been observed. Gold (40) found that alloxan diabetes results in a loss of activity of this enzyme which can be restored by insulin treatment. Bishop (41) has observed that infusion of insulin-plus-glucose into pancreatectomized dogs maintained with insulin produces a rapid increase in phosphatase activity.

VII.   ACKNOWLEDGEMENTS
This work was supported in part by Program Project Grant AM 07462 and Grant 15988 from the National Institutes of Health and by Diabetes-Endocrinology Center Grant P17 17026. One investigator, J. D. C. , is an investigator of the Howard Hughes Medical Institute; S. L. K. is a postdoctoral fellow of the Middle Tennessee Heart Association; and P. H. S. is a N. A. T. O. postdoctoral fellow of the United Kingdom Science Research Council. T. R. S. has been the recipient of a Research and Development Award from the American Diabetes Association. We are grateful to Ms. Maureen McRedmond for excellent technical assistance and to Mr. Lewe West for developing the cAMP-binding assay.

VIII.   REFERENCES
1.   Krebs, E. G. (1972) Curr. Top. Cell. Regul. 5, 99-133

2.   Friedman, D. L. , and Larner, J. (1965) Biochemistry 4, 2261-2264

3.   Soderling, T. R. , Hickenbottom, J. P. , Reimann, E. M. , Hunkeler, F. L. , Walsh, D. A. , and Krebs, E. G. (1970) J. Biol. Chem. 245, 6317-6328

4.   Walsh, D. A. , Perkins, J. P. , and Krebs, E. G. (1968) J. Biol. Chem. 243, 3763-3765

5.   Langan, T. A. (1968) Science 162, 579-580

6.   Corbin, J. D. , Reimann, E. M. , Walsh, D. A. , and Krebs, E. G. (1970) J. Biol. Chem. 245, 4849-4851

7. Huttunen, J. K. , Steinberg, D. , and Mayer, S. E.   (1970)
    Proc. Natl. Acad. Sci. U.S.   67, 290-295

8. Kuo, J. F. , and Greengard, P.   (1969) Proc. Natl. Acad.
    Sci. U.S.   64, 1349-1355

9. Corbin, J. D. , and Reimann, E. M.   (1974) Methods Enzymol.
    38, 287-290

10. Ashby, C. D. , and Walsh, D. A.   (1973) J. Biol. Chem. 248,
    1255-1261

11. Brostrom, C. O. , Corbin, J. D. , King, C. A. , and Krebs,
    E. G. (1971) Proc. Natl. Acad. Sci. U.S.   68, 2444-2447

12. Rosen, O. M. , Rubin, C. S. , and Erlichman, J.   (1973)
    Proc. Miami Winter Symp.   5, 67-82

13. Bechtel, P. J. and Beavo, J. A.   (1974) Fed. Proc.   33, 786

14. Soderling, T. R. , and Park, C. R.   (1974) Adv. Cyclic Nucleo-
    tide Res.   4, 283-333

15. Swillens, S. , Van Cauter, E. , and Dumont, J. E.   (1974)
    Biochem. Biophys. Acta 364, 250-259

16. Butcher, R. W. , Sneyd, J. G. T. , Park, C. R. , and Sutherland,
    E. W. (1966) J. Biol. Chem.   241, 1652-1653

17. Gilman, A. G. (1970) Proc. Natl. Acad. Sci. U.S.   67, 305-
    312

18. Wastila, W. B. , Stull, J. T. , Mayer, S. E. , and Walsh, D. A.
    (1971) J. Biol. Chem.   246, 1996-2003

19. Sutherland, E. W. , and Rall, T. W.   (1958) J. Biol. Chem.
    232, 1077-1091

20. Corbin, J. D. , Soderling, T. R. , and Park, C. R.   (1973)
    J. Biol. Chem.   248, 1813-1821

21. Soderling, T. R. , Corbin, J. D. , and Park, C. R.   (1973)
    J. Biol. Chem.   248, 1822-1829

22. Corbin, J. D. , Keely, S. L. , Soderling, T. R. , and Park, C. R. (1975) Adv. Cyclic Nucleotide Res. 5, 265-279

23. Reimann, E. M. , Walsh, D. A. , and Krebs, E. G. (1971) J. Biol. Chem. 246, 1986-1995

24. Corbin, J. D. , Brostrom, C. O. , King, C. A. , and Krebs, E. G. (1972) J. Biol. Chem. 247, 7790-7797

25. Corbin, J. D. , Keely, S. L. , and Park, C. R. (1974) J. Biol. Chem. 250, 218-225

26. Means, A. R. , MacDougall, E. , Soderling, T. R. , and Corbin, J. D. (1974) J. Biol. Chem. 249, 1231-1237

27. Haddox, M. K. , Newton, N. E. , Hartle, D. K. , and Goldberg, N. D. (1972) Biochem. Biophys. Res. Commun. 47, 653-661

28. Keely, S. L. , Corbin, J. D. , and Park, C. R. (1975) Proc. Natl. Acad. Sci. U. S. 72, 1501-1504

29. Jungmann, R. A. , Hiestand, P. C. , and Schweppe, J. S. (1974) Endocrinology 94, 168-183

30. Korenman, S. G. , Bhalla, R. C. , Sanborn, B. M. , and Stevens, R. H. (1974) Science 183, 430-432

31. Palmer, W. K. , Castagna, M. , and Walsh, D. A. (1974) Biochem. J. 143, 469-471

32. Zieve, F. J. , and Glinsmann, W. H. (1973) Biochem. Biophys. Res. Commun. 50, 872-878

33. Kato, K. , and Bishop, J. S. (1972) J. Biol. Chem. 247, 7420-7429

34. Riley, W. D. , DeLange, R. J. , Bratvold, G. E. , and Krebs, E. G. (1968) J. Biol. Chem. 243, 2209-2215

35. Villar-Palasi, C. (1969) Ann. N. Y. Acad. Sci. 166, 719-730

36. Nakai, C. , and Thomas, J. A. (1973) Biochem. Biophys. Res. Commun. 52, 530-536

37. Killilea, S. D. , Brandt, H. , Lee, E. Y. C. and Whelan, W. F.
     (1974) <u>Fed. Proc.</u> 33, 1431

38. Hayakawa, T. , Perkins, J. P. , and Krebs, E. G. (1973)
     <u>Biochemistry</u> 12, 574-579

39. Soderling, T. R. (1975) <u>J. Biol. Chem.</u> , in press

40. Gold, A. H. (1970) <u>J. Biol. Chem.</u> 245, 903-906

41. Bishop, J. S. (1970) <u>Biochim. Biophys. Acta</u> 208, 208-218

CYCLIC AMP AND CYCLIC GMP BINDING IN TISSUES

Simone Harbon
Lien Do Khac

Institut de Biochimie
Université de Paris-Sud
91405 Orsay (France)

Contents

INTRODUCTION

In an attempt to characterize the initial molecular events, after generation of cyclic AMP, experiments were performed which revealed the presence of intracellular sites, capable of binding cyclic AMP (1, 2). These cyclic AMP binding fractions were considered to be involved in the action of the cyclic nucleotide. Then, following the first discovery by Walsh *et al.* (3) that certain protein kinases could be directly activated by cyclic AMP, Kuo and Greengard (4), using histone as substrate, established that cyclic

----

Figures 1 to 6 and Table IV to VI are reproduced by permission of the European Journal of Biochemistry.

AMP dependent protein kinases are widely distributed in animal
tissues and postulated that all cyclic AMP activities could be
mediated through regulation of these protein kinases.

Molecular interrelationships between the cyclic AMP binding
proteins and the cyclic AMP dependent protein kinases became evident : both activities appeared to be enriched in parallel through
all purification steps, except in the presence of cyclic AMP where
they could be physically separated. The mechanism of activation of
the protein kinases by cyclic AMP has been proposed concurrently by
Tao *et al*. (5) with the reticulocyte protein kinases, Gill and Garren
(6) with adrenal gland protein kinase, and then found to be applicable with protein kinases of other sources (7 - 10) : cyclic AMP
dependent protein kinases are composed of two dissimilar subunits,
a regulator (R) and a catalytic (C) subunit. Cyclic AMP regulates
the enzyme activity by binding to the regulatory unit, with the concomittant release of the free catalytic subunit for enzyme activity.

This activation by cyclic AMP has been expressed by Brostrom
et al. (11) according to the following equation :

$$\{R.C\} + \text{cyclic AMP} \rightleftharpoons R\text{-cyclic AMP} + C$$

(inactive holoenzyme)   (active)

C, the catalytically active kinase subunit, is cyclic AMP independent
and does not bind cyclic AMP. R is invariably referred to as the
cyclic AMP binding protein, regulatory subunit, or cyclic AMP receptor protein; R exhibits two activities, *viz*. it binds cyclic AMP, and
if added to the isolated C, in the absence of cyclic AMP, it sup-
presses its activity and restores cyclic AMP responsiveness.

At least in animal cells, it appears that the only structure
found up to the present time that is capable of binding cyclic AMP
is the R subunit associated with the protein kinase. No evidence for
the existence of other binding structures has ever been obtained.

In this article, discussion will first concern some general aspects of cyclic nucleotide binding to receptors, with particular emphasis on evidence from the literature which may be of some
importance in understanding the mechanism of action of cyclic AMP
and more recently that of cyclic GMP. It is not, however, an exhaustive bibliography in this area. Finally, some recent experiments (12) from our own work, essentially performed with rat diaphragm, will be discussed. Evidence is presented that the hormonal
effect can promote changes in the degree of saturation of the intracellular receptor by cyclic AMP, which occur subsequent to hormone-
induced variations in cyclic AMP concentration. The data obtained

demonstrate that in the intact cell correlations could be established between the level of intracellular cyclic AMP and the extent to which it is bound to its specific receptor protein under well-defined physiological conditions.

CHARACTERISTICS OF THE CYCLIC AMP BINDING SYSTEM

General Properties of the Binding Reaction

Measurement of cyclic AMP binding activity. The assay for cyclic AMP binding includes two different steps *viz.* incubation of the protein fractions in the presence of ^{3}H-cyclic AMP under conditions which allow maximal binding of the cyclic nucleotide, followed by a suitable technique for the separation of the protein bound cyclic AMP from the free (unbound) ligand.

The conditions most commonly employed for the binding reaction are those first described by Gilman (13) : incubation is performed at 0° at pH 4.0, in the presence of ^{3}H-cyclic AMP at saturating concentrations, which vary from 30 nM - 200 nM according to the source of the binding protein. Binding equilibrium under these conditions, is usually attained within 60 minutes. Some minor modifications are sometimes made : binding reaction being performed at pH 5.0 (10) or at the more physiological pH 7-7.5 (12, 14-18); with buffer at pH 7.0, 6-8 mM theophylline is usually present so as to prevent any contaminating phosphodiesterase activity. Binding of cyclic AMP can also be carried out at 30° (15, 19) and in this case, the reaction is complete within 5 to 10 minutes. Reactions are usually initiated by the addition of the binding protein preparation, and depending on the purification stage, this may represent from 2-200 μg of protein, the final volume of the reaction mixture, varying from 50-250 μl. In all cases, the solutions are kept at 0°, at the end of the incubation.

A rapid and quantitative separation of protein bound cyclic AMP from the free cyclic nucleotide is accomplished by the use of cellulose ester Millipore filters (0.45 μ) which have been found to have an affinity for the cyclic AMP binding protein (13, 14) : at the end of the binding reaction, the chilled mixture is diluted (5-10 fold) with cold buffer (phosphate pH 6.0 or Tris HCl pH 7.0) containing 20 mM MgCl$_2$, and passed through filters which have been previously rinsed with the same buffer. The filter is immediately washed 2-3 times with 5-10 ml of the cold buffer and placed in a counting vial for determination of radioactivity. This simple method forms the basis of the sensitive assay developed for the determination of cyclic AMP levels in various tissues (13, 14, 20).

Binding of cyclic AMP has also been determined using equilibrium dialysis (1, 21) : protein solution was dialyzed against a large volume of buffer containing ^{3}H-cyclic AMP for 16 hours at 4°. In some instances, gel filtration through Sephadex G 50 proved satisfactory in separating free from protein bound cyclic AMP (11, 22). Brown *et al.* (23) have demonstrated that activated charcoal (Norit GS X) may sufficiently differentiate free from bound cyclic AMP. The cyclic nucleotide-protein complex remain in solution whereas the free cyclic AMP is quantitatively adsorbed by the charcoal. This method enabled these authors to design an assay system for cyclic AMP (23, and article by Brown *et al.* these proceedings).

Stability of the ^{3}H-cyclic AMP-receptor complex. The early report by Gilman (13) that the complex formed between ^{3}H-cyclic AMP and its binding protein was extremely stable and poorly dissociable at 0° (5 % decline in the bound radioactivity per hour), has also been confirmed by Odea *et al.* (17) for bovine skeletal muscle protein kinase preparations. Walton and Garren (14) also noticed with adrenal cortex binding protein that the binding once established was poorly reversible : after 96 hours of dialysis against buffer alone, only 25 % of bound cyclic AMP was reported to be released. ^{3}H-cyclic AMP bound to its receptor could be released when enzyme preparations are denatured by heat, urea, 0.1 N NaOH, 5 % TCA or 32 % ethanol, and in all these cases the released radioactivity has always been identified as authentic cyclic AMP.

Optimum pH and binding constant[x]. (See review by Swillens *et al.*, these proceedings). The effect of pH on the binding is critical : for skeletal muscle preparation the highest affinity was at pH 4.0 in acetate buffer. Gilman (13) reported a binding constant for cyclic AMP of 2-3 nM at pH 4.0 at 0°, while the value at pH 6.0 was 10-20 nM, which is very similar to the binding constant found by Walsh *et al.* (22) at the same pH. These binding constants are very comparable to those described for protein kinases of different sources, as well as for the membrane bound erythrocyte enzyme (10, 14, 24) (Table I). With the endometrial enzyme the binding constant measured at 20° was 40 nM, compared to 60 nM at 0°; however, the number of binding sites/mg protein did not change with the temperature.

---

[x]Apparent binding constant (Kd) is usually referred to the concentration of cyclic AMP needed to half saturate total binding sites, under the experimental conditions.

TABLE I : Cyclic AMP Binding Constants (nM)

pH	4.0	5.0	6.0	7.0
Skeletal Muscle	3		($_{18}^{15}$	
Adrenals				13
Uterus		($_{40(20°)}^{60}$		
Heart				22
Erytrocytes				3.3

Data from Gilman (13), Walsh et al. (22), Walton and Garren (14), Sanborn et al. (10), Rosen et al. (24).

Specificity of the binding reaction. When a variety of nucleotides were added to the binding reaction mixture in order to test
their ability to compete with cyclic AMP for the binding sites (10,
13, 14, 23) it appeared that unlabelled cyclic AMP effectively com-
peted with the labelled form and that the other nucleotides which
inhibited the binding, though less effectively were the 3',5' cyclic
nucleotides in the following order of potency I > G > U > C. Cyclic
GMP at a concentration 100-fold greater than that of cyclic AMP inhibited ^{3}H-cyclic AMP binding by 30-40 %. The 2',3', cyclic nucleotides did not appear to cross react significantly with the binding
system. Other nucleotides did not interfere unless at a concentration of 1 mM and had no effect at 0.1 mM. At 1 mM, UTP, CTP, 5'AMP,
ADP did not inhibit more than 20 % while adenosine and theophylline
had no effect. The specific effect of MgATP will be discussed
below.

Factors which influence the binding reaction.

- *Effect of the heat stable protein kinase inhibitor (I).*Walsh *et
al.* (22) examined the effect of the inhibitor on the binding of
cyclic AMP to a partially purified preparation of skeletal muscle
protein kinase. The binding constant for cyclic AMP was found to
be decreased 5-fold in the presence of the inhibitor; changing
from 14 nM in the absence of I to 2.8 nM in its presence. Although

the binding of cyclic AMP to the receptor protein was increased in
the presence of I, for all the concentrations of the cyclic nucleotide examined, there was almost no difference in the maximal cyclic
AMP binding. These observations were also mentioned by Gilman (13)
who noticed not only an increase in affinity of the binding protein
for cyclic AMP but also a greater stability of the cyclic AMP-
receptor complex in the presence of I.

     Some aspects of the mechanism of action of I has been studied
by Ashby and Walsh (25) and will be discussed later.

- *Effect of ATP (Mg^{2+})*. Evidence has been presented by Haddox *et*
al. (26) that binding of cyclic AMP to its receptor may be influenced by ATP : exposure of skeletal muscle protein kinase to μmolar
concentration of ATP in the presence of Mg^{2+} before initiating the
binding reaction, inhibited the binding of ^{3}H-cyclic AMP (1-10 nM)
and increased the Kd value from 20 nM to 200 nM. 50 % inhibition
of cyclic AMP binding (10 nM) occurred at approximately 200 nM ATP,
a concentration which also induced impairment of the kinase activation by cyclic AMP. Binding of ATP to the protein kinase has
been found to take place and to parallel its inhibitory effect.
Similarly Beavo *et al*. (57) reported in the case of purified
skeletal muscle protein kinase that the dissociation constant for
cyclic AMP was nearly 50-fold higher in the presence of 4 mM MgATP,
while maximal binding was not affected.

          Subcellular distribution of cyclic AMP binding activity

     Substantial quantities of cyclic AMP binding protein appear to
be present in the cytosol of all cellular homogenates which exhibit
cyclic AMP binding activity. However, subcellular localization of
the binding subunit has been highly variable, but in all cases, both
protein kinase and binding activities follow the same distribution
pattern.

     In some instances, such as the uterus (10), mammary glands (27),
skeletal muscle (3), liver (28), heart (24), diaphragm (12) about
90 % of the cyclic AMP binding activity is located almost exclusively
in the cytosol soluble fractions. In contrast, in the adrenal cortex
(1, 29) cyclic AMP receptor protein is found in both the cytosol and
endoplasmic reticulum, and in human erythrocytes (30), about 70 %
of the binding activity is bound to the cell membrane. Cyclic AMP
binding has also been demonstrated in liver microsomes (21), rabbit
reticulocyte ribosomes (31) and nuclei (32), but these activities
represented only a small percentage of the total cyclic AMP binding
activity which was present mainly in the cytosol.

In many other tissues, protein kinase activity itself and its responsiveness to cyclic AMP has been the main parameter examined in different subcellular fractions. In these cases, activation by cyclic AMP has been considered as an evidence for the presence of cyclic AMP binding protein in the fractions under investigation : in brain (33) and the anterior pituitary (34) cyclic AMP dependent protein kinases were located in particulate fractions and could be released by detergents; however, 50 % of this activity was still found in the cytosol.

In general, highly purified preparations of protein kinases from which the regulatory subunits have been derived, were prepared from the cytosol fractions.

Preparation of Cyclic Binding Fractions (R) Free
from Catalytic Kinase Activity

Initially the most commonly used method for preparing regulatory subunits was based on the property of cyclic AMP to dissociate the holoenzyme into regulatory (R) and C active subunits; various attempts were then made to physically separate the two functionally distinct subunits. Partial but not complete separations have been obtained using sucrose gradient analyses, with protein kinases isolated from red blood cells (5) and adrenal glands (6). In the latter case, satisfactory separation was further obtained by electrophoresis on polyacrylamide gels (35).

Substrate affinity chromatography. With rabbit muscle protein kinase, Reimann *et al.* (8) described the separation and isolation of regulatory and catalytic subunits using a casein Sepharose 4B column in the presence of cyclic AMP : the protein kinase was first incubated with ^{3}H-cyclic AMP at 0° before application to the column which was then washed with buffer containing ^{3}H-cyclic AMP and developed using NaCl gradient. Under these conditions all the cyclic AMP binding fractions devoid of catalytic activity, were recovered as a R-^{3}H-cyclic AMP complex which passed through the column while the kinase activity was retained, could be eluted with 0.15 M NaCl and was completely cyclic AMP independent. When the cyclic AMP dependent protein kinase from adipose tissue was applied under the same conditions to the casein sepharose column, dissociation also occurred with the concomittant separation of the cyclic AMP independent or C subunit; however, attempts to demonstrate the presence of the cyclic AMP receptor protein (R) have been unsuccessful. This result was interpreted by Corbin *et al.* (36) as being due to instability of R subunit in this enzyme. On the other hand, separation of the cyclic AMP receptor protein from endometrial protein kinase, in the form of a binding protein cyclic

AMP complex has been obtained by Sanborn *et al.* (10), using a casein Sepharose 4B column.

Affinity chromatography on columns containing covalently bound protamine (enzite CM-cellulose protamine) has been used by Miyamoto *et al.* (37) to separately obtain (R) and (C) from brain protein kinases.

Dissociation of protein kinase by substrates. Regulatory subunit free of bound cyclic AMP was prepared from brain protein kinase by taking advantage of the ability of histone to cause dissociation of the enzyme into its subunits : preincubation of the enzyme at 30° for 10 minutes in the presence of histone was followed by a chromatography on hydroxylapatite which resulted in the separation of a cyclic AMP binding protein, which retained the binding activity but showed insignificant catalytic protein kinase activity (37, 38).

Tao (39) and Tao and Hachet (40) also described the dissociation of rabbit erythrocyte cyclic AMP dependent protein kinase by protamine (but not histone) into a cyclic AMP independent C unit which can be separated by sucrose gradient centrifugation. In this case, no cyclic AMP binding protein activity could be detected unless cyclic AMP was included in the gradient : the presence of cyclic AMP apparently enhanced the stability of the R unit which, under these conditions, was isolated as a heavy R-cyclic AMP protamine complex.

DEAE-cyclic AMP procedure. Cyclic AMP receptor subunit free of bound cyclic AMP has been purified from bovine heart protein kinase according to Erlichman *et al.* (9) and Rubin *et al.* (16) : purified protein kinase was applied to the DEAE cellulose column equilibrated in 0.05 M potassium phosphate : the C subunit could be eluted with the buffer containing 10^{-5}M cyclic AMP, residual free cyclic AMP was washed from the resin with 0.12 M potassium phosphate buffer and the cyclic AMP binding protein eluted with buffer of increasing molarity up to 0.25 M. This DEAE-cyclic AMP procedure has been slightly modified by Sanborn *et al.* (10) for the isolation of cyclic AMP binding protein from endometrial protein kinase.

Affinity chromatography with immobilized cyclic AMP. In a recent publication Ramseyer *et al.* (41) described the purification of the cyclic AMP receptor protein, from bovine adrenal cortices and porcine skeletal muscle, using 8-(6-aminohexyl) amino-adenosine 3',5'-monophosphate coupled to sepharose as an affinity chromatography medium. The specific retention of the receptor protein by immobilized cyclic AMP resulted in separation of the subunits and passage of the catalytic kinase subunit; the receptor protein

could then be eluted with 7 M urea. Binding activity was inhibited
by urea but this inhibition was reversed upon removal of urea by
dialysis or dilution, resulting in recovery of full receptor activity. Using an almost identical immobilized cyclic AMP sepharose
column, Jergil *et al.* (42) while succeeding in activating protein
kinase from trout testis, could not recover any cyclic AMP receptor protein. However, in this case elution with urea was not used.
Furthermore, Wilchek *et al.* (43) reported previously the use of N^6-
caproyl cyclic AMP sepharose as an affinity column which activated
protein kinases from skeletal muscle and parotid preparations, but
from which recovery of cyclic AMP receptor protein could not be
achieved.

Reverse Reaction – Dissociation of ^{3}H–Cyclic AMP

from ^{3}H–Cyclic AMP Protein Complex

     As already mentioned, cyclic AMP bound to the protein kinase
could not be easily liberated at 0°. Dissociation of the cyclic
nucleotide from the protein complex could however be studied in
the presence of large excess of unlabelled cyclic AMP. This type
of exchange reaction has been carried out with ^{3}H–cyclic AMP bound
to the protein kinase complex, (*i.e.* in the simultaneous presence
of R–^{3}H–cyclic AMP and C subunits) or with purified R–^{3}H–cyclic
AMP.

     Dissociation of ^{3}H–cyclic AMP from the protein kinase complex.
Table II summarizes the results, adapted from different publications,
of a series of experiments which were aimed at determining the rate
of cyclic AMP dissociation from its binding protein, using protein
kinase preparations from various sources. Binding was first
allowed to take place at 0° in the presence of ^{3}H–cyclic AMP (10–
30 nM), a 100–fold or more excess unlabelled cyclic AMP was then
added, and after further incubations for different times, the dissociation reaction was stopped by isolating the cyclic AMP receptor
protein on Millipore filters. As was first noticed by Gilman (13)
and subsequently confirmed by others (10, 14, 17), the reverse
reaction is very slow at 0°, and usually there is an initial rapid
rate of cyclic AMP dissociation which is followed by a secondary
rate. Dissociation is highly temperature dependent, the rate of
dissociation increasing progressively from 0° to 37° with a half
time varying from 7 to 20 hours at 0° but which is approximately
2.5 – 3.5 minutes at 37°.

     While Mg^{2+} had little effect on the binding constant at pH
4.0, it increased the rate of dissociation of ^{3}H–cyclic AMP bound
to protein kinase (13).

TABLE II : Dissociation of ^{3}H-Cyclic AMP-Protein Complex
$(t(\frac{1}{2}))$.

Temperatures		$0°$	$10°$	$20°$	$30°$	$37°$	pH
			hours		minutes		
Skeletal Muscle	(a)	7					4.0
− holoenzyme							
	(b)			0.5	10	<3	7.5
Endometrium	(c)						
− holoenzyme		20	10	2.8			5.0
− R-^{3}H-cyclic AMP		19	5.8	1.9			
Adrenal	(d)						
− R-^{3}H-cyclic AMP						2.5	7.0

Data from (a) Gilman (13), (b) O'Dea et al. (17), (c) Sanborn et al. (10), (d) Gill et al. (44).

Wilchek *et al.* (43) discussed the role of both ATP and Mg^{2+} in the dissociation of ^{3}H-cyclic AMP bound to a supernatant extract of rat parotid and to a partially purified preparation of rabbit skeletal muscle protein kinase. In both cases the exchange reaction was very slow at pH 7.5 even at 30° unless ATP + Mg^{2+} were present in the reaction mixture. Under the latter conditions, ^{3}H-cyclic AMP bound to muscle protein kinase was almost completely exchanged within 10 minutes incubation. This effect of ATP and Mg^{2+} had also been described for the dissociation of ^{3}H-cyclic AMP bound to soluble diaphragm extract proteins (12).

Liberation of ^{3}H-cyclic AMP from purified R-^{3}H-cyclic AMP. It is evident from the experiments of Brostrom *et al.* (11) that in the absence of any catalytic subunit, the binding of cyclic AMP to the purified R-cyclic AMP complex from skeletal muscle, was completely irreversible. Unlabelled cyclic AMP did not exchange with ^{3}H-cyclic AMP bound to the receptor and only prolonged dialysis of R-^{3}H-cyclic AMP complex against Norit, removed any substantial amount of ^{3}H-cyclic AMP. However, this treatment was accompanied by denaturation of the cyclic AMP receptor.

It is possible that cyclic AMP is bound particularly tightly to the R subunit of the skeletal muscle, compared with that prepared from liver (19), heart (9) or endometrium (10), since these regulatory subunits isolated after protein kinase dissociation with unlabelled cyclic AMP can still bind ^{3}H-cyclic AMP. There is of course no evidence that even in these cases, complete removal of unlabelled cyclic AMP took place. However, results presented in Table II show that ^{3}H-cyclic AMP bound to endrometrial protein kinase, or its isolated R subunit, can dissociate at almost identical rate in the presence of unlabelled cyclic AMP. Under these conditions, ^{3}H-cyclic AMP bound to the purified adrenal receptor protein, free of catalytic kinase activity, could readily exchange with the unlabelled cyclic nucleotide (44).

Effect of the catalytic subunit and protein kinase inhibitor on the liberation of ^{3}H-cyclic AMP from R-^{3}H-cyclic AMP of skeletal muscle. The experiments of Brostrom *et al.* (11) have further demonstrated that with R-^{3}H-cyclic AMP from skeletal muscle, addition of adequate concentrations of C subunit, in the presence of ATP and Mg^2, resulted in an almost complete release reaction (measured by Sephadex G25 gel filtration which separated free from protein bound cyclic AMP). It is interesting to note from the experiments of Ashby and Walsh (25) that prior addition of protein kinase inhibitor (I) to catalytic (C) subunit prevented the promoted release of ^{3}H-cyclic AMP from R-^{3}H-cyclic AMP. The concentration of C in this latter case induced 40 % release in the absence of I (Table III).

TABLE III : Release of ^{3}H-Cyclic AMP from the Isolated R-^{3}H-Cyclic AMP Complex of Skeletal Muscle. Effect of the Catalytic Subunit (C) and the Protein Kinase Inhibitor (I)

	Addition		cpm released	Conditions
	(C)	(I)	%	
(a)	−		3	30°, 5 min.
	+		88	
(b)	−	−	2	
	+	−	40	30°, 7 min.
	−	+	2	
	+	+	2.5	

Data from (a) Brostrom et al. (11), (b) Ashby and Walsh (25).

Purified R-^{3}H-cyclic AMP complex obtained from skeletal muscle protein kinase was incubated at 30° in the presence or absence of (C) and/or (I). Liberated ^{3}H-cyclic AMP was determined by gel filtration.

This effect of I is readily explained (25) since interaction appears to occur between the catalytic subunit and I leading to the formation of a complex CI. Free C would not then be available to mediate the release of cyclic AMP from R-^{3}H-cyclic AMP.

Interaction of Phosphodiesterase with Bound Cyclic AMP

The only physiological mechanism known to terminate the action of cyclic AMP is through its hydrolysis to 5'AMP catalyzed by the 3',5' cyclic nucleotide phosphodiesterase. The question arises as to whether the bound form of cyclic AMP is susceptible to attack by the phosphodiesterase. Using holoenzyme protein kinase from bovine skeletal muscle (17) and kidney (45), it has been demonstrated that if cyclic AMP was incubated with protein kinase, under conditions where essentially all of the cyclic AMP became bound to receptor protein, addition of phosphodiesterase at 0° resulted in almost no hydrolysis of the cyclic nucleotide. Inhibition of phosphodiesterase action in the presence of the protein kinase was less pronounced but still observed at 30°. It was concluded from these results that cyclic AMP bound to the receptor protein is not hydrolyzed and that it becomes accessible to the action of phosphodiesterase only when dissociated from the protein. The stability of cyclic AMP protein complex being greater at 0° than at 30°, explains the fact that some bound cyclic nucleotide could be hydrolyzed by phosphodiesterase at 30°.

In a similar manner, Brostrom *et al.* (11) performed an experiment using a purified binding fraction from skeletal muscle obtained as R-^{3}H-cyclic AMP, which was free of catalytic kinase subunit but was contaminated with a phosphodiesterase activity : upon incubation of R-^{3}H-cyclic AMP at 30° in the presence of Mg^{2+}, no significant hydrolysis of the cyclic nucleotide could be detected. When the C subunit was added, 50 % of the cyclic AMP present was converted to 5'AMP in 30 minutes incubation. The authors came to the same conclusion as O'Dea *et al.* (17) and Cheung (45) *viz.* : in the absence of C, cyclic AMP is tightly bound to R and is therefore not attacked by the phosphodiesterase, but addition of C subunit promotes the liberation of cyclic AMP which then becomes accessible to the phosphodiesterase.

CYCLIC GMP BINDING SYSTEM

Several lines of evidence published recently suggest that cyclic GMP may be under controls which are different from and sometimes opposite to those affecting cyclic AMP. This problem will be discussed elsewhere. However, compared to the body of knowledge that has accumulated concerning the mode of action of

cyclic AMP, little evidence is at present available for cyclic GMP.
By analogy with the hypothesis that biochemical effects of cyclic
AMP are mediated via activation of cyclic AMP dependent protein
kinases, it seemed reasonable to postulate and to look for protein
kinase activity dependent on cyclic GMP (46-48) and for intracellular cyclic GMP receptors.

Cyclic GMP Receptor

The existence of cyclic GMP receptor proteins in lobster
muscle extracts, which also contained a cyclic GMP dependent protein kinase activity, has been described by Murad et $al.$ (49).
Dialyzed $(NH_4)_2SO_4$ preparations, incubated at 0°, pH 4.0 in
the presence of ^{3}H-cyclic GMP have been shown to bind significant amounts of cyclic GMP. ^{3}H-cyclic GMP complex can be retained
on Millipore filters as under the conditions described by Gilman
(13). Binding was maximal after 75 minutes incubation at 0° and
was constant for at least 45 minutes thereafter. Binding constant
for cyclic GMP has been found to be in the range of 2-10 nM, and
saturation of binding was usually observed at 60 nM with optimal
binding at pH 4.0. When the binding reaction was carried out
with ^{3}H-cyclic GMP at 0.1 µM, the presence of equimolar amounts
of cyclic AMP inhibited the binding 5-7 %, and addition of cyclic
AMP in a 10-fold excess produced 15-20 % inhibition. The binding
constant for cyclic AMP was 15-20 fold higher than that of cyclic
GMP. High concentrations (10 µM) of cyclic IMP interfered with
the binding of cyclic GMP while other nucleotides tested by Murad
et $al.$ (49) including GTP, GDP, and guanosine (1 mM) had little or
no effect. The authors also reported that the inhibitor of protein
kinase which enhances cyclic AMP binding and decreases the binding
constant for cyclic AMP did not alter the cyclic GMP binding.

The use of cyclic GMP binding protein preparations from
lobster muscle allowed the development of analytical procedures
for the measurement of tissue cyclic GMP based on competition with
^{3}H-cyclic GMP (49, 50).

Cyclic GMP Dependent Protein Kinases

Protein kinases controlled by cyclic GMP have been found in
large quantities in various tissues and species of arthropoda and
the enzyme purified from lobster muscle (46, 47). Some mammalian
tissue protein kinases with relative specificity for cyclic GMP
have been mentioned (48) and Hofmann and Sold (51) recently
reported that an extract of rat cerebellum contains protein kinase
activity which can be stimulated by low concentrations of cyclic
GMP (Ka 0.038 µM) as well as high concentrations of cyclic AMP
(Ka 0.9 µM).

The mechanism of activation of the protein kinase by cyclic GMP has been studied with the lobster muscle preparation : cyclic GMP and histone caused the dissociation of the holoenzyme from a fraction sedimenting at 7.7 S to a catalytic unit independent of cyclic GMP with a sedimentation constant of 3.6 S. However, all attempts to recover cyclic GMP binding fractions have been unsuccessful, probably due to the lability of the receptor subunit.

It is of interest that the regulatory subunit of the cyclic AMP dependent protein kinase from mammalian brain, inhibited the catalytic activity of the subunit prepared from the lobster muscle cyclic GMP dependent protein kinase. This resulted in the reconstitution of a "hybrid" holoenzyme which was preferentially activated by cyclic AMP rather than cyclic GMP, indicating that the cyclic nucleotide specificity of the receptor protein was not modified by its combination with the heterologous C subunit.

Cyclic GMP Binding in Mammelian Tissues

In a recent report, Sold and Hofmann (52) investigated the ability of several mammalian tissues to bind cyclic AMP as well as cyclic GMP, when incubated, at pH 4.0 in the presence of the corresponding cyclic nucleotide (0.1 µM). The ratio of bound cyclic AMP to bound cyclic GMP varied from 2.9 for the cerebellum to 7.2 for the cerebrum. Skeletal and cardiac muscles, adrenal glands, and the thymus gave intermediate ratios.

Cyclic GMP binding was further studied in more detail in the cerebellar extract : it appeared that cyclic GMP was bound by a different protein than that of cyclic AMP. Two different types of binding sites for cyclic GMP were observed; one non specific from which cyclic GMP could be displaced by low concentrations of cyclic AMP, and another which was specific for cyclic GMP. The apparent Kd for the cyclic GMP specific site was 12 nM and at saturating concentrations (0.1 µM), the maximal binding capacity reached a value of 1.5 pmole bound cyclic GMP/mg extracted proteins.

Several attempts to purify the protein which specifically binds cyclic GMP and to separate it from the cyclic AMP binding protein, resulted in an almost complete loss of cyclic GMP binding activity and yielded only a cyclic AMP dependent protein kinase. A partial separation of cyclic AMP and cyclic GMP binding activities has been achieved by fractionation with ammonium suffate : cyclic AMP binding as well as cyclic AMP dependent kinase activities were mostly found in the 35 % fraction, whereas the specific cyclic GMP binding activity was recovered in the 35–55 % ammonium sulfate fraction. The latter precipitate contained in addition, a protein kinase activity which was stimulated more by cyclic GMP (5.4 x) than by cyclic AMP (3.3x).

It still remains to establish if this cyclic GMP binding protein is part of a cyclic GMP dependent protein kinase, or is not related to this class of enzyme and has a rather different intracellular function.

An interesting finding has recently been reported by Haddox *et al.* (53) who demonstrated that the binding of cyclic GMP to some classes of cyclic AMP dependent protein kinases may become markedly increased at acidic pH : in a binding reaction of ^{3}H-cyclic AMP (20 nM), carried out at pH 4.0 with a skeletal muscle protein kinase, obtained as a simple peak from DEAE cellulose, cyclic GMP at a concentration of 40 nM, could diplace 50 % of the bound labelled cyclic AMP. Cyclic GMP, in this case, exhibited one-fifth of the apparent reactivity observed with cyclic AMP. The ability of cyclic GMP to act as a competitor for ^{3}H-cyclic AMP binding was pH dependent, being much more pronounced at pH 4.0 than at pH 7.0. This inhibition of ^{3}H-cyclic AMP binding, was also reflected by an increased capacity of the enzyme to bind cyclic GMP. With this form of skeletal muscle protein kinase, the apparent binding constant for cyclic GMP varied from 125 nM at pH 7.5 to 20 nM at pH 4.0, while the changes in pH did not affect the binding of cyclic AMP.

If this increased effectiveness of cyclic GMP for binding at acidic pH to some but not all forms of cyclic AMP dependent protein kinases, has any particular physiological significance, is at present unknown.

HORMONAL REGULATION - INTRACELLULAR TITRATION OF CYCLIC AMP BOUND TO RECEPTOR PROTEINS IN RAT DIAPHRAGM

In the preceding sections, general considerations for cyclic AMP binding have been outlined, from various observations established *in vitro* with purified or partially purified protein preparations. It became important to demonstrate to what extent, in the intact cells, binding of cyclic AMP to its receptor would reflect the true intracellular concentration of the cyclic nucleotide and how modulations in levels of cyclic AMP promoted by various effectors would be paralleled by variations in endogenous R-cyclic AMP complex.

From the equation, postulated by Brostrom *et al.* (11) to represent protein kinase activation by cyclic AMP :

$$RC + \text{cyclic AMP} \rightleftharpoons R\text{-cyclic AMP} + C$$

it could be expected that variations in intracellular cyclic AMP

levels must be accompanied by opposite changes in non saturated
cyclic AMP binding sites : the higher the level of cyclic AMP in
the cell, the more saturated would be the receptor. Consequently
the ability of the extracted proteins to bind exogenous ^{3}H-cyclic
AMP would be reduced as compared to proteins extracted from non
stimulated cells with low endogenous levels of cyclic AMP. Experimental verification of this hypothesis has been obtained in the
case of rat diaphragm (12).

As a basis for studying any hormonal effect in intact tissue,
the properties of the binding reaction using ^{3}H-cyclic AMP were
investigated in diaphragm extracts obtained after different tissue
incubations : diaphragms were incubated at 37° in Brebs Ringer
bicarbonate, with or without the addition of theophylline and/or
epinephrine 5 µM. At the end of incubation, the tissue was rapidly
chilled and extracted with cold Tris-HCl buffer pH 7.0 containing
6mM theophylline. The proteins recovered in the 50,000 x supernatant of the homogenates, were used for the cyclic AMP binding
assay which was carried out at 0°, pH 7.5 in the presence of ^{3}H-
cyclic AMP. Bound ^{3}H-cyclic AMP retained on Millipore filters
represented the binding capacity of the corresponding extract.

Kinetics and Concentration Dependence of Exogenous Cyclic

AMP Binding in the Soluble Extracts

When various concentrations of ^{3}H-cyclic AMP were added to
proteins extracted from diaphragm incubated in the absence of hormone, and the binding reaction carried out for different incubation
times at 0°, it can be seen (Figure 1) that saturation was obtained
at a concentration of 80 nM cyclic AMP and that the binding equilibrium was reached in less than 60 minutes incubation. From a reciprocal plot of cyclic AMP binding *versus* cyclic AMP concentration,
an apparent dissociation constant (Kd) of 33 nM can be calculated
for the cyclic nucleotide. This value is very similar to the
apparent Kd for cyclic AMP which have been described for protein
kinases of various tissues other than the diaphragm.

It has also been verified that with the protein concentration
used (70-200 µg in 250 µl reaction mixture), binding of cyclic AMP
was directly proportional to the amount of added proteins. In
addition, when the bound radioactivity was extracted from the Millipore filters with cold TCA and chromatographed on cellulose thin
layer sheets in ethanol : M ammonium acetate solvent (75:30, v/v)
all the extracted radioactive material could be identified as
unmodified cyclic AMP.

Specificity of cyclic AMP binding has been assessed by dilution experiments of ^{3}H-cyclic AMP (100 nM) with unlabelled adenine

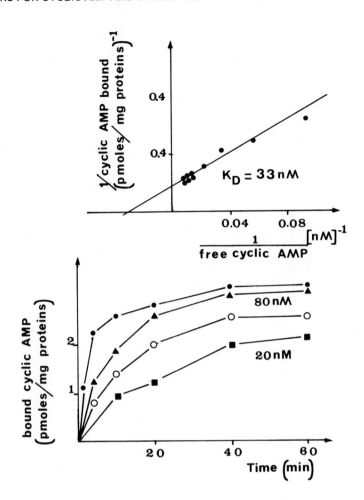

Figure 1 : *Time course and cyclic AMP concentration dependence of cyclic AMP binding in rat diaphragm extract.*
Figure taken from Do Khac et al. (12)

A) Cyclic AMP binding was estimated in the presence of various concentrations of ^3H-cyclic AMP : 20 nM ■; 60 nM 0; 80 nM ▲; 100 nM ● at 0° and for different times.

B) Data obtained from similar experiments where binding for cyclic AMP was performed at 0° for 1 hour in the presence of ^3H-cyclic AMP ranging from 12 nM to 110 nM. Double reciprocal plots.

In (A) and (B) bound ^3H-cyclic AMP was estimated by the Millipore filter technique.

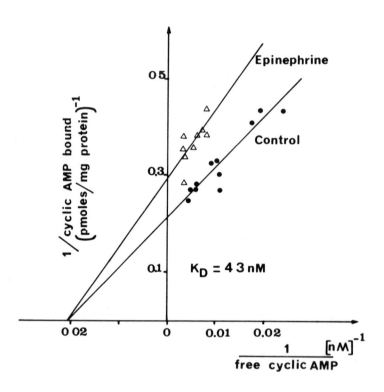

Figure 2. Cyclic AMP concentration dependence of cyclic AMP binding in rat diaphragm extracts (Method B). Effect of epinephrine.
Figure taken from Do Khac et al. (12).

Various concentrations of ³H-cyclic AMP ranging from 12 nM to 200 nM were added directly to the homogenizing medium for preparing extracts from epinephrine treated and untreated diaphragms. Aliquots of the extracts were filtered through Millipore Filters.

nucleotides (adenine, AMP, ATP, cyclic AMP) at 0.1 mM concentrations. In no case, except with unlabelled cyclic AMP, was the amount of radioactive material bound to the proteins and retained on the filter significantly reduced.

Location of Total Cyclic AMP and Cyclic AMP Binding Fractions

As shown in Table IV, when the diaphragms were treated in the presence of epinephrine 5 µM, there was the expected rise in total tissue cyclic AMP, as extracted by cold 7 % TCA and estimated according to Gilman (13). It is interesting to note that if cyclic AMP was assayed in the 50,000 x g soluble diaphragm extract, either the acetate extract or Tris extract, after deproteinization with TCA, the values for cyclic AMP levels were identical to those found when the diaphragms were directly extracted with TCA. This is the case for the untreated as well as for the epinephrine treated diaphragm. Hence almost none of the cyclic nucleotide in these extracts appeared to be tightly associated with membrane fractions.

TABLE IV : Location of Cyclic AMP in Different Extracts obtained from Epinephrine-treated and untreated Rat Diaphragms

Total cyclic AMP	pmoles/100 mg wet tissue					
		in				
Fractions	TCA		20 mM acetate		20 mM Tris	
Tissue incubation with epinephrine	−	+	−	+	−	+
Extract	57	280	45	242	48	212
Pellet	−	−	8.5	8.5	9.5	2.0

Data from Do Khac et al. (12).

After incubation with 10 nM theophylline, in the presence or absence of 5 µM epinephrine diaphragms were homogenized in three different solutions : cold 7 % TCA, Tris-HCL pH 7.5 or acetate pH 7.5. Centrifugation was carried out at 50,000 x g Soluble Tris extract acetate extract and their corresponding sediments were deproteinized by 7 % TCA before cyclic AMP assay.

When the distribution of ^{3}H-cyclic AMP binding activities was analyzed in various fractions of rat diaphragm homogenates, it was found (Table V) that in all cases more than 90 % of this activity was recovered in the 50,000 x g supernatant, almost no cyclic AMP binding occurred in the pellets. Preincubation of the diaphragms with epinephrine did not modify the percentage distribution of the radioactive cyclic nucleotide. However, it was evident that for the epinephrine-treated diaphragm, less exogenous labelled cyclic AMP (about 50-60 %) was bound to the various fractions, indicating a decrease in the binding capacity of the extracts as compared to the untreated diaphragm. Clearly in the latter case, the concentration of unlabelled cyclic AMP has been taken into account for the estimation of the specific activity of ^{3}H-cyclic AMP.

TABLE V : Distribution of ^{3}H-cyclic AMP binding fractions in different homogenates from epinephrine-treated and untreated rat diaphragms

Bound ^{3}H-cyclic AMP			pmoles/100 wet tissue	
Extracts	4 mM EDTA	20 mM acetate	20 mM Tris	
Tissue incubated with epinephrine	−	−	−	+
Supernatant 50,000 x g	17.17	16.44	16.65	10.20
Pellet 3,000 x g	1.49	1.50	1.10	0.39
Pellet 50,000 x g	0.76	0.83	0.80	0.44

Data adapted from Do Khac et al. (12).

Incubation as described in Table IV. Tissue homogenization in 4mM EDTA, 20 nM acetate or 20 mM Tris-HCl. Cyclic AMP binding activity determined in various fractions after centrifugation. The reaction mixture for the binding assay contained in a final volume of 250 µl 20 mM Tris-HCl buffer pH 7.5, 10 nM MgCl$_2$, 6.7 mM theophylline 100 nM ^{3}H-cyclic AMP and aliquots of the corresponding protein fractions. After 1 hour incubation at 0°, binding of ^{3}H-cyclic AMP was measured by the Millipore filter technique.

Effect of Theophylline and Epinephrine Treatment on

the Binding of Exogeneous Cyclic AMP by Rat Diaphragm Extracts

In the experiments described above for the estimation of
residual binding capacities of the epinephrine treated and untreated diaphragm extracts, the possibility existed that the bulk
of cyclic AMP if sequestered in the cell might be released during
homogenization and centrifugation steps, giving rise to additional
binding of unlabelled cyclic AMP. This may then result in an
underestimate of the exogeneous binding. In order to avoid this
artefactual error, similar experiments were performed by adding
^{3}H-cyclic AMP into the homogenizing medium, allowing therefore the
labelled nucleotide to become directly accessible to the binding
proteins, at the moment the hormonal effect was stopped. Table VI
also shows that with method B the effect of epinephrine, $i.e.$ a
decrease in the residual binding of ^{3}H-cyclic AMP as compared to
the control, was still evident. It appears however that with this
Method (B) higher values were obtained both with eprinephrine-
treated and untreated diaphragms than with the previous method
(A). This demonstrated that some additional (25 %) binding of
endogenous cyclic AMP actually occurred during the homogenization
procedure and hence the values obtained with method B seem to
reflect intracellular conditions more accurately. Method B has
then been currently employed for the estimation of exogeneous
cyclic AMP binding. Using this method, the affinity for cyclic
AMP has been determined by adding various concentrations of ^{3}H-
cyclic AMP to the homogenizing medium of diaphragms which have
been incubated in the presence and absence of epinephrine : the
double reciprocal plots obtained in Figure 2 allow the calculation
of apparent Kd values equal to 43 nM which are in the same range as
that described in Figure 1. The Figure also shows that epinephrine
treatment did not modify the affinity of the binding proteins for
the cyclic nucleotide. However, for all the concentrations of ^{3}H-
cyclic AMP which have been added, epinephrine treatment resulted
in a decrease in the amount of exogenous cyclic AMP which can be
bound to the extract proteins.

Figure 3 shows the result of a typical experiment in which
diaphragms have been incubated in the absence or presence of theophylline and/or epinephrine. After each incubation half a diaphragm was extracted with TCA for total cyclic AMP estimation;
the other half was homogenized with Tris buffer containing 100 nM
3H-cyclic AMP, the centrifugation time kept to a minimum (10 minutes) and the binding capacity for ^{3}H-cyclic AMP determined at
different times. During the whole titration period, ^{3}H-cyclic AMP
binding was inversely related to the amount of endogenous cyclic
AMP present in the relevant extract. It must also be emphasized
that if propranolol was added to the incubated diaphragms prior to
the addition of epinephrine, there was almost complete inhibition

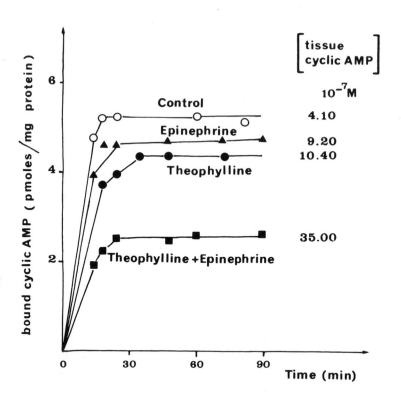

<u>*Figure 3*</u> : *Time course of ^{3}H-cyclic AMP binding in extracts from diaphragms incubated in the absence or presence of theophylline and epinephrine. Correlation with intracellular cyclic AMP concentrations.*
Data from Do Khac et al. (12)

Incubation of the diaphragms in the absence or presence of 10 mM theophylline and/or 5 μM epinephrine (5 minutes) at 37° :

a) half diaphragm was extracted by cold TCA for the estimation of cyclic AMP level in the tissue,
b) and half diaphragm was homogenized in Tris-HCl buffer containing 100 nM ^{3}H-cyclic AMP and centrifuged at 5,000 x g for 10 minutes. Binding of ^{3}H-cyclic AMP was measured in aliquots of the supernatant.

of the hormonal effect as far as cyclic AMP accumulation is concerned, and under these conditions no effect of epinephrine could
be demonstrated at the level of the binding capacities of the
extract. Therefore the agents which increase intracellular cyclic
AMP level appear to decrease the amount of binding sites available
for exogenous ^{3}H-cyclic AMP. It remained to demonstrate that this
latter decrease was the consequence of an increase in the endogenous
cyclic AMP-receptor complex. A simple method for determining the
true value of endogenous cyclic AMP binding necessitates the precise
evaluation of total binding capacities of the extract. Then the
difference between total binding capacities and residual binding
activity will reflect the endogenous cyclic AMP binding at the
moment when the tissues were homogenized.

TABLE VI : Comparison of Exogenous Binding of ^{3}H-Cyclic AMP to
Diaphragm Extracts by Method A and B.
Effect of Epinephrine.

	Bound cyclic-AMP pmoles/mg protein	
	− Epinephrine	+ Epinephrine 5 µM
Extract A	4.0 ± 0.34	2.0 ± 0.13
Extract B	4.8 ± 0.20	3.0 ± 0.19

Data from Do Khac et al. (12)

*After incubation in the presence or absence of epinephrine,
diaphragms were extracted with Tris-HCl buffer, 10 mM theophylline for subsequent binding of ^{3}H-cyclic AMP (100 nM) 1 hour
at 0° (4). A second series of extracts were prepared in the same
way but in the presence of 100 nM ^{3}H-cyclic AMP in the homogenizing
medium (B).*

Cyclic AMP Exchange and Determination of Maximal

Binding Capacities

To estimate the maximal binding capacities of the extract,
it was necessary to devise experimental conditions which allow
not only binding of labelled cyclic AMP to the unoccupied sites
of the receptor protein, but in addition, permit the complete
exchange of endogenous bound cyclic AMP with added radioactively
labelled cyclic AMP. Experiments showed that this exchange can

readily be obtained under the conditions defined by Wilchek *et al.* (43) : extracts from both epinephrine treated and untreated diaphragms were first incubated at 0° with ^{3}H-cyclic AMP (100 nM) under binding conditions, and then allowed to exchange with 1 μM unlabelled cyclic AMP at 20° in the presence of 100 μM ATP and 10 mM MgCl$_2$. Almost complete exchange of bound radioactivity readily occurred within 30 minutes. Total binding capacities of the proteins could thus be measured by incubating the extracts first with unlabelled cyclic AMP at 0° and carrying out the exchange reaction in the presence of large quantities (1 μM) ^{3}H-cyclic AMP at 20°. As shown in Figure 4, maximal exchange can be obtained with a plateau value reached at 60 minutes and remaining stable for at least 2 hours. The values for total cyclic AMP binding averaged 8.5 - 9.5 pmoles ^{3}H-cyclic AMP/mg soluble protein, both with epinephrine treated and untreated diaphragms. These values can be confirmed by direct assay of bound cyclic AMP : extracts were first saturated with unlabelled cyclic AMP, filtered on Millipore filters, and bound cyclic AMP was extracted with cold TCA and assayed according to Gilman (13). The average values obtained were also 9.8 ± 0.4 pmoles cyclic AMP/mg soluble proteins[*]. These results also demonstrate that epinephrine treatment did not introduce any modification in the maximal binding capacity of the extracted proteins.

Titration of Endogenous Cyclic AMP Binding in Rat
Diaphragm. Effect of Theophylline and Epinephrine.

Since total binding capacities of the receptor protein in the extracts and the amount of exogenous ^{3}H-cyclic AMP bound by these extracts after homogenisation may be estimated it became possible to calculate the endogenous cyclic AMP bound in intact cells. However an additional experimental control appeared important namely to try to find out if there was any simultaneous exchange of cyclic AMP under the binding conditions (0°, 1 hour, 100 nM cyclic AMP) and if this did occur, to try to evaluate the extent of this exchange. Extracts of rat diaphragm were first saturated with 100 nM unlabelled cyclic AMP (binding conditions) and then exchanged with 1 μM ^{3}H-cyclic AMP but at 0°. After 2 hours, 100 μM ATP and Mg^{2+} were added the temperature raised to 20° and completion of the exchange measured after 1-2 hours further incubation. The results of such an experiment (Figure 5)

---

[*] The values for maximal cyclic AMP binding capacities may also be expressed as pmoles/Kg wet tissue. An intracellular concentration for total cyclic AMP binding sites in rat diaphragm is then found to be 0.25 μM which is quite similar to the value of 0.46 μM reported by Beavo *et al.* (57) in the case of skeletal muscle.

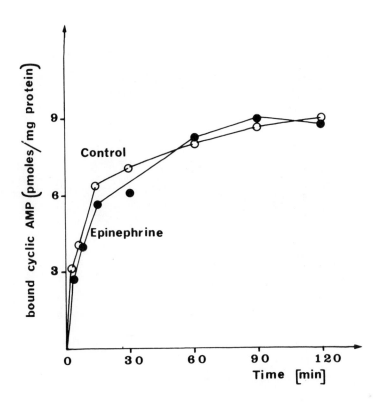

Figure 4 : Exchange of bound cyclic AMP in the presence of
³H-cyclic AMP 1 μM. Maximal binding capacity.

Data from Do Khac et al. (12).

    Extracts prepared from epinephrine treated and untreated
tissue were first incubated with unlabelled 200 nM cyclic AMP
(2 hours at 0°). 1 μM ³H-cyclic AMP was then added and the
reaction mixtures were kept at 20°. At the different times
indicated on the figure, aliquots were filtered for the estimation
of bound ³H-cyclic AMP.

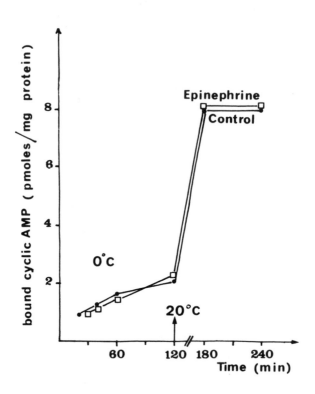

Figure 5 : Cyclic AMP exchange under binding (0°) and exchange (20° + ATP Mg^2) conditions.

Figure taken from Do Khac et al. (12).

Extracts from epinephrine treated and untreated tissue were incubated at 0°C, first with 100 nM unlabelled cyclic AMP for 1 hour, then with additional 100 nM ^{3}H-cyclic AMP for 2 hours. At the end of the binding reaction, 1 μM ^{3}H-cyclic AMP together with 1.00 μM ATP was added (arrow) and the reaction mixtures were maintained at 20° for 2 more hours. At the different times indicated in the figure, aliquots were filtered for the estimation of bound ^{3}H-cyclic AMP.

show that, at 0° within 1 hour incubation, about 20 % of sites are exchangeable as compared to total exchange capacities determined at 20°. Hence in evaluating the endogenous R-cyclic AMP complex, a correction for this 20 % exchange under binding conditions, has always been considered.

Table VII summarizes the results of a series of experiments where diaphragms have been incubated under different conditions which modify cellular levels of cyclic AMP. At the end of the incubation half a diaphragm was extracted for cyclic AMP assay, and the other half for the estimation of residual binding and total cyclic AMP binding capacities. From the latter experimental data, the corresponding endogenous binding has been calculated. It appears that :

a) Various treatments did not modify the maximal cyclic AMP binding capacities of the extracts.

b) The rise in tissue cyclic AMP content induced by theophylline or epinephrine or both agonists was accompanied in all cases by an increase in endogenous R-cyclic AMP complex. In the unstimulated diaphragm about 50 % of the available binding sites were occupied by endogenous cyclic AMP, this value increasing to almost 90 % when the diaphragm was fully stimulated.

c) A comment on the cyclic AMP binding capacities should also be made. The values obtained were very low as compared to total endogenous cyclic AMP present in the extract : while the tissue could be stimulated with intracellular values for cyclic AMP reaching 170 pmoles/mg protein, the maximal binding capacity of the receptor did not exceed 8-9 pmoles cyclic AMP/mg proteins.

Finally similar experiments were performed under more varied incubation conditions (different epinephrine concentrations or incubation times, etc.), in order to get various values for the intracellular concentration of cyclic AMP and of the corresponding endogenous R-cyclic AMP complex. A double reciprocal plot of intracellular binding *versus* intracellular cyclic AMP (Figure 6) showed that this correlation closely fitted simple saturation kinetics. The apparent Kd value for intracellular binding according to this plot was estimated to be 330 nM $\pm$ 50. Maximal binding capacities calculated from the intercept of the plot with the ordinate axis gave a value of 8.9 pmoles/mg protein, which coincided with the values measured by the previous techniques. On the other hand, it is evident that the binding constant for cyclic AMP within the cell was 10 times higher when compared with crude extracts of broken cell preparations. This clearly indicates that the binding constant measured with purified protein kinases do not reflect true intracellular conditions. It has been repeatedly pointed out that cyclic AMP concentration even in the

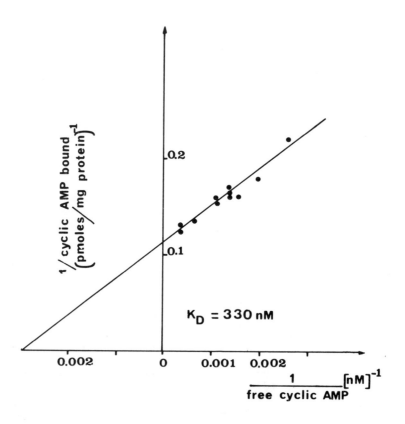

<u>Figure 6</u> : Reciprocal plot of intracellular cyclic AMP
level and intracellular cyclic AMP binding

Data from Do Khac et al. (12)

TABLE VII : Relationship between Intracellular Cyclic AMP Levels and Intracellular Cyclic AMP bound to its Receptor (Endogenous R-Cyclic AMP)

Incubation conditions

Cyclic AMP pmoles / mg proteins

Theophylline	Epinephrine	Time min.	Total level	Binding Maximal (a)	Binding Exogeneous (b)	Endogenous R-cyclic AMP (a − b) *
−	−	0	20.5 ± 4.7	9.6 ± 0.9	5.35 ± 0.40	5.31
−	+	2	52 ± 0.47	9.4 ± 0.1	4.50 ± 0.133	6.13
−	+	10	43	9.20	4.40	6
−	+	30	38	9.40	4.70	5.85
+	−	5	46 ± 2	8.9 ± 0.73	4.46 ± 0.20	5.53
+	+	5	170 ± 10.7	8.9 ± 0.85	2.7 ± 0.224	7.77

* Values corrected for 20 % exchange under binding conditions.

Data from Do Khac et al. (12)

unstimulated cell was far in excess of the concentration which
should result in maximal stimulation of protein kinases. Compartmentation of the cyclic nucleotide within the cell has been
postulated to explain this contradiction (18, 54-56). If this was
the case, the simple saturation kinetics obtained in Figure 6 would
indicate that the various pools of cyclic AMP attain equilibrium
very rapidly. However, this compartmentation hypothesis may
be considered oversimplified : indeed if the equilibrium reaction
described by the equation 1 may be applied within the cell, without any modification, then a decrease in the apparent Kd could be
merely a consequence of the dilution (about 10-fold) of the
protein components during extraction of the tissue, while cyclic
AMP concentrations are maintained constant by the addition of
^{3}H-cyclic AMP. The effect of protein dilution on the cyclic AMP
activation constant measured has been pointed out by Beavo *et al.*
(57). More recently, Swillens *et al.* (58 and these proceedings)
considered on theoretical grounds that the discrepancies observed
for activation or binding constant in intact cell as compared to
broken cell conditions, may just be due to the fact that protein
kinase activation by cyclic AMP is much more complex than the
simple binding of a ligand to a specific protein.

In addition, one must also bear in mind that some factors
such as the intracellular concentrations of the heat-stable
kinase inhibitor (22, 25) and ATP-Mg^{2+} (26, 43) may seriously
affect intracellular cyclic AMP binding. It is still difficult,
at the present time, to decide which of these interpretations is
most likely to reflect true intracellular conditions.

These experiments have, however, demonstrated a hormonal
control at the level of cyclic AMP-receptor protein interaction in
an identical manner to the one first described by Corbin *et al.*
(59) and Soderling *et al.* (60) at the level of the activated state
of the protein kinase. The latter results will be discussed in
the section on protein kinases (see Corbin *et al.*, these proceedings).

Some recent experiments, with the aim of correlating modulations in levels of cyclic AMP secondary to hormonal stimulation
with a decrease in residual cyclic AMP binding sites of the receptor protein have been performed with the diaphragm (61), uterus
(62, 63) and liver (64).

CONCLUSIONS

This review has summarized some of the information available at present concerning *in vitro* cyclic AMP and cyclic GMP binding to receptor proteins obtained from various animal tissues. It appears, at least for cyclic AMP, since far fewer experiments have been performed with cyclic GMP that the binding reaction is not only controlled by variations in the concentrations of the cyclic nucleotide available to its binding protein, but that other intracellular factors may influence the binding reaction as well as the rate of dissociation of cyclic AMP bound to its receptor. The only protein component, found to the present time, which is able to bind cyclic AMP is the R subunit associated with protein kinase. One report (18) has mentioned in liver extracts the presence of a cyclic AMP binding protein of high molecular weight, which was devoid of any catalytic kinase activity; however, this fraction has not been tested for its ability to reassociate with the free C subunit. Moreover, Filler and Litwack (65) reported the presence in rat liver cytosol, of two different protein fractions, one which binds cyclic AMP and the other that binds dibutyryl-cyclic AMP. The significance of this intracellular dibutyryl-cyclic AMP binding protein is at the present time merely speculative. Antonoff and Ferguson (66), using photoaffinity labelling technique, have described experiments indicating that ^{3}H-cyclic AMP, upon irradiation with ultra violet light, forms a covalent bond with receptors in extracts of testis and adrenals. Cyclic GMP can also be tightly bound to the extracted proteins. The question of whether the receptors which are labelled by this method are the R subunits of cyclic nucleotide dependent protein kinases has not, as yet, been resolved.

Finally, experiments reported with intact diaphragm revealed that rises in cyclic AMP levels evoked by theophylline and/or epinephrine are accompanied by a corresponding increase in the degree of saturation of endogenous receptor protein, *i.e.* an increase in the quantity of endogenous R-cyclic AMP. Accurate estimations of intracellular binding of cyclic AMP have been correlated with level of cyclic AMP in the tissue : the reaction seems to obey simple saturation kinetics, an apparent intracellular Kd for cyclic AMP being evaluated as 330 nM. Different hypotheses (some theoretical and some derived from experimental data) have been advanced to explain the discrepancy between the binding constant for cyclic AMP in intact cell and that measured in extracts (33-43 nM). No definite explanation can yet be considered to reflect, any more accurately, intracellular conditions.

The results obtained have, however, demonstrated that hormonal controls can be obtained not only at the level of cyclic AMP formation but also at the level of cyclic AMP receptor interaction.

In many regulatory mechanisms, completely satisfactory correlations have been difficult to obtain between levels of intracellular cyclic AMP and the final hormone induced metabolic effect (67–72). In all these cases, cyclic AMP levels may be elevated without eliciting the expected metabolic responses and hence a regulatory control could be exerted at a step beyond cyclic AMP formation. The data reported provide a suitable means for investigating this type of hormonal regulation.

REFERENCES

(1)   GILL, G.N. and GARREN, L.D. (1969) Proc. Natl. Acad. Sci. US, 63, 512

(2)   SALOMON, Y. and SCHRAMM, M. (1970) Biochem. Biophys. Res. Comm., 38, 106

(3)   WALSH, D.A., PARKINS, J.P. and KREBS, E.G. (1968) J. Biol. Chem., 243, 3763

(4)   KUO, J.F., and GREENGARD, P. (1969) Proc. Natl. Acad. Sci. US, 64, 1349

(5)   TAO, M., SALAS, M.L. and LIPMANN, F. (1970) Proc. Natl. Acad. Sci. US, 67, 408

(6)   GILL, G.N. and GARREN, L.D. (1970) Biochem. Biophys. Res. Comm., 39, 335

(7)   KUMON, A., YAMAMURA, H. and NISHIZUKA, Y. (1970) Biochem. Biophys. Res. Comm. 41, 1290

(8)   REIMANN, E.M., BROSTROM, C.O., CORBIN, J.D., KING, C.A. and KREBS, E.G. (1971) Biochem. Biophys. Res. Comm. 42, 187

(9)   ERLICHMAN, J., HIRSCH, A.H. and ROSEN, O.M. (1971) Proc. Natl. Acad. Sci. 68, 731

(10) SANBORN, B.M., BHALLA, R.C. and KORENMAN,S.G., (1973) J. Biol. Chem. 248, 3593

(11) BROSTROM, C.O., CORBIN, J.D., KING, C.A., and KREBS, E.G. (1971) Proc. Natl. Acad. Sci. 68, 2444

(12) DO KRAC, L. HARBON, S. and CLAUSER, H. (1973) Euro. J. Biochem. 40, 177

(13) GILMAN, A. (1970) Proc. Natl. Acad. Sci. 67, 305

(14)   WALTON, G.M. and GARREN, L.D. (1970) Biochemistry 9, 4223

(15)   TAO, M. (1971) Arch. Biochem. Biophys. 143, 151

(16)   RUBIN, C.S., ERLICHMAN, J. and ROSEN, O.M. (1972) J. Biol.
       Chem. 247, 36

(17)   O'DEA, R.F., HADDOX, M.K. and GOLDBERG, N.D. (1971) J. Biol.
       Chem. 246, 6183

(18)   CHAMBAUT, A.M., LERAY, F. and HANOUNE, J. (1971) FEBS Letters
       15, 328

(19)   KUMON, A., NISHIYAMA, K., YAMAMURA, H. and NISHISUKA, Y.
       (1972) J. Biol. Chem. 247, 3726

(20)   WELLER, M., RODNIGHT, R., and CARRERA, D. (1972) Biochem. J.
       129, 113

(21)   DONOVAN, G. and OLIVER, I.T. (1972) Biochemistry 11, 3904

(22)   WALSH, D.A., ASHBY, C.D., GONZALEZ, C., CALKINS, D.,
       FISHER, E.H. and KREBS, E.G. (1971) J. Biol Chem. 246, 1977

(23)   BROWN, B.L., ALBANO, J.D.M., EKINS, R.P. and SGHERZI, A.M.
       (1971) Biochem. J. 121, 561

(24)   ROSEN, O.M., RUBIN, C.S. and ERLICHMAN, J. (1973) Miami
       Winter Symposia, Vol. 5, 67, Ed. by F. Huijing and E.Y.C.
       Lee
(25)   ASHBY, D.C. and WALSH, D.A. (1972) J. Biol. Chem. 247, 6637

(26)   HADDOX, M.K., NEWTON, N.E., HARTLE, D.K. and GOLDBERG, N.D.
       (1972) Biochem. Biophys. Res. Comm. 47, 653

(27)   MAJUNDER, G.C. and TURKINGTON, R.W. (1971) J. Biol. Chem.
       246, 2650

(28)   CHEN, L.J. and WALSH, D.A. (1971) Biochemistry 10, 3614

(29)   WALTON, G.M., GILL, G.N., ABRASS, I.B. and GARREN, L.D.
       (1971) Proc. Natl. Acad. Sci. 68, 880

(30)   RUBIN, C.S., ERLICHMAN, J. and ROSEN, O.M. (1972) J. Biol
       Chem. 247, 6135

(31)   FONTANA, J.A., PICCIANO, D. and LOVENBERG, W. (1972) Bio-
       chem. Biophys. Res. Comm. 49, 1225

(32) PIERRE, M. and LOEB, J.E. (1971) BIOCHIMIE 53, 727

(33) MAENO, H., JOHNSON, E.M. and GREENGARD, P. (1971) J. Biol.
      Chem. 246, 134

(34) LEMAIRE, S., PELLETIER, G. and LABRIE, F. (1971) J. Biol.
      Chem. 246, 7303

(35) GILL, G.N. and GARREN, L.D. (1971) Proc. Natl. Acad. Sci.
      US, 68, 786

(36) CORBIN, J.D., BROSTROM, C.O., ALEXANDER, R.L. and KREBS, E.G.
      (1972) J. Biol. Chem. 247, 3736

(37) MIYAMOTO, E., PETZOLD, G.L., KUO, J.F. and GREENGARD, P.
      (1973) J. Biol. Chem. 248, 179

(38) MIYAMOTO, E. PETZOLD, G.L., HARRIS, J.S. and GREENGARD, P.
      (1971) Biochem. Biophys. Res. Comm. 44, 305

(39) TAO, M. (1972) Biochem. Biophys. Res. Comm. 46, 56

(40) TAO, M. and HACKETT, P. (1973) J. Biol. Chem. 248, 5324

(41) RAMSEYER, J., KASLOW, H.R. and GILL, G.N. (1974) Biochem.
      Biophys. Res. Comm. 59, 813

(42) JERGIL, G., GUILFORD, H. and MOSBACH, K. (1974) Biochem. J.
      139, 441

(43) WILCHEK, M., SALOMON, Y., LOWE, M. and SELLINGER, Z. (1970)
      Biochem. Biophys. Res. Comm. 45, 1177

(44) GILL, G.N., WALTON, G.M., HOLDY, K.E. MARIASH, C.N. and
      KALSTROM, J.B. (1973) Miami Winter Symposia, Vol. 5, 175,
      Ed. by F. Huijing and E.Y. Lee

(45) CHEUNG, W.Y. (1972) Biochem. Biophys. Res. Comm. 46, 99

(46) KUO, J.F. and GREENGARD, P. (1970) J. Biol. Chem. 245, 2493

(47) KUO, J.F., WHYATT, G.R., GREENGARD, P. (1971) J. Biol. Chem.
      246, 7159

(48) GREENGARD, P., KUO, J.F. in Role of Cyclic AMP in cell
      function (Greengard, P. and Costa, E. Eds.) 302, Raven
      Press, New York

(49) MURAD, F., MANGANIELLO, V., VAUGHAN, M. (1971) Proc. Natl.
      Acad. Sci. US 68, 736

(50) MURAD, F. and GILMAN, A.G. (1971) Biochim. Biophys. Acta 252,
      397

(51) HOFMANN, F. and SOLD, G. (1972) Biochem. Biophys. Res. Comm.
      49, 1100

(52) SOLD, G. and HOFMANN, F. (1974) Eur. J. Biochem. 44, 143

(53) HADDOX, M.K., NICOL, S.E. and GOLDBERG, N.D.(1973), Biochem.
      Biophys. Res. Comm. 54, 1444

(54) EXTON, J.H., LEWIS, S.B., HO, R.J., ROBISON, G.A. and PARK,
      C.R. (1971) Ann. N.Y. Acad. Sci. 185, 85

(55) RALL, T.W. (1972) Pharmacol. Rev. 24, 399

(56) MONTAGUE, W. and HOWELL, S.L. (1973) Biochem. J. 134, 321

(57) BEAVO, J.A., BECHTEL, P.J. and KREBS, E.G. (1974) Proc. Nat.
      Acad. Sci. 71, 3580

(58) SWILLENS, S., VANTAUTER, E. and DUMONT, J.E., (1974) Biochim.
      Biophys. Acta 364, 250

(59) CORBIN, J.D., SODERLING, T.R. and PARK, C.R. (1973) J. Biol.
      Chem. 248, 1813

(60) SODERLING, T.R., CORBIN, J.D. and PARK, C.R. (1973) J. Biol.
      Chem. 248, 1822

(61) WALAAS, O., WALAAS, E. and GRUNNERUD, O. (1973) Eur. J. Bio-
      chem. 40, 465

(62) KORENMAN, S.G., BHALLA, R.C., SANBORN, B.M. and STEVENS,
      R.H. (1974) Science, 183, 430

(63) HARBON, S. and DO KHAC. L., manuscript in preparation

(64) SUDILOVSKY, O. (1974) Biochem. Biophys. Res. Comm. 58, 85

(65) FILLER, R. and LITWACK, G. (1973) Biochem. Diophys. Res.
      Comm. 52, 159

(66) ANTONOFF, R.S. and FERGUSON, S.J. Jr. (1974) J. Biol. Chem.
      249, 3319

(67)   CRAIG, J.W., RALL, T.W. and LARNER, J. (1969) Biochim.
       Biophys. Acta, 177, 213

(68)   STULL, J. and MAJER, S.E. (1971) J. Biol. Chem. 246, 5716

(69)   MILLER, T.B., EXTON, J.H. and PARK, C.R. (1971) J. Biol.
       Chem. 246, 3672

(70)   HARBON, S. and CLAUSER, H. (1971) Biochem. Biophys. Res.
       Comm. 44, 1496

(71)   KHOO, J.C., STEINBERG, D., THOMPSON, B. and MAYER, S.E.
       (1973) J. Biol. Chem. 248, 3823

(72)   VESIN, M.F. and HARBON, S. (1974) Mol. Pharmacol. 10, 457

THE ASSAY OF CYCLIC AMP IN BIOLOGICAL MATERIAL

B.L. Brown,[a] J.D.M. Albano,[b] G.D. Barnes,[a]
D.V. Maudsley,[c] and R.P. Ekins[a]

[a]Department of Nuclear Medicine
 The Middlesex Hospital Medical School
 Thorn Institute of Clinical Science
 Mortimer Street, London W1N 8AA (United Kingdom)
[b]Department of Medicine, Bristol Royal Infirmary
 Bristol B52 8HW (United Kingdom)
[c]The Worcester Foundation for Experimental Biology
 Shrewsbury, Massachusetts 01545 (USA)

Contents

INTRODUCTION

The assay of cyclic nucleotide concentrations in biological material represents a considerable analytical challenge.
This is due both to the low concentrations normally present in
most cells and to the presence of other structurally similar
compounds in much higher concentrations. With the advent over the
last decade of numerous analytical procedures, the investigator
is now faced with an almost bewildering choice of assay techniques.
It is clearly beyond the scope of this paper to discuss each
method in detail. It is equally impossible to identify a preferred
method since the available procedures each have advantages and
disadvantages, and so the method of choice in each laboratory will
usually depend on special factors related to the system under

investigation and on the particular expertise of the investigators.
Particular assay parameters to be considered in making this choice
include sensitivity, specificity, precision and practicability.

Fortunately, most of the methods in current use have been
published in detail elsewhere and there have been a number of
excellent reviews (e.g. 1); the reader is directed particularly
towards Volume II of "Advances in Cyclic Nucelotide Research" (2),
"Cyclic AMP" (3), "Methods in Molecular Biology" (4) and "Methods
of Biochemical Analysis" (5). Since it would be inappropriate to
cover the same ground this article will deal primarily with the
advances that have occurred in the last two or three years, and
more particularly with the saturation assay systems.

METHOD OF CYCLIC AMP ANALYSIS

Initially, cyclic AMP determinations were based on the
ability of the nucleotide to increase the rate of conversion of
inactive liver phosphorylase to its active form (3.6). Later,
a number of assay techniques based on the conversion of cyclic
AMP to 5'AMP and then to ATP were developed. Various means for
detecting the ATP formed were employed, e.g. enzymatic cycling
and fluorometric detection (7), a radioactive phosphate exchange
reaction (8) or the use of the firefly luciferin-luciferase
reaction (2,9). These assay methods have the advantages of reproducibility and considerable sensitivity (5 x 10^{-14} moles cyclic AMP
may be detected), moreover the luciferase technique gives a linear
response over a fourfold concentration range. However, for best
results, it is essential that the samples and the enzymes used are
purified to remove other nucleotides which are normally present in
excess.

The principles of radioenzymatic assay were exploited by
Brooker and his colleagues (2, 10) for the assay of cyclic AMP.
Unfortunately, the Km for the phosphodiesterase, a factor
determining the sensitivity of this assay system is quite low.
High pressure ion exchange chromatography has been applied
successfully to the analysis of cyclic AMP concentrations, the
nucleotide being detected by an ultrasensitive 254nm absorption
flow cell (2,11). This technique has not been widely used despite claims that it is particularly reproducible and produces a
consistently linear response.

An assay technique based on the ability of low concentrations of cyclic AMP to activate cyclic AMP-dependent protein kinase, which catalyses the transfer of the terminal phosphate of ATP to protein substrates was developed by Kuo and
Greengard (2,12). Under certain conditions the extent of
histone phosphorylation is directly proportional to the, cyclic
AMP concentration. The minimum detectable concentration of
cyclic AMP in this method is approximately 0.3pmole.

A major advance in this field was the development in 1969 by Steiner and his coworkers of a radioimmunoassay procedure for cyclic AMP (13). These authors subsequently described similar assays for other cyclic nucleotides (14). These techniques are based on the saturation assay principle (15), and rely on the competition of the cyclic nucleotide with an isotopically labelled derivative for a limited number of binding sites on a specific antibody. In the original technique, cyclic AMP was succinylated at the 2'0 position and the free carboxyl group of this derivative was then coupled to protein (human serum albumin, keyhole limpet haemocyanin) or poly-L-lysine polymers. The resulting conjugate when injected into rabbits led to the production of extremely specific antisera after as little as 6 weeks. The tracer ligand used to reflect the extent of competitive cyclic AMP binding was a radio-iodinated tyrosyl derivative of the 2-O succinyl cyclic AMP. This material labelled with (^{125}I) can be prepared with high specific activities ($\sim$ 150 Ci/mmole), but it is relatively labile and has a fairly short half-life (60 days). It is possible to use (^{3}H)-cyclic AMP as the tracer ligand in radioimmunoassays. The advantages associated with the use of this tracer are its radiochemical stability, long half-life and relatively low cost. However, it can be prepared at only relatively low specific activities: approximately 28Ci/mmole of (8-^{3}H) cyclic AMP and approximately 50 Ci/mole of (2,8-^{3}H) cyclic AMP. In addition, considerably more antibody is necessary than with the (^{125}I)-succinyl cyclic AMP as tracer. This is probably due to the fact that the succinyl derivative more closely resembles the initial antigen, and thus may react with a higher avidity. When this results in higher sensitivity is dependent on the relationship between the avidity of the labelled derivative and that of the native molecule. In practice, it appears that this relationship and the higher specific activity attainable with the iodinated derivative do lead to higher sensitivity in many cases. One avenue not yet fully explored is the use of (^{3}H)-succinyl cyclic AMP which also reacts with a higher affinity towards the antibody.

The various techniques which have been used to separate the free nucleotide from that bound to the antiserum include precipitation of the bound with a second antibody, filtration through cellulose ester filters and precipitation with ammonium sulphate or polyethylene glycol. The sensitivity of this system is less than 0.1 pmole per incubation tube.

The sensitivity and specificity of the immunoassay system have permitted the measurement of cyclic AMP in small quantities of tissue normally without the need for sample purification (2, 16). The method is reproducible and simple to perform, the only obvious drawbacks being the preparation of the antigen and the labelled derivative (which has to be prepared every few months) and the fact that not all animals will produce usable antisera.

The fact that many antisera raised against succinyl cyclic AMP display a greater affinity for this derivative than for the unreacted nucleotide led Cailla et al. (17) to develop a radioimmunoassay method based on the systematic succinylation of assay samples. This reaction is reported to occur with a near 100% yield and their assay system has a sensitivity of about 10^{-15} mole cyclic AMP, but is clearly a little more tedious than the standard Steiner radioimmunoassay.

In the first years of this decade, three groups of workers developed the so-called "competitive protein binding assays" for cyclic AMP (18-20). The basic simplicity of these methods together with the high sensitivity and specificity rapidly resulted in their general acceptance. This type of assay, similar in principle to the radioimmunoassays, relies on endogenous binding proteins as the saturable reagent, and (^{3}H) cyclic AMP as the tracer. In practice this binding reagent (presumably the regulatory subunit of protein kinase) may be obtained from various tissues, e.g. skeletal muscle (18), adrenal glands (19,20), ovaries (21) and cerebral cortex (22). The question as to whether it is necessary to purify and characterise the binding agent has not been universally resolved - some arguing that it is a necessary prerequisite (e.g. 5) while others disagree (20,23). An interesting comparison may be made with radioimmunoassays where it is not normally regarded as necessary to isolate specific antibody populations from an antiserum for a reliable assay; albeit such isolation may, under certain circumstances, increase both sensitivity and specificity. The binding constants for the various kinase preparations used are similar at approximately $5 \times 10^{-10} - 1 \times 10^{-9}$M. In addition, the specificity characteristics are also similar from preparation to preparation and, while often lower than that of the radioimmunoassay, are probably adequate for most applications. A number of methods have been used to separate the protein bound and free moieties including filtration through cellulose ester filters (18), adsorption of the free nucleotide to charcoal (20) or ion exchange resin (24), and ammonium sulphate precipitation (21). A number of investigators (e.g. 6,25) have successfully combined the binding protein prepared as described by Gilman (18) with the charcoal separation step of Brown et al.   An interesting variation was introduced by Pliska et al. (26). They covalently attached cyclic AMP binding protein to sepharose 2B; the resulting insoluble compound retained all of the binding characteristics of the original protein mixture. This technique facilitated the separation step since the moieties could be easily separated by filtration or centrifugation.

The lower limit of detection of protein binding assays of cyclic AMP is normally less than 0.1 pmole (e.g. 18,20) but may be further lowered by the technique of 'disequilibrium' assay (or late addition of label assay) (see 27,28).

ASSAY OF CYCLIC AMP IN BIOLOGICAL SAMPLES

The following discussion is primarily concerned with the use of saturation assay techniques for the determination of cyclic AMP concentrations in biological samples. However, many of the matters raised and conclusions drawn may be equally applicable to other assay systems.

1. Extraction

Since it is clear that cyclic AMP concentrations in tissue can change rapidly after hormonal stimulation (and also possibly artefactually on handling the tissue), rapid fixation of the tissue is of the utmost importance if the measured cyclic AMP is to reflect accurately the physiological situation. Conventionally, the tissue has been subjected to quick-freezing to the temperature of liquid nitrogen (or isopentane cooled by liquid nitrogen) or to clamping between large metal blocks previously cooled in liquid nitrogen. Another technique is that of microwave irradiation which is particularly useful when the tissue is not readily accessible. However, certain reservations have been expressed regarding this procedure (5).

Once the tissue has been fixed, it is necessary to deproteinise the sample prior to assay. This is normally achieved by homogenisation in either trichloracetic acid (TCA) or perchloric acid (PCA). The addition of radioactively labelled cyclic AMP at this stage allows for the correction for any loss of the cyclic AMP during extraction and subsequent manipulations. The trichloracetic acid is removed by ether extraction and the perchloric acid by precipitation as the potassium salt. The cyclic AMP content of isolated cells may be extracted using the above methods or by the use of ethanol (29). These techniques serve both for fixation and extraction. In certain circumstances, it is possible to use 80% ethanol to extract cyclic AMP from tissues (30). The extraction of cyclic nucleotides from blood may be achieved with TCA or PCA (see ref. 31 for a discussion of the handling of blood samples), but it is also possible to assay cyclic AMP directly in diluted plasma (25,32). Urinary cyclic AMP assays pose few problems, the determinations being performed on diluted urine specimens. (31,32)

2. Sample Purification and Assay Interference

The extent to which purification procedures should be carried is dependent largely on the biological material under test and on the assay technique used. In many cases, extracts of biological specimens may be assayed directly by radioimmunoassay or protein binding assay without purification. This is due, in

part, to the specificity characteristics of the antisera and
binding proteins employed, and to the sensitivity attainable
relative to the concentration of cyclic AMP in the sample. Thus,
extensive dilution of the sample prior to assay is often possible
with consequent minimisation of 'non-specific' interference. True
cross-reaction with related compounds has not proven to be a
major problem (2,13,20). Even ATP does not interfere since it
reacts with cyclic AMP binding sites (on both antibodies and
binding proteins) with an energy at least four orders of magnitude
lower than the reaction energy of cyclic AMP.

Nevertheless, certain tissue extracts contain substances
which interfere with protein binding and radioimmunoassays. This
appears to be a particularly major problem with extracts of brain
(22,33). In addition, in the inevitable quest for higher sensitivity in response to the necessity to measure cyclic AMP in ever
decreasing amounts of material, non-specific interference (or
blank effects) have been observed with various samples (34). The
non-specific interference observed in saturation assays may be
manifest via an effect on the primary binding reaction between
cyclic AMP and its receptor protein, or antibody, either by alterations in the number of available binding sites or by affecting
the equilibrium constant of the reaction. Additionally, the
efficiency of the separation procedure for sequestering free from
bound nucleotide may be modified by substances in extracts. In
instances where low levels of cyclic AMP are being measured or
the changes are small, this interference may attain some significance and failure to eliminate its effect can give rise to misleading data. The usual solution to problems of this nature is
to extend the extraction procedures in an attempt to isolate
cyclic AMP and thereby eliminate any interference in the assay.
Probably the most commonly used technique in this context is ion
exchange column chromatography. Both anion (Dowex 1 or Dowex 2)
and cation (Dowex 50) exchange resins have been successfully
employed (see 5,22). Column chromatography on alumina (35) and
on PEI cellulose (see article by Jakobs et al. : this volume)
have also proved valuable either alone or in combination with
other techniques. Thin layer chromatography on various supports
has also been employed albeit less frequently. (The chapter by
Jakobs, Bohme and Schultz in this volume provides a more comprehensive review of these methods and they will not be considered
in detail here). Another popular purification procedure is the
$BaSO_4$ co-precipitation method originally described by Krishna
et al. (36) for adenylate cyclase determinations. It is worth
re-emphasising that this method - in which the $BaSO_4$ is generated
from $ZnSO_4$ and $Ba(OH)_2$, - is unsuitable for use on unpurified
extracts. This is due to the non-enzymic generation of cyclic
AMP from ATP under the conditions used. Moreover, the use of

this method after purification may also be contraindicated since
zinc ions markedly affect some saturation assay systems (34).
Although these purification techniques clearly have a place in
cyclic AMP methodology, it should be noted that such procedures
often result in a significant reduction in the recovery of cyclic
AMP from the initial starting material (although it is possible
to apply a correction); they are not always successful in completely eliminating interference (blanks) in the assay; they
often contribute their own blank effects, and furthermore, they
do not always lend themselves to routine analysis of large
numbers of samples.

Various techniques have been devised for eliminating the
effects of interfering substances. For example, Weller et al.
(33) developed a method involving the assay of each sample with
and without internal standards. Tovey et al. (25) have, by
adapting the published saturation assay systems (18,20), developed
an assay system that is relatively free of interference problems
but with slightly lower sensitivity. Since the magnitude of non-
specific effects depends inter alia on the degree of sample
dilution and on the inherent sensitivity of the assay; an assay
set up with low sensitivity (i.e. high detection limit) will be
normally less prone to the effects of interfering substances.
We have adhered to the principle, common in hormone assays, that
valid assays are those in which the standards and unknowns differ
(as far as is possible) only in their cyclic AMP content. Thus,
unknown samples are compared with standards set up in a milieu
supplemented with an equivalent amount of reagent, incubation
medium, nucleotide-free plasma, etc. It is important that complete response curves are set up in this way since, when expressed
in terms of an incremental concentration of cyclic AMP, the
magnitude of non-specific effects is extremely dependent on the
concentration of cyclic AMP under assay. It follows that it is
not generally legitimate to subtract 'blank' values measured at
zero added nucleotide from measurements of the unknown sample.
As noted earlier, purification procedures often give rise to blank
effects and therefore it is necessary to add an amount of 'reagent
blank' (e.g. chromatographic eluate) to the standards which is
equivalent to that in the unknown sample. Only if it can be
shown beyond doubt that the response curves with and without
'reagent blank' are identical, is it reasonable to dispense with
this procedure. It is also well worth ascertaining whether added
substances (e.g. hormones, catecholamines, inhibitors, etc.)
interfere in the assay. Some of these compounds may co-chromato-
graph with cyclic AMP, and so again it is advisable to take the
various incubation media used through the entire extraction and
purification procedure and to add equivalent amounts to assay
standards.

However, the assay of samples before and after purification is a useful test of validity, particularly if the foregoing comments are borne in mind. Other tests of validity include sample dilution and recovery of exogenous nucleotide although both may be open to criticism under certain circumstances (34). The complete hydrolysis of cyclic AMP by phosphodiesterase is also an important check on the validity of the measurements - again amended reagent blank curves may be necessary (34).

SUMMARY

It has not been our purpose in this article to present recipes for valid cyclic AMP assays; this has been very success-fully achieved by others (see Introduction). Rather to outline the various procedures available to investigators in this field and, more particularly, to concentrate on the saturation assay systems which seem to have become the methods of choice in a large number of laboratories. (The reason for this emphasis has been largely dictated by our own rather limited experience.) In addition, we considered that it was probably worth re-emphasing that there are pitfalls associated with the use of these tech-niques. Of course, we have been able only to discuss those pro-blems that we have encountered or that have been communicated to us, but at least some of the pitfalls have been identified and solutions proposed. Alternative solutions can be, and indeed have been, suggested. It is to be hoped that such re-appraisals of techniques lead to continual refinement of assay protocols.

REFERENCES

(1) BRECKENRIDGE, B.McL. (1971), Ann. N.Y., Acad. Sci. 185, 10

(2) Advances in Cyclic Nucleotide Research, Volume 2 (1972), Edited by Greengard, P. and Robison, G.A., Raven Press, New York

(3) Cyclic AMP (1971), Edited by Robison, G.A., Butcher, R.W., Sutherland, E.W., Academic Press, New York and London

(4) Methods in Molecular Biology, Volume 3 (1972), Edited by Chasin, M., Marcel Dekker, Inc., New York

(5) BROOKER, G. (1974). Methods in Biochemical Analysis, 22, 95

(6) RALL, T.W., and SUTHERLAND, E.W., (1958) J. Biol. Chem., 232, 1065

(7)   GOLDBERG, N.D., LARNER, J., SASKO, H., and O'TOOLE, A.G.
      (1969). Anal. Biochem., 28, 523

(8)   AURBACH, G.D., and HOUSTON, B.A. (1968), J. Biol. Chem., 243,
      5935

(9)   JOHNSON, R.A., HARDMAN, J.G., BROADUS, A.E., and SUTHERLAND,
      E.W. (1970), Anal. Biochem., 35, 91

(10) BROOKER, G., THOMAS, L.J., and APPLEMAN, M.M. (1968), Bio-
      chemistry, 7, 4177

(11) BROOKER, G. (1971), J. Biol. Chem., 246, 7810

(12) KUO, J.F., and GREENGARD, P. (1970), J. Biol. Chem., 245,
      4067

(13) STEINER, A.L., KIPNIS, D.M., UTIGER, R., and PARKER, C.
      (1969), Proc. Nat. Acad. Sci. (USA), 64, 367

(14) STEINER, A.L., PARKER, C.W., and KIPNIS, D.M. (1972), J.
      Biol. Chem., 247, 1106

(15) EKINS, R.P., NEWMAN, G.B., and O'RIORDAN, J.L.H. (1968),
      Radioisotopes in Medicine: In Vitro Studies 59, Edited by
      Hayes, R.L., Goswitz, F.A., and Pearson Murphy, B.E.

(16) STEINER, A.L., WEHMANN, R.E., PARKER, C.W., and KIPNIS, D.M.
      (1972). Advances in Cyclic Nucleotide Research 2, 51,
      Edited by Greengard, P., and Robison, G.A., Raven Press, New
      York

(17) CAILLA, H.L., RACINE-WEISBUCH, M.S., and DeLAAGE, M.A.
      (1973), Anal. Biochem., 56, 394

(18) GILMAN, A.G. (1970). Proc. Nat. Acad. Sci. (USA), 67, 305

(19) WALTON, G.M., and GARREN, L.D. (1970), Biochemistry, 9, 4233

(20) BROWN, B.L., ALBANO, J.D.M., EKINS, R.P., SGHERZI, A.M., and
      TAMPION, W. (1971), Biochem. J., 121, 561

(21) SANBORN, B.M., BHALLA, R.C., and KORENMAN, S.G. (1973).
      Endocrinology, 92, 494

(22) WEINRYB, I. (1972), Methods in Molecular Biology, 3, 29,
      Edited by Chasin, M. Marcel Dekker, Inc., New York

(23) BROWN, B.L., EKINS, R.P., and ALBANO, J.D.M. (1972). Advances in Cyclic Nucleotide Research, 2, 25. Edited by Greengard, P. and Robison, G.A., Raven Press, New York

(24) TSANG, C.P.W., LEHOTAY, D.C., and PEARSON MURPHY, B.E. (1972) J. Clinc. Endocrinol. Metabol. 35, 809

(25) TOVEY, K.C., OLDHAM, K.G., and WHELAN, J.A.M. (1974). Clinica Chimica Acta, 56, 221

(26) FISCH, H.U., PLISKA, V., and SCHWYZER, R. (1972). Experientia 28, 630

(27) COOPER, R.H., ASHCROFT, S.J.H., RANDLE, P.J. (1973), Biochem. J., 134, 599

(28) BROWN, B.L., ALBANO, J.D.M., BARNES, G.D., and EKINS, R.P., (1974), Biochem. Soc. Trans., 2, 388

(29) ALBANO, J.D.M., BROWN, B.L., EKINS, R.P., TAIT, S.A.S., and TAIT, J.F. (1974), Biochem. J., 142, 391

(30) ALBANO, J.D.M., and BROWN, B.L. Unpublished observations.

(31) BROADUS, A.E., HARDMAN, J.G., KAMINSKY, N.I., BALL, J.H., SUTHERLAND, E.W., and LIDDLE, G.W. (1971). Ann. N.Y. Acad. Sci. 185, 50

(32) TOMLINSON, S., BARLING, R.M., ALBANO, J.D.M., BROWN, B.L., and O'RIORDAN, J.L.H. (1974), Clin. Sci. and Mol. Med., 47, 481

(33) WELLER, M., RODNIGHT, R., and CARRERA, D. (1972), Biochem. J. 129, 113

(34) ALBANO, J.D.M., BARNES, G.D., MAUDSLEY, D.V., BROWN, B.L., and EKINS, R.P. (1974). Anal. Biochem., 60, 130

(35) RAMACHANDRAN, J. (1971), Anal. Biochem., 43, 227

(36) KRISHNA, G., WEISS, B., and BRODIE, B.B. (1968), J. Pharma. Exper. Therap., 163, 379

DETERMINATION OF CYCLIC GMP IN BIOLOGICAL MATERIAL

Karl Heinrich Jakobs
Eycke Böhme
Günter Schultz

Department of Pharmacology
University of Heidelberg
D-6900 Heidelberg (Germany)

Contents

Determination of cyclic GMP
Application to biological material

INTRODUCTION

Guanosine 3',5'-monophosphate (cGMP) has been detected in most animal (11) and plant (12) tissues and in bacteria (1). Its concentration generally varies between 10^{-8} and 10^{-7} mol/kg wet weight, although in some cases it can be as high as 10^{-6} mol/kg (11). This is very low compared to the concentrations of related nucleotides and of cAMP.

In the last few years remarkable progress has been made in analyzing cGMP levels in biological material. The presently available methods are reviewed in this paper.

DETERMINATION OF CYCLIC GMP

A variety of assays for cGMP has been published in the last few years (Table I). The basis of the first two assays published was enzymatic cycling (9, 13, 14). Both assays being too laborious are not used anymore. An enzymatic isotope displacement procedure using high affinity cyclic nucleotide phosphodiesterase

TABLE I. Published assays for cGMP

AUTHORS	PRINCIPLE	SENSITIVITY (pmol/tube)
Hardman et al., 1966, 1969	enzymatic cycling	>1
Brooker et al., 1968	enzymatic isotope displacement	20
Goldberg et al., 1969	enzymatic cycling	0.1
Steiner et al., 1969, 1972	radioimmunoassay	<0.1
Murad et al., 1971, Dinnendahl, 1974	protein binding (protein kinase)	0.1 – 1
Brooker, 1972	high pressure anion-exchange chromatography, UV absorption	
Kuo et al., 1972	protein kinase activation	1
Schultz et al., 1973	enzymatic conversion	<0.1

(4) was used for cAMP determinations, but has not been applied to
cGMP determinations; the theoretical sensitivity, which highly
depends on the K_m of the phosphodiesterase used, is low as compared to other available assays for cGMP. The high pressure
chromatography technique described (3) for separation and determination of cAMP has not been used for the determination of cGMP
in tissues.

Kuo, Greengard and their associates (18, 19) described the
occurrence of protein kinases stimulated by cGMP in various arthropoda. cGMP-dependent protein kinases isolated from lobster tail
muscle and from the fat body of silkmoth pupae have been used for
cGMP determination using the following principle (20) :

$$\text{histone} + \{\gamma\text{-}^{32}P\} \text{ ATP} \xrightarrow[\text{protein kinase}]{\text{cGMP}} {}^{32}P\text{-histone} + \text{ADP}$$

Under appropriate conditions, the formation of ^{32}P-histone is
directly proportional to the concentration of cGMP in the assay
tubes. The sensitivity of the assay is about 1 pmol of cGMP per
tube.

cGMP-stimulated protein kinases from lobster tail muscle and
from silkmoth have also been used for competitive binding assays
cGMP[1] (7, 22, 32). In these assays, cGMP competes with tritiated
cGMP for binding sites on the regulatory subunit ("binding protein")
of the protein kinases. The assay can be performed under equilibrium conditions; the sensitivity is about 1 pmol/tube with the
lobster protein and may be slightly better with the protein kinase
prepared from silkmoth. The sensitivity of the assay can be
increased by disequilibrium conditions (Figure 1) or by using the
sequential saturation technique (33) which has been applied so far
only to the binding assay of cAMP (6). For separation of protein
kinase-bound from free cyclic nucleotide, various methods have
successfully been used. These include filtration through cellulose
ester filters, ammonium sulfate precipitation and adsorption to
Dextran- or to albumin-coated charcoal.

Steiner et al. (28, 29) have described a radioimmunoassay for
cGMP in which cGMP competes with ^{125}I- or ^{131}I-labelled 2'0-
succinyl tyrosyl methyl ester of cGMP for binding sites on an antibody against succinyl cGMP. The ^{125}I-succinyl cGMP tyrosyl methyl

----

[1]Kits for cGMP determination based on binding proteins isolated
from lobster tail muscle and from silkmoth will be available from
the Radiochemical Centre, Amersham, and from Boehringer Mannheim
Corporation, respectively.

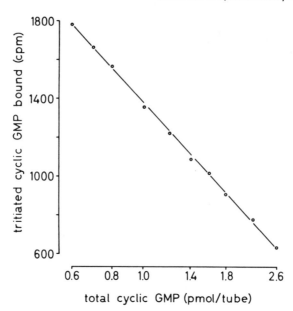

FIGURE 1. *Standard curve for cGMP in a protein-binding assay. Various amounts of cGMP were incubated with 0.6 pmol of tritiated cGMP (corresponding to 4,500 cpm) and an amount of cyclic GMP-stimulated silkmoth protein kinase that was capable of binding 40 % of the tritiated cGMP within 20 minutes at 0°C. The incubation was performed in 200 µl of a 50 mM sodium acetate buffer, pH 4.0. Bound cyclic GMP was separated from the free nucleotide by ammonium sulfate precipitation.*

ester – antibody complex is separated from free ^{125}I-succinyl cGMP tyrosyl methyl ester by filtration, ammonium sulfate or polyethylene glycol precipitation or by charcoal adsorption. Antibody[1] is obtained by immunization against succinyl cGMP coupled to human serum albumin (28, 29).

The sensitivity of the radioimmunoassay for cGMP is usually a little better than 0.1 pmol/tube when equilibrium conditions

---

[1]Succinyl cGMP and its tyrosyl methyl ester have become commercially available from Boehinger Mannheim Corporation and Sigma; cGMP antibody and ^{125}I-succinyl cGMP tyrosyl methyl ester from Collaborative Research and from Schwarz-Mann.

are used (Figure 2). The sensitivity is possibly increased by
applying a sequential saturation technique (33). Cailla *et al.*
(5) recently showed that the sensitivity of the cAMP radioimmunoassay can be increased markedly by succinylation of the
cAMP in the tissue extracts. Since cGMP can similarly be succinylated in aqueous solution, this technique will also be applicable
to cGMP radioimmunoassays. Although the use of the sequential
saturation technique and of cyclic nucleotide succinylation increase the sensitivity of the method, these modifications also make
the determination more complex and thus more liable to additional
error potential.

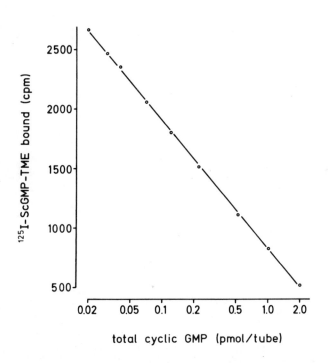

total cyclic GMP (pmol/tube)

FIGURE 2. *Standard curve for cGMP in a radioimmunoassay.*
Various amounts of cGMP were incubated with 0.02 pmol of [125]I-
tyrosol methyl ester of succinyl cGMP (^{125}I-ScGMP-TME*) corres-*
ponding to 8,400 cpm and an amount of cGMP antibody that was
sufficient to bind 32 % of the ^{125}I-ScGMP-TME. *The incubation*
was performed in 200 µl of a 50 mM imidazole buffer, pH 7.0, for
18 hours at 0°C. Bound cGMP was separated from the free nucleo-
tide by polyethylene glycol precipitation.

Another relatively sensitive assay for cGMP was recently described by Schultz *et al.* (25, 27). It is based on the following enzymatic steps:

$$cGMP \xrightarrow{\text{phosphodiesterase}} GMP$$

$$GMP + \{\gamma -{}^{32}P\}\ ATP \xrightarrow{\text{GMP kinase}} \{\beta -{}^{32}P\}\ GDP + ADP$$

The remaining labelled ATP is degraded :

$$\{\gamma -{}^{32}P\} \xrightarrow{\text{myosin}} {}^{32}P_i + ADP$$

and the labelled inorganic phosphate is precipitated as phosphate-molybdate-triethylamine complex. ^{32}P-GDP formed proportionally to the amount of cyclic GMP remains in the supernatant fluid and is counted. The sensitivity of this assay depends on the materials used, especially on the specific activity and purity of the $\{\gamma -{}^{32}P\}$ ATP and on the purity of the enzymes. The standard curve represents a direct proportional relationship between cGMP concentration from about 0.02 to 1 or 2 pmol/tube and the ^{32}P counted (Figure 3). Thereby, detection of very small amounts of cGMP and of small differences in cGMP levels is possible.

APPLICATION TO BIOLOGICAL MATERIAL

The determination of cyclic nucleotide levels in biological material requires some provisions to prevent the interference by enzymes and other tissue constituents (for review see: 10). To avoid changes of cyclic nucleotide levels during handling of the tissue, rapid fixation is accomplished by freezing of the material in a Wollenberger-type of aluminium clamp or in Freon 12 or iso-pentane cooled in liquid nitrogen. Fixation can also be accomplishe by microwave radiation (24). Tissues and cells must be dis-integrated (by various types of homogenizers) for extraction of cyclic nucleotides. To denature and remove enzymes from the tissue extracts, acids are usually added before or after tissue disinte-gration. Most frequently used are trichloroacetic acid and per-chloric acid which can easily be removed by ether or chloroform extraction and by precipitation as potassium salt, respectively. When anion-exchange procedures are used for cyclic nucleotide purification, homogenization in 50 % ethanol containing 50 mM zinc acetate is useful (25). Besides inhibiting and removing enzymes, the zinc salt can be used for an easy purification step removing 5'-nucleotides (see below).

Most if not all cyclic nucleotide assays require the preceding purification of biological material to remove endogenous or exogen-ous substances that can interfere with the assay. Although some

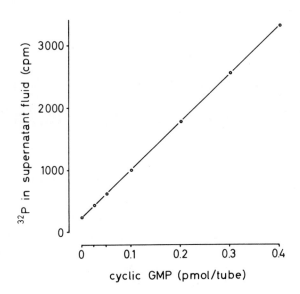

<u>FIGURE 3</u>.   *Standard curve for cGMP in an enzymatic assay.   Various
amounts of cGMP were incubated with phosphodiesterase, ATP : GMP
phosphotransferase and {γ $-^{32}$P} ATP (0.1 pmol corresponding to
24,000 cpm per tube).   The conditions were as previously described
(25, 27) except for the addition of 0.3 mM dithiothreitol and 0.1
mg/ml of bovine serum albumin for the 18 hours' incubation period
with ATP:GMP phosphotransferase.*

methods for cyclic nucleotide determination have recently been
introduced that seem to require no or only little purification of
tissue extracts, it is still necessary to prove by control experiments that no purification is required for the tissue or system
under study. Therefore, it may be better to purify tissue samples
routinely, especially since relatively easy and effective methods
for cyclic nucleotide purification have become available.

Besides enzymes, which are capable of altering the amount of
cyclic nucleotides in tissue extracts, a variety of compounds can
interfere with cyclic nucleotide determinations. Various cations
and anions present in tissue extracts can affect all types of
cyclic nucleotide assays. Purine nucleotides occurring in much
higher concentrations than cGMP especially interfere with enzymatic
assays of this cyclic nucleotide, but can also affect binding
assays of cGMP. The present useful possibilities to purify cyclic
nucleotides can be summarized as follows :

1. co-precipitation of 5'-nucleotides by $ZnCO_3$ or $CdCO_3$,

2. nucleotide adsorption to charcoal,

3. thin-layer chromatography on silica gel, aluminium oxide,
    cellulose or anion-exchange celluloses, e.g. polyethyleneimine
    (PEI) cellulose,

4. column chromatography on cation-exchange resin (Dowex-50), on
    anion-exchange materials (Dowex-1, QAE-Sephadex, PEI cellulose),
    or an aluminium oxide and

5. batch procedures employing aluminium oxide or anion exchange
    materials.

An easy but effective way to reduce the concentration of 5'-
nucleotides in tissue extracts is provided by inorganic salt precipitation steps. The $BaSO_4$ co-precipitation procedure of 5'-nucleo-
tides, which was described by Krishna *et al.* (17) and which should
not be applied to unpurified tissue extracts in any case, is not
applicable to cGMP purification (cGMP is largely precipitated by
$BaSO_4$). In contrast, $ZnCO_3$ (25) and $CdCO_3$ (15) only slightly
affect cyclic nucleotides while effectively co-precipitating 5'-
nucleotides (Table II). These carbonates can be generated from
Na_2CO_3, K_2CO_3 or $(NH_4)_2CO_3$ and any zinc or cadmium salt :

$$Zn^{++} + CO_3^{--} \longrightarrow ZnCO_3 \downarrow$$

$$Cd^{++} + CO_3^{--} \longrightarrow CdCO_3 \downarrow$$

TABLE II. Co-precipitation of 5'-nucleotides by $ZnCO_3$, $CdCO_3$ and Al_2O_3.

In 50 mM triethanolamine buffer, pH 7.0, containing nucleotides or nucleosides (about 20 μM), $ZnCO_3$ or $CdCO_3$ (50 mM) were formed by the addition of $Zn(CH_3COO)_2$ or $CdCl_2$ and Na_2CO_3. When Al_2O_3 (neutral) was added, its concentration was 100 mg/ml. After sedimentation of the carbonate or of the Al_2O_3, the amount of nucleotide or nucleoside remaining in the supernatant fluid was determined.

	% non-precipitated or non-adsorbed		
	$ZnCO_3$	$CdCO_3$	Al_2O_3
ATP, ADP	<1	<1	<1
5'-AMP	<10	<10	<1
cAMP	~100	~100	~100
Ado	~100	~100	~90
GTP, GDP	<1	<1	<1
5'-GMP	<10	<10	<1
cGMP	>80	>80	~100
Guo	>80	>80	~90

The $ZnCO_3$ or $CdCO_3$ concentration should be about 50 mM, the pH about neutral. The use of Zn offers the additional advantage of precipitating proteins, the use of zinc acetate rather than of the chloride or sulfate is preferable when anion-exchange chromatography steps follow.

For the determination of cyclic nucleotides in large volumes of biological media or tissue extracts, removal of salts and reduction of the volume may be required. Nucleotide adsorption to charcoal (in batch or as column) under acid conditions and desorption by alcohol and ammonia (30) is a helpful procedure.

Thin-layer chromatography has been applied to cyclic nucleotide purification (2), but column chromatography offers advantages especially in routine work. Thin-layer plates coated with silica gel (8), aluminium oxide (8), cellulose and anion-exchange celluloses, especially PEI cellulose (2), have been used.

The first material used in column chromatographic purification of cyclic nucleotides was the cation-exchange resin Dowex-50 (14, 26). This material developed with acid solvents (e.g. 0.1 N HCl) is especially useful if the samples contain large amounts of electrolytes (e.g. tissue or medium constituents and acid used for extraction), and the reproducibility is high. The sample volume, however, is limited; the resolution is poorer than that of some anion-exchange materials, and developing these columns is relatively time-consuming.

Anion-exchange columns have been used more recently for cyclic nucleotide purification. The application of anion-exchange materials to purification of cyclic nucleotides from tissue extracts is complicated and limited by the amount of electrolytes in the samples. Small columns of Dowex-1 developed with formic acid (22) or hydrochloric acid (4) have been used for the separation of cAMP and cGMP with relatively poor purification from other nucleotides. Small QAE-Sephadex columns developed with ammonium formate (25) give a better separation of the cyclic nucleotides from 5'-nucleotides. PEI cellulose developed with acetic acid and ammonium acetate (Figure 4) (16, 26) gives a better resolution than any other material mentioned, but requires preceding electrolyte removal in most cases.

Column chromatography of cyclic nucleotides on aluminium oxide developed with neutral solvents was originally used for adenylate and guanylate cyclase determinations (23, 31) and appears to be valuable for cyclic nucleotide purification from tissue extracts (21), especially for the separation from 5'-nucleotides. The preceding use of acid solvents results in a more extensive purification (Figure 5). cAMP and cGMP cochromatographing on aluminium oxide columns are separated from each other on a subsequent short anion- or cation-exchange column.

Batch procedures applying the compounds mentioned above to cyclic nucleotide purification have not been published yet except for aluminium oxide (7) but appear to be potentially valuable techniques (Table II).

Each step in the treatment of biological material results in some loss of cyclic nucleotide. To monitor the overall recovery, tritiated cyclic nucleotides are usually added as tracers as early as in the extraction step. The specific activity of the tritiated cGMP that is currently available[1] requires the addition of an amount of labelled cGMP that can be in the same order of

----

[1] The highest specific activity of tritiated cGMP presently available is about 20 Ci/mmol.

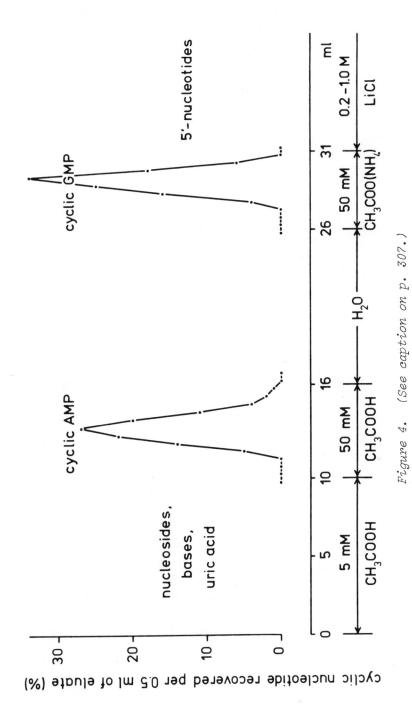

Figure 4. (See caption on p. 307.)

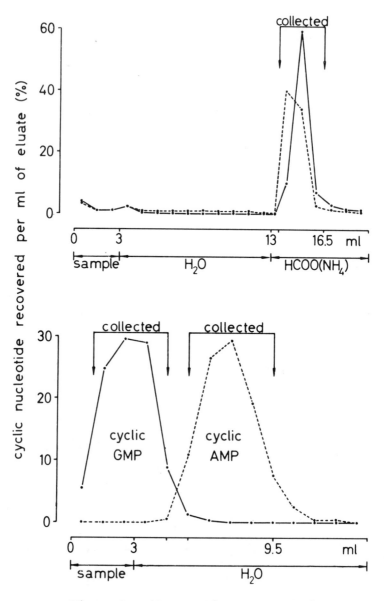

Figure 5.   (See caption on p. 307.)

FIGURE 4. *Elution profiles of cAMP and cGMP on PEI cellulose columns. Cyclic nucleotides (0.2 μmol of each) were applied in water, dilute acetic or formic acid to 6.5 x 0.5 cm columns of PEI cellulose. Nucleosides, bases and uric acid were eluted with 10 ml of 5 mM acetic acid, cAMP with 6 ml of 50 mM acetic acid followed by 10 ml of water. cGMP was eluted with 5 ml of 50 mM ammonium acetate. The elution of purine 5'-nucleotides required salt solutions of higher concentration (16, 26).*

FIGURE 5. *Elution profiles of cAMP (dotted line) and cGMP (solid line) on successive columns of aluminium oxide (upper panel) and Dowex-50 (lower panel). Cyclic nucleotides (0.2 μmol of each) were applied in 0.5 M perchloric acid (PCA) to 2.2 x 0.65 cm columns of neutral aluminium oxide. After application of 10 ml of distilled water, the solvent was changed to 0.2 M ammonium formate, pH 6.0. The first 0.5 ml was discarded, and the following 3 ml containing cAMP and cGMP were collected. 5'-nucleotides were retained by the column. For separation of cAMP and cGMP, the 3 ml - fraction containing the cyclic nucleotides was then applied to a 4 x 0.75 cm column of Dowex-50 W-X 8, 100 - 200 mesh, in H^+ form, followed by distilled water as solvent. The first ml of the eluate was discarded, and the following 3.5 ml containing cGMP were collected. After discarding the next 1 ml of the eluate, the following 4 - 5 ml containing cAMP were collected.*
For purification of cyclic nucleotides from tissue or plasma extracts prepared in 1 M PCA, the tissue sample should be followed by about 10 ml of 1 M PCA before the aluminium oxide column is developed with water and buffer.

magnitude as the endogenous cyclic nucleotide. Therefore, it is important to know the specific activity of the tritiated cyclic nucleotide exactly, considering that tritiated guanine nucleotides are particularly labile. This requires the repurification of the cyclic nucleotide from time to time and the determination of the molar amount of tritiated cGMP added which may need to be considered in calculating the endogenous amount of cyclic nucleotide.

The sufficiency of a certain purification procedure for biological samples is checked by including individual control tubes in the assay (see, e.g. 10, 27). In enzymatic assays of cGMP, the degradability by cyclic nucleotide phosphodiesterase is an important criterion, and besides the regular phosphodiesterase-containing tubes phosphodiesterase-free control tubes are generally used to

monitor the efficiency of the purification in each sample. To
check the validity of the determination of each sample, another
set of control tubes is generally included in which an internal
standard is added or the sample is assayed at another dilution.
In binding assays of cGMP, the reliability of the determination is
greatly validated by control tubes equivalent to those outlined
above for enzymatic assays. The possible induction of "blanks" by
the chromatographic procedure should be considered when using
binding assays for cyclic nucleotides.

In general, how much purification is necessary will depend on
the tissue and on the assay used. Enzymatic assays generally
require much more sample purification with regard to related nucleotides. The sufficiency of the purification procedure used must be
proven in each system.

Acknowledgments

The authors greatly appreciate valuable suggestions and criticism by Dr. Joel G. Hardman and skilful technical assistance of
Mrs. S. Mocikat and Mrs. E. Smend. The authors' studies
presented in this review were supported by grants of the
Deutsche Forschungsgemeinschaft. Cyclic GMP-stimulated protein
kinase from silkmoth pupae as part of the kit for cyclic GMP
determination was kindly supplied by Dr. P. Wunderwald,
Boehringer Mannheim GmbH, Tutzing, Germany.

REFERENCES

(1)   BERNLOHR, R.W., HADDOX, M.K. and GOLDBERG, N.D. (1974)
      Cyclic guanosine 3':5'-monophosphate in Escherichia coli
      and Bacillus licheniformis, J. Biol. Chem. 249, 4329

(2)   BÖHME, E., and SCHULTZ, G., (1974), Separation of cyclic
      nucleotides by thin layer chromatography on polyethylene-
      imine cellulose, in "Methods in Enzymology", ed. by S.P.
      Colowick and N.O. Kaplan, 38, 27

(3)   BROOKER, G. (1972), High pressure anion exchange chromato-
      graphy and enzymatic isotope displacement assays for cyclic
      AMP and cyclic GMP, Adv. Cyclic Nucl. Research 2, 111

(4)   BROOKER, G., THOMAS, L.J. and APPLEMAN, M.M. (1968), The
      assay of adenosine 3':5'-cyclic monophosphate and guanosine
      3':5'-cyclic monophosphate in biological materials by enzyma-
      tic radioisotopic displacement, Biochemistry 7, 4177

(5)   CAILLA, H.L., RACINE-WEISBUCH, M.S. and DeLAAGE, M.A.
      (1973), Adenosine 3', 5' cyclic monophosphate assay at 10^{-15}
      mole level. Analyt. Biochem. 56, 394

(6)   COOPER, R.H., ASHCROFT, S.J.H., and RANDLE, P.J. (1973)
      Concentration of adenosine 3':5'-cyclic monophosphate in
      mouse pancreatic islets measured by a protein-binding radio-
      assay. Biochem. J. 134, 599

(7)   DINNENDAHL, V. (1974) A rapid and simple procedure for the
      determination of guanosine 3', 5'-monophosphate by use of
      the protein-binding method. Naunyn-Schmiedeberg's Arch.
      Pharmacol. 284, 55

(8)   FLOURET, G., and HECHTER, O (1974) Adsorption chromatography
      of cyclic nucleotides on silica gel and alumina thin-layer
      sheets. Analyt. Biochem. 58, 276

(9)   GOLDBERG, N.D., DIETZ, S.B. and O'TOOLE, A.G. (1969) Cyclic
      guanosine 3':5'-monophosphate in mammalian tissues and urine
      J. Biol. Chem. 244, 4458

(10) GOLDBERG, N.D. and O'TOOLE, A.G. (1971) Analysis of cyclic
      3',5'-adenosine monophosphate and cyclic 3'5'-guanosine mono-
      phosphate, in "Methods Biochem. Anal.", ed. by D. Glick,
      Vol. 20, 1

(11) GOLDBERG, N.D., O'DEA, R.F. and HADDOX, M.K. (1973), Cyclic
      GMP, Adv. Cycl. Nucl. Res. 3, 155

(12) HADDOX, M.K., STEPHENSON, J.H., and GOLDBERG, N.D. (1974)
      Cyclic GMP in meristematic and elongating regions of bean
      root. Fed. Proc. 33, 522

(13) HARDMAN, J.G., DAVIS, J.W. and SUTHERLAND, E.W. (1966).
      Measurement of guanosine 3', 5'-monophosphate and other
      cyclic nucleotides. Variations in urinary excretion with
      hormonal state of the rat. J. Biol. Chem. 241, 4812

(14) HARDMAN, J.G., DAVIS, J.W. and SUTHERLAND, E.W. (1969).
      Effects of some hormonal and other facts on the excretion of
      guanosine 3', 5'-monophosphate and adenosine 3',5'-mono-
      phosphate in rat urine. J. Biol. Chem. 244, 6354

(15) JAKOBS, K.H., BÖHME, E., MOCIKAT, S. (1974). Cyclic GMP forma-
      tion in human platelets. Naunyn-Schmiedeberg's Arch.
      Pharmacol. 282, R 40

(16) JAKOBS, K.H., BÖHME, E., SCHULTZ, G. (1974). Determination
      of cyclic GMP and cyclic AMP in human platelets. Second
      International Conference on Cyclic AMP, Vancouver 1974,
      Abstracts, 51

(17) KRISHNA, G., WEISS, B. and BRODIE, B.B. (1968) A simple
      sensitive method for the assay of adenyl cyclase. J.
      Pharmacol. exper. Therap. 163, 379

(18) KUO, J.F., and GREENGARD, P. (1970) Cyclic nucleotide-
      dependent protein kinases. VI. Isolation and partial puri-
      fication of a protein kinase activated by guanosine 3',5'-
      monophosphate. J. Biol. Chem. 245, 2493

(19) KUO, J.F., WYATT, G.R. and GREENGARD, P. (1971) Cyclic
      nucleotide-dependent protein kinases. IX. Partial puri-
      fication and some properties of guanosine 3',5'-mono-
      phosphate-dependent and adenosine 3',5'-monophosphate-de-
      pendent protein kinases from various tissues and species
      of arthropoda. J. Biol. Chem. 246, 7159

(20) KUO, J.F., LEE, T.P., REYES, P.L., WALTON, K.G. DONNELLY,
      T.E., and GREENGARD, P. (1972) Cyclic nucleotide-dependent
      protein kinases. X. Assay method for measurement of
      guanosine 3',5'-monophosphate in various biological
      materials and a study of agents regulating its levels in
      heart and brain. J. Biol. Chem. 247, 16

(21) MAO, C.C., and GUIDOTTI, A. (1974) Simultaneous isolation
      of adenosine 3',5'-cyclic monophosphate (cAMP) and guanosine
      3',5'-cyclic monophosphate (cGMP) in small tissue samples.
      Analyt. Biochem. 59, 63

(22) MURAD, F., MANGANIELLO, V., and VAUGHAN, M. (1971). A simple,
      sensitive protein-binding assay for guanosine 3',5'-
      monophosphate. Proc.Nat.Acad.Sci. US, 88, 736

(23) NAKAZAWA, K., and SANO, M. (1974). Studies on guanylate
      cyclase. A new assay method for guanylate cyclase and pro-
      perties of the cyclase from rat brain. J. Biol. Chem. 249,
      4207

(24) SCHMIDT, M.J., SCHMIDT, D.E., and ROBISON, G.A. (1971)
      Cyclic adenosine monophosphate in brain areas : Microwave
      irradiation as a means of tissue fixation. Science 173,
      1142

(25) SCHULTZ, G., HARDMAN, J.G., SCHULTZ, K., DAVIS, J.W. and
      SUTHERLAND, E.W. (1973). A new enzymatic assay for guanosine
      3':5'-cyclic monophosphate and its application to the ductus
      deferens of the rat. Proc.Nat.Acad.Sci. US, 70, 1721

(26) SCHULTZ, G., BÖHME, E., and HARDMAN, J.G. (1974). Separation
      and purification of cyclic nucleotides by ion-exchange resin
      column chromatography, in "Methods in Enzymology", ed. by
      S.P. Colowick and N.O. Kaplan, 38, 9

(27) SCHULTZ, G., and HARDMAN, J.G. (1974). Determination of cyclic
      GMP by formation of (β-^{32}P) GDP, in "Methods in Enzymology",
      ed. by S.P. Colowick and N.O. Kaplan, 38, 106

(28) STEINER, A.L., KIPNIS, D.M., UTIGER, R.D. and PARKER, C.W.
      (1969), Radioimmunoassay for the measurement of adenosine
      3',5'-cyclic phosphate. Proc. Nat. Acad. Sci. US, 64, 367

(29) STEINER, A.L., PARKET, C.W. and KIPNIS, D.M. (1972) Radio-
      immunoassay for cyclic nucleotides. I. Preparation of anti-
      bodies and iodinated cyclic nucleotides. J. Biol. Chem. 247,
      1106

(30) TSUBOI, K.K., and PRICE, T.D. (1959). Isolation, detection
      and measure of microgram quantities of labeled tissue
      nucleotides. Arch. Biochem. Biophys. 81, 223

(31) WHITE, A.A., ZENSER, T.V. (1971) Separation of cyclic 3',5'-
      nucleotide monophosphates from other nucleotides on aluminum
      oxide columns. Application to the assay of adenyl cyclase
      and guanyl cyclase. Analyt. Biochem. 41, 372

(32) WUNDERWALD, P., and MICHAL, G. (1974), personal communication

(33) ZETTNER, A., and DULY, P.E. (1974). Principles of competitive
      binding assays (Saturation analyses). II. Sequential
      saturation. Clin. Chem. 20, 5

METHODS FOR THE STUDY OF CYCLIC AMP METABOLISM IN INTACT CELLS

John P. Perkins, Ying-Fu Su, Gary L. Johnson,
Rainer Ortmann, and Ben H. Leichtling

Department of Pharmacology
University of Colorado Medical School
Denver, Colorado 80220

Table of Contents

INTRODUCTION

The concentration of adenosine $3':5'$ -monophosphate (cAMP) in cells is determined predominantly by the relative rates of synthesis by adenylate cyclase and degradation by phosphodiesterase; although other contributing factors may exist. For example, a significant portion of the cAMP content under basal conditions may exist in a protein-bound form that is not susceptible to hydrolysis by phosphodiesterase activity (1). Also, in certain cases the rate of secretion of cAMP from hormon-ally-stimulated cells can be a major factor in determining the intracellular content (2,3). It is usually assumed that hormones elicit a rise in cellular cAMP levels by activation of adenylate cyclase. However, if some degree of turnover of cAMP occurs under basal conditions, then theoretically, the steady state level of cAMP could be raised by either an increase in its rate of synthesis or a decrease in its rate of degradation.

Attempts to account for changes in cellular cAMP content or for changes in the magnitude of response to a hormone by measuring changes in adenylate cyclase and phosphodiesterase activities in homogenates is usually a fruitless effort. Alterations in the integrity of the fragile adenylate cyclase systems is probably the basis for the often observed differences in hormonal respon-siveness of whole cells and their homogenates (4). Under certain circumstances changes in the responsiveness of cells to hormones may well be caused by factors which result in altered phos-phodiesterase activity (5,6,7). However, the existence of multiple forms of this enzyme (8,9) makes it difficult to detect changes in the activity of the single form that may be responsi-ble for the observed change in hormonal responsiveness.

Such circumstances make it advantageous to have at hand methods for the analysis of rates of synthesis, degradation and turnover of cAMP in whole cells. In this article, we discuss certain procedures currently used in our laboratory for such analyses.

METHODS

Experimental Incubation Conditions

Slices of rat cerebral cortex. The methodology utilized for estimating the effects of catecholamines on the cAMP content of brain slices has been described in detail previously (22,23).

Astrocytoma cells in culture. If changes in cAMP were to be determined by the pre-labeling technique (21), the cultures (4-5 x 10^5 cells per 35 mm dish) were incubated with 10 µCi ^{3}H-adenine (14 Ci/mmole) for 1 or more hr in complete growth medium. The medium was then aspirated and the attached cells washed and incubated with test agents in 2.0 ml of growth medium minus serum. A detailed description of the labeling conditions

and the kinetic characteristics of the incorporation of label into
ATP and cAMP has been presented elsewhere (19,20).

Measurement of ^{3}H-cAMP or cAMP content

Trichloracetic acid extracts of cells or brain slices containing cAMP were applied directly to Dowex-50w-x8 columns previously washed with 1.0 N HCl then water. A fraction containing
primarily ATP (90% of radioactivity) and ADP (8% of radioactivity)
as determined by chromatography on DEAE-81 ion-exchange paper, was
eluted by the sequential addition to the column of 1.5 ml of 0.1 N
HCl and 1.5 ml water. Cyclic AMP was then eluted from the column
with 3 x 1.0 ml water. An aliquot of this fraction could be used
to determine the cAMP content of the cells by the Gilman (12)
binding assay. If the cells were prelabeled, the ^{3}H-cAMP was
further purified. The cAMP-containing fraction eluted from Dowex
columns was brought to pH 8.0 with Trisma base and passed over
columns of neutral alumina (Woelm) (20). Recovery of cAMP
throughout the purification procedure was determined by the use of
standards and all values reported below have been corrected based
on recovery standards. In some cases the results are reported as
"% conversion". Such values represent dpm of (^{3}H-cAMP x 100)/dpm
of (^{3}H-ADP + ^{3}H-ADP + ^{3}H-cAMP).

Determination of ATP

ATP content was measured in the Dowex-50w-x8 fractions by
the luciferin-luciferase method using a liquid scintillation
counter as described by Stanley and Williams (28).

RESULTS

Determination of Changes in Cellular cAMP Content

The determination of changes in cAMP levels in cells is
readily accomplished by a number of procedures which have been
described in detail by others (10-14). Binding of cAMP to
specific proteins and the quantitation of such binding by isotope
dilution analysis is the most commonly used procedure. The
binding protein employed is usually the regulatory subunit of
protein kinase (12,15) or an antibody to cAMP (13). Such procedures allow an estimation of the absolute amount of cAMP in a
tissue sample. An alternate procedure, involving radioisotopic
labeling of cellular cAMP, allows the detection of changes in
cAMP content but does not provide an estimation of the absolute
amount of cAMP (16,17). This method is briefly described here

as we have used it for the analysis of changes in the cAMP content of human astrocytoma cells (1321N1) in cultures (18-20).

When monolayer cultures of 1321N1 cells are incubated in the presence of ^{3}H-adenine or ^{3}H-adenosine, the labeled precursors are taken into the cell and converted largely to ATP (Fig. 1). If the culture is washed free of excess ^{3}H-adenine and the incubation continued, the amount of ^{3}H-ATP in the cells declines only slowly (Fig. 1B). If the cells are exposed to norepinephrine (NE), there is a rapid rise in the cellular content of ^{3}H-cAMP whether the

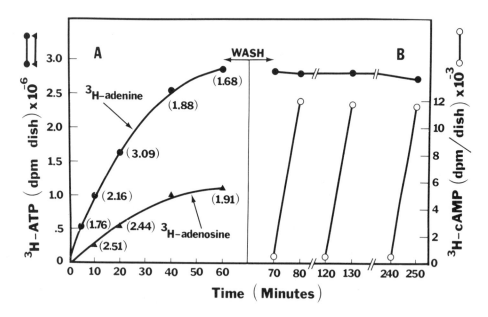

Fig. 1.   Kinetics of labeling of 1321N1 cells with ^{3}H-adenine and ^{3}H-adenosine.   (A) Cells were incubated with ^{3}H-adenine or ^{3}H-adenosine (5 µCi; 0.5 nmoles) in 2.0 ml of medium containing 5% serum.   At the times indicated the incubations were terminated, ^{3}H-ATP extracted, and purified on Dowex-50 columns.   In parallel experiments cultures labeled for the times indicated were washed free of exogenous labeled precursor and then incubated in the presence of 100 µM NE for 5 min.   The ^{3}H-cAMP formed was extracted and purified by the standard procedure.   The values in brackets represent the percentage conversion of ^{3}H-ATP to ^{3}H-cAMP.   (B) Cells labeled as in (A) with ^{3}H-adenine were washed free of exogenous label and the incubation continued in the absence of label. At the times indicated 100 µM NE was added for 10 min.   The ^{3}H-ATP and ^{3}H-cAMP were extracted and purified by standard procedures.

cells are stimulated immediately after washing (70 min) or 3 hrs later (Fig. 1B). These observations suggest that the ^{3}H-ATP pool serving as substrate for adenylate cyclase is reasonably stable.

If NE is added to cultures at various points during the course of labeling with ^{3}H-adenine or ^{3}H-adenosine, the same percentage of the ^{3}H-ATP is converted to ^{3}H-cAMP (Fig. 1A). The numbers in brackets indicate the percentage conversion of ^{3}H-ATP to ^{3}H-cAMP. Such results indicate that the ATP pool is not expanded during labeling and suggest that both precursors are labeling the same pool of ATP, albeit at different rates.

Two other observations indicate that most of the cellular ATP is available to adenylate cyclase in these cells.   (1) The specific

Table 1. The specific activity of ATP and cyclic AMP in 1321N1 cells during the time course response to 100 μM NE.

Time addition of NE (min.)	ATP			Cyclic AMP
	Radioactivity[1]	Concentration[2]	Sp. Act[3]	Sp. Act[3]
0 (Basal)	7.0×10^6	30.3	231	209
10	7.1×10^6	28.1	252	183
30	6.2×10^6	29.8	207	205
60	7.3×10^6	32.5	225	194
90	6.3×10^6	29.9	210	198
			225	198

1. total dpm/petri dish of cells
2. total nmol/petri dish of cells
3. dpm/pmol

Table 2. The per cent conversion of total cell content of ATP and radioactive ATP to cyclic AMP and the fold increases of cyclic AMP in 1321N1 cells during the time course of response to 100 μM NE.

Time after addition of NE (min)	Total Content		Radioisotope Pre-labeling	
	% Conv.	Fold Increase	% Conv.	Fold Increase
0 (Basal)	0.04	1	0.04	1
10	1.33	29.8	1.21	29.3
30	0.66	14.2	0.68	16.2
60	0.45	9.2	0.43	10.5
90	0.31	7.7	0.30	7.3

activity of the cAMP formed in the presence of NE is about the
same as the specific activity of total ATP (TCA-extractable ATP)
(Table 1). (2) The percentage conversion of total ATP to cAMP
in the presence of NE is the same as the percentage conversion of
[3]H-ATP to ^{3}H-cAMP (Table 2). In contrast, Shimizu and Daly (21)
have suggested that in guinea pig brain slices specific, unique-
labeled pools of ATP might serve as precursors for adenylate
cyclase.

When the changes in cAMP content elicited by NE in 1321N1 cells
are measured simultaneously by the pre-labeling method and the
Gilman binding assay, quite good agreement is obtained (19,20)
(Fig. 2A). Similar agreement of the two assays has been obtained
using slices of rat cerebral cortex as the test system (22,23)
(Fig. 2B). Of interest is the observation that the specific
activity of the cAMP formed in response to NE in the cortex slices
is the same as the specific activity of cAMP prior to stimulation.
This suggests that under basal conditions sufficient turnover of
cAMP occurs to allow incorporation of label into cAMP even though
the total level of cAMP does not change.

Although the pre-labeling technique is applicable to many
experimental systems, one should be wary of conditions which
might lead to changes in the specific activity of the ATP serving
as precursor which would result in artifactual, "apparent"
changes in cAMP content. When properly validated this procedure
provides a simple and highly reproducible assay for changes in
cAMP content. Of course, adequate purification of the ^{3}H-cAMP
is required for the use of the pre-labeling assay. Ion exchange
chromatography on Dowex 50 followed by chromatography on columns
of alumina (19,24) appears to provide sufficient purification.

Determination of the Rate of Synthesis of cAMP in Whole Cells

If the level of cAMP in cells represents a steady state due
to a balance of its rates of synthesis and degradation, then
activation of adenylate cyclase by a hormone would be expected to
cause a rise in cAMP content to a new steady state level (Fig. 3).
For this discussion we will assume that the rate of synthesis is
zero order with respect to the concentration of cAMP and that for
all levels of activation of adenylate cyclase saturating levels of
ATP exist. The rate of degradation will be assumed to be first
order and, in fact, can be shown to approximate first order
kinetics over a wide range of cellular cAMP concentrations (see
below). Thus, the velocity of the synthetic reaction (V_s) may
be described by equation [1] and the velocity of the degradative
reaction (V_d) by equation [2].

$$V_s = \frac{d[cAMP]}{dt} = k_s \qquad\qquad [1]$$

$$V_d = -\frac{d[cAMP]}{dt} = k_d [cAMP] \qquad\qquad [2]$$

The velocity of net accumulation of cAMP would be the resultant of both reactions and is described by equation [3].

$$V_{accum} = \frac{d[cAMP]}{dt} = k_s - k_d [cAMP] \qquad\qquad [3]$$

Integration of equation [3] yields equation [4],

$$[cAMP]_t = \frac{k_s}{k_d}(1-e^{k_d t}) \qquad\qquad [4]$$

where t is the time after the addition of the hormone and [cAMP]$_t$ is the concentration of cAMP at that point in time. It is apparent from equation [4] and Figure 3 that, upon addition of a hormone, the level of cAMP should assymptotically approach a new steady state level. The rate at which the new steady state is approached is determined only by the rate constant of degradation. The time taken to increase to one-half of the ultimate increase at the new steady state can be shown to be equal to the half-life of cAMP and is related to the rate constant of degradation as shown in equation [5].

$$t_{\frac{1}{2}} = \frac{0.693}{k_d} \qquad\qquad [5]$$

The magnitude of the new steady state level is determined by the ratio of the rate constant of synthesis to the rate constant of degradation. At steady state, by definition, $d[cAMP]/dt = 0$ and $k_s = k_d [cAMP]$; therefore, the concentration at steady state, [cAMP]ss, is equal to k_s/k_d.

This theoretical response is seldom observed upon addition of hormones to tissue preparations or cells in culture. Usually, the level of cAMP rises to a new level that is maintained only transiently and then the cAMP content slowly declines back toward basal levels even in the continued presence of active hormone (for example see Fig. 2A, ref. 20). In order to determine the basis for this biphasic response to hormones we have attempted to measure directly the rates of synthesis and degradation of cAMP in whole cells. From such measurements we hoped to determine if the decline from the hormone-induced transient steady state is due to a decrease in the rate of synthesis or an increase in the rate of degradation.

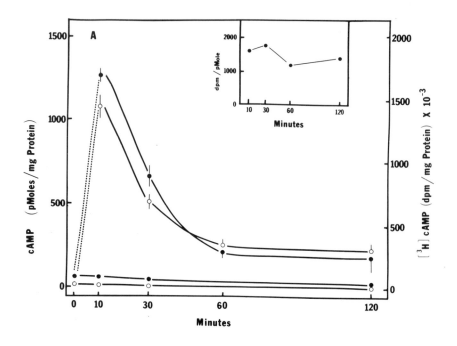

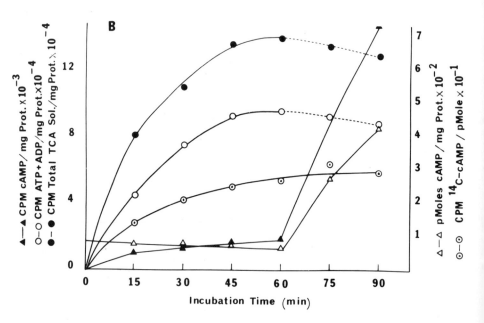

Fig. 2. The time course of change in cAMP and labeled cAMP in (A)
1321N1 cells and in (B) slices of rat cerebral cortex, after addition of 100 μM NE. (A) The open symbols represent pmoles cAMP per
mg protein and the closed symbols dpm ^{3}H-cAMP per mg protein. The
vertical bars represent S.E.M. of three determinations. The insert
illustrates the specific activity of the ^{3}H-cAMP formed during incubation. The two lower curves indicate cAMP and ^{3}H-cAMP content
in absence of NE. (B) Cortex slices were incubated with ^{14}C-adenine
(58 Ci/mmole; 15 μM). At the times indicated the slices were washed
free of exogenous ^{14}C-adenine and homogenized in 5% TCA. ATP and
cAMP were purified by standard procedures. After 60 min 100 μM NE
was added and the incubation continued for 15 or 30 min. The symbols represent the average of duplicate determinations: ●, total
TCA-soluble radioactivity; ○, ^{14}C-ATP; ▲, ^{14}C-cAMP; △, total cAMP
and ⊙ specific activity of ^{14}C-cAMP.

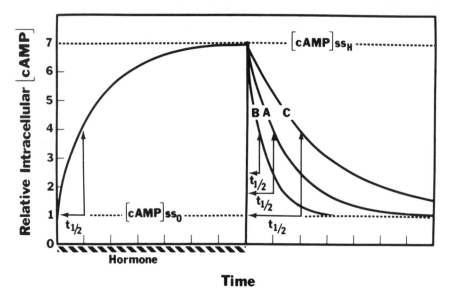

Fig. 3. *Theoretical time course for the changes in the steady state level of cAMP during hormonal stimulation and after subsequent removal of hormone. The basal cAMP level is represented by the broken line and the period of hormonal stimulation by the hatched bar. Time is expressed in units of half time ($t_{1/2}$) which is the time required for the cAMP level to rise from the basal level to half of the maximally stimulated level, or the time required to decline from the maximally stimulated level to 50% of maximal. Curve A represents the rate of decline if the hormone only increased k_S during exposure. Curve B represents the rate of decline if the hormone increased k_S but also decreased k_d during exposure. Curve C represents the rate of decline if the hormone increased k_S but also increased k_d during exposure.*

Since degradation is a first order process the initial rate of accumulation of cAMP upon addition of a hormone should approximate the actual rate of synthesis. The experiment shown in Fig. 4 suggests that this assumption is correct. The initial rate of accumulation of cAMP is not affected by a concentration (1.0 mM) of isobutylmethylxanthine (IBMX) that can be shown to cause about 80% inhibition of phosphodiesterase activity in intact cells (see Fig. 6). The rate constant of synthesis (k_S) can be assigned a minimal value from such data. Thus, from Fig. 4 cAMP is initially synthesized at 1,750 cpm/min/mg protein. From the relationship, [cAMP]ss = k_S/k_d and a knowledge of k_d (see Fig. 6) the predicted

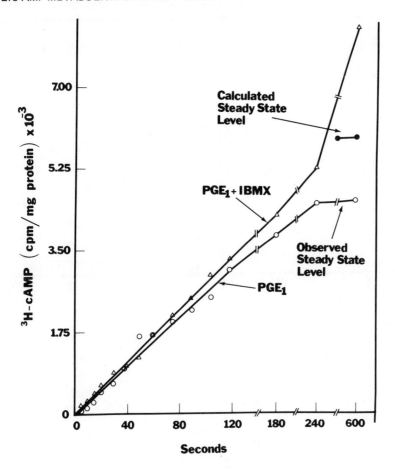

Fig. 4. *Initial velocity of accumulation of ^{3}H-cAMP in 1321N1 cells upon addition of 10 μM PGE$_1$ in the presence and absence of 1.0 mM IBMX. Cells were pre-labeled with ^{3}H-adenine then suspended and stirred in a temperature controlled (37°) vessel. At zero time PGE$_1$ was added and thereafter at the times indicated aliquots of cells were removed and mixed with TCA (final dilution 5%). ^{3}H-cAMP was purified by the standard procedure. The ^{3}H-cAMP formed in the cells prior to addition of PGE$_1$ was subtracted from all values.*

steady state concentration of cAMP (5,800 cpm/mg protein) can be calculated. As shown in Fig. 4 and as is usually the case, the experimentally observed, transient steady state concentration of cAMP is significantly less than the value predicted from initial rate data. Such results indicate that either k_s declines rapidly during exposure to the hormone or that k_d increases rapidly.

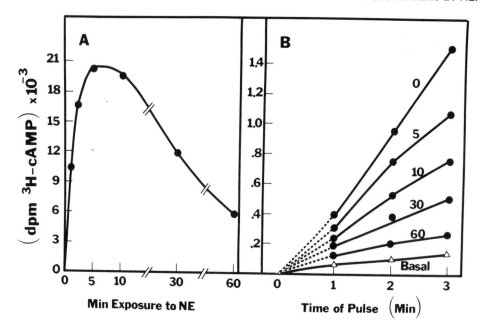

Fig. 5. *The rate of incorporation of ^3H-adenine into cAMP during the time course of exposure to 100 μM NE. Cells (1321N1) were exposed to NE at 0 time and ^3H-adenine was added at 0, 5, 10, 30, and 60 min after addition of NE. ^3H-cAMP was determined in samples taken from cells at 1, 2 and 3 min. after addition of ^3H-adenine. The symbols represent the average of duplicate determinations. The time course of <u>accumulation</u> of ^3H-cAMP was measured in a parallel experiment by the pre-labeling method and is shown in panel A.*

We also have attempted to measure rates of synthesis by pulse-labeling cultures with ^3H-adenine at various times after addition of NE. The rate of incorporation of label into cAMP is measured at 60 sec intervals during a 3 min pulse (Fig. 5). The rate of incorporation was found to decline with increasing time of exposure of the culture to NE. In fact, the rate of incorporation usually declines significantly by 5-10 min. Interpretation of this kind of experiment is fraught with potential pitfalls since there are numerous metabolic steps involved in the conversion of adenine to cAMP. Thus, hormone-induced changes in the rate of incorporation of label into cAMP could occur by an effect of the hormone at a step other than the conversion of ATP to cAMP. However, we have observed that the rate of incorporation of label into ATP does not change with increasing time of exposure to NE (not illustrated). Also, it can be shown in experiments like that

illustrated in Table 1, in which total cAMP and ^{3}H-cAMP are determined simultaneously, that the specific activity of the cAMP
formed after 60 min of exposure to NE is at least 90% of that of
the cAMP formed during the first 5 min of exposure. Taken together
these two observations suggest that NE has little effect on reactions involved in the formation of ATP and that the declining rate
of incorporation of label into cAMP is a valid measure of the
change in the rate of synthesis of cAMP.

Determination of the Rate of Degradation of cAMP in Whole Cells

     The rate of degradation of cAMP was measured in cells, pre-
labeled with ^{3}H-adenine and then exposed to NE to raise the cAMP
content. After addition of sufficient propranolol to completely
block the effect of NE, the rate of decline of cellular ^{3}H-cAMP
was determined (Fig. 6). The data are plotted as natural log of
the fraction of ^{3}H-cAMP remaining in the cells versus the time
after addition of propranolol. The slope of the resulting
straight lines indicate the rate constant of degradation (k_d). It
is clear from the graph that the value for k_d (0.30/min) does not
change significantly during a 60 min exposure to NE (Fig. 6A).

     After more than 60 min of exposure to catecholamines or
prostaglandins the amount of cAMP in the cells declines to levels
insufficient to allow the analysis of rates of degradation by the
method just described. However, since the cells respond to both
catecholamines and prostaglandins and the desensitization process
is somewhat agonist-specific, it is possible to increase the cAMP
content in cells treated for greater than 60 min with NE or
isoproterenol (ISO) by adding PGE$_1$, and vice-versa. When such experiments are carried out the rate constant for degradation is
observed to increase significantly after 90 min of exposure to
PGE$_1$ and is increased 2-fold after 180 min of exposure (Fig. 6).
In other studies we have shown that growth of 1321N1 cells in the
presence of low concentrations of PGE$_1$ (0.01 μM to 1.0 μM) for 72
hrs can lead to a 2-fold increase in the rate constant of
degradation.

     We also have used this procedure to test the effect of
putative inhibitors of phosphodiesterase as inhibitors of the
degradation of cAMP in whole cells. Under these conditions 1.0
mM IBMX causes about 80% inhibition of the rate of degradation of
cAMP (Fig. 6C).

Turnover of cAMP in Whole Cells

     The turnover of cAMP at steady state can be assessed from
a knowledge of either the rate constant of synthesis or of degra-

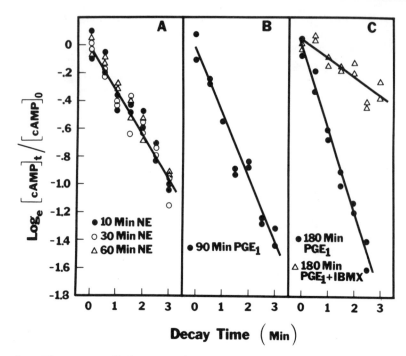

Fig. 6. The rate of degradation of cAMP after increasing time of exposure of 1321N1 cells to NE or PGE₁. (A) Cells were incubated with 100 μM NE. After 10, 30 or 60 min of incubation, propranolol (0.1 mM) was added and the cAMP content of the cells determined during the subsequent 3 min. (B,C) Cells were incubated with PGE₁ (3 μM) for 90 or 180 min then washed and incubated for 15 min in the absence of hormones. The cultures were then exposed to iso-proterenol (10 μM) for 5 min to raise the cAMP content. At 5 min propranolol (0.1 mM) was added and the cAMP content of the cells determined during the subsequent 3 min. IBMX (1.0 mM) was present during exposure to isoproterenol and during the 3 min after addition of propranolol (panel C). The results are expressed as the natural logarithm of the fraction of ³H-cAMP remaining after the addition of propranolol, versus time. The symbols represent the average of duplicate determinations. The time course of accumulation of ³H-cAMP was determined in parallel experiments and was similar to that shown in Fig. 7 for isoproterenol.

dation and the relationship, $k_s = [cAMP]ss\ k_d$. For cultures of 1321N1 cells exposed to 100 μM NE, the concentration of cAMP during the transient steady state is usually about 800 pmoles/mg protein. Thus, if k_d is 0.30/min, the turnover rate at steady would be about 240 pmoles/min/mg protein.

As shown in Figure 3, k_d also can be determined from a knowledge of the half-life of cAMP and equation [5]. The half-life can be determined by measuring the time required to proceed one-half of the way to the hormone-induced steady state. For this relationship to hold the hormone must cause a rapid increase in the rate of synthesis that is maintained until the new steady state is reached. Furthermore, the hormone should not alter the rate constant for degradation. Figure 3 illustrates the theoretical determination of the half-life of cAMP from the time course of change in cAMP after addition of a hormone and from the time course of decay after removal of the hormone. This type of analysis may be of use in determining if the hormone, in fact, alters only k_s or alters k_d as well. Thus if the $t_{1/2}$ of increase from basal levels to [cAMP]ss is the same as the $t_{1/2}$ for the return to basal levels (Fig. 3, curve A), then the hormone has probably only affected k_s. If the $t_{1/2}$ for decay, measured after removal of hormone, is less than for the approach to steady state (curve B) then the hormone may also have decreased the rate constant of degradation during exposure to the cells. Conversely, if the $t_{1/2}$ for decay is greater than the $t_{1/2}$ for the approach to steady state (curve C) then the hormone may also have increased k_d during exposure to the cells. Such conclusions can be drawn if the hormone-effects are assumed to be instantaneously reversible upon removal of the hormone or blockade of its action with inhibitors. Actual calculations based on experiments such as shown in Figures 4 and 6 indicate a $t_{1/2}$ of 2.3 min from decay data and a $t_{1/2}$ of 1.0 to 1.5 min based on the rate of approach to maximal accumulation.

The theoretical possibilities for differing values of $t_{1/2}$ (Fig. 3) assume that the effect of the hormone on either k_s or k_d is instantaneous, constant during the time of exposure, and instantaneously reversible. Thus, for either example of deviation (curve B or C) the approach to the hormone-induced steady state would be assymptotic. In either situation (curve B or C) the steady state level of accumulation would be accurately predicted from a measure of the initial rate of accumulation. Our observations indicate that the approach to steady state is not assymptotic and that the maximal level of accumulation is less than the value predicted from the initial rate of accumulation. (Fig. 4).

An alternate explanation for the lower $t_{1/2}$ observed for the approach to the NE-induced steady state is that after an initial abrupt increase, k_s actually declines during the exposure to NE. Our evidence to date would favor this explanation. As indicated in the pulse-labeling experiments k_s is not maintained at the same value even during the initial few minutes of exposure of 1321N1 cells to NE (Fig. 5) or PGE_1 (not illustrated). If indeed, k_s is declining with time and k_d does not change, then the $t_{1/2}$

for the approach to the observed, transient steady state would be shorter than the $t\frac{1}{2}$ for decay back to basal.

We have tentatively concluded that the biphasic change of cAMP induced in 1321N1 cells by NE and PGE_1 is due to an initial rapid rise in k_s followed within 5 min by a decline in k_s even in the continued presence of active hormone. Neither NE nor PGE_1 appear to have an effect on k_d until after 60-90 min. The increase in k_d observed after 90 min should act in addition to the decline in k_s to reduce responsiveness of the cells to the hormones. A detailed analysis of the desensitization phenomenon will be presented elsewhere (25-27).

CONCLUSIONS

We have attempted to demonstrate that kinetic constants for the rates of synthesis and degradation of cAMP in intact cell can be estimated by rather simple experimental procedures. Such determinations allow an assessment of the validity of adenylate cyclase and phosphodiesterase activities determined in homogenates as indicators of the synthetic and degradative capacities of whole cells.

It should be clear that the rate of approach to a new steady state level of cAMP is determined by the magnitude of the rate constant for degradation, i.e., the level of phosphodiesterase activity in the cell. The absolute level of cAMP at the new steady state is determined by the ratio k_s/k_d. Thus, for cells with low phosphodiesterase activity relative to the maximally stimulated adenylate cyclase activity, the response to a hormone will be large and the approach to steady state will be relatively slow. Conversely, cells with high levels of phosphodiesterase activity will exhibit a smaller rise in cAMP but will attain steady state more rapidly. In either situation co-addition of an inhibitor of phosphodiesterase with the hormone will cause a large increase in cAMP with a slower approach to steady state (Fig. 7). It is clear that the apparent magnitude of effect of IBMX is a variable that depends on the point in time at which the comparison is made (Fig. 7). This fact has apparently not been appreciated in numerous previous studies in which the effects of phosphodiesterase inhibitors on the response to hormones have been measured at the time that is optimum for the response to the hormone alone.

The magnitude of the effect of an inhibitor of phosphodiesterase on basal cAMP levels will be directly proportional to the percentage inhibition of the enzyme. However, for an equal change in the ratio of k_s/k_d elicited by a hormone on the

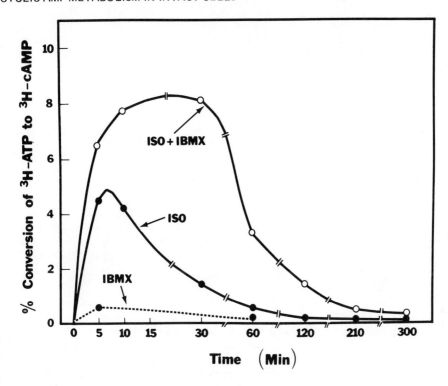

Fig. 7. Time course of the change in ^{3}H-cAMP in the presence of isoproterenol or isoproterenol and IBMX. Cells (1321N1) were exposed to either 10 μM isoproterenol, 10 μM isoproterenol plus 1.0 mM IBMX or 1.0 mM IBMX alone. The symbols represent the average of triplicate determinations. ^{3}H-cAMP was extracted and purified by the standard procedures.

Table 3. Comparison of the $t_{1/2}$ for approach to a new steady state initiated by activation of adenylate cyclase (Δk_s) or inhibition of phosphodiesterase (Δk_d) (simulated data).

Condition	k_s/k_d	Relative steady state [cAMP]	Relative $t_{1/2}$
Basal	$100/100$	1	–
NE (Δk_s)	$1000/100$	10	100
IBMX (Δk_d)	$100/10$	10	1000

one hand and an inhibitor of phosphodiesterase on the other there would be a marked difference in the rates of approach to the same eventual steady state (Table 3). Of course, cells that are not synthesizing cAMP under basal conditions will not respond at all to the addition of phosphodiesterase inhibitors. Conversely, cells that respond with a marked rise in cAMP content upon addition of such inhibitors must have been turning over cAMP at a high rate.

We have not discussed in detail other possibilities for the disposition of cAMP such as binding to macromolecules to give phosphodiesterase-resistant pools (1) or excretion of cAMP from cells to provide a non-phosphodiesterase pathway for the elimination of cAMP (2,3). The magnitude of the latter pathway can be determined by analysis of the incubation medium for cAMP. The existance of large reservoirs of phosphodiesterase-resistant cAMP may be indicated by a marked deviation from first order kinetics in the rate of degradation of cAMP.

A perusal of the literature reveals that marked differences in the metabolism of cAMP can be observed in different tissues and cell types. Not only are there large differences in the ratio of synthetic to degradative capacities, but also in the absolute capacities. The physiological significance of this variation is not readily apparent. However, cognisance of such variations is important for the proper interpretation of experiments involving the response of tissues to hormones. The methods described here should be useful in analyzing some of the complexities of the cAMP-second messenger system.

ACKNOWLEDGEMENTS

This work was supported in part by USPHS grant NS 10233. J.P.P. is the recipient of Research Career Development Award 6K04 CA70466. G.L.J. is a pre-doctoral fellow supported by USPHS training grant 5T01 GM01983. R.O. is a visiting fellow of the Deutsche Forschungsgemeinschaft.

REFERENCES

1 O'Dea, R.F., Haddox, M.K. and Goldberg, N.D. (1971) J. Biol. Chem. 246, 6183.
2 Kelly, L.A., Hall, M.S. and Butcher, R.W. (1974) J. Biol. Chem. 249, 5182.
3 Davoren, P.R. and Sutherland, E.W. (1963) J. Biol. Chem. 238, 3009.

4   Perkins, J.P. (1973) Adenyl Cyclase in Advances in Cyclic
    Nucleotide Research Vol. 3 pp. 1-64, eds. P. Greengard and
    G.A. Robison, Raven Press, New York.
5   Loten, E.G. and Sneyd, J.G.T. (1970) Biochem. J. 120, 187.
6   Armstrong, K.J., Stouffer, J.E., VanInwegen, R.G., Thompson,
    W.J. and Robison, G.A. (1974) J. Biol. Chem. 249, 4226.
7   D'Armiento, M., Johnson, G.S. and Pastan, I. (1972) Proc. Nat.
    Acad. Sci. 69, 459.
8   Brooker, G., Thomas, L., Jr. and Appleman, M.M. (1968) Bio-
    chemistry 7, 4177.
9   Thompson, W.J. and Appleman, M.M. (1971) Biochemistry 10, 311.
10 Butcher, R.W., Ho, R.J., Meng, H.C. and Sutherland, E.W.
    (1965) J. Biol. Chem. 240, 4515.
11 Goldberg, N.D., Larner, J., Sasko, H. and O'Toole, A,G, (1969)
    Anal. Biochem. 28, 523.
12 Gilman, A.G. (1970) Proc. Nat. Acad. Sci. 67, 305.
13 Steiner, A.L., Kipnis, D.M., Utiger, R. and Parker, C. (1969)
    Proc. Nat. Acad. Sci. 64, 367.
14 Greengard, P. and Robison, G.A. eds. (1972) New Assay Methods
    for Cyclic Nucleotides in Advances in Cyclic Nucleotide
    Research Vol. 2, Raven Press, New York.
15 Krebs, E.G. (1972) Protein Kinases in Current Topics in
    Cellular Regulation Vol. 5, eds. Horecker, B.L. and Stadtman,
    E.R. pp. 99-133, Academic Press, New York.
16 Kuo, J.F. and DeRenzo, E.C. (1969) J. Biol. Chem. 244, 2252.
17 Shimizu, H., Daly, J.W. and Creveling, C.R. (1969) J.
    Neurochem. 16, 1609.
18 Clark, R.B. and Perkins, J.P. (1971) Proc. Nat. Acad. Sci. 68,
    2757.
19 Clark, R.B., Su, Y-F., Gross, R. and Perkins, J.P. (1974) J.
    Biol. Chem. 249, 5296.
20 Clark, R.B., Su, Y-F., Ortmann, R., Cubeddu, L.X., Johnson,
    G.L. and Perkins, J.P. (1975) Metabolism 24, 343.
21 Shimizu, H. and Daly, J.W. (1970) Biochim. Biophys. Acta. 222,
    465.
22 Perkins, J.P. and Moore, M.M. (1973) J. Pharmacol. Exp. Therap.
    185, 371.
23 Perkins, J.P. and Moore, M.M. (1973) Mol. Pharmacol. 9, 774.
24 Saloman, Y., Londos, C. and Rodbell, M. (1974) Biochem. 58,
    451.
25 Su, Y-F., Cubeddu, L.X. and Perkins, J.P. (1975)

26 Su, Y-F., Johnson, G.L., Cubeddu, L.X., Ortmann, R. and Perkins,
    J.P. (1975)
27 Leichtling, B., Drotar, A., Ortmann, R. and Perkins, J.P.
    (1975)
28 Stanley, P.E. and Williams, S.G. (1969) Anal. Biochem. 29, 381.

THE ACTIONS OF NUCLEOTIDES ON ADENYLYL CYCLASE SYSTEMS

L. Birnbaumer, T. Nakahara, and M. Hunzicker-Dunn

Department of Physiology, Northwestern University
Medical School, Chicago, Illinois   60611 and
Department of Molecular Medicine, Mayo Clinic,
Rochester, Minnesota   55901

CONTENTS

1. INTRODUCTION AND BASIC OBSERVATIONS

In recent years it has become increasingly clear that the hormonal activation of adenylyl cyclase systems is under regulation by
nucleotides and nucleosides. The original finding leading to this
recognition (1,2) was that under stringent assay conditions (using
as substrate either low ATP or AMP-PNP) the liver plasma membrane
adenylyl cyclase exhibited an almost total requirement for GTP (or
ATP) to show activation by glucagon. Similar findings were soon
reported for other adenylyl cyclase systems activated by other hormones (3,4) and led to the early conclusion that a nucleotide dependent step is involved in hormonal activation in an obligatory
manner (5). Further experimentation, however, has shown that the
situation is more complex and that nucleotides rather than inter-
vening in an obligatory fashion, play a more subtle role and modulate hormonal stimulation of adenylyl cyclase systems either posi-

tively or negatively. They appear to do so by affecting not only
the degree of hormonal stimulation, but also the basal activity of
the system and the receptor-hormone interaction. We shall review
the experimental evidence relating to these effects and discuss the
possibility that nucleotides interact with adenylyl cyclase systems
at more than one site, providing a plausible explanation as to why
the effects of nucleotides are complex and often difficult to interpret from a kinetic point of view.

    Important for our current view of modulation of adenylyl cyclas-
es by nucleotides and nucleosides was our finding (6,7) that GTP
not always promoted or enhanced hormonal stimulation but that it
could also inhibit the expression of hormonal stimulation. This
finding emerged from a detailed study on the ATP dependency of a
vasopressin-sensitive adenylyl cyclase present in membranes of beef
renal medulla. As can be seen in Fig. 1, in this system ATP has both
a stimulatory and an inhibitory effect on vasopressin action. The
stimulatory effect becomes maximal between 0.07 and 0.10 mM and the
inhibitory effect becomes apparent when the concentration of ATP is
further increased to levels of 1.0 mM and above. GTP, when tested
at an ATP concentration giving optimal vasopressin stimulation, was
clearly inhibitory to hormone-stimulated activity without apparently
affecting basal activity to a significant extent (Fig. 2). Other
experiments showed (7) that GTP had little or no effect at ATP concentrations about 1.5 mM, probably because of a GTP-like effect of
ATP. While GTP inhibited the degree to which adenylyl cyclase is
stimulated by vasopressin, adenosine and AMP enhanced hormone stimulation when tested at concentrations lower than 0.08 mM ATP (shown

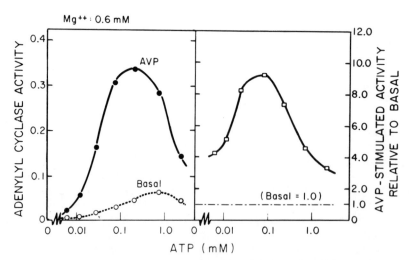

Fig. 1. Effect of varying ATP concentration on responsiveness of th
beef renal adenylyl cyclase to arginine vasopressin (AVP). For details of membrane preparation and of incubation conditions see ref.7

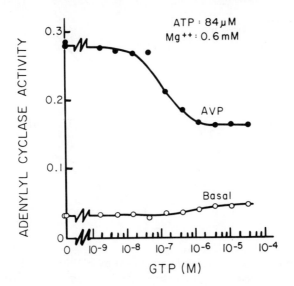

Fig. 2.   Inhibitory effect of GTP on stimulation of beef renal medullary adenylyl cyclase by arginine vasopressin (AVP).   For details
see refs. 6 and 7.

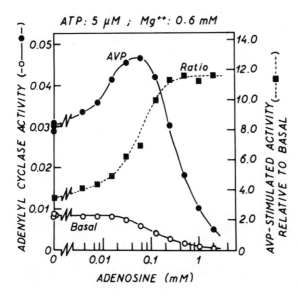

Fig. 3.   Effect of adenosine on hormonal stimulation of beef renal
medullary adenylyl cyclase.   For details see refs. 6 and 7.

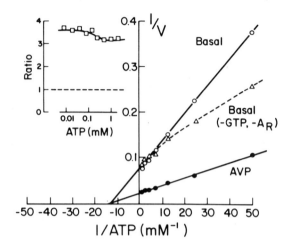

Fig. 4. Dependency of the beef renal adenylyl cyclase on substrate concentration. The reaction mixtures contained the indicated concentrations of ATP (varying from 0.02 mM to 0.7 mM), 2.0 mM $MgCl_2$, 1.2 mM EDTA, 1.0 mM cyclic AMP, 20 mM creatine phosphate, 0.2 mg per ml of creatine kinase, 25 mM Bis-tris-propane-HCL buffer (Sigma) pH 8.0, and when present (continuous lines) 10^{-5} M GTP and 2×10^{-4} M adenosine (A_R). Ratio of AVP-stimulated activity to basal as a function of ATP concentration. The relative constancy of this value over the entire range of ATP used in this experiment is indicative that allosteric regulatory interaction sites have been occupied by GTP and adenosine. The apparent K_m of this system for ATP calculated from this experiment was 0.08 mM.

for adenosine in Fig. 3), indicating that the hormonal responsiveness of beef renal system is not only under negative control by GTP but also under positive control by adenine nucleosides and nucleotides (adenosine, AMP and ATP).

A study of the ATP dependency of this system carried out in presence of maximally effective concentrations of both adenosine and GTP eliminated the "regulatory" effects of ATP (led to relatively constant hormonal stimulation regardless of the ATP concentration tested) and yielded "Michaelis-Menten" type kinetics for the catalytic unit (Fig. 4). This indicated that the sites with which nu-

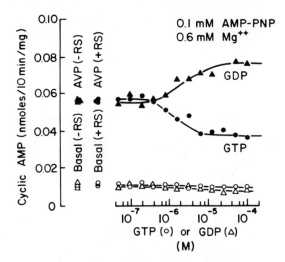

Fig. 5. Opposing effects of GTP and GDP on hormonal stimulation of the beef renal medullary adenylyl cyclase system. Reactions were carried out using AMP-PNP as substrate and omitting the nucleotide triphosphate regenerating system (RS) when the nucleoside diphosphate was tested. For details see ref. 8.

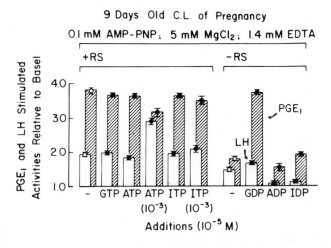

Fig. 6. Effects of nucleotides on hormonal stimulation of corpus luteum adenylyl cyclase. Note opposing effects of ATP on stimulation by LH and enhancing effect of GDP on stimulation by PGE_1. As in the experiment of the previous figure AMP-PNP was used as substrate and the nucleoside triphosphate regenerating system (RS) was omitted when nucleoside diphosphates were tested. Corpora lutea of pseudopregnant (PSP) rabbits were used. For rest of details see ref. 8.

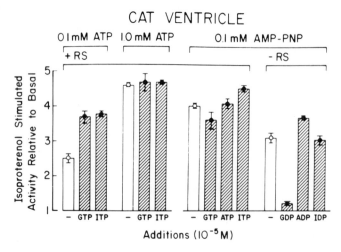

Fig. 7. Effects of nucleotides on catecholamine stimulation of cat myocardio adenylyl cyclase activity. Note the profound inhibitory action of GDP (seen in the absence of regenerating system (RS) with AMP-PNP as substrate) and the positive effect of GTP (seen in the presence of regenerating system with 0.1 mM ATP as substrate). The presence of low concentrations of GDP coupled to a relatively strong enhancing effect of AMP-PNP itself, is probably responsible for an apparent lack of a positive effect of GTP when tested with AMP-PNP as substrate in the presence of regenerating system. The regenerating system used (creatine kinase/creatine phosphate) is not totally effective in converting nucleoside diphosphates to the triphosphate state when the substrate levels are below 10^{-6}M. For rest of details see ref. 8.

cleotides and nucleosides interact to exert their actions are allosteric to the catalytic site, and provided strong evidence that hormonal stimulation is the result of a change in the catalytic capacity of the adenylyl cyclase rather than of an increase in the affinity of the enzyme's catalytic site for the substrate.

Modulation of hormone action by nucleotides appear to be complex and variable, depending on the systems studied. Figs. 5 to 7 present some examples in which either positive or negative effects of either nucleoside triphosphates or nucleoside diphosphates are seen. In systems where nucleoside triphosphates and nucleoside diphosphates appear to have opposite effects (GDP/GTP in renal membranes on vasopressin action, ATP/ADP in corpus luteum membranes on luteinizing hormone (LH) action, and GTP/GDP in myocardial membranes on catecholamine action it is not known whether they interact competitively at one site or whether there are respective "stimulatory" and "inhibitory" sites. Table I presents examples of effects of nucleotides in various systems.

Table I

Examples of positive and negative modulation by nucleotides of hormonal stimulation (relative to basal) of adenylyl cyclase systems.

1. Enhancement:

GTP: Glucagon in rat liver (1), in hamster β cell (24), in rat heart (25).
       Prostaglandins in human platelets (3), in beef thyroid gland (23), in beef renal medulla (8).
       Catecholamines in rat liver (4), in rat adipose tissue (11), in kitten myocardium (8).
       ACTH in rat adipose cell (11).
       Oxytocin in frog bladder epithelium (26).

ITP: TSH in beef thyroid gland (23), in horse thyroid gland (21).

ATP: LH in corpus luteum of pregnant rabbit (8).
       AVP, LVP and oxytocin in beef renal medulla (8).

GDP: Prostaglandins in corpus luteum of pregnant rabbits (8).
       AVP, LVP and oxytocin in beef renal medulla (8).

2. Inhibition:

GTP: AVP, LVP and oxytocin in beef renal medulla (7)

GDP: Catecholamines in kitten myocardium (8), in rat adipose cell (11).

ADP: LH in corpus luteum of pregnant rabbit (8).

During the following discussion we shall assume that adenylyl cyclase systems are composed of one or more catalytic units, responsible for cyclic AMP formation, and one or more regulatory units or hormone receptors, capable of affecting, under the influence (binding) of the hormone, the conformation of the catalytic part of the enzyme, thereby modulating or regulating its catalytic capacity. Having established unequivocally that hormonal stimulation of adenylyl cyclases can be modulated either positively or negatively by nucleotides it became of interest to explore in detail the mode or modes by which nucleotides exerted their effects.

2.   EFFECT OF NUCLEOTIDES ON THE BEHAVIOR OF THE CATALYTIC UNIT (S)

Detailed investigation of the time courses of cyclic AMP accumulation by beef renal medullary membranes either in the absence (basal) or in the presence of vasopressin (hormone-stimulated) under conditions giving maximal hormone stimulation (0.08 to 0.10 mM ATP) revealed the presence of a burst phenomenon, i.e. that the initial rate of cyclic AMP formation is greater than that obtained after

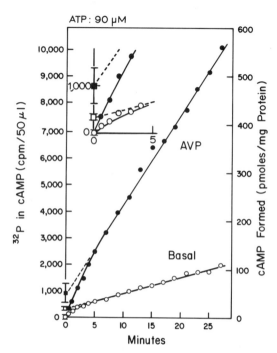

Fig. 8 Time course of adenylyl cyclase activities (cyclic AMP accumulation) in beef renal medullary membranes tested under conditions that allow for optimal hormonal response.---, extrapolations of rates of accumulation obtained after 7 min. of incubation calculated by least squares regression analysis of the data points; squares, calculated y-intercepts ± 2 standard deviations; circle at origin: reaction blank ± 2 standard deviations (the reaction blank has been subtracted from all data points, hence its place at the origin). Inset: Same as main graph but with expanded scale. For rest of details see ref. 7.

the enzyme has reached an apparent steady state of activity as seen by a continuous linear rate of cyclic AMP accumulation (Fig. 8).

If, as it is reasonable to assume, substrate and ligands (hormone in the case of the experiment of Fig. 8) established rapid equilibrium with membrane bound adenylyl cyclase, then the nonlinear time course of cyclic AMP accumulation is an indication of a slow isomerization of the catalytic unit of the enzyme from a more active conformational state to a less active conformational state (activity). This change in conformation may be induced by the binding of substrate (MgATP) to the catalytic site or by binding of a ligand (Mg?) to an allosteric regulatory site. In this context the renal adenylyl cyclase serves to fit the description of an histeretic enzyme as defined by Frieden (9), i.e. of an enzyme that responds slowly to rapid changes in ligand concentration.

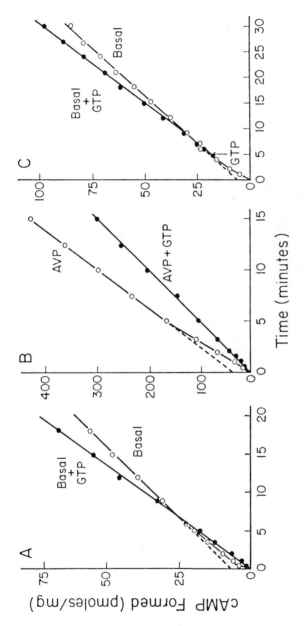

Fig. 9. Effect of GTP addition on the time course of adenylyl cyclase activities (basal and arginine vasopressin (AVP)-stimulated) in beef renal medullary membranes. For rest of details see ref. 7.

It is clear from the data of Fig. 8 that the initial, transient and more active state of the enzyme, as well as the final, stable and less active state of the enzyme are susceptible to hormonal stimulation, the degree of stimulation being about the same. Thus, the presence of hormone did not seem to influence to a significant extent the process(es) responsible for the transition of states. GTP, on the other hand, abolished the burst phenomenon and induced rapid formation of stable states of activity (basal and hormone-stimulated) that are distinct from those seen in its absence.

Initial, stable and GTP-induced states of activity seem to be interconvertible. As shown in Figs. 9 and 10, the GTP states can be formed by adding GTP at the beginning of the incubation (transition of transient state to stable GTP state) or after stable states of activity have been obtained (transition of stable basal or stable hormone-stimulated states to stable GTP of stable hormone-stimulated GTP states). It is also possible to switch from a stable GTP state to a stable hormone-stimulated GTP state by the post-addition of hormone to the system. Washing of membranes containing an adenylyl cyclase system in the stable hormone-stimulated GTP state of acti-vity (i.e. incubated for vasopressin-stimulated activity in the presence of GTP) results (not shown) in the re-establishment

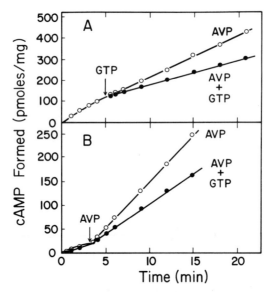

Fig. 10 Effect of post-addition of GTP or of arginine vasopressin (AVP) on time course of adenylyl cyclase activities in beef renal medullary membranes. Inhibition of AVP-stimulated activity by GTP was about the same whether resulting from post-addition of GTP (39% inhibition) or AVP (37% inhibition). For rest of details see ref. 7.

of a state of the adenylyl cyclase system that exhibits bursting
basal and hormone-stimulated activities that are susceptible to the
influence of GTP in the same manner as described above (for details
see ref. 7).

Although not specifically commented on, non-linear time courses
of cyclic AMP accumulation suggestive of the existence of transient
conformational forms of activity have been reported by Murad et al.
for fluoride-stimulated activity in rat testis (10) and more recently by Harwood et al. (11) for basal as well as for epinephrine-
stimulated adenylyl cyclase activity in fat cell membranes. Bursts
of this kind, although of somewhat shorter duration, have been described for more "orthodox" enzymes such as homoserine dehydrogenase
from E. coli (12), threonine deaminase from B. subtilis (13) and
hexokinase from yeast (14). Finally, more recent experiments in
our laboratory on the properties of the LH-sensitive adenylyl cyclase system of pig Graafian follicles showed the existence of discrete states of activity, and hence discrete conformations, also
in this system. As can be seen in Fig. 11, cAMP accumulation with
membranes obtained from Graafian follicles of the pig exhibited an
initial non-linear component, necessitating 6 to 9 min. to reach
linearity. However, in contrast to findings with renal membranes
(Figs. 9 and 10) the initial and transient basal state is less
active than the final stable basal state and GTP addition does not
result in obliteration of the transient states, thus allowing the
effect of GTP on these forms of adenylyl cyclase to be visualized.
The following scheme describes the interconversions of states
found:

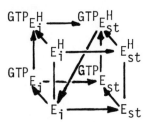

where E stands for enzyme and the sub- and superscripts i, st, GTP
and H stands for initial, stable, GTP and hormonal states of activity, respectively. The initial GTP states ($^{GTP}E_i$ and $^{GTP}E^H_i$) were
only observed in the LH-sensitive system.

Note that while the catalytic capacities of the various conformational states (from less active to the most active) form the series

$$E_{st} < {}^{GTP}E_{st} < E_i < {}^{GTP}E^H_{st} < E^H_{st} < E^H_i$$

in renal membranes, in membranes from the Graafian follicle of the
pig they align differently:

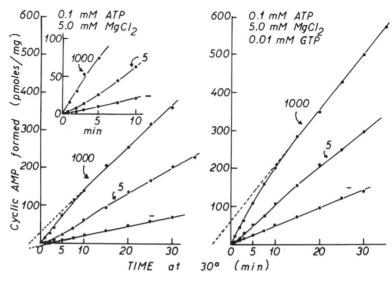

Fig. 11. Time course of adenylyl cyclase activities (basal and luteinizing hormone (LH)-stimulated) in membrane particles from Graafian follicles of the pig. Adenylyl cyclase activity was determined
at 30° for the indicated times in a medium containing: 0.1 mM ATP,
5.0 mM $MgCl_2$, 1.0 mM EDTA, 1.0 mM EGTA, 1.0 mM cyclic AMP, 20 mM creatine phosphate, 0.2 mg per ml of creatine kinase, 25 mM Tris-HCl pH
7.5, ca. 20 ug membrane particles, and when present in either 5 or
1000 ng per ml LH (LER #1347) and 10^{-5}M GTP. Membrane particles were
prepared from Graafian follicles larger than 6 mm in the following
way: dissected follicles (kept in iced KRB medium) were cut into
small pieces, weighed and homogenized in 10 volumes of 27% sucrose,
1 mM EDTA and 10 mM Tris-HCl, pH 7.5 using a Dounce homogenizer.
The homogenate was filtered through #12 silk screen and centrifuged
at 12,000 xg for 20 min at 4° yielding a first pellet of membrane
particles. These particles were resuspended in 20 volumes of 10 mM
Tris-HCl, pH 7.5 and 1 mM EDTA and repelleted as above. The washing procedure was repeated twice more. The final pellet was resuspended in 5 volumes of the original homogenizing medium and kept frozen until used in the study described on the figure.---,extrapola-
tions of the linear portions of the cyclic AMP accumulation curves.
Note that as shown for beef renal membranes below, submaximally stimulating concentrations of hormone do not lead to "instantaneous"
activation of the system; rather, a lag period between hormone addition and "steady state" of increased activity can be seen. The vi-
sualization of this lag period is complicated by the existence of
the burst phase in the accumulation curves, leading to an apparent
oscillatory 10 min after initiation of the adenylyl cyclase reaction
(be it in the absence or the presence of GTP),at which time the enzyme has reached its stable state conformation (not shown). It should
be pointed out that the decay of activity seen in the presence of LH
during the first five min of incubation is not due to stimulation

$$E_i < E_{st} < {}^{GTP}E_{st} = {}^{GTP}E_i < E_{st}^H < E_i^H \approx {}^{GTP}E_{st}^H < E_i^H$$

The fact that the activity of the GTP state in renal membranes induced in the absence of hormone $\left({}^{GTP}E_{st}\right)$ lies in between the activities of the initial (E_i) and the stable (E_{st}) states, with a resulting crossover in the cyclic AMP accumulation curves after about 10 min. of incubation, is responsible for the apparent "lack" of effect of GTP on the renal basal adenylyl cyclase activity seen in initial experiments (cf. Fig. 2 and ref. 2). From the above the following can be inferred:

1) The beef renal medullary adenylyl cyclase system exists in several discrete conformational states which, under appropriate conditions, can be shown to be in equilibrium with each other (reversal to bursting state after having been in a stable state).

2) GTP affects adenylyl cyclase systems in the absence of hormonal stimulus, i.e. has an effect on the behavior of the catalytic unit regardless of the presence of stimulating hormones.

3) One mechanism by which nucleotides affect expression of hormonal stimulation of adenylyl cyclase systems is by (allosterically?) inducing an enzymatic conformation whose catalytic capacity is either less (negative modulation or more) (positive modulation) apt to be increased by the stimulatory hormone-receptor.

3. EFFECT OF NUCLEOTIDES ON THE BEHAVIOR OF THE HORMONE RECEPTOR

As shown by Bockaert et al. (15) working with a vasopressin-sensitive adenylyl cyclase from pig renal medulla, and by Rodbell et al. (16) working under stringent (low nucleotide) assay conditions with the glucagon-sensitive adenylyl cyclase from rat liver plasma membranes, and by us (17) working with the vasopressin-sensitive adenylyl cyclase from beef renal medulla, submaximally stimulating concentrations of hormone may activate adenylyl cyclase slowly. This was inferred from the fact that cyclic AMP accumulation curves obtained at low hormone concentrations showed lag periods between hormone addition and attainment of steady state rates of

---

Fig. 11 (cont'd)

by LH of a densitization mechanism, such as seen in membranes from pig Graafian follicles, because addition of LH after 10 min. of incubation under basal assay conditions leads immediately to an activity (slope) that is equal to the linear portion of the cyclic AMP accumulation curve obtained when LH was added at time zero, (not shown).

accumulation. In each of these systems it was concluded that the
lag periods observed are due to the time necessary for the hormone
to establish equilibrium of binding. Bockaert et al. (15) and
Rodbell et al. (16) based their arguments on comparative studies
of hormone binding (for a detailed discussion, however, see ref.
18) and we based ours (17) on a kinetic analysis of the lag period.
Since the interpretation of the effects of nucleotides at the receptor level depend on some of the assumptions made and on the
meaning of the lag periods observed we shall present our evidence
that the lag periods are dependent on and a reflection of the time
necessary for hormones to bind to the receptor.

We made two basic assumptions: 1) that the hormone-receptor
complex formation is the rate limiting step of the process that
activates adenylyl cyclases, and 2) that there is a linear relation between receptor occupation and adenylyl cyclase activation.
We then investigated whether experimentally obtained data would
fit a model with these assumptions. Thus if:

$$H + R \underset{k_2}{\overset{k_1}{\rightleftharpoons}} HR \dashrightarrow \text{Effect} \tag{1}$$

then
$$d[HR]/dt = k_1[H][R] - k_2[HR] \tag{2}$$

with
$$[R_t] = [R] + [HR] \tag{3}$$

At equilibrium:

$$p_e = [HR]/[R_t] = x/(x + k_2/k_1) \tag{4}$$

where p is the fractional occupancy of receptors, subscript e denotes
equilibrium condition and x is concentration of free hormone $[H]$ in
equations (1) and (2). Receptor occupation short of equilibrium is
derived from equation (2). Substitution of $[R_t] - [HR]$ for $[R]$, rearrangement, division by $-(k_1x + k_2)$, and final arrangement yields:

$$d[HR]/ ([HR] - \frac{k_1[R_t]}{k_1x + k_2}) = d[HR]/([HR] - [R_t]p_e)=$$
$$= -(k_1x + k_2)dt \tag{5}$$

and analytical integration according to formula II of Table II, followed by antilog and appropriate rearrangement yields:

$$p = p_e(1 - e^{-(k_1x + k_2)t}) \tag{6}$$

If, as assumed, coupling between receptor and adenylyl cyclase
is linear (a "must" if the cyclase system is formed by a single catalytic unit coupled to a single receptor molecule, but only a "maybe"
if the system is polymeric, i.e. formed by a complex arrangement of
several catalytic units coupled to several receptor molecules), then

Table II
Some integration formulae

$$\int e^x dx = e^x + C \qquad (I)$$

$$\int e^{ax} dx = \frac{1}{x} e^{ax} + C \qquad II)$$

$$\int \frac{1}{x} dx = \ln(x) + C \qquad (III)$$

$$\int \frac{1}{x + a} dx = \ln(x + a) + C \qquad (IV)$$

v, the rate of cyclic AMP formation at any given receptor occupation p is:

$$v = V_m p \qquad (7)$$

where V_m is the rate of the enzyme at full receptor occupancy, i.e. at $p = 1$.

Accumulation of cyclic AMP as a function of time will then be:

$$cAMP_{acc} = \int_0^t v \, dt = V_m \int_0^t p \, dt = V_m P_e \int_0^t (1 - e^{-(k_1 x + k_2)t}) dt =$$
$$= V_m P_e \int_0^t dt - V_m P_e \int_0^t e^{-(k_1 x + k_2)t} dt \qquad (8)$$

which after analytical integration according to formula IV of Table II and appropriate rearrangement yields:

$$cAMP_{acc} = V_m P_e + \frac{V_m P_e}{k_1 x + k_2} e^{-(k_1 x + k_2)t} - \frac{V_m P_e}{k_1 x + k_2} \qquad (9)$$

At equilibrium:

$$\frac{V_m P_e}{k_1 x + k_2} e^{-(k_1 x + k_2)t} \approx 0 \qquad (10)$$

and

$$cAMP_{acc} \approx s = V_m P_e t - \frac{V_m P_e}{k_1 x + k_2} \qquad (11)$$

Thus, the y-intercept extrapolated from the progress curve obtained after equilibrium of binding has been reached (linear portion of the progress curve) differs from 0 by $(V_m P_e / k_1 x + k_2)$. Since $V_m P_e$ is the slope of the progress curve at equilibrium of binding, it is possible to calculate $k_1 x + k_2$. Equation 10 describes the difference between the extrapolation from equilibrium conditions and the real cyclic AMP accumulation, and indicates that that difference should diminish exponentially with a time constant also of $k_1 x + k_2$.

It follows that the term $k_1 x + k_2$ can be approximated both from

the linear portion of the progress curve (the position of which depends on the extent of the lag) and the non-linear portion of the
progress curve (the form of which should be exponential). Determination of $k_1x + k_2$, as a function of x (hormone concentration)
should yield a straight line with k_1 as a slope and k_2 at the y-intercept, allowing for determination of the rate constants of the hormone-receptor interaction. Furthermore, $k_1x + k_2$ determined from
the linear portion of the progress curve should be the same as when
determined from the non-linear portion, thus providing for an internal check of the approximation used.

In practice, due to the existence of a basal adenylyl cyclase
activity (v_b) and the presence of the burst phenomenon in renal
plasma membranes, which made it necessary to delay hormone addition
by 5 min, i.e. until a stable steady state of activity had been on-
tained, equations (9) and (10) were corrected to:

$$cAMP_{acc} = (V_mP_e + v_b)t + \frac{V_mP_e}{k_1x + k_2} e^{-(k_1x + k_2)t} - \frac{V_mP_e}{k_1x + k_2} + b \qquad (12)$$

and,

$$cAMP_{acc} \simeq s = (V_mP_e + v_b)t - \frac{V_mP_e}{k_1x + k_2} + b \qquad (13)$$

where b is the amount of cyclic AMP present in the incubation at the
moment of hormone addition. A typical accumulation curve, and the
way calculations were performed as shown in Fig. 12.

Fig. 13 shows experimental data (circles) and calculated progress curves individually optimized for each of the hormone concentrations used (dotted lines); Fig. 14 shows the dependence on
hormone concentration of the calculated time constants (obtained
separately from the linear and non-linear (exponential) portions
of the progress curves); and Fig. 15 shows again the experimental
data, but this time with progress curves calculated using a single
set of constants derived from the plots shown in Fig. 14.

From this it was concluded that the beef renal medullary system
fits the theoretical model presented at the beginning of this
section, with the hormone-receptor interaction being the rate limiting step at maximally stimulating hormone concentrations, and
with coupling between receptor occupancy and adenylyl cyclase activation being linear.

Addition of GTP either prior to (as shown in Fig. 16) or together with hormone (not shown) resulted in obliteration of the lag
period in the hormone-stimulated progress curve, indicating that
the rate limiting step of the activating process (i.e. the rate of
interaction of hormone with adenylyl cyclase-coupled receptor) is
accelerated by the nucleotide. A possible change in the coupling

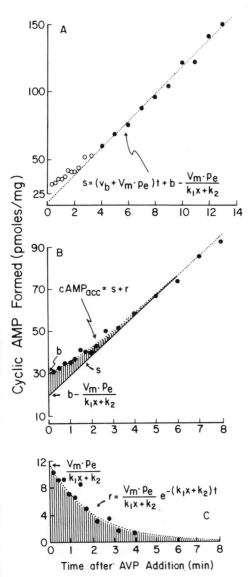

Fig. 12 Non-linearity of cyclic AMP accumulation and mode of determination of velocity parameters of stimulation by AVP of been renal medullary adenylyl cyclase. Experimental: membrane particles were added to complete adenylyl cyclase incubation medium and incubated for 5 min. to allow for formation of steady (stable) state of activity. At 5 min, time zero on figure, 0.6 mM AVP was added, and the incubation continued for the indicated times. The reaction was then stopped and the cyclic AMP formed determined. In all panels the circles represent experimental points of single incubations. Calculations: Panel A; Data obtained after 4 min of incubation (filled circles) corresponding to the linear portion of the progress curve, were subjected, to least square regression analysis yielding the dotted line; $y = a_1 + a_0$. According to our theoretical assumptions (see text) a_1 sould correspond to $v_b + V_m P_e$ and a_0 to $b - [V_m Pe/(k_1 + k_2)]$. Panel B: Shaded area represents the deviation of initial data points (open circle in panel A) from linearity and is determined by the difference between line y derived in A (——) and the experimental data points. (o). Panel C: Evaluation of the time constant with which the non-linear portion of the progress. curve approaches linearity: •••••, best fit of deviation of progress curve from linearity (as determined in B) according to $y = ae^{bt}$ obtained by least square regression analysis where a is assumed to correspond to $(V_m P_e / k_1 x + k_2)$ and b to $-(k_1 x + k_2)$: Panel B: •••••, total calculation of progress curve according to $\overline{cAMP_{acc}} = y(A) + y(C)$, where $y(A)$ was derived in A from best fit of the linear portion of the progress curve and $y(C)$ was derived in C from the best fit of the non-linear portion of the progress curve. For other details see ref. 17.

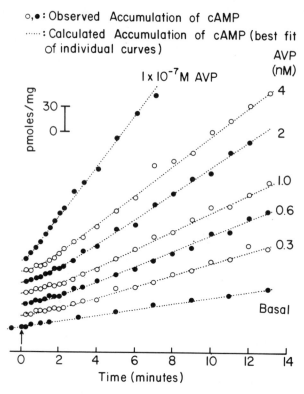

Fig. 13. Same experiment as in Fig. 12, only that now all data points obtained are shown including those where no hormone was added, allowing for calculation of b (cyclic AMP present in the incubation at the moment of hormone addition) and V_b (the basal rate of cyclic AMP accumulation). Circles: experimental data points (curves are displaced vertically and represented in an alternate pattern of closed and open circles for clarity of vision);..., best fits of the individual progress curves calculated as described in the legend to Fig. 12. For rest of experimental details see ref.17.

Fig. 14. (top of next page) Linear dependence on hormone concentration of the time constants used for calculation of the progress curves shown in Fig. 13 and calculation of k_1 and k_2. Circles: values of $k_1x + k_2$ obtained from calculations described in the legend to Fig. 12.

Fig. 15. (bottom of next page) Simulation of progress curves for activation of the beef renal medullary adenylyl cyclase by varying concentrations of arginine vasopressin (AVP) using a single set of parameters derived from the final calculations shown in Fig. 14 and equation 12 of text b = 29.4 pmoles and V_b = 4.62 pmoles per min per mg. Circles: experimental data points (same as in Fig. 13);···, fit of data points to equation 12.

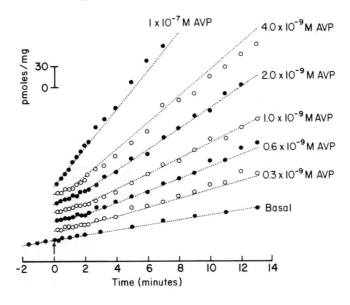

Fig. 14

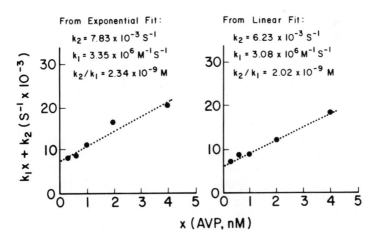

Fig. 15

function (eg. from linear to hyperbolic-like) may also occur; however, since GTP addition did not result in a concomitant shift of the dose response curve (for details see ref. 7) relating vasopressin concentration to adenylyl cyclase activation, such a change must be small in this system and cannot account for the altered rate of activation seen upon GTP addition.

Shortly before we observed an effect of GTP on the rate of hormonal activation in the beef renal system, Rodbell and his collaborators (16) had seen a similar effect in the liver plasma membrane adenylyl cyclase. However, in the liver system GTP has the additional effect of shifting the dose response curve towards lower concentrations of glucagon (the effective hormone) making it difficult to distinguish whether GTP is affecting the binding behavior of the receptor unit or the **function** that couples receptor occupancy to adenyl yl cyclase activation. If findings from one system can be extrapolated to another, then our data obtained with the beef renal system would indicate that the effect of GTP on the liver system is due, at least in part, to enhancement of the rates at which the adenylyl cyclase-coupled glucagon receptor interacts with its hormone.

In the vasopressin-sensitive system from beef kidney medulla as well as in the glucagon sensitive system from rat liver, high concentrations (mM) of ATP mimic the actions of GTP not only on catalytic activity but also on the rate at which the system can be stimulated by low hormone concentrations. Thus while in both systems the hormonal activation is slow at low ATP concentration or when AMP-PNP is used as substrate, it becomes practically instantaneous at high concentrations of ATP (larger than 1.0 mM). It was under this "nucleotide-dominated" condition that the original experiments on the reversibility of the hormonal activation of the liver adenylyl cyclase (2) and on the possible correlation between rate of activation and **rate of** binding of glucagon to specific acceptor sites (19) were performed.

4. EFFECTS OF NUCLEOTIDES ON THE COUPLING (OR TRANSDUCTION) PROCESS AND MULTIPLICITY OF SITES OF NUCLEOTIDE INTERACTION.

Perhaps the most striking evidence for GTP having an effect on the coupling of hormone receptor to adenylyl cyclase stems from recent studies of Rodbell's group on the mode of action of GTP and glucagon on liver plasma membranes. In their experiments, Rodbell et al (16) found that glucagon increases the apparent affinity of the system for GTP and that GTP increases the apparent affinity of the system for glucagon, indicating that GTP and glucagon do not interact with the membranes independently of each other. Accordingly Rodbell et al. interpreted these findings as evidence for an interdependent action of hormone and nucleotide with GTP increasing the efficacy with which multiple receptor sites affect, upon occupation, a cluster of multiple catalytic units, i.e. with the

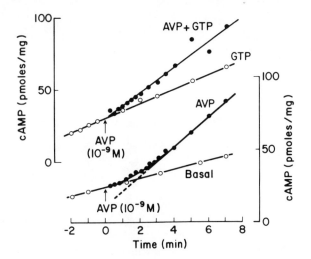

Fig. 16. Effect of GTP (10^{-5}M) on the rate of activation of the beef renal medullary adenylyl cyclase by arginine vasopressin (AVP). For rest of details see ref. 17.

coupling function that relates receptor occupation to adenylyl cyclase activation being variable and under the control of both the nucleotide and the hormone. Since involvement of a polymeric enzyme formed by multiple receptors and catalytic units was necessary mainly to account for variations in the behavior of glucagon-specific binding sites assumed to be representative or receptor binging, and since this latter assumption may not be applicable (18), the interdependent actions of GTP and glucagon can also be explained by assuming that the adenylyl cyclase system is formed by only one catalytic unit, where the hormone binds to a specific receptor site (distal from the catalytic site) and affects the conformation of the GTP binding site and where GTP binds to its site of action (be it on the catalytic unit, or the receptor or between the two, each subunit contributing to the nucleotide specific cleft) and affects allosterically the conformation (and behavior) of both the receptor and the catalytic unit.

The mechanism of action of guanyl nucleotides may even be more complex than that suggested by the experiments presented thus far. Up to this point all of the observed effects can be explained by interaction of, say, GTP with a single type of site of the system. There may, however, be more than one type of sites involved, especially in systems affected by more than one type of nucleotide. Evidence suggesting the existance of at least two sites of nucleotide interactions stems from our studies on the mode of action of luteinizing hormone (LH) in corpus luteum as well as of vasopressin in kidney. Adenylyl cyclase from corpora lutea of pseudopregnant rabbits is affected by both GTP and ATP (8 and unpublished). In

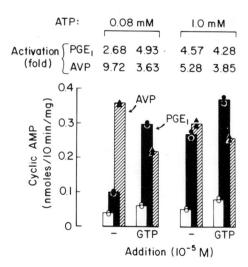

ATP:	0.08 mM		1.0 mM	
Activation (fold) PGE$_1$	2.68	4.93	4.57	4.28
AVP	9.72	3.63	5.28	3.85

Fig. 17. Dual effect of ATP and GTP on corpus luteum adenylyl cyclase. Incubations were carried out at 37° for 10 min. in medium containing the indicated concentrations of ATP (labelled in the α position with ^{32}P), 5.0 mM $MgCl_2$, 1.0 mM EDTA, 1.0 mM cAMP, 20 mM creatine phosphate, 0.2 mM per ml of creatine kinase, 25 mM Tris-HCL, pH 7.5 ca. 80 μg of membrane particle protein, and when present, 10 μg per ml of LH (NIB-LH-B8) of PGE$_1$ (Upjohn) and 10^{-5}M GTP. Membrane particles were prepared from corpora lutea dissected from ovaries of pregnant rabbits. Open bars, activities determined in the absence of either LH or PGE$_1$. For rest of details see ref. 8.

contrast to other adenylyl cyclase systems ATP and GTP act differently and GTP does not mimic the regulatory effects of ATP. As shown in Fig. 17, the response of this system to LH is almost totally dependent on the addition of higher concentrations of ATP (1.0 to 3.0 mM). Addition of GTP does not exert this effect of ATP even though it does interact with the system as indicated by a 2.5 **fold** increase of both the basal and the LH-stimulated activities (without alteration of the stimulation) when tested at low (0.08 mM) ATP and by an about 35% increase of both activities when tested at the high (3.0mM) concentration of ATP. In some ways this system is re miniscent of the vasopressin sensitive system of beef renal medullary membranes. In both systems there appear to be ATP (or adenosine) and GTP specific effects and in neither does GTP either mimic or interfere with the action of adenine derivatives. The systems differ of course in terms of mode of regulation in that the inhibitory effect of GTP on hormonal stimulation seen in the renal system appears to be absent in the corpus luteum system and in that much higher concentrations of ATP are necessary in the corpus luteum system to maximize the

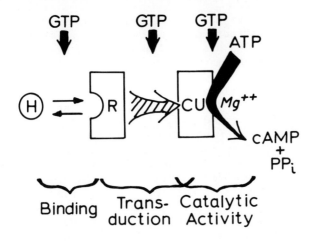

<u>Fig. 18.</u> Functional levels at which GTP has been found to affect adenylyl cyclase systems.

hormonal response. A solution to which of the above explanations, if any, is applicable has to come from further experimentation determining whether adenylyl cyclases are monomeric or polymeric in structure and establishing the role of slowly reacting binding hormone-specific binding in rapidly activated adenylyl cyclases (18,19). The recent findings by Helmreich's group (20) that a factor or a fraction responsible for the action of GTP on catalytic activity can be removed by affinity chromatography from the liver adenylyl cyclase system after detergent solubilization indicate that additional subunits, responsible for nucleotide regulation, also have to be con - sidered.

The possible existence of more than one site of nucleotide interaction, one responsible for modulation of receptor-hormone interaction and the other responsible for regulation of the stimulatory activity of the occupied receptor, may explain some of the complex kinetics of ITP (shift of a hormone dependence curve from negatively cooperative to positively cooperative coupled to simultaneous enhancement of the stimulating effect of the hormone) seen recently by Dumont and collaborators in their studies on the mechanism of action of thyroid stimulating hormone (TSH) in horse thyroid membranes (21,22). ITP had previously been shown by Wolff and Cook to increase the stimulatory action of TSH in beef thyroid membranes (23).

In conclusion, we have presented our view of how nucleotides (and nucleosides) affect adenylyl cyclases and their response to hormones. In so doing we discussed many of the more recently discovered properties of these enzymes (bursts, lags, histeretic enzyme concept) and our current views of the receptor occupancy-adenylyl cyclase activation relationship (linear vs non-linear, structural features required for non-linear coupling). We also speculated as to the number of nucleotide-specific sites involved in the action of nucleotides, but in view of the fact that the actual structural features of adenylyl cyclases are still unknown, we restricted ourselves primarily to defining the functional aspects affected by nucleotides. As represented in Fig. 18, it is clear that nucleotides affect all known levels of adenylyl cyclase function: receptor, tranduction (coupling) and catalytic activity. Detailed investigation of any one of the affected functions should eventually lead to disclosure of the mechanism (how and where) by which nucleotides exert their action.

5. NOMENCLATURE USED

The term adenylyl rather than the original adenyl or the more often used adenylate has been used throughout this article. We prefer this name because it more accurately relates to the reaction catalyzed by the enzyme: the intramolecular transfer of the 5'-adenylyl group to its 3' position, and because it accurately describes the substrates of the reaction: 5'-adenylyl pyrophosphate (ATP) and 5'-adenylyl imidodiphosphate (AMP/PNP). AMP, an adenylate is therefore automatically excluded as substrate.

6. ABBREVIATIONS

ACTH, adrenocorticotropin; AMP_PNP, 5'-adenylyl imidodiphosphat A_R, adenosine; AVP, arginine vasopressin; LH, luteinizing hormone; LVP, lysine vasopressin; PG, prostaglandin; PSP, pseudopregnancy or pseudopregnant; RS, ATP regenerating system (creatine kinase - creatine phosphate); TSH, thyroid stimulating hormone.

7. ACKNOWLEDGEMENTS AND PRESENT ADDRESSES

We wish to express our appreciation for the excellent technical assistance of Mr. Po-Chang Yang, who carried out many of the experiments reported above. This research was supported in part by Grants HD-06513 and HD-06723 from the United States Public Health Service. Present addresses: L.B.: Department of Cell Biology, Baylor Colleg of Medicine, Houston, Texas 77025; T.N.: Department of Chemistry, Faculty of Science, Kyusyu University, Fukuoka, Japan; and M.H.-D.: Department of Biochemistry, Northwestern University Medical School, Chicago, Illinois, 60611.

8.   REFERENCES

1.   Rodbell, M., Birnbaumer, L., Pohl, S.L. and Krans, H.M.J. (1974)
     J. Biol. Chem. 246, 1877.
2.   Birnbaumer, L., Pohl, S.L., Rodbell, M. and Sundby, F. (1972)
     J. Biol. Chem. 247, 2038.
3.   Krishna, G., Harwood, J.P., Barber, A.J. and Jamieson, G.A.
     (1972) J. Biol. Chem. 247, 2253.
4.   Leray, F., Chambaut, A.-M. and Hanoune, J. (1972) Biochem.
     Biophys. Res. Commun. 48, 1385.
5.   Rodbell, M., Birnbaumer, L., Pohl, S.L. and Krans, H.M.J. (1971)
     Excerpta Medica Int. Congr. Ser. No. 241, Vol. 1, 199.
6.   Birnbaumer, L. (1973) Biochim. Biophys. Acta. (Reviews on Bio-
     membranes) 300, 129.
7.   Birnbaumer, L., Nakahara, T. and Yang, P. Ch. (1974) J. Biol.
     Chem. 249, 7857.
8.   Birnbaumer, l., and Yang, Ph. Ch. (1974) J. Biol. Chem 249,
     7867.
9.   Frieden, C. (1970) J. Biol. Chem. 245, 5788.
10. Murad, F., Strauch, B.S. and Vaughan, M. (1969) Biochim. Biophys.
     Acta. 177, 591.
11. Harwood, J.P., Low, H. and Rodbell, M. (1973) J. Biol. Chem.
     248, 6239.
12. Barber, E.D. and Bright, H.J. (1968) Proc. Nat. Acad. Sci. U.S.
     60, 1363.
13. Hatfield, G.W. and Umbarger, H.E. (1970) J. Biol. Chem 245, 1742.
14. Shill, J.P. and Neet, K.E. (1971) Biochem. J. 123, 283.
15. Bockaert, J., Roy, Ch., Rajerison, R. and Jard, S. (1973) J.
     Biol. Chem. 248, 5922.
16. Rodbell, M., Lin, M.C. and Salomon, Y. (1974) J. Biol. Chem.
     249, 59-65.
17. Nakahara, T. and Birnbaumer, L. (1974) J. Biol. Chem. 249, 7886.
18. Birnbaumer, L., Pohl, S.L. and Kaumann, A.J. (1974) In, "Ad-
     vances in Cyclic Nucleotide Research," (Greengard, P. and
     Robison, G.A., eds.) Raven Press, New York, vol. 4, pp. 239.
19. Birnbaumer, L. and Pohl, S.L. 1973) J. Biol. Chem 248, 2056.
20. Pfeuffer, T. and Helmreich, E.T.M. (1975) J. Biol. Chem. 250,
     867.
21. Boeynaems, J.M., Van Sande, J., Pochet, R. and Dumont, J.E.
     (1974) Mol. Cell. Endocrinology 1, 139.
22. Pochet, R., Boeynaems, J.M. and Dumont, J.E. (1974) Biochem.
     Biophys. Res. Commun. 58, 446.
23. Wolff, J. and Cook, G.H. (1973) J. Biol. Chem. 248, 350.
24. Goldfine, I.D., Roth, J. and Birnbaumer, L. (1972) J. Biol. Chem.
     247, 1211.
25. Lefkowitz, R.J. (1974) J. Biol. Chem. 248, 350.
26. Bockaert, J., Roy, Ch. and Jard, S. (1972) J. Biol. Chem 247,
     7073.

CYCLIC AMP METABOLISM OF SOME FIBROBLASTIC AND EPITHELIAL CELLS IN VITRO

Francis J. Chlapowski and Reginald W. Butcher

Department of Biochemistry, University of Massachusetts

Medical School, Worcester, MA, USA 01605

LIST OF CONTENTS

In the second messenger concept, adenylate cyclase and its hormonal receptors translate specific extracellular signals into intracellular cyclic adenosine 3':5'-monophosphate (cyclic AMP) production. Cyclic AMP, in turn, interacts with the regulatory subunits of protein kinase, and also is degraded into 5'-AMP by cyclic nucleotide 3':5'-phosphodiesterase (phosphodiesterase) (1). For these reasons it is common to use measurements of adenylate cyclase activities and phosphodiesterase activities in cell-free preparations as indicators of the kinetics of cyclic AMP metabolism in intact cells. Alternatively, the accumulation of cyclic AMP in intact cells often is viewed as a measure of the rate of intracellular production and destruction of cyclic

AMP. In this report we would like to discuss these notions.

It is our contention that while enzyme measurements in broken cells and determinations of cyclic AMP levels in intact cells can give evidence of the existence of cyclic AMP metabolism and the hormonal specificity of the system, studies with cell-free preparations do not necessarily represent what may occur in living cells and vice versa. Furthermore, measurements of cyclic AMP accumulation in intact cells is not simply the resultant sum of adenylate cyclase production and phosphodiesterase degradation of cyclic AMP.

To illustrate the latter points, data obtained with four different cell types are selectively summarized. The cells were: WI-38, human diploid lung fibroblasts (obtained from Dr. L. Hayflick); WI-38-VA13-2RA, SV40-transformed WI-38 cells (obtained from Dr. A. Girardi and hereafter referred to as VA-13); HEp-2, human laryngeal epithelial carcinoma cells (obtained from Dr. D. Merchant); and freshly isolated transitional epithelium from the urinary bladders of adult male rabbits. While the cells used were pairs of normal and neoplastic fibroblastic and epithelial cells, it was not our intent to draw conclusions about neoplasia and cyclic AMP metabolism. Rather, these cells were chosen to represent a wide range of responses to similar hormonal signals.

METHODS

The experimental incubations for the 3 monolayer cultures (WI-38, VA13, and HEp-2) as well as the freshly isolated, homogeneous, transitional epithelium preparations were essentially identical, except that brief low speed centrifugations were carried out to separate the transitional epithelium from the incubation medium before fixation of the cells and medium separately in intact cell studies (1-6). Briefly summarized, the procedure was similar to that described by Gilman and Nirenberg (7). Cells were rinsed and equilibrated for a short time in fresh, serum-free Eagle's minimal essential medium (Grand Island Biological Co.) at $37°$ in humidified 95% air/5% CO_2. Experimental incubations were begun with the addition of appropriate agonists or phosphodiesterase inhibitors. The incubations were terminated by aspirating or centrifuging the medium, which was fixed by the addition of trichloroacetic acid or HCl containing a small amount of high specific activity ^{3}H-cyclic AMP to monitor recovery. The cell sheet or tissue pellet was fixed in a similar manner. The cells appeared to be fixed essentially instantaneously and the recovery of cyclic AMP appeared to be quantitative in all cases as verified by ^{3}H-cyclic AMP recovery, exhaustive extraction, and comparison of the results to identical

TABLE 1. *Effects of epinephrine, PGE₁ and phosphodiesterase inhibitors on cyclic AMP levels of cells in vitro.* - *Intact WI-38, VA13, HEp-2, and transitional epithelial cells were prepared for experiments in 90 mm plastic petri dishes as described (2-5). Cells were rinsed and preincubated briefly in serum-free Eagle's minimal essential medium. Incubations were carried out in the presence of the indicated additions for 10 min. The additions were distilled water (Control), 10 μM epinephrine, or 5.7 μM PGE₁. In the indicated experiments 2 mM theophylline was added to the incubation media of WI-38 and VA13 cells, while 2 mM MIX was added to the media of HEp-2 and transitional epithelial cells. Trichloroacetic acid extracts of the cells were analyzed for cyclic AMP as previously described (2-5). Each value is an average based upon 3 to 10 experiments.*

Additions	Phosphodiesterase Inhibitor	pmoles cyclic AMP/mg cell protein			
		WI-38	VA13	HEp-2	Transitional Epithelium
Control	−	55	30	17	12
	+	55	30	20	89
Epinephrine	−	600	2000	35	20
	+	800	3000	500	975
PGE₁	−	800	2100	17	27
	+	1500	3500	20	1400

experiments in which the acid was added directly to the medium plus cells. The acid extracts were fractionated to purify cyclic AMP on Dowex-50 and Dowex-2 columns as described (1-6). Adenylate cyclase activities and phosphodiesterase activities were determined in cell-free homogenates prepared and assayed essentially as described by Chlapowski and Butcher (8). Samples of purified cyclic AMP from intact cell studies and adenylate cyclase experiments were treated with purified beef heart cyclic nucleotide 3', 5'-phosphodiesterase to test the validity of the binding assay.

LACK OF CORRELATION BETWEEN INTACT CELL STUDIES AND CELL-FREE ENZYME STUDIES

As shown in Table 1, all of the cells tested in the presence of 10 μM epinephrine plus a phosphodiesterase inhibitor responded with an increase in intracellular cyclic AMP levels. Since WI-38 cells lose the ability to respond well to epinephrine with increasing cell density (2), only cells of densities appropriate to give substantial responses were used in the present experiments. All of the cells, except HEp-2, also responded in a more dramatic manner to 5.7 μM PGE$_1$ in the presence of a phosphodiesterase inhibitor. However, in absence of either 2 mM theophylline or 2 mM l-methyl, 3-isobutylxanthine (MIX) the responses of HEp-2 and transitional epithelial cells were slight, while those of WI-38 and VA13 were still quite substantial.

The levels of cyclic AMP accumulated after a 10 min stimulation of transitional epithelial cells with either epinephrine or PGE$_1$ in the presence of MIX were about 50-fold greater than values obtained in the absence of MIX. The potentiation of the epinephrine response of HEp-2 cells was approximately 15-fold. In contrast, 2 mM theophylline rarely potentiated the responses of either WI-38 or VA13 greater than 2-fold as shown in Table 1. Although 2 mM MIX potentiated the intracellular accumulation of cyclic AMP in WI-38 and VA13 cells to a greater extent than theophylline (L. Kelly, personal communication), such potentiation

TABLE 2.   *A comparison of adenylate cyclase and phosphodiesterase activities in homogenates of cells.* - *Cells were prepared, homogenized, and assayed for adenylate cyclase and phosphodiesterase activities using slight modifications (3,4,6) of the method of Chlapowski and Butcher (8). Phosphodiesterase activities were determined at cyclic AMP concentrations of 100 μM and 1 μM and are presented as pmoles cyclic AMP destroyed/mg protein/min. Adenylate cyclase activities were determined in the presence of additions containing distilled water (Control), 10 μM epinephrine, or 5.7 μM PGE$_1$ and are expressed as pmoles cyclic AMP produced/mg protein/min. Adenylate cyclase activities were assayed in the presence of 6.7 mM caffeine. Each value presented is the average of 3 to 5 experiments.*

Enzyme Assayed	Additions	Specific Activity			
		WI-38	VA13	HEp-2	Transitional Epithelium
Adenylate cyclase	Control	8	6	3	30
	Epinephrine	25	75	45	185
	PGE$_1$	65	35	3	170
Phospho-diesterase	100 μM cyclic AMP	4.50	0.25	1.10	0.25
	1 μM cyclic AMP	0.11	0.02	0.06	0.02

TABLE 3. Accumulation of cyclic AMP in cells and in incubation media after exposure to epinephrine or PGE$_1$. - Cells were prepared and incubated as described in Table 1, in the presence of 2 mM theophylline (WI-38 and VA13 cells), or 2 mM MIX (HEp-2 and transitional epithelium). Following a 60 min incubation period, the media and the cells were fixed separately as previously described (2-5). Values are the average of at least three determinations in one experiment and representative of similar experiments.

Additions	pmoles cyclic AMP/mg cell protein	
	Cells	Media
WI-38		
PGE$_1$ (5.7 μM)	1300	5200 (<40)[a]
VA13		
PGE$_1$ (5.7 μM)	3600	4400 (<40)
HEp-2		
Epinephrine (10 μM)	80	125 (20)
Transitional epithelium		
Epinephrine (10 μM)	750	500 (150)
PGE$_1$ (10 μM)	1400	1200 (150)

[a]Control media levels of cyclic AMP are shown in parentheses.

was only on the average about 5-fold for WI-38 cells and much less for VA13.

Based upon the latter data, it might be predicted that cell-free studies of the enzymes of cyclic AMP production and destruction would reveal that adenylate cyclase activities would be low and/or that phosphodiesterase activities would be high in transitional epithelial cells and HEp-2 cells in comparison to WI-38 and VA13 cells. In fact, as shown in Table 2, such is not the case. Transitional epithelial cells demonstrated the highest adenylate cyclase activity and the lowest phosphodiesterase activity under the conditions of these experiments. HEp-2 cells also had a greater epinephrine-stimulated adenylate cyclase activity and a lesser phosphodiesterase activity than WI-38 cells.

RELEASE OF CYCLIC AMP FROM CELLS

Following prolonged stimulation of cells, substantial levels of cyclic AMP accumulated in the incubation media as shown in

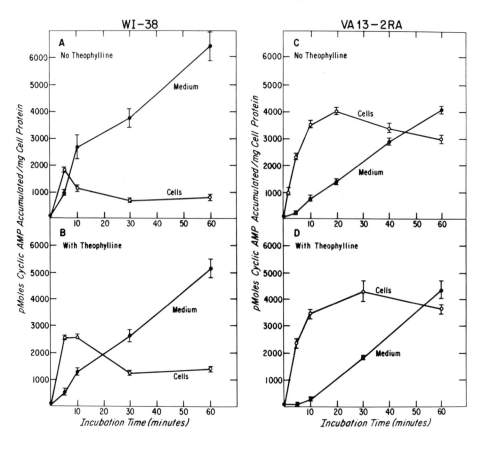

Figure 1. *The effect of 5.7 μM* PGE_1 *on the accumulation of cyclic AMP in the cells and incubation media of WI-38 (A & B) and VA13 cells (C & D), in the presence or absence of 2 mM theophylline. Incubation media and cells were fixed as previously described (3). Reprinted with permission from Kelly, Hall and Butcher (3).*

Table 3. While this phenomenon was not seen to any great extent in HEp-2 and transitional epithelial cells in the absence of 2 mM MIX, the escape of cyclic AMP from WI-38 and VA13 cells to the medium occurred to a greater extent in the absence of a phosphodiesterase inhibitor (Fig. 1). In fact, the primary effect of theophylline on both WI-38 and VA13 cells seemed to be in delaying the onset of release of cyclic AMP. In WI-38 cells theophylline also seemed to reduce the amount of cyclic AMP released. In fact, in WI-38 cells the "phosphodiesterase inhibitor" appeared to

increase intracellular levels of cyclic AMP by partially inhibiting
cell escape and not by substantially affecting the rate of cyclic
AMP destruction. If the sums of intracellular and medium cyclic
AMP levels are compared at each time point shown in Fig. 1, it can
be seen that there is little difference.

However, unlike theophylline, the phosphodiesterase inhibitors
MIX, R020-1724, and papaverine did substantially increase total
cyclic AMP levels of cells plus medium (not shown). Nonetheless,
like theophylline, the latter phosphodiesterase inhibitors also
inhibited release of cyclic AMP (L. Kelly, personal communication).

The results obtained with WI-38 and VA13 may be contrasted to
those observed with HEp-2 and transitional epithelial cells. In
both types of epithelial cells neither substantial intracellular
accumulations of cyclic AMP nor release of cyclic AMP into the
medium was observed, unless a phosphodiesterase inhibitor was
utilized.

COMMENTS

The lack of correlation between experiments with intact cells
and enzyme measurements of cell-free preparations is demonstrated
by a comparison of Tables 1 and 2. If the data obtained from the
enzyme measurements shown in Table 2 were used to predict the
magnitude of intracellular cyclic AMP responses to epinephrine,
the order of the cells, placed according to decreasing responsiveness, would be transitional epithelium > VA13 > HEp-2 > WI-38.
The actual order of responsiveness illustrated in Table 1 was
VA13 > WI-38 > transitional epithelium > HEp-2. There are a
plethoria of possible explanations for this lack of correspondence
ranging from our ignorance of the kinetics of cyclic AMP metabolism
in intact cells to the very stylized conditions of enzyme measurements in broken cell preparations. While it is important to determine the reasons for the disparities between broken cell and intact
cell experiments, it is equally as important to keep in mind that
such differences in fact exist.

Similarly, as shown in Table 3 and Fig. 1, there was little
correlation between the intracellular accumulation of cyclic AMP
and the actual rate of cyclic AMP production, due to the release
of cyclic AMP into the media of stimulated cells. The decrease
and leveling off of intracellular levels of cyclic AMP during
prolonged PGE_1 stimulation of WI-38 and VA13 cells was not due
simply to increased intracellular degradation by phosphodiesterase,
but in large part was a result of steady and continuing release of
cyclic AMP from the cells. In this light, our observations were
similar to those of Exton et al. (10), who reported that the
increased glucose production of perfused liver stimulated by

glucagon was better correlated to measurements of cyclic AMP in the liver plus the perfusion medium, rather than just the liver alone. Franklin and Foster (9) also have reported the appearance of cyclic AMP in the culture medium of human diploid lung fibroblasts stimulated with PGE₁ or isoprenaline.

A major effect upon cyclic AMP accumulation in WI-38 cells of all the phosphodiesterase inhibitors examined appeared to be a partial inhibition of cell escape of cyclic AMP. Theophylline did not seem to have any other major effect, while RO20-1724, papaverine, and particularly MIX, did potentiate total cyclic AMP accumulation in the cells plus the media.

In contrast, hormonally-stimulated cyclic AMP accumulation in HEp-2 and transitional epithelium cells or their incubation media was slight in the absence of a phosphodiesterase inhibitor, perhaps indicating that phosphodiesterase control of cyclic AMP levels was more stringent in these cells. Nonetheless, release of cyclic AMP into the surrounding media of these cells was observed in the presence of MIX, and was quite substantial in the case of transitional epithelium (5). Thus, even in these cells, a more accurate measurement of the rate of cyclic AMP production in the presence of a phosphodiesterase inhibitor would entail measurement of medium as well as cellular cyclic AMP levels.

REFERENCES

1. Robison, G.A., Butcher, R.W., and Sutherland, E.W. (1971) Cyclic AMP, Academic Press, New York.
2. Kelly, L.A., and Butcher, R.W. (1974) The effects of epinephrine and prostaglandin E₁ on cyclic adenosine 3':5'-monophosphate levels in WI-38 fibroblasts. J. Biol. Chem., 249:3098-3102.
3. Kelly, L.A., Hall, M.S., and Butcher, R.W. (1974) Cyclic adenosine 3':5'-monophosphate metabolism in normal and SV40-transformed WI-38 cells. J. Biol. Chem., 249:5182-5187.
4. Kelly, L.A., and Butcher, R.W. (1975) Studies on cyclic AMP metabolism in human epidermoid carcinoma (HEp-2) cells. Metabolism, 24:359-368.
5. Chlapowski, F.J. (1975) The effects of hormones on cyclic adenosine 3':5'-monophosphate accumulation in transitional epithelium of the urinary bladder. J. Cyclic Nucleotide Research, in press.
6. Chlapowski, F.J. (1975) Adenylyl cyclase and phosphodiesterase in transitional epithelium of the urinary bladder. Manuscript in preparation.

7. Gilman, A.G., and Nirenberg, M. (1971) Effect of catechola-
      mine on the adenosine 3':5'-cyclic monophosphate con-
      centrations of clonal satellite cells of neurons.
      Proc. Nat. Acad. Sci. U.S.A., 68:2165-2168.
8. Chlapowski, F.J., and Butcher, R.W. (1973) Subcellular
      distribution of adenylyl cyclase and phosphodiesterase
      in Acanthamoeba palestinensis. Biochim. Biophys. Acta,
      309:138-148.
9. Franklin, T.J., and Foster, S.J. (1973) Leakage of cyclic
      AMP from human diploid fibroblasts in tissue culture.
      Nature New Biol., 246:119-120.
10. Exton, J.H., Lewis, S.B., Ho, R.J., Robison, G.A., and
      Park, C.R. (1971) The role of cyclic AMP in the inter-
      action of glucagon and insulin in the control of liver
      metabolism. Ann. N.Y. Acad. Sci., 185:85-100.
11. This work was supported by research grants AM-13904 and
      GM-18332 from the National Institutes of Health, United
      States Public Health Service.

METABOLISM OF CYCLIC GMP IN VASCULAR SMOOTH MUSCLE, LEUKOCYTES,

AND LUNG

Martha Vaughan

Laboratory of Cellular Metabolism
National Heart and Lung Institute
National Institutes of Health
Bethesda, Maryland 20014, USA

Contents

There are obvious historical reasons for the fact that our understanding of cyclic GMP metabolism in 1974 is far more limited than that relating to cyclic AMP. Over the almost 20 years that cyclic AMP has been known, the methodology has been consistently improved and refined whereas experience in the extraction, purification and measurement of cyclic GMP from tissues is much less extensive. The radioimmunoassay of Steiner et al. (1) with its sensitivity and specificity is obviously an extremely powerful tool. Nevertheless, perhaps in large part because of the low cyclic GMP content of most mammalian cells, there are often technical problems encountered in attempting to apply the assay successfully with tissue extracts (2,3). In our laboratory it has been invariably necessary to purify cyclic GMP samples before assay, and to modify the purification procedures depending on the system studied.

In several tissues, cholinergic agents, evidently acting through muscarinic receptors, can cause accumulation of cyclic GMP, and typically cholinergic physiological responses to other stimuli may be accompanied by increases in cyclic GMP content. Less is known about other ways in which cyclic GMP metabolism can be regulated and the types of functions that may be influenced by this nucleotide. Much of the available information has been reviewed by Goldberg et al. (4). This presentation deals only with certain specific aspects of cyclic GMP metabolism, and is divided into three parts:

(1) a consideration of the relationship between cyclic GMP and contraction in vascular smooth muscle,

(2) a summary of some information concerning factors that can alter cyclic GMP metabolism in leukocytes and possible functional roles for this nucleotide in different types of white blood cells,

(3) an outline of the results of studies with lung slices that have led to the suggestion that cyclic GMP may play a part in the regulation of prostaglandin synthesis and release.

It will be noted that there is no discussion of the mechanisms by which the several agonists mentioned below bring about accumulation of cyclic GMP in these and other tissues. Although it seems probable that acetylcholine, bradykinin, histamine and serotonin elevate cyclic GMP in specific cells as a consequence of increasing its synthesis, i.e., by increasing guanylate cyclase activity, this remains to be established.

VASCULAR SMOOTH MUSCLE

Evidence of several types is consistent with the view that relaxation of smooth muscle is associated with elevation in the cyclic AMP content of this tissue and a role for cyclic GMP in smooth muscle contraction has been suggested [see review by Schultz et al. (5)]. In vein segments (bovine and canine), Dunham et al. (6) found that both isoproterenol and PGE_1,[1] which cause vasodilatation, produced elevation of cyclic AMP while, associated with the vasoconstriction caused by $PGF_{2\alpha}$, there was an increase in the cyclic GMP content of the vein. Some other factors that can influence cyclic GMP metabolism in human umbilical artery have recently been investigated (7).

In umbilical artery segments incubated in air the cyclic GMP content was almost twice as high as the cyclic AMP content (7), whereas in all other mammalian tissues thus far studied the cyclic

---

[1]Abbreviations: PGA_1, PGA_2, PGE_1, $PGF_{2\alpha}$, prostaglandins A_1, A_2, E_1, and $F_{2\alpha}$.

AMP concentration is greater, often many times greater than that of cyclic GMP (4). It is tempting to speculate that the relatively high cyclic GMP content of the umbilical artery under these conditions is in some way related to the physiological importance of contraction at this stage of development.

One particularly interesting and physiologically important characteristic of the umbilical artery is its ability to close completely relatively soon after birth. Bradykinin, serotonin, histamine, acetylcholine, prostaglandins A_1 and $F_{2\alpha}$, as well as oxygen, have been suggested as possible factors in this process. All of these stimuli can cause constriction of the umbilical artery in vitro (8-10) and several of the chemical mediators have been reported to induce accumulation of cyclic GMP in other tissues (4,5,11). It has now been shown (7) that bradykinin, serotonin, histamine, and acetylcholine, as well as K^+ ion in concentrations that cause contraction of the artery (9,10) can increase the cyclic GMP content of the human umbilical artery without affecting its cyclic AMP content. Bradykinin, histamine, acetylcholine and K^+ raised cyclic GMP only when Ca^{++} was present in the incubation medium, but the effects of serotonin were undiminished in the Ca^{++}-depleted artery.

Of the agents tested known to cause constriction of the umbilical artery in vitro, only PGA_2 and $PGF_{2\alpha}$ failed to cause accumulation of cyclic GMP (7). They also had no effect on cyclic AMP. PGE_1 did induce accumulation of cyclic AMP (7) and is known to cause relaxation (12), whereas isoproterenol, which does not (9,13), had no effect on cyclic AMP (7), consistent with the view that the human umbilical artery lacks functional β-adrenergic receptors.

The effects of acetylcholine on cyclic GMP in several tissues are apparently mediated through muscarinic receptors and in the umbilical artery the effect of acetylcholine was completely prevented by atropine, which did not interfere with the effects of bradykinin, histamine, serotonin, or K^+ ion (7). The effects of histamine were prevented by pyrilamine, an inhibitor of the so-called H1 histamine receptor (14), and all data were consistent with the conclusion that histamine increases cyclic GMP in the artery as a result of its interaction with H1 receptors (7). There was no evidence that histamine, acting through H2 receptors, could influence the metabolism of cyclic GMP or of cyclic AMP in the umbilical artery.

It appears that, in the umbilical artery as in many tissues, the concentrations of cyclic AMP and cyclic GMP are independently controlled. In addition, the observations are consistent with data obtained in other systems, that chemical stimuli that cause contraction of smooth muscle also cause accumulation of cyclic GMP.

The mechanisms by which acetylcholine, histamine, serotonin, bradykinin, and K^+ ions produce these two effects and the nature of the
relationship between them remains to be elucidated. Although it
seems probable that the increase in cyclic GMP occurs in the smooth
muscle cells of the artery it should be recognized that not all
of these cells are necessarily responsive to each of the stimuli.

LEUKOCYTES

Cyclic nucleotides have been implicated in several aspects of
leukocyte function. Kaliner and Austen (15) have recently reviewed
the evidence relating to the role of cyclic nucleotides in the
inflammatory response. We shall attempt to summarize here the
limited information available concerning factors that can alter
cyclic GMP metabolism in human leukocytes and possible physiological
roles for cyclic GMP in specific types of white blood cells. Many
experiments have been carried out with preparations of cells separated from human peripheral blood and in only a few cases have more
or less homogeneous populations of cells been studied. Thus, when
changes in cyclic GMP content are observed, it is often difficult
to attribute them with any degree of certainty to a specific type
of cell.

Effects of Cholinergic Agonists on Cyclic GMP Metabolism

The selective release of lysosomal enzymes from human polymorphonuclear leukocytes without concomitant release of cytoplasmic enzymes can be induced in several ways, in some instances
accompanied by phagocytosis and in others not (16-20). Cyclic AMP
and agents that can cause its accumulation, such as theophylline,
PGE_1 and epinephrine, interfere with lysosomal enzyme release,
whereas cyclic GMP or cholinergic agents can increase it (2,20-24).
Zurier et al. (2) reported that carbamylcholine increased the
cyclic GMP content (but not the cyclic AMP content) of human
leukocyte suspensions incubated in the presence of cytochalasin B,
serum and zymosan. Ignarro and George (24) found that zymosan
(treated with serum from patients with rheumatoid arthritis),
after a delay of about 1 minute, caused accumulation of cyclic GMP
which continued to increase for at least 10 minutes. The addition
of acetylcholine accelerated the initial accumulation but in the
absence of zymosan, acetylcholine was without effect on cyclic GMP.
The effects of acetylcholine both on lysosomal enzyme release and
on cyclic GMP were prevented by atropine but not by hexamethonium
(24). Thus in these cells as in many other tissues, accumulation
of cyclic GMP caused by cholinergic agents is evidently mediated
through a muscarinic receptor and is associated with effects on cell
function that are apparently opposite to those associated with elevation of cell cyclic AMP content.

Lymphocyte-mediated cytotoxicity is a phenomenon that occurs in animals that have received incompatible tissue grafts. The graft recipient develops a population of T lymphocytes that, when brought in contact with cells bearing the appropriate antigenic determinants, induces lysis of these target cells (25). It was found by Henny et al. (26,27) that lymphocyte-mediated cytotoxicity could be counteracted by agents capable of causing accumulation of cyclic AMP and it has now been shown that theophylline, PGE_1, iso-proterenol and cholera toxin, all can interfere with this process (26-29). Cholinergic agents cause accumulation of cyclic GMP in lymphocytes (31,32) and they, as well as 8-bromo cyclic GMP, enhance lymphocyte mediated cytotoxicity (28,29,32). It has been reported that the cyclic GMP content of lymphocytes is increased by phyto-haemoglutinin and by concanavalin A (31,33) but whether these agents act on the same population of cells as do the cholinergic agents or whether they can influence lymphocyte-mediated cyto-toxicity is unknown. It is known that the modification of cyto-toxicity by cyclic nucleotides occurs at a very early stage in the process (15), but elucidation of the precise mechanism through which the nucleotides produce their effects will probably await a better understanding of the nature of the phenomenon itself. In any case it appears that in lymphocytes also, muscarinic agonists can cause accumulation of cyclic GMP and produce functional changes that are opposite to those associated with elevation of intracellu-lar cyclic AMP content.

Effects of Serotonin and Melatonin on Cyclic GMP Metabolism

While investigating the effects of phagocytosis and of several putative mediators of the inflammatory response on cyclic GMP and cyclic AMP metabolism in leukocytes in our laboratory, it was found that serotonin can cause accumulation of cyclic GMP but not cyclic AMP in monocytes from human peripheral blood (34). In these cells, serotonin and cyclic GMP may play a role in the regulation of chemotaxis and/or cell motility.

In preparations of mixed leukocytes from human peripheral blood, the cyclic GMP content was consistently elevated after exposure for 5 minutes to 100 µM serotonin (a maximally effective concentration) (34). The magnitude of the effect was, however, extremely variable. When unfractionated leukocytes from a single donor were compared with fractions enriched respectively in mono-nuclear cells and in polymorphonuclear cells, serotonin caused a much greater accumulation of cyclic GMP in the mononuclear fraction than it did in the unfractionated leukocytes and was essentially without effect on the polymorphonuclear cells. By incubating the mononuclear cell preparations for 24 hours in plastic dishes, it is possible to separate two populations of cells, those which adhere to the surface (in our experience >90% monocytes) and those which do not. The cyclic GMP content and the effect of serotonin on it was much greater in the adherent monocytes, or circulating macrophages than it was in the non-adherent cells. In fact, it was calculated that the observed increment in cyclic GMP produced by serotonin in the non-adherent cell fractions could be accounted for entirely by the response of the monocytes contained in them (34).

Melatonin and certain other derivatives of 5-hydroxytryptamine were as effective as serotonin in causing accumulation of cyclic GMP in monocytes but tryptamine itself had little or no effect. Other potential mediators of the inflammatory response, histamine and kinins (bradykinin, lysyl bradykinin, and methionyl lysyl brady-kinin) had no effect on cyclic GMP in the mononuclear cells (34). Serotonin can increase the cyclic GMP content of uterine smooth muscle (30) and, as mentioned above, it causes accumulation of cyclic GMP in the human umbilical artery (7) but no effects of melatonin on cyclic GMP metabolism have previously been reported. It has been found that carbamylcholine (35) as well as ascorbic acid (36) can enhance leukocyte migration. In preliminary experiments (37) both significantly elevated the cyclic GMP content of human monocytes while serotonin (like ascorbate and carbamylcholine) increased the movement of monocytes in response to a chemotactic stimulus. Histamine and bradykinin had no effect under the same conditions. When current experiments are completed, it may be possible to define more clearly the relationship between cyclic GMP metabolism and monocyte function, and to evaluate the physiological or pathological significance of the effects of serotonin (and melatonin) on cyclic GMP in human monocytes.

LUNG

Compared to several other tissues in the rat, the lung contains rather large amounts of cyclic GMP (38). Accumulation of cyclic GMP induced by acetylcholine has been shown in lung from several species (3,4,30,39). In slices of guinea pig lung, acetylcholine caused a rapid transient increase in the cyclic GMP content and, in addition, parallel changes in cyclic AMP content (3). In the other tissues discussed thus far, increases in cyclic GMP produced by acetylcholine or other stimuli were not accompanied by increases in cyclic AMP. Bradykinin likewise caused a rapid rise in both cyclic GMP and cyclic AMP in the guinea pig lung slices (11). The effects of bradykinin were very similar to those of acetylcholine but were evidently not secondary to release of endogenous acetylcholine since they were not inhibited by atropine which inhibited the effects of acetylcholine on both cyclic nucleotides. Histamine also increased cyclic GMP as well as cyclic AMP (40) in guinea pig lung slices. Thus, in this tissue in contrast

to others, each of the agonists that caused accumulation of cyclic
GMP also increased cyclic AMP.

On investigating the possibility that the increase in cyclic
AMP caused by bradykinin was a result of the induced release of
another agonist, it was found that neither promethazine, an anti-
histamine, nor propranolol, a beta adrenergic blocking agent,
modified the effects of bradykinin on either nucleotide. Indomethacin, or aspirin, on the other hand, completely prevented
the rise in cyclic AMP but had no effect on the accumulation of
cyclic GMP in response to bradykinin (11). These drugs can
inhibit the synthesis of prostaglandins in homogenates of lung
and inhibit the release of prostaglandins from perfused lung when
it is induced by bradykinin (41,42). All of these observations
were consistent with the hypothesis that the effect of bradykinin
on cyclic AMP in guinea pig lung was indirect and secondary to
the induced release of prostaglandins (11).

Indomethacin likewise abolished the effect of acetylcholine
on cyclic AMP without altering its effect on cyclic GMP. Acetylcholine can cause release of prostaglandins from the adrenal (43)
and it seems likely that this occurs also in lung, accounting for
the rise in cyclic AMP produced by acetylcholine. The guinea pig
lung is the only tissue in which increased cyclic GMP has been
reported to be accompanied by an increase in cyclic AMP content.
In the studies of Kuo and Kuo (39) with rat lung, acetylcholine
increased cyclic GMP levels but alone had no effect on cyclic AMP.
Whether this is a reflection of species differences or is related
to differences in experimental conditions remains to be determined.
Clearly, prostaglandins synthesized and released in response to an
elevation of intracellular cyclic GMP concentration, would have no
demonstrable effect on the cyclic AMP content of a tissue unless
there were cells in that tissue capable of responding to prostaglandins of the amount and type present with an increase in
cyclic AMP formation. Thus far, the evidence is circumstantial
but consistent with the suggestion that agents that cause accumulation of cyclic GMP may thereby enhance the synthesis and release
of prostaglandins in certain types of cells.

As the lung slices contain a heterogeneous population of
cells, it will be difficult to determine directly whether acetylcholine, bradykinin and histamine all act on the same cells to
increase cyclic GMP and whether the accumulation of the two nucleotides in response to any of these agents occurs in the same or in
different cells. Perhaps, through studies with homogeneous populations of separated cells or with other model systems, it will be
possible to localize the effects of the several agonists and the
changes in nucleotide concentrations to specific types of cells and
thereby gain some clues to the functions served by cyclic GMP in
lung.

REFERENCES

1.   Steiner, A.L., Parker, C.W. and Kipnis, D.M.   (1972)
J. Biol. Chem. 247: 1106.

2.   Zurier, R.B., Weissman, G., Hoffstein, S., Kammerman, S.
and Tai, H.H.   (1974)   J. Clin. Invest. 53: 297.

3.   Stoner, J., Manganiello, V.C. and Vaughan, M.   (1974)
Mol. Pharmacol. 10: 155.

4.   Goldberg, N.D., O'Dea, R.F. and Haddox, M.K.   (1973), in
Advances in Cyclic Nucleotide Res., P. Greengard and G.A. Robison,
eds., Raven Press, N.Y., p 155-223.

5.   Schultz, G., Hardman, J.G. and Sutherland, E.W.   (1973),
in Asthma: Physiology, Immunopharmacology and Treatment, K. F.
Austen and L. M. Lichtenstein, eds., Academic Press, N.Y.,
p 123-137.

6.   Dunham, E.W., Haddox, M.K. and Goldberg, N.D.   (1974)
Proc. Nat. Acad. Sci. U.S.A. 71: 815.

7.   Clyman, R.I., Sandler, J.A., Manganiello, V.C. and
Vaughan, M. (1975)   J. Clin. Invest. **55: 1020.**

8.   Bor, I. and Guntheroth, W.G.   (1970)   Canad. J. Physiol.
Pharm. 48: 500.

9.   Eltherington, L.G., Stoff, J., Hughes, T. and Melmon, K.L.
(1968)   Circ. Res. 22: 747.

10.   Altura, B.M., Malaviya, D. Reich, C.F. and Orkin, L.R.
(1972)   Am. J. Physiol. 222: 345.

11.   Stoner, J., Manganiello, V.C. and Vaughan, M.   (1973).
Proc. Nat. Acad. Sci. USA 70: 3830.

12.   Karim, S.M.M.   (1967)   Brit. J. Pharmacol. Chemother.
29: 230.

13.   Somlyo, A.V., Woo, C.Y. and Somlyo, A.P.   (1965)
Am. J. Physiol. 208: 748.

14.   Ash, A.S.F. and Schild, H.O.   (1966)   Brit. J. Pharmacol.
Chemother. 27: 427.

15. Kaliner, M. and Austen, K.F.   (1974)   Biochem. Pharmacol.
23: 763.

16. Weissman, G., Zurier, R.B., Spieler, P.J. and Goldstein, I.
(1971)   J. Exp. Med. 134: 149s.

17. Henson, .P.M.   (1971)   J. Immunol. 107: 1535.

18. Hawkins, D.   (1972)   J. Immunol. 108: 310.

19. Oronsky, A.L., Ignarro, L.J. and Perper, R.J.   (1973)
J. Exp. Med. 138: 461.

20. Weissman, G., Dukor, P. and Zurier, R.B.   (1971)   Nature,
New Biol. 231: 131.

21. Ignarro, L. J.   (1973)   Nature, New Biol. 245: 151.

22. Ignarro, L. J.   (1974)   J. Immunol. 112: 210.

23. Goldstein, I., Hoffstein, S., Gallin, J. and Weissman, G.
(1973)   Proc. Nat. Acad. Sci. USA 70: 2916.

24. Ignarro, L. J. and George, W. J.   (1974)   Proc. Nat.
Acad. Sci. USA 71: 2027.

25. Brunner, K.T., Manuel, J., Rudolf, H.L. and Chapnis, B.
(1970)   Immunology 18: 501.

26. Henney, C.S. and Lichtenstein, L.M.   (1971)   J. Immunol.
107: 610.

27. Henney, C.S., Bourne, H.E. and Lichtenstein, L.M.   (1972)
J. Immunol. 108: 1526.

28. Strom, T.B., Deisseroth, A., Morganroth, J., Carpenter,
C.B. and Merrill, J.P.   (1972)   Proc. Nat. Acad. Sci. USA 69: 2995.

29. Strom, T.B., Carpenter, C.B., Garovoy, M.R., Austen, K.F.,
Merrill, J.P. and Kaliner, M.   (1973)   J. Exp. Med. 138: 381.

30. Goldberg, N.D., Haddox, M.K., Hartle, D.K. and Hadden, J.W.
(1973), in Pharmacology and the Future of Man, Karger, Basle, p. 146.

31. Illiano, G., Tell, G.P.E., Siegel, M.I. and Cuatrecasas, P.
(1973)   Proc. Nat. Acad. Sci. USA 70: 2443.

32.   Strom, T.B., Sytkowski, A.J., Carpenter, C.B. and Merrill, J.P.   (1974)   Proc. Nat. Acad. Sci. USA 71: 1330.

33.   Hadden, J.W., Hadden, E.M., Haddox, M.K. and Goldberg, N.D. (1972)   Proc. Nat. Acad. Sci. USA 69: 3024.

34.   Sandler, J.A., Clyman, R.I., Manganiello, V.C. and Vaughan, M.   (1975)   J. Clin. Invest. 55:431.

35.   Estensen, R.D., Hill, H.R., Quie, P.G., Hogan, N. and Goldberg, N.D.   (1973)   Nature 245: 458.

36.   G oetzl, E.J., Wasserman, S.I., Gigli, I. and Austen, F.K. (1974)   J. Clin. Invest. 53: 813.

37.   Sandler, J.A., Gallin, J.I. and Vaughan, M., unpublished observations.

38.   Murad, F., Manganiello, V.C. and Vaughan, M. (1971) Proc. Nat. Acad. Sci. USA 68: 736.

39.   Kuo, J.F. and Kuo, W.-N.   (1973)   Biochem. Biophys. Res. Commun. 55: 660.

40.   Palmer, G.C.   (1972)   Biochem. Pharmacol. 21: 2907.

41.   Vane, J.R.   (1971)   Nature, New Biol. 231: 232.

42.   Piper, P.J. and Vane, J.R.   (1969)   Nature 223: 29.

43.   Ramwell, P.W., Shaw, J.E., Douglas, W.W. and Poisner, A.M. (1966)   Nature 210: 273.

CYCLIC NUCLEOTIDE ANALOGUES

B. Jastorff

University of Bremen
Studienbereich Biologie/Chemie
28 Bremen 33, Achterstrasse
Federal Republic of Germany

Contents

INTRODUCTION

The first report on chemical modifications of cyclic
AMP was published in 1962 by Sutherland and co-workers. Since
1970 the number of studies dealing with the biological properties
of cyclic AMP has increased rapidly. Then research groups at
universities, research institutes and especially in the laboratories of the pharmaceutical industry began to modify cyclic AMP
and other cyclic nucleotides systematically. More than 150

derivatives of cyclic AMP have been described. What justifies
such a great interest in chemical derivatives of cyclic nucleotides ? The most important reason depends on the central role
that cyclic AMP plays in numerous hormone induced metabloic
processes. Diseases that result from disorders in cyclic AMP
metabolism could probably be treated by substitution therapy
with cyclic nucleotides and their derivatives. The use of the
naturally occurring cyclic nucleotides, however, suffers from
the potential drawback of lack of specificity, since these second
messengers must be able to influence all cyclic nucleotide
dependent processes. Additionally the application of exogenous
cyclic AMP to isolated tissues or organs at physiological
(10^{-8}-10^{-6}M) or even higher concentrations (10^{-6}-10^{-4}M) does not
produce the desired response in most instances. This seems to be
due to the poor permeability of the membranes of intact cells and
to rapid destruction by intracellular or extracellular phosphodiesterases. These problems might be eliminated by selective use
of derivatives. Therefore, by modification of the basic structure
chemists have tried to change the following properties of cyclic
nucleotides:

- specificity
- activity
- stability against enzymes
- permeability
- toxicity

All these factors are not only of great interest for
the pharmacologist, who hopes to obtain terapeutically useful
substances. They are valuable also for the molecular biologist
to obtain new information about the molecular mechanism of action
of cyclic nucleotides in different systems.

Using analogues with structural elements which have been
determined one could also investigate the molecular mechanisms of
the interaction of cyclic nucleotides and their specific protein
receptors, i.e. structure-activity relationships. So one may, for
instance, answer the question whether cyclic AMP binds
identically to all of the binding sites in the protein receptors.
But these biological or biochemical questions could not alone
justify the synthesis of such a large number of analogues.

This paper will not review all known chemical or biochemical information on cyclic nucleotide analogues, as this has
been done recently in great detail by Simon et al. (1). Here
only the following chemical and biochemical aspects of nucleotides
will be discussed:

- general synthetic principles, demonstrating how it was possible to synthesize more than 150 derivatives;

- a short review on the types of structural elements which have been introduced;

- structure – activity relationships using as an example the influence of modifications of cyclic AMP on the activity of protein kinase;

- cyclic AMP analogues – useful therapeutical agents?

SYNTHETIC PRINCIPLES

Cyclic AMP can be divided into three regions – the heterocyclic base, the ribose and the cyclic phosphate moiety. These regions differ specifically in their chemical properties. One may theoretically substitute every atom or group in each of these regions. Furthermore, one can add different residues and last but not least, derivatives can be synthesized in which groups are completely missing. As you will see later on, all these possibilities have been investigated.

Without going into synthetic details the most important modification pathways will be discussed (s. loc. sit. (1)), the most important and mostly-used synthetic principles will be outlined.

Substitution Reactions

Starting with cyclic AMP the different functional groups of the molecule are reacted with specific reagents to obtain the modified derivative in one step.

Figure 1 indicates schematically those positions which can be modified by the following types of reactions:

(a)   acylation at N-6 and/or 2'-OH
(b)   bromination at C-8
(c)   N-oxidation with following alkylation at N-1
(d)   esterification or acid amide preparation

As the residue R can be varied the chemist is able to influence the steric and electronic properties in the positions 1,6,8,2' and the phosphate OH-groups. He can introduce long-chained, short-chained or branched residues of aliphatic, aromatic or hetero-cyclic nature. The basic molecule can be

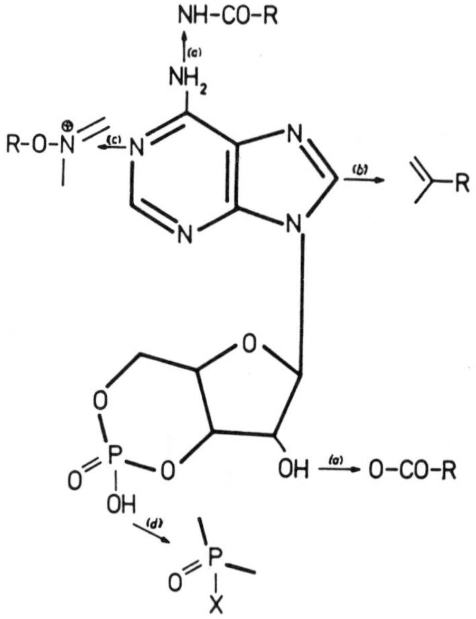

Figure 1: Schematic description of substitution reactions at the function groups of cyclic AMP. For explanation see text ($X = OR$, $N (R_2)$).

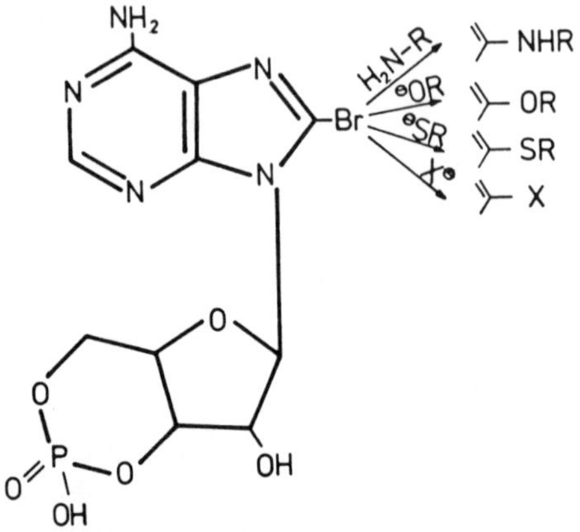

Figure 2: Schematic description of substitution reactions at 8-bromo cyclic AMP.

substituted ad libitum and can have either hydrophilic or hydrophobic character. In this way a radioactive and fluroescent
marker or a spin label can be introduced.

Thus, there is almost no limit for the scope of modification of the chemist. In cooperation with biologists, bio-
chemists or pharmacologists the chemist may therefore synthesize
derivatives that are suitable for further studies. A quite
similar type of reaction is shown in Figure 2, starting with an
analogue of cyclic AMP which bears already a highly reactive
functional group. In this example, it is the 8-bromo group,
which can be introduced as shown before. By nucleophilic substitution of this atom it is possible to introduce amines,
alcohols, mercaptides or small anions. Positions 6 and 2 can be
modified in the same way. In these cases the reactive chloro-
group is used. The synthesis of these intermediates is, however,
somewhat more complicated (1).

Total Synthesis

This type of synthesis is the most expensive way of preparation as every modification requires several reaction steps
if a modification of the same position of the molecule is required.
Figure 3 schematically indicates what steps are necessary.

Firstly, the modified nucleoside is synthesized, often
in several steps. This is phosphorylated to the 5'-monophosphate
and subsequently converted to 3'. 5'-cyclic phosphate. There
exists no general synthetic principle.

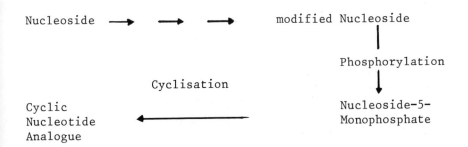

Figure 3. *Schematic description of a total synthesis of cyclic
nucleotide analogue*

Even for phosphorylation and cyclisation a special method is often necessary depending either on the chemical properties of the nucleoside or on the position that is to be modified. Lastly it should be mentioned that most, but not all, of the cyclic-analogues have been synthetised by the pathways described.

STRUCTURE OF MODIFICATIONS

As has been mentioned in the introduction the number of modifications of cyclic AMP and other cyclic nucleotides is unusually high. But considering the synthetic possibilities this great number becomes understandable. Figure 4 shows schematically that attempts have been made to modify nearly all the positions of the molecule. A selection of these modifications is shown in Table 1, to illustrate the different structural elements that have been introduced.

Due to ease of access positions 6,8 and 2' have been modified to a greater extent than for instance position 3'-0 or 7, which may be modified by de novo synthesis.

But modification of the cyclic AMP molecule need not be restricted to one position: several analogues exist in which

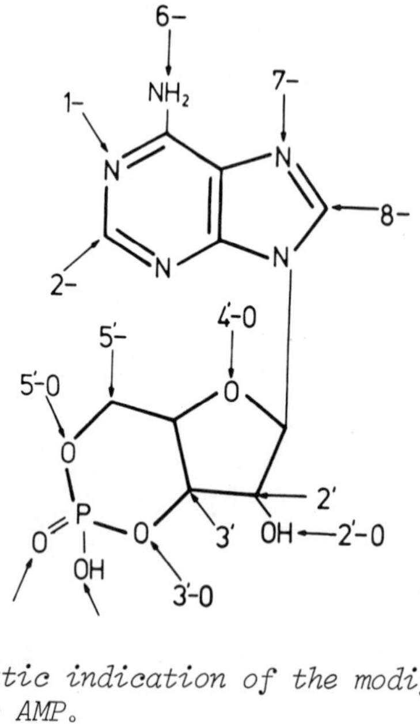

Figure 4.   *Schematic indication of the modified positions of cyclic AMP.*

Table 1. Atoms or groups introduced to different positions of cyclic AMP.

Position:

8	: Br, Cl, J, N_3, SH, OH, NH_2, SR, OR, NHR ($R = CH_3$, C_2H_5, CH_2COOH, $CH_2-C_6H_5$, CH_2CH_2OH, $CH_2CH_2NH_2$, etc.)
6	: Cl; SH; OH; $HN-R$, NR_2, SR ($R = CH_3$, C_2H_5, C_3H_7, C_4H_9, $CH_2C_6H_5$ etc.); $NH-CO-R'$ ($R' = C_2H_5$, C_3H_7, C_4H_9, C_6H_5, $CH_2C_6H_5$)
2'-O	: $-COR$ ($R = CH_3$, C_2H_5, C_3H_7, C_4H_9, C_8H_{17} etc.); $-R'$ ($R' = CH_3$, C_6H_5 $(NO_2)_2$)
2	: NH_2; Cl; Br; SH; OH, SCH_3; CH_3
1	: O; OR ($R = CH_3$, C_2H_5, $CH_2C_6H_5$), CH_3
7	: $>CH$; $>C-CN$; $>C-CONH_2$
4'-O	: S, CH_2
5'-O	: CH_2, NH, NR ($R = CH_3$, C_4H_9, C_8H_{17}, $CH_2O_6H_5$), S
3'-O	: CH_2, NH, NR ($R = CH_2C_6H_5$)
P=X	: $X = S$
P-Y	: $Y = OCH_3$, OC_2H_5, $N(CH_3)_2$

two or even more positions are changed. Dibutyryl–cyclic AMP, the most famour cyclic AMP analogue, is an example; in this N - 6 and 2^{1}O are substituted by a butyryl group ($-COC_3H_7$).

STRUCTURE–ACTIVITY–RELATIONS

Influence of Structure–Modifications on Chemical Properties

For structure–activity–relationship studies it is necessary to summarize the chemical properties of the molecule that may be changed by a given modification and discuss how this might influence the interaction with the biological receptors (2):

- the shape of the molecule is changed by protruding residues. This is the case with nearly all analogues. By changing the molecule this way, the interaction with the active side must be influenced by steric hindrance;

- by introduction of bulky residues to the 8-position the conformation of the base is fixed in syn;

- by substitution of the nitrogen atoms in position 1, 6 and 7, as well as by substitution of the oxygen atoms 2'-0, 3'-0 or 5'-0, possible hydrogen bonding to the active site of the protein is disturbed;

- the electron density of the base or of the phosphate moiety is influenced by introduction of more electronegative or more electropositive substituents (3) and this might change the binding constant;

- the whole molecule can become either more lipophilic or more hydrophylic. This property should strongly influence the ability of the molecule to penetrate membranes.

Relating the chemical properties to the biological activity should lead to a more rational selection of analogues with defined biological properties.

Influence of Modifications on Biological Activity
Example: Protein Kinase System

Most of the analogues have been tested in vitro with respect to interactions with the two enzyme systems which, besides adenyl cyclase, are the key enzymes in cyclic AMP metabolism: i.e. protein kinase and phosphodiesterase. Structure-activity relationships for these enzymes should yield information on how analogues might act in intact cells. This paper will be concerned only with studies on protein kinase.

Nearly all tissues in an organism contain cyclic AMP dependent protein kinases. For an exact comparison of structure-activity relationship it would be necessary to use a highly purified enzyme from one tissue and to test all analogues under the same conditions. This has not yet been done.

In most cases data on the protein chemical characterisation of their system was not published. Only the type of tissue and the steps of purification were mentioned. Therefore an exact quantitative comparison of the published results is impossible. However, it seems possible to make a comparison

relating the results with analogues with those with cyclic AMP.
Nearly all authors determined K-values (the concentration at which
the enzyme is activated halfmaximally) for cyclic AMP and the
analogues tested. A relative activation can be determined by
dividing K_a of cyclic AMP by the K_a of the analogue (1).

$$K'_a = \frac{K_a \text{ cyclic AMP}}{K_a \text{ Analogue}}$$

K'_a- values should be comparable even if the enzymes
have been prepared in different laboratories (see article by
Swillens; this book).

Most of the K'_a- values are published for the "protein
kinase from bovine brain" (1). We used our (4) and published
results (1) to study the following: How does modification in the
base, sugar or phosphate moiety influence the activation capacity
K'_a ? The data are summarized in Table 2 and are discussed
below:

Base Moiety. If one compares the K'_a- values of analogues which
have been modified in the base region one finds that structural
variations in this part of the molecule influences its activating capacity only marginally. Table 2 only shows a very small
fraction of those analogues.

But this fraction is typical for all the other analogues.
Moreover, there does not seem to be a position which might be
preferred for substitution nor a substituent which preferentially
raises the activating capacity of the molecule.

In spite of the great number of results with base
modified cyclic AMP analogues it is not yet possible to predict
the influence of a distinct modification on the activating
capacity. All one can say is, that a modification in the base
region of cyclic AMP will not result in a complete loss of
activating capacity.

From all the results we reason that there are no interactions between distinct atoms of the base and the active site
of the protein which are essential for the activating process.
There must be enough space in the active site for even very bulky
substituents and there is evidence that cyclic AMP binds to the
enzyme in its syn-conformation.

Table 2. K'$_a$- values of an assortment of analogues (1) (4)
          modified in the different regions of cyclic AMP
          (base, phosphate moiety). Enzyme system: Protein
          Kinase from bovine brain (the preparations are from
          different laboratories).

	X	K'a	Y	K'a	Z	K'a
	SH	0.56	SH	3.8	CH	1.5
	SC$_2$H$_5$	2.0	SCH$_2$C$_6$H$_5$	1.7	C-CH	0.52
	NHC$_2$H$_5$	0.50	NH CH$_2$C$_6$H$_5$	0.023	C-CONH$_2$	0.23
	S	0.50			OCH$_3$	inactive
	NH	0.007	NH	0.0008		
	NR	inactive			N(CH$_3$)$_2$	inactive
	CH$_2$	0.012	CH$_2$	inactive		
			H	0.01		
	S	~1	OCH$_3$	0.002		
			arabino	0.001		

Phosphate Moeity. Distinct structural variations in the cyclic
phosphate moiety affect the interaction with the kinase so
severely that the molecule is no longer able to activate the
enzyme. For instance, a negative charge on phosphorus is
essential for stimulating properties. The phosphate triesters
as well as the phosphor amidates of cyclic AMP are inactive. The
geometry of the ribose is also essential: a xylose cyclic
phosphate is inactive.

     The stimulating properties are also abolished if the
shape of the ring is changed by protruding substituents, as the
5'-N substituted cyclic AMP analogues show. Obviously the interaction of the phosphate ring is so disturbed by protruding
groups that an activation of the kinase is no longer possible.
Also inactive surprisingly, is the 3' methylene analogue, in which

the 3'-oxygen is substituted by a CH_2-group. In this case the
conformation of the cyclic phosphate ring is not influenced, but
the electronic properties are changed.

As the Table shows, there are no cyclic AMP derivatives
modified in the phosphate moiety, that are more active than the
parent compound. Even the substitution of the 3'- or 5'-oxygen
by a NH-group lowers the activating capacity to a great extent.
Similar results were found for the 5'-methylene analogue. The
substitution of 5'-oxygen by sulphur changes the stimulating
properties slightly. So we may conclude that a sterically and
electronically intact cyclic phosphate ring is essential for
optimal interaction with the active site and for the subsequent
activation of the catalytic unit.

Ribose Moiety. The influence of the 2'-hydroxy group on activation is still not clear. Some authors found that the stimulating properties were lost when this group was absent or was
substituted while other authors found only a slight influence on
the activating capacity. To clarify this question it is
necessary to use identical enzyme systems.

The comparison of K'_a- values has shown that the three
regions of the molecule must be involved in binding to and in
subsequent activation of protein kinase. While optimal binding
of the cyclic phosphate moiety to the active site of the protein
is essential for the activation process, optimal interaction with
the rest of the molecule is not essential.

From these results one could predict the following
properties of the different types of analogues in intact cell
systems:

- all derivatives modified in the base should be able to control
  cyclic AMP dependent processes in a similar way to cyclic AMP
  itself and therefore none of them would be able to control
  selectively only a single process;

- all derivatives modified in the phosphate moiety will have
  little or no influence on cyclic AMP processes.

The published results on the effects of some cyclic AMP-
analogues in the isolated tissues confirm that prediction (1).
But to clarify how a distinct analogue interferes with cyclic AMP
processes in vivo, it is necessary to perform similar structure-
activity relationship studies with the phosphodiesterase system
and for membrane permeability.

CYCLIC ANALOGUES – USEFUL THERAPEUTICAL AGENTS?

The question whether cyclic nucleotides might become useful as therapeutical agents cannot be answered yet. Only a small number of the synthesized compounds have been tested in <u>in vivo</u> systems. None of them had exceptional properties, i.e. a specific influence on a single cyclic AMP dependent process. In all cases several processes were influenced simultaneously (for example glucose metabolism, steroidogenesis and lipolysis) and one can be sure that other processes which have not been measured, were influenced, too. The number of systematic tests is too small to give a final answer to the question whether one of the numerous analogues may have the desired properties. Only a careful and systematic screening of all representative derivatives would clarify this definitely. But concerning the structure–activity relationship studies it seems to become more and more doubtful, whether one of the synthesized analogues or one still to be synthesized could be useful in the desired way.

REFERENCES

(1) SIMON, L.N., SHUMAN, D.A. and ROBINS, R.K. (1973) in Advances in Cyclic Nucleotide Research Volume 3, P. Greengard and G.A. Robison, Editors, 225, Raven Press Publishers New York – North Holland Publishing Company Amsterdam

(2) WEBB, J.L. (1963), Enzyme and Metabolic Inhibitors Volume 1, Academic Press, New York and London

(3) HUG, W. and TINOCO, J., Jr., (1974) J. Amer. Chem. Soc. 96, 665

(4) JASTORFF, B. and BAER, H.P., (1973) Europ. J. Biochem., 37, 491; N. Panitz, E. Rieke, K.G. Wagner, M. Morr, G. Roesler and B. Jastorff, manuscript in preparation.

MICROTUBULE MORPHOLOGY

Pierre Nève

Laboratories of Experimental Medicine,
Pathology and Electron Microscopy
University of Brussels, Belgium

Contents

INTRODUCTION

Before we knew the structures of microtubules, or had even named them, we were aware of their presence in cells from birefringence studies.

Indeed, microtubules correspond to structures well-known for several years like the fibres of the mitotic spindle (1, 2, 3) and fibres in neurons (4). Electron microscopy has revealed the fine structure of these so-called microtubules. Introduced by Slautterback in 1963 (5), the term of microtubule has been extensively used by everybody who found these structures in his own material.

During the last ten years, these microtubules have been recognized as ubiquitous organelles in all the eukaryotes. Prior to 1963 (6), the most commonly used fixative in electron microscopy was osmium tetroxide, that destroys most of the microtubules. Therefore it is not surprising that these microtubules became studied extensively only after the introduction of glutaraldehyde as fixative : the latter does not appear to interfere with the morphology of the microtubules. The aim of the present work is to give a general review of microtubules and their properties from the standpoint of morphology. We plan to consider first the fundamental morphology of microtubules, and then to show some morphological evidence related to the functional properties of these organelles. For this purpose, it will be necessary to integrate some biochemical knowledge (see next paper by J. Nunez) which probably will be extensively taken in account by the next communication, devoted to the biochemistry of the microtubules.

SUBSTRUCTURE OF THE MICROTUBULES

As already mentioned, microtubules are commonly observed in the cytoplasm of both animal and plant cells (for literature see reviews : 7, 8, 9, 10, 11, 12, 13). Biochemical techniques have isolated the major constituant protein that is called tubulin, the properties of which it will be discussed in the next lecture : let us confine our comments at present to saying that tubulin is a dimer composed of two distinct globular molecules called α- and β-tubulins the interconnections of which are rigid in the microtubule (see 14). The conclusion has been reached, using immunological techniques, that a common antigenic determinant is present in microtubules from all great groups of vertebrates, although the tubulin itself was not necessarily identical (15).

Microtubules appear as long and narrow dense-walled cylinders with a hollow core 220-250 Å in diameter and often surrounded by a clear zone which may contain mucopolysaccharides (Fig. 1) (16, 17). This has been suggested by studies with electron-scattering lanthanum (18) which strongly stains the microtubules in their clear zones and which is known to bind to anionic groups and mucopolysaccharide (19). This clear area surrounding the core of the microtubules is approximately 100 Å wide ; it always clearly separates the microtubules from the other cellular organelles and therefore facilitates the identification in the cells of microtubules in cross section. Some microtubules are very long and in axons their length would attain more than one metre (7, 20). Microtubules are straight and rigid structures : usually they do not bend and, when observed after biochemical isolation, they do not flex or split longitudinally, but break, the broken microtubules forming sharp angles. At high magnification, when viewed in transverse section, the wall of each microtubule is 45 Å thick and appears composed of subunits. The number of these subunits has

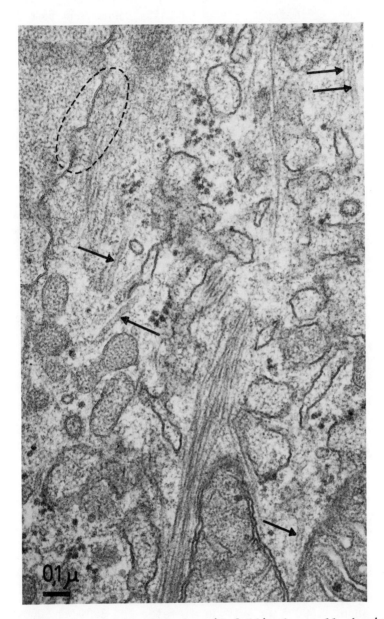

Fig. 1. Apical part of a dog thyroid follicular cell showing microtubules (arrows) in longitudinal section and microfilaments.
Two kinds of microfilaments are encountered. The first, 100 Å
thick, are associated in bundles whereas the second type is thinner, constituting a filamentous network in the subcortical area
(dotted zone). × 73,000.

been conclusively demonstrated to be 13 in different cells of various tissues : in fact, these subunits correspond to cross sections of 13 protofilaments aligned parallel to the long axis of the tubule (21). In longitudinal sections, at high magnification and principally when negative staining is achieved with sodium phosphotungstate, the margins of the microtubules appear saw-toothed or crinkled and often the microtubules appear crossbanded. The crossbands are usually slightly oblique and these aspects correspond to the fact that microtubules are made up of the helical arrangement of tubulin dimers, each turn of spiral containing 13 subunits. Polymerization of microtubules has been obtained *in vitro* (22) and calcium inhibits this polymerization (22, 23). X-ray diffraction patterns of sea urchin microtubules have suggested that the microtubules consisted of roughly spherical subunits arranged in 13 protofilaments (24).

There has been growing interest in the spatial relationship between microtubules and the cytoplasm which surrounds them. Microtubule to microtubule cross connections have been observed in a number of situations (25, 26, 27, 28). Lanthanum staining strongly delineates these filamentous elements interconnecting the microtubules (18). In the axons of the ventral nerve cord of the crayfish, connexions also exist between microtubules and the plasma membrane to form a 3-dimensional latticework (18). The biochemical nature of these lateral expansions or side-arms is unsettled : Mooseker and Tilney (29) have suggested that they could be dynein which has the size of the side-arms (150 Å) ; others think that these connexions are formed by tubulin (30) or by mucopolysaccharides (18).

Since the majority of evidence as to the structure of microtubules comes from observations of fixed material, the question arises, how does this structure so described relate to that in the living cell ? The answer has been given by a study of freeze-etched microtubules from the ovaries of the insect Notonecta : the observations reported from this investigation correspond in many ways with the picture of microtubules, which have been subjected to chemical fixation (16).

ASSOCIATED STRUCTURES : THE CENTRIOLES AND THE CILIA

Using the electron microscope, centrioles appear as small cylinders about 1500 Å in outside diameter and 3000 to 5000 Å long. Their wall is formed by nine groups of three microtubules so closely apposed that they seem to share common walls (1). Starting with the innermost, the microtubules of each triplet are designated the A-, B- and C-subfibrils. Pericentriolar bodies or satellites are small masses with striation patterns forming two superimposed pericentriolar crowns , each satellite being connected to a triplet of microtubules (31, 32).   Microtubules are very often found in association with centrioles : they seem to arise from the pericentriolar bodies and in three dimensional space, they constitute the typical "aster", that is generally surrounded by the Golgi apparatus.

Cilia and flagella in cross section have a structure that recalls that of the centriole but instead of being formed by 9 triplets of microtubules, they contain 9 peripheral doublets of microtubules surrounding two central microtubules : this 9 + 2 complex is called the axoneme.   The nine peripheral doublet microtubules of the axoneme of cilia and flagella are directly continuous with the A and B microtubules of centriolar triplets constituting the kinetosome or centriolar-like structure seen at the base of each cilium.   The central axonemal microtubules arise in a dense granule or plate just distal to the kinetosome. These dense plates appear as "nucleation sites" which would play a major role in the assembly of tubulin into microtubule.   Fulton and collaborators (33) have demonstrated a serological similarity between flagellar and mitotic microtubules.   Like microtubules, centrioles and cilia are self-assembling structures and probably arise from the same pool of monomers (34).   Isolating gill cilia from a mussel, Warner and Satir (35) demonstrated that thirteen protofilaments made up the wall of both the central pair microtubules and subfibre A of each doublet, whereas subfibre B of the doublet consisted of 10 protofilaments.   All these arguments show that the usual microtubules are closely related to the constitutive microtubules of centrioles, kinetosomes and cilia.   However, neither centrioles, nor the basal bodies and cilia are generally affected by treatments which usually destroy the microtubules.   This does not necessarily indicate that different types of tubulin are present in both structures (36) as the increase of microtubular antagonist's concentration very often induces the destruction of the ciliary microtubules (37) ;   indeed, it might be explained by the slow penetration of the drug in these cells or by differences in the proteins associated with the tubules.

AGENTS ACTING ON MICROTUBULES

Recent years have witnessed major advances in the elucidation of functions of the microtubules.   This accumulation of publications has been due largely to the existence of different agents which, acting on microtubules, produce morphological changes at the same time as interfering with cellular function or shape.

We do not intend to give here an exhaustive review of what is known about the microtubules and their antagonists.   We shall only give a brief enumeration of the various agents used and underline their morphological effects on the microtubules with respect to their functional effects on the cells concerned. For illustration, we shall use our own material i.e. the thyroid cell assuming that the morphological effects observed at the level of microtubules in the thyroid are similar to those produced by the same agents in other systems.

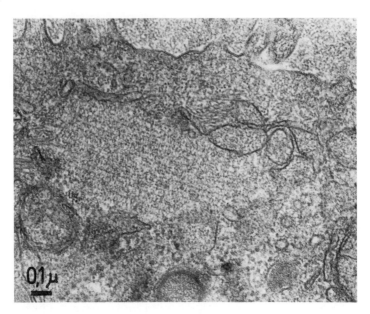

Fig. 2.   Typical crystalline structure induced by vincristine in dog thyroid cell.   × 60,000.

    Firstly one should consider change induced by alteration of the physical environment.   Cold and hydrostatic pressure cause microtubules to disassemble.   These agents were used in pioneering studies (38) which served as the starting point for much work increasing our   knowledge   of   microtubular functions.   Tilney showed that the axopodia of *Actinosphaerium nucleofilum* were unable to reform if the microtubules were kept in the disassembled state with hydrostatic pressure and low temperature (39, 40). Colchicine is the best known antagonist for microtubules (41, 42, 43) : it decreases the number of microtubules and binds with a microtubular protein (44).   It is suggested that colchicine acts by preventing microtubule assembly (45) and that the microtubules already assembled, undergoing a rapid turn-over, are transformed into monomers or dimers.   However, a recent report shows that colchicine also interacts with plasma membranes and in that case one cannot attribute colchicine-induced alterations of membranes solely to microtubule involvement (46).   An other recent work suggests that colchicine plays a role in the distribution of lectin-binding sites on cell surfaces (47).

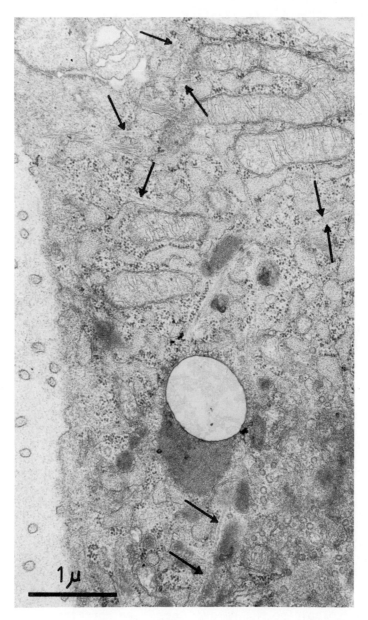

Fig. 3. Part of a follicular cell in a dog thyroid slice incubated in presence thyrotropin and of D_2O. Microtubules (arrows) are stabilized but biochemical data show that thyroid hormone secretion induced by thyrotropin has been inhibited. × 27,000.

Vinca alkaloids such as vincristine and vinblastine also destroy microtubules and result in the formation of crystalline
structures within the cells after treatment with these agents (48)
(Fig. 2).   These crystalline structures are made of tubules which
have a diameter greater than that of microtubules (350 Å) ;   they
share a common antigenicity with microtubules and remain able to
bind colchicine (49, 50).

Other drugs do not disassemble the microtubules but stabilize
them resulting in interference with their normal function. Hexy-
leneglycol, ethanol and D_2O stabilize the microtubules (51, 52)
(Fig. 3).   Other less-known substances react with the microtubules : podophyllotoxin (53), griseofulvin (54), general anesthe-
tic gases, chlorate hydrate, sulfhydryl reagents and copper (55).
Most of these antimicrotubular agents have been used to probe the
possible role of the microtubular system in different cellular
functions.

MORPHOLOGICAL EVIDENCES OF MICROTUBULAR FUNCTIONS

During the last 4 years, there have been a considerable number of papers published providing evidence that microtubules might
play several roles in the cells. From this literature, it is worth
selecting some pertinent examples in order to demonstrate how microtubules may be contributing to cellular function.

Mitotic Movements

In mitotic spindles, microtubules bind chromosomal kinetocho-
res to pericentriolar masses. The microtubule reacting agents
block the mitoses before metaphase and induce the afore-mentioned
changes at the level of the microtubules. It becomes logical therefore that in anaphase, microtubules interference with chromosome
movement to the spindle decreases. However, the exact role of the
microtubules in mitosis remains unknown (12, 56, 57, 58, 59).

Cytoskeletal Role of the Microtubules

Tilney has reported that the axial rods of *Echinosphaerium*
contain highly structured arrays of parallel microtubules (38).
The microtubule breakdown by colchicine and subsequent reassembly
when the colchicine is removed has been correlated with the re-
traction and elongation of the cell processes. These observations
are in agreement with the development and maintenance of asymmetric cell shapes mediated through the microtubular system.

The circulating human platelet is disc-shaped. This peculiar

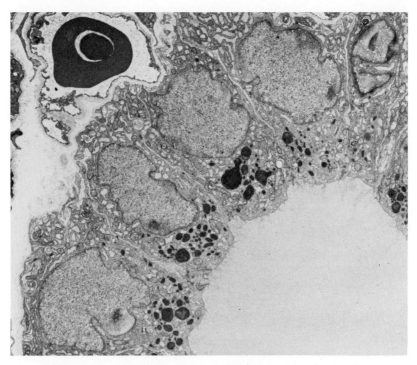

Fig. 4.   Part of a follicle in the cream hamster thyroid.   The
follicular cells display a stratification of their organelles.
× 3,100.

shape is likely to be due to bundles of microtubules lying all
around the cell's periphery, just beneath the plasma membrane.
Exposure of the platelet to almost any stimulus turns the disc-
shaped platelet into a spiny sphere, during which process the microtubules move towards the centre of the cell and the granules
become centralised (60).

   Normal thyroid cells of the cream hamster (Fig. 4) are characterized by an abundance of microtubules and a stratification of
their organelles (61). In these cells, it might be that the microtubules would play a role of cytoskeleton maintaining the stratification of the organelles. When such glands are incubated in presence of vincristine the follicular cells loose this stratification of their organelles and concurrently crystalline microtubular
structures appear and normal microtubules vanish (Figs. 5 and 6).

   Orci et al. (62) have observed linear columns of granules separated by rows of microtubules in the beta cells of cultured rat
pancreas.

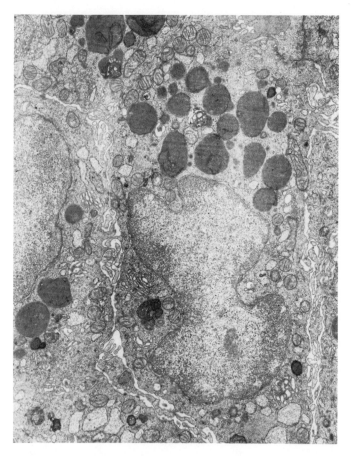

Fig. 5. Follicular cell of a cream hamster thyroid incubated in presence of 6.10^{-4} M of vincristine. Paracrystalline structures (arrows). Lysosomes and Golgi cisternae are observed near the base of the cell. Stratification of organelles is not as obvious as in reference glands (Fig. 4). × 9,000.

Microtubules and Cell Elongation or Movements

Lens fibre differentiation of the chick involves the elongation of epithelial cells. Piatigorsky et al. (63) have demonstrated that early stage of cell elongation requires the assembly and organization of microtubules which probably cooperate with other factors to promote cell elongation.

Extensive morphological investigations of the presence and orientation of microtubules during avian gastrulation (64) and during neurulation in *Xenopus* (65) have been made. Experiments with antimicrotubular agents which block both processes have suggested

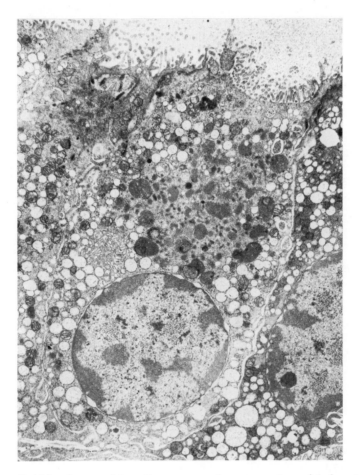

Fig. 6.   Follicular cell of a cream hamster thyroid incubated in presence of 9.10^{-4} M of vincristine.   Besides changes noted in the preceeding figure, rounded rough endoplasmic cisternae occupy the whole cytoplasm.   × 5,500.

that microtubules were responsible for the elongation of the cells occurring during gastrulation and neurulation.

Microtubules and Axonal Transport

Microtubules or neurotubules are so abundant in the neuronal axons that the brain is the organ most frequently used as a source of tubulin.   A recent *in vitro* study suggests that derivatives of cAMP enhance neuron maturation via some pathway that stimulates microtubule assembly (66).

Noradrenaline and acetylcholine are synthesized in cell bodies of noradrenergic and cholinergic neurons and transported with varying rapidity down the axons to the nerve terminals. Fluorescence and electron microscopy, in studies on rat sympathetic ganglia and interganglionic interconnecting nerves treated with colchicine or vinblastine, has shown that granular vesicles accumulated in the cell bodies with a reduction in the number of microtubules : this demonstrated that microtubule antagonists interrupted the centrifugal transport of noradrenaline granules (67).

Flament-Durand and Dustin (68) using colchicine after labelling of the hormones with ^{35}S-cysteine have shown that antimicrotubular agents blocked the migration of the neurosecretary granules from the paraventricular and supraoptic hypothalamic nuclei to the posterior lobe of the hypophysis, although the microtubules did not appear to be destroyed.

Microtubules and Secretion

The microtubule reacting agents have been shown to inhibit the release of insulin granules from pancreatic beta cells (69, 70) ; to inhibit the release of catecholamines from the adrenal medulla (71) to inhibit thyroid secretion (72, 73). The latter inhibitory effect on secretion after acute thyrotropin stimulation is due to the inhibition of the first step of thyroid secretion i.e. formation of apical pseudopods. There would normally phagocytose thyroglobulin-containing colloid droplets which would thereafter fuse with lysosomes and release thyroxine after the action of hydrolytic enzymes. Scanning electron microscope studies (72, 73) on dog thyroid slices in presence of antimicrotubular agents and thyrotropin have demonstrated the total absence of pseudopod formation (74, 75). This inhibition of secretion *in vitro* has been confirmed by the works of Williams and Wolff (76, 77) ; similar results have been obtained *in vivo* (78). The microtubule reacting agents *in vitro* also block pseudopod formation and thyroid secretion after stimulation of the thyroid slices by cAMP or dibutyryl-cAMP. However, in the same experimental conditions, the same inhibitory effects on thyroid secretion have been obtained with a non-reacting microtubule agent such as cytochalasin, which is suspected to react solely with microfilaments (79, 80). These features call attention to other organelles which while being different from microtubules are frequently associated with them, namely microfilaments (81). In the dog thyroid it is possible to distinguish two different morphological populations of microfilaments. The first, and most easily visible variety, is made up of 80-100 Å wide microfilaments often associated in bundles widely dispersed throughout the cytoplasm. The microfilaments of the second type are principally located in the subcortical area of the cells ; they are thinner (50 Å wide) and seem shorter : they frequently appear as a fine filamentous network that appears to be inserted in the inner surface of the plasma membrane. At high magnification, the matrix of the apical pseudopods formed in TSH-stimulated cells is composed of a filamentous network similar to that of the cytoplasmic subcortical area.

Microfilaments are being increasingly recognized in different systems where microtubules have been observed (82) and where different roles have been suggested to be promoted by the microtubules. The frequent association of both organelles makes it difficult to dissociate the functions of microtubules and microfilaments in the cells since antimicrotubular agents could also react with microfilaments (55, 83).

Therefore, it is still impossible to distinguish cell functions which are mediated by microtubules from those which are mediated by microfilaments. From the recent literature (84, 85, 86, 87) it increasingly appears that microtubules and microfilaments are closely involved in cell movements : it is suggested that microfilaments play an active role in cytokinesis whereas microtubules remain passive. In melanophores of frog or *Xenopus*, cAMP causes reversible dispersion of the melanosomes : this dispersion is reversibly inhibited by cytochalasin whereas colchicine alone causes irreversible melanosomal dispersion. These experiments suggest that cAMP is closely related to microtubules and microfilaments perhaps through the stimulation of a cAMP-dependent protein-kinase associated with these organelles (85, 88).

Work realized thanks to grant 20013 of the "Fonds de la Recherche Scientifique Médicale" and under contract of the "Ministère de la Programmation Scientifique" within the framework of the Association Euratom - University of Brussels - University of Pisa.

References

1. de Harven, E. and Bernhard, W. (1956) Z. Zellforsch. 45, 378
2. Mazia, D. (1961) In: The Cell, (Brachet, J. and Mirsky, A.E., eds) vol. III, pp. 77-412, Academic Press, New York
3. Kane, R.E. (1962) J. Cell Biol. 15, 279
4. Palay, S.L. (1956) J. Biophys. Biochem. Cytol. 2 (suppl.), 193
5. Slautterback, D.B. (1963) J. Cell Biol. 18, 367
6. Sabatini, D.D., Bensch, K. and Barrnett, R.J. (1963) J. Cell Biol. 17, 19
7. Porter, K.R. (1966) In: Ciba Foundation Symposium on principles of biomolecular organization, pp. 308-345, Churchill, London
8. Faure-Fremiet, F. (1970) Ann. Biol. 9, 1

9. Tilney, L.G. (1971) In: Origin and continuity of cell organelles, (Reinert, U. and Ursprung, H., eds) pp. 222-260, Springer-
   Verlag
10. Dustin, P. (1972) Arch. Biol. 83, 419
11. Dustin, P. (1974) Arch. Biol. 85, 263
12. Rebhun, L.I. (1972) Int. Rev. Cytol. 32, 93
13. Olmsted, J.B. and Borisy, G.G. (1973) Ann. Rev. Biochem. 42,
    507
14. Bryan, J. (1974) Fed. Proc. 33, 152
15. Dales, S. (1972) J. Cell Biol. 52, 748
16. Stebbings, H. and Willison, J.H.M. (1973) Z. Zellforsch. 138,
    387
17. Kwiatkowska, M. (1973) Histochemie 37, 107
18. Burton, P.R. and Fernandez, H.L. (1973) J. Cell Sci. 12, 567
19. Lane, N.J. and Treherne, J.E. (1970) J. Cell Sci. 7, 217
20. Weiss, P.A. and Mayr, R. (1971) Acta neuropathol. suppl. 5,
    198
21. Tilney, L.G., Bryan, J., Bush, D.J., Fujiwra, K., Mooseker,
    M.S., Murphy, D.B. and Snyder,D.H. (1973) J. Cell Biol. 59, 267
22. Weisenberg, R.C. (1972) Science 177, 1104
23. Borisy, G.G., Olmsted, J.B., Marcum, J.M. and Allen, C. (1974)
    Fed. Proc. 33, 167
24. Cohen, C., De Rosier, D., Harrison, S.C., Stephens, R.E. and
    Thomas, J. (1974) Conference on the biology of cytoplasmic mi-
    crotubules, N.Y. Acad. Sci., abstr. n° 3, New York
25. Grimstone, A.V. and Cleveland, L.R. (1965) J. Cell Biol. 24,
    387
26. Tucker, J.B. (1968) J. Cell Sci. 3, 494
27. Tilney, L.G. and Byers, B. (1969) J. Cell Biol. 43, 148
28. McIntosh, J.R. (1974) J. Cell Biol. 61, 166
29. Mooseker, M.S. and Tilney, L.G. (1973) J. Cell Biol. 56, 13
30. Burkholder, G.D., Okada, T.A. and Comings, D.E. (1972) J. Cell
    Biol. 55, 32a
31. Stubblefield, E. and Brinkley, B.R. (1967) In: Formation and
    fate of cell organelles, (Warren, K.B., ed) Symp. Internat.
    Soc. Cell.Biology, vol. 6, p. 175, Academic Press, New York
32. Pitelka, D.R. (1969) In: Handbook of Molecular Cytology, (Lima-
    De-Faria, A., ed) pp. 1199-1218, North Holland Publishing Com-
    pany, Amsterdam - London
33. Fulton, C., Kane, R.E. and Stephens, R.E. (1971) J. Cell Biol.
    50, 762
34. Dirksen, E.R. (1971) J. Cell Biol. 51, 286
35. Warner, F.D. and Satir, P. (1973) J. Cell Sci. 12, 313
36. Brown, D.L. and Bouck, G.B. (1973) J. Cell Biol. 58, 96
37. Tilney, L.G. (1968) J. Cell Sci. 3, 549
38. Tilney, L.G. (1965) J. Cell Biol. 27, 107A
39. Tilney, L.G., Hiramoto, Y. and Marsland, D.A. (1966) J. Cell
    Biol. 29, 77
40. Tilney, L.G. and Porter, K.R. (1967) J. Cell Biol. 34, 327

41. Robbins, E. and Gonatas, N.K. (1964) J. Histochem. Cytochem. 12, 704
42. Malawista, S.E. and Bensch, K.G. (1967) Science 156, 521
43. Holmes, K.V. and Choppin, P.W. (1968) J. Cell Biol. 39, 526
44. Borisy, G.G. and Taylor, E.W. (1967) J. Cell Biol. 34, 525
45. Wilson, L. (1974) Abstracts of the Conference on the Biology of cytoplasmic microtubules, N.Y. Acad. Sci., New York
46. Wunderlich, F., Müller, R. and Speth, V. (1973) Science 182, 1136
47. Oliver, J.M., Ukena, T.E. and Berlin, R.D. (1974) Proc. Natl. Acad. Sci. U.S. 71, 394
48. Bensch, K.G. and Malawista, S.E. (1968) Nature 218, 1176
49. Krishan, A. and Hsu, D. (1969) J. Cell Biol. 43, 553
50. Shelanski, M.L. and Ventilla, M. (1970) Proc. VIth Int. Congr. Neuropathol., pp. 84-85, Masson et Cie, Paris
51. Kirkpatrick, J.P. (1969) Science 163, 187
52. Marsland, D. and Hecht, R. (1968) Exp. Cell Res. 51, 602
53. Wilson, L. and Friedkin, M. (1967) Biochemistry 6, 3126
54. Wilson, L. (1970) Biochemistry 9, 4999
55. Wilson, L., Bamburg, J.R., Mizel, S.B., Grisham, L.M. and Creswell, K.M. (1974) Fed. Proc. 33, 158
56. Brinkley, B.R. and Cartwright, J. Jr. (1971) J. Cell Biol. 50, 416
57. McIntosch, J.R., Hepler, P.K. and Van Wie, D.G. (1969) Nature 224, 659
58. McIntosch, J.R., Cande, Z., Snyder, J. and Vandeslice, K. (1974) Abstracts of the Conference on the Biology of cytoplasmic microtubules, N.Y. Acad. Sci., New York
59. Bajer, A.S. and Mole-Bajer, J. (1972) Int. Rev. Cytol. suppl. 3, 1
60. Behnke, O. (1970) J. Ultrastruct. Res. 31, 61
61. Nève, P. and Wollman, S.H. (1971) Anat. Rec. 168, 23
62. Orci, L., Like, A.A., Amherdt, M., Blondel, B., Kanazawa, Y., Marliss, E.B., Lambert, A.E., Wollheim, C.B. and Renold, A.E. (1973) J. Ultrastruct. Res. 43, 270
63. Piatigorsky, J., Webster, H. de F. and Wollberg, M. (1972) J. Cell Biol. 55, 82
64. Granholm, N.H. and Baker, J.R. (1970) Developmental Biology 23, 563
65. Karfunkel, P. (1971) Developmental Biology 25, 30
66. Roisen, F.J. (1974) Abstracts of the Conference on the Biology of cytoplasmic microtubules, N.Y. Acad. Sci.. New York
67. Hökfelt, T. and Dahlström, A. (1971) Z. Zellforsch. 119, 460
68. Flament-Durand, J. and Dustin, P. (1972) Z. Zellforsch. 130, 440.
69. Lacy, P.E., Howell, S.L., Young, D.A. and Finck, C.J. (1968) Nature 219, 1177
70. Malaisse,W.J., Malaisse-Lagae, F., Walker, M.O. and Lacy, P.E. (1971) Diabetes 20, 257

71. Poisner, A.M. and Bernstein, J. (1971) J. Pharmacol. Exp. Ther. 177, 102
72. Nève, P., Willems, C. and Dumont, J.E. (1970) Exp. Cell Res. 63, 457
73. Nève, P., Ketelbant-Balasse, P., Willems, C. and Dumont, J.E. (1972) Exp. Cell Res. 74, 227
74. Ketelbant-Balasse,P., Rodesch, F., Nève, P. and Pasteels, J.M. (1973) Exp. Cell Res. 79, 111
75. Ketelbant-Balasse, P. and Nève, P. (1974) Proc. of the Workshop on Advances in Biomedical Applications of the SEM, Part III, IIT Research Institute, Chicago, pp. 761-768
76. Williams, J.A. and Wolff, J. (1970) Proc. Natl. Acad. Sci. U.S. 67, 1901
77. Williams, J.A. and Wolff, J. (1972) J. Cell Biol. 54, 157
78. Ekholm, R., Ericson, L.E., Josefsson, J.O. and Melander, A. (1974) Endocrinology 94, 641
79. Spooner, B.S. and Wessells, N.K. (1970) Proc. Natl. Acad. Sci. U.S. 66, 360
80. Spudich, J.A. and Lin, S. (1972) Proc. Natl. Acad. Sci. U.S. 69, 442
81. Hinkley, R.E. Jr. (1973) J. Cell Sci. 13, 753
82. Reaven, E.P. and Axline, S.G. (1973) J. Cell Biol. 59, 12
83. Wilson, L., Bryan, J., Ruby, A. and Mazia, D. (1970) Proc. Natl. Acad. Sci. U.S. 66, 807
84. Taylor, A., Mamelak, M., Reaven, E. and Maffly, R. (1973) Science 181, 347
85. Magun, B. (1973) J. Cell Biol. 57, 845
86. Fisher, M. and Lyerla, T.A. (1974) J. Cell Physiol. 83, 117
87. Allison, A.C. and Davies, P. (1974) In: Advances in Cytopharmacology, (Ceccarelli, B., Clementi, F. and Meldolesi, J., eds) vol. 2, pp. 237-248, Raven Press, New York
88. Goodman, D., Rasmussen, H., Dibella, F. and Guthrow, C.E. (1970) Proc. Natl. Acad. Sci. U.S. 67, 652

CYCLIC AMP AND MICROTUBULES

J. Nunez
L. Rappaport
J.F. Leterrier

Unité de Recherche sur la Glande Thyroide et la
 Régulation Hormonale I.N.S.E.R.M.
et Equipe de Recherche Associée N° 449 du C.N.R.S.
78, avenue du Général Leclerc
Hôpital de Bicêtre
94270 Bicêtre (France)

Contents

INTRODUCTION

Microtubules, tubular structures of 240 Å diameter, are widely distributed in plant and animal cells (for a review see (1)). These organelles are present in different sites of the cell; they make up the spindle fibres of the mitotic cells and they are prominent in the axons and dendrites of neurons. The axonemal complex of the cilia and flagella is composed of microtubules; they are also present near the plasmia membrane of the cell and the endoplasmic reticulum.

Although the precise function of microtubules is unknown, they have been implicated in several functions such as ciliary motion, secretion and transport of molecules in the cell body and the axon, maintenance of the form of the cell, cell differentiation, neurite outgrowth, movement of the chromosomes during mitosis, etc.

The spindle apparatus of the mitotic cell may be disrupted by different drugs such as colchicine and the Vinca alkaloids (anti-mitotic drugs). Colchicine specifically binds to the microtubules. This property has been widely used to study the function of micro-tubules and to isolate their structural protein, tubulin. Micro-tubules are disrupted by colchicine treatment or exposure to low temperature (2) into their basic subunit, tubulin; these effects are reversible. Colchicine is able to inhibit several cell pro-cesses : cell division, cell differentiation, neurite extension and axonal elongation, intracellular movements of lysosomes and several types of transport and secretory processes. These effects have been attributed to the specific disruptive action of this agent on the microtubular system.

Several authors have also noted that many of these processes, which are inhibited by colchicine, are on the contrary activated by cyclic AMP (or its dibutyryl derivative) or by agents such as hormones or neurotransmitters which exert their intracellular effects by activating the membrane adenylate cyclase and producing an increase in the intracellular cyclic AMP content. Moreover, in eukaryotic cells, most if not all of the effects of cyclic AMP depend on the activation of cyclic AMP dependent protein kinases, enzymes which catalyse the phosphorylation of protein substrates. In 1970 Goodman *et al.* (3) reported that tubulin is phosphorylated by a cyclic AMP dependent "intrinsic" protein-kinase; these authors have also postulated that this phosphorylation reaction could have some importance in the microtubule-dependent secretory processes. These assumptions have been widely accepted and further studies have been devoted to *in vitro* or *in vivo* phosphorylation of tubulin and to the protein-kinase activity which is always co-puri-fied with tubulin.

In this paper we will review the biochemical properties of tubulin. We will then discuss the problems related to the protein kinase activity which is copurified with tubulin, the nature of the substrate which is phosphorylated *in vitro* and the possible relationship between the phosphorylation reaction and the *in vitro* microtubule assembly.

SUBUNITS AND STRUCTURE OF TUBULIN

Microtubules prepared from different sources are formed by the assembly of a dimeric protein with a molecular weight of 110,000 and a sedimentation coefficient of 6 S, for brain (4 - 9), cilia and sperm tail (10 - 13), Chlamydomonas flagella (14), thyroid (15, 16), tubulin, etc.   This molecule is composed of two peptide chains of molecular weight 56,000 and 53,000 (6 - 8, 17). These two chains (α and β) are present in equimolecular amounts and may be easily separated by polyacrylamide gel electrophoresis (8, 18) after denaturation, reduction and alkylation as described by Renaud *et al*. (12). Significant differences were found for several aminoacids of these chains, although similarities were also observed (7, 18). Several authors (8, 19) have also shown that the peptide maps of the α and β chains are very similar but not identical. The partial sequence analysis, recently obtained by Luduena and Woodward (20) for the molecules prepared from chick embryo brain and sea urchin sperm outer doublets, indicates that α and β chains are very similar; in the first 24 positions there are no differences between the two α tubulin-chains and only one difference between the two β chains. Ten positions were identical in all four proteins. These results imply that α and β chains evolve from a single ancestral protein.

Several authors have reported that the microtubular protein is a glycoprotein (3, 8, 19, 21). However, further purification, performed by Eipper (9) eliminates most of the carbohydrate and nucleic acid material which contaminates the tubulin when it is prepared by the method of Weisenberg (4).

BINDING SITES OF TUBULIN

Purified tubulin binds several ligands including guanine nucleotides, colchicine, and vinblastine.

Purified tubulin from brain has one mole of tightly bound guanine nucleotide per mole of protein and is capable of binding another mole of readily exchangeable GTP per mole(4). Isolated flagellar outer doublet microtubules contain two moles of guanine nucleotide per mole of tubulin (22). Berry and Shelanski (23)

have shown that transphosphorylation occurs between the terminal
phosphate of the exchangeable nucleotide and the tightly bound
nucleotide. Tightly bound nucleotide is found chiefly as GDP (23).

   Colchicine and to a lesser extent other antimitotics such as
vinblastine, podophyllotoxin, etc. have been extensively used both
to characterize and to study the tubulin molecule and to show,
indirectly, that microtubules are involved in different cell functions (24). Colchicine is best known as an inhibitor of mitosis
whose action appears to be on the organization of the spindle microtubules (25 - 28).

   One mole of colchicine is bound to one mole of tubulin (4)
provided that tubulin is freshly prepared. The binding of colchicine may be easily assessed by a filter paper assay (4, 29).
Colchicine binding decays (first order reaction) on exposure at 37°
(4, 24, 28, 29). GTP largely prevents the loss of colchicine
activity; binding of colchicine also protects against the loss of
GTP binding activity. Weisenberg et $al.$ assume that colchicine and
GTP, though bound to different sites, both require the native configuration of the protein. Finally, vinblastine stabilizes colchicine binding activity as does GTP (10^{-3} M) but vinblastine
(3 x 10^{-4} M) is more potent than GTP (29).

   Native tubulin at 4° and pH 6.5 contains approximately 22 %
α helix, 30 % β structure and 48 % random coil (30). At 37° when
colchicine binding is optimal, the protein undergoes a slow conformational change resulting primarily in loss of α helix. This
change increases the lability of the protein to irreversible
denaturation accompanied by aggregation.

   The Vinca alkaloids, known for their metaphase blocking
antimitotic activity (31 - 35),   induce the formation of microtubular cristals in the cytoplasm of various types of cells (36 -
40). Precipitation of microtubule proteins can be induced by vinblastine (1 mg/ml) (41 - 44). However, precipitation of microtubule protein by vinblastine is not very specific, a number of
proteins being precipitated in addition to the microtubular protein
(45). Those proteins which precipitate with vinblastine sulfate
also precipitate with Ca^{2+} ions. Wilson et $al.$ (45) have suggested
that vinblastine sulfate, presumably acting as a cation, precipitates
proteins by combining with sites which can also combine with Ca^{2+}
ions. Tubulin binds half a mole of vinblastine per mole of tubulin
(23, 46), $i.e.$ one vinblastine per two tubulin dimers. Berry and
Shelanski (23) have shown that one half of the exchangeable GTP is
protected from exchange during vinblastine induced precipitation,
thus clearly reflecting the interaction of dimers.

PURIFICATION AND POLYMERIZATION OF TUBULIN

The first procedure proposed by Weisenberg *et al.* (4) was based on a batch adsorption on DEAE-Sephadex; thus the time required to obtain as much as 100 mg of purified brain tubulin is minimized, an important fact because of the lability of the protein. However, amorphous or 36-40 S aggregates are formed which are not microtubules and which could represent partially denatured tubulin. In the Weisenberg procedure (4) GTP (10^{-4} M), necessary to protect the protein, was added to the medium in which the minced brain was suspended before homogeneization. On the contrary, long exposure to 0.8 M KCl, which is used for the elution from the DEAE-Sephadex batch, appears to accelerate denaturation and must be removed as soon as possible by $(NH_4)_2SO_4$ precipitation. The purity of the preparation is 90-95 % judging by disk-gel electrophoresis. An additional purification step, precipitation by $MgCl_2$ (final concentration 0.05 M) (47) is generally omitted as it increases the proportion of aggregates.

Eipper (9) modified the method of Weisenberg *et al.* (4), by using pyrophosphate buffers throughout to minimize the interaction of microtubular protein with nucleic acids which are contaminants of the preparation of Weisenberg *et al.* (4). Further purification on Bio-gel A 15 m was performed (9).

Another type of purification procedure is based on the observation (48) that isolated brain tubulin can be repolymerized *in vitro* in solutions containing ATP or GTP (10^{-3} M), Mg^{2+} ions (0.5 mM) and a calcium chelator (EGTA 1mM). MES (2-(N-morpholino) ethane sulfonic acid) buffer (0.1 M) pH 6.4 was used which appears to protect microtubule protein. Shelanski *et al.* (49) were able to purify tubulin directly from brain supernatants by an assembly-disassembly procedure. The brain supernatant was prepared in the reassembly buffer of Weisenberg (48) at 4° and then mixed with an equal volume of 8 M glycerol in the same buffer. Upon incubation at 37° for 20 minutes, tubulin polymerizes to give reconstitued microtubules which are collected by centrifugation at 25° *i.e.* a temperature where the microtubules are not disassembled; lowering the temperature to 4° results in disassembly of the microtubules. Further purification may be obtained after a new addition of 8 M glycerol-reassembly buffer in another assembly cycle. Brain tubulin thus obtained is 80-90 % pure. However, this procedure cannot be easily applied to the purification of tubulin from other sources as a minimum concentration of protein (1-5 mg/ml) is necessary for assembly (49, 50). For other tissues such as thyroid (16, 51) or liver (52) where the tubulin content is much lower (0.2 mg/g of tissue), when compared to brain ($\sim$ 15 %) or flagella, Weisenberg's procedure (4, 47) has been applied but with some modifications such as the use of MES buffer which markedly improves the result.

Other methods of purification have employed vinblastine (40,43), calcium precipitation (53), affinity chromatography (54). In this last procedure a mixture of deacetylcolchicine and iso-deacetylcolchicine were allowed to react with activated Sepharose. This procedure allows the preparation of 2 mg of tubulin which was 90-95 % pure.

Great interest has been devoted to the *in vitro* polymerization reaction (48 - 50). The effect of Ca^{2+} (mM) as an inhibitor of polymerization has been studied by Olmsted and Borisy (56) and Haga *et al.* (57). However, Ca^{2+} when at μM concentration is an activator of polymerization (58). Another important problem is the existence of nucleation centres in the polymerization process, and of possible intermediates of polymerization between the 6 S subunit and the microtubule. Gaskin *et al.* (59) have made the observation that short pieces of microtubules obtained by sonication act as nucleation sites for the assembly. Borisy *et al.* (50) have isolated disk-type structures (rings) which appear to be required for microtubule assembly *in vitro* and to act as nucleation centres for the polymerization of microtubule protein. In a more recent report Kirshner *et al.* (60) postulate that 6 S tubulin exists in two states; the first is able to aggregate readily into a 36 S intermediate structure, the second being unable to polymerize alone. Finally, other types of aggregation figures may be observed *in vitro*, aster like structures (61), double rings and spirals (62) etc. It is not clear at the present time if these figures are actually significant for the polymerization process.

ATPASES AND NUCLEOTIDE TRANSPHOSPHORYLASE ACTIVITIES
"ASSOCIATED" WITH TUBULIN

One or more ATPases such as dynein (59, 63 - 66), a cyclic AMP dependent protein kinase (3, 16, 51, 67 - 72), and a nucleotide transphosphorylase (23, 73) are found in most of the tubulin preparations.

Summers and Gibbons (74) have shown that the tubules and dynein interact in a "sliding filament" mechanism to produce flagellar bending which is dependent on ATP as an energy source. Dynein is an EDTA-inhibited, divalent ion activated ATPase which is present as arms in the tubule of the flagella (63, 64). Gaskin *et al.* (59) have shown that brain neurotubules show an active MgATPase activity; most of this activity can be separated from the tubules and dynein by sucrose gradient ultracentrifugation. When compared to flagella dynein, the ATPase activity of brain dynein is very low.

Transphosphorylase activity is also associated with microtubules but does not appear to be an "intrinsic" property of tubulin (73). As indicated above, tubulin contains two nucleotide binding sites (4, 23, 73), one of which is readily exchangeable with the medium (E site); the other site binds GDP or GTP tightly (N site). An enzymatic activity "associated" with purified tubulin is involved in the binding of ATP or GTP for transfer of a γ-phosphate to GDP on the N site. The E site is saturated with GTP in less than one second and on the N site GDP is transphosphorylated by GTP with a half life of 5-10 minutes. Polymerization of tubulin with bound GTP on the E and N sites is accompanied by hydrolysis of both γ-phosphates and the microtubules formed have two moles of bound GDP/mole of tubulin. Morgan and Seeds (55) have reported that the polymerization of tubulin to microtubules is inhibited by the non-β, γ-hydrolyzable GTP analogues GMPPCP and GMPPNP.

CYCLIC AMP AND TUBULIN

Protein kinase activity (3, 16, 18, 51, 67 - 72) is consistently co-purified with tubulin regardless of the purification method used.

The substrate used to test protein kinase activity was either histone II A or the proteins which are present in the 90-95 % pure tubulin preparation. Although Soifer et al. (69) and Eipper (75) were unable to find any stimulation of the kinase activity by cyclic AMP, three criteria show (72) that, according to Goodman et al. (3) the protein kinase associated with tubulin is cyclic AMP dependent. Figure 1 shows a clear stimulation by cyclic AMP; Figure 2 depicts the binding of ^{3}H-c-AMP at the level of the protein kinase activity peak and finally the thermostable muscle inhibitor protein (76) inhibits both the basal and the cyclic AMP stimulated protein kinase activities present in brain tubulin preparations (Figure 3).

Both brain and thyroid protein kinase activities associated with tubulin were eluted from a DEAE Sephadex column by a KCl solution of molarity higher than 0.4 M, whereas the main peaks of soluble protein kinases from both tissues were eluted at a lower molarity ($\simeq$ 0.3 M). The enzymatic activity eluted at 0.5 - 0.6 M KCl represents only a very small fraction of the total soluble protein kinase activity. It might therefore result from a contamination by the main soluble protein kinases. Several criteria have been used to try to solve this problem (51 - 72). Firstly the "associated" protein kinase and the entity which is eluted by 0.37 M KCl exhibit different substrate specificities (cassein, histone, phosphvitine, protamine) (51). From these results it might be concluded that "associated" protein kinase is not a contamination from the main brain or thyroid soluble cyclic AMP-dependent protein kinase.

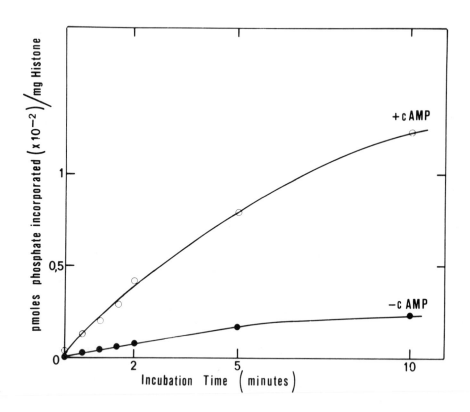

Figure 1. Kinetics of phosphorylation of Histone II A by the protein-kinase "associated" with brain tubulin. Protein kinase
activity was measured according to the procedure of Reimann et al.
(87). Experimental conditions used were : 600 µg histone/200 µl
of incubation medium, 190 µg brain tubulin, γ-^{32}P-ATP 20µM, c-AMP
5 µM (when added). The incubation was performed at 30°C.

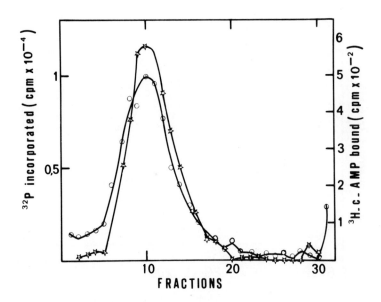

Figure 2. Sucrose gradient (5 –20%) ultracentriguation of the purified brain tubulin preparation (obtained by the batch method of Weisenberg, (4, 47), $MgCl_2$ precipitation being omitted) for 14 hours at 50 000 rpm at $4°C$, SW 50 L rotor, Spinco L_250. The sucrose solutions for the gradients were buffered with sodium phosphate 10 mM pH 6.8 and contained $MgCl_2$ 10 mM and GTP 10^{-4}M. Protein kinase activity (O———O) was measured as described in Figure 1 in the presence of c-AMP 5 μM; ^{3}H-c-AMP binding capacity (✻———✻) was measured by the method of Walton and Garren (88).

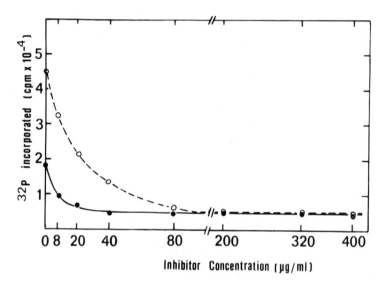

<u>Figure 3.</u>   *Inhibition of the brain associated tubulin protein-*
kinase activity in presence (0-----0) or absence (●——●) of
c-AMP (5 μM) with increasing amount of rabbit muscle thermo-
stable inhibitor (76).   Conditions are those of Figure 1.

Secondly the same conclusion might be deduced from the "Km" value for both enzyme preparations and from Ca^{2+} effects on their activities (Table I). As previously shown by Goodman *et al.* (3), the apparent Km for cyclic AMP differs by an order of magnitude when brain "associated" and "soluble" enzymes are compared. For the thyroid preparation the difference was even greater.* Soluble and tubular protein kinases do not exhibit the same behaviour towards calcium; Ca^{2+} 10 mM in the presence of Mg^{2+} (10 mM) strongly inhibits the "soluble" enzyme activities but inhibits to a lesser extent the enzymatic activity associated with brain tubulin. All these data suggest that the two kinase activities might be distinct entities.

In addition it has been shown (18, 51, 72, 77) that the associated protein kinase activity is not "intrinsic" to the tubulin as has been concluded by several authors (3, 70, 78, 79). By ultracentrifugation on a sucrose (5-20 %) gradient (Figure 4) neurotubulin may be partially separated from the kinase activity (72). Tubulin was identified by a ^{3}H-colchicine binding assay or by protein analysis. Protein kinase was followed by phosphorylation of histone II A. The sedimentation coefficients of "associated" protein kinase and neurotubulin were respectively 7.1 S and 6.1 S. Finally, the brain tubulin preparation was also submitted to ultracentrifugation on a 20 - 50 % sucrose gradient in order to separate the 6 S subunit from the (30 - 40 S) tubulin aggregates (Figure 5). Under these conditions it may be seen that no enzymatic activity could be found at the level of the tubulin aggregates. These results strongly suggest that "associated" protein kinase activity is not an "intrinsic" property of the tubulin molecule. Eipper (18) using different techniques of column chromatography has also shown that no form of tubulin has protein kinase activity.

Highly purified tubulin preparations therefore contain several enzymatic activities which are most probably not "intrinsic" properties of the molecule. ATPase (and dynein) and nucleotides transphosphorylase ATPase(s) are probably involved in some aspect of microtubule assembly and (or) function. The same possibility may exist for the "associated" protein kinase and several authors have assumed that tubulin is a substrate for this enzyme. Moreover, Goodman *et al.* (3) have reported that the neurotubular subunits serve as a substrate for this enzyme suggesting that this reaction could explain the role of microtubules and cyclic AMP to secretory processes.

----

* However, such differences in apparent Km for cyclic AMP may only reflect differences in protein kinase concentrations (80).

Table I

Protein-kinases and tissue	% inhibition by Ca^{++} (10 mM) of protein kinase activity		Apparent Km for c-AMP
	Minus c-AMP	Plus c-AMP	
Thyroid "Associated"	45	70	6×10^{-7} (a)
"Soluble"	70	80	2.5×10^{-8} (a)
Brain "Neurotubular"	24	27	2×10^{-6} (b)
"Soluble"	30(a)	65(a)	2.5×10^{-7} (c)

(a) from J.F. Leterrier et al.(82)

(b) from D. Goodman et al. (3)

(c) from E. Miyamoto et al. (89)

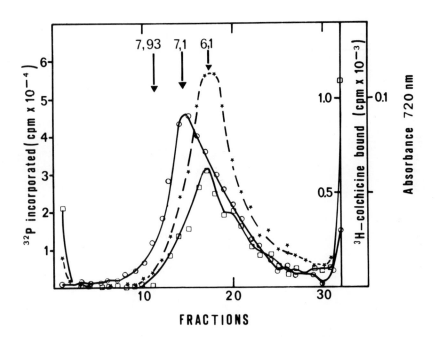

<u>Figure 4.</u>   Sucrose gradient (5-20%) ultracentrifugation of the puri-
fied brain tubulin preparation.   Conditions are those of Figure 2.
Tubulin was determined by bound ^{3}H-colchicine (*————*) and by protein concentration (□————□).   Protein kinase activity (○————○) was
measured as described in Figure 1 in the presence of c-AMP 5 μM.
Sedimentation coefficient was evaluated using glucose oxidase as
an internal marker.   Colchicine binding to tubulin : freshly prepared tubulin (3.4 mg/ml) was incubated at 37°C for 1 hour with
^{3}H-colchicine 2 μM (4 μCi/ml).   The incubation medium was filtered
on Sephadex G50 to remove free colchicine.   An aliquot was layered
on the sucrose gradient together with the tubulin preparation to be
analyzed.

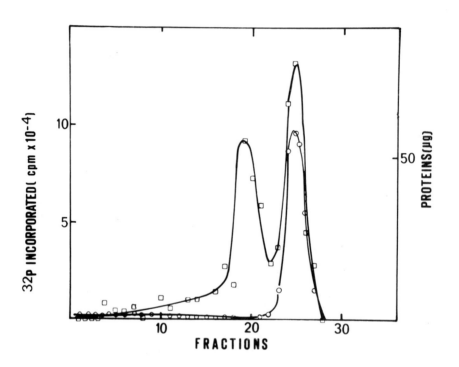

Figure 5. Sucrose gradient (20-50% in buffer as in Figure 2) ultracentrifugation of brain tubulin after a 1-hour incubation at 30°C. Protein-kinase activity (O——O) was measured using the conditions described under Figure 1. Protein concentration (□——□). Ultracentrifugation 3 hours at 4°C, 50 000 rpm, SW 50 L rotor, Spinco $L_2$50.

"IN VITRO" AND "IN VIVO" PHOSPHORYLATION REACTIONS
CATALYZED BY "ASSOCIATED" PROTEIN KINASE

Results concerning tubulin phospohorylation differ markedly depending on the method used to purify the protein. From results previously reported (16, 72) which were obtained with tubulin purified using the batch procedure of Weisenberg *et al.* (4), it may be concluded that a small percentage of the tubulin molecules are phosphorylated *in vitro* but only when present as 40 S aggregates. These aggregates, however, cannot be considered as reconstituted microtubules, as they may only be obtained in the presence of higher GTP concentrations and (or) in different mediums (48 - 50, 81).

The problem of tubulin phosphorylation has therefore been studied (51, 82) using tubulin purified by the aggregation-disaggregation procedure (49) which has the advantage of yielding molecules which are able to reconstitute, *in vitro*, large microtubules. Polyacrylamide disc-gel electrophoresis of tubulin prepared by this method revealed that tubulin is not labelled with ^{32}P *in vitro* (Figure 6). Further analysis (Figure 7) showed that no ^{32}P is present at the level of the tubulin cleaved chains, obtained after SDS-MSH treatment and alkylation. On the contrary, several peaks of radioactivity are observed near the origin, where heavy molecular weight material migrates, and between the origin and the tubulin chains. These constituents may be separated into at least five peaks by DEAE-Sephadex column chromatography (Figure 8). The first three ^{32}P labelled peaks are clearly separated from tubulin, which is eluted between peak IV and V.

These results suggest that tubulin is not phosphorylated when the conditions of preparation allow maintenance of the native structure which is also essential to obtain reassembly of microtubules. Purification of tubulin by the batch procedure must therefore introduce some denaturation, and the formation of aggregates, which would permit phosphorylation of seryl residues of the protein normally unavailable to the protein-kinase. The true substrates for *in vitro* phosphorylation of tubulin seem to be the proteins which are co-purified with tubulin. Since these components are present in low concentration with respect to tubulin (dynein for example represents 4 to 12 % of total proteins (59)), it is possible to account for the low amount of phosphate incorporated *in vitro* per mole of tubulin (0.1-0.8%) which was always much lower than that expected from stoichiometry (72).

However, several authors have reported data suggesting that neurotubulin is phosphorylated in brain slices or *in vivo* (9, 71, 75, 77, 79, 83). Eipper (9) after incubation of rat brain slices for 10 hours with ^{32}P orthophosphate found that the neurotubulin

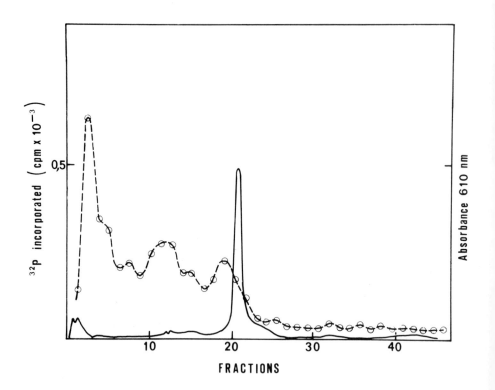

Figure 6. *7.5% polyacrylamide gel electrophoresis (pH 8.5 in 6.5 M urea 0.1% SDS) of phosphorylated brain tubulin prepared by the aggregation-disaggregation method of Shelanski et al. (49). Microtubules were isolated by centrifugation (105 000 g for 1 hour at 4°C) through a layer of buffer A mixed with the same volume of 8 M glycerol, dissociated at 4°C during 30 minutes and dialyzed against 8 % urea, 0.12 M MSH. The preparation was reduced by the method of Renaud et al. (12); 4 mA per tube were applied during 3 hours. The densitometer tracing (⸺) of the stained gel (amido black) was performed using a Gilford scanning densitometer. The gel was sliced into 1 mm fractions and the radioactivity counted (O-----O).*
Buffer A : 100 mM MES (2-(N-morpholino) ethanesulfonic acid) pH 6.4, MgCl$_2$ 0.5 mM ; EGTA 1 mM ; GTP 1 mM.

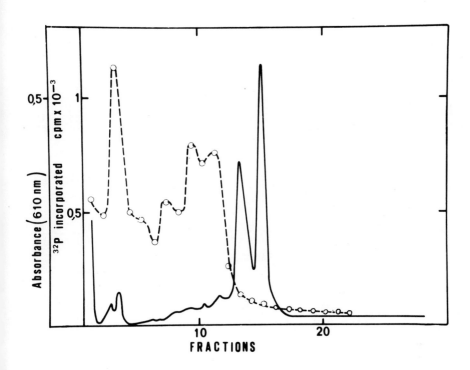

Figure 7. 7.5% polyacrylamide gel electrophoresis of phosphorylated brain tubulin reduced and alkylated by iodacetamide. Conditions are those of Figure 6.

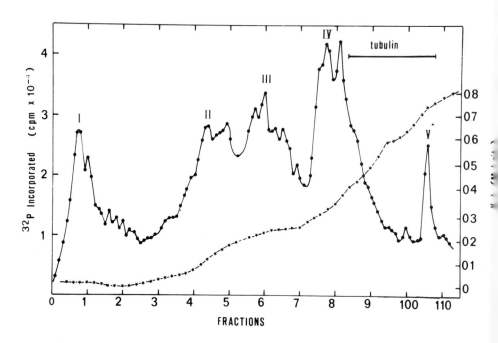

Figure 8. *DEAE Sephadex A50 column chromatography of brain phosphorylated microtubules disassembled by exposure to cold. 10 ml of
tubulin (6.8 mg/ml) purified as described in Figure 6 were phosphorylated during a 30-minute incubation period at 37°C in buffer
A (see Figure 6) with 0.6 mC of ^{32}P-ATP 0.1 mM and c-AMP 5μM.
This preparation was maintained at 4° for 1 hour and analyzed on a
DEAE Sephadex A50 column equilibrated with 100 mM MES pH 6.5, EGTA
1 mM, MgCl$_2$ 0.5 mM, dithiothreitol 2.5 mM. After washing the column
with 50 ml of the same buffer, a first KCl molarity gradient (0 to
0.3 M) was applied (300 ml) (59). A second KCl molarity gradient
(0.3 to 0.8 M) was applied (200 ml) and the column was washed with
50 ml of KCl 0.8 M. Aliquots (01 ml) of each fraction (3 ml) were
layered on 31 ET chromatography papers which were then washed three
times with TCA and two times with alcohol ether. ^{32}P radioactivity
was counted (●——●) and KCl molarity was measured using a monitored
conductimeter (×——×).*

purified by a modification of the method of Weisenberg *et al.* (4) is phosphorylated *in vivo* on a serine residue(s) in the β chain. The stoichiometry was 0.8 mole of phosphate per 6 S subunit. In a further study the same author (84) analyzed ^{32}P labelled tubulin after *in vivo* performic oxidation and trypsin digestion, confirming that *in vivo* phosphorylation of serine residues in the β chain occurs. Moreover, the tryptic map of *in vivo* ^{32}P labelled tubulin showed one ^{32}P peptide suggesting to Eipper that the phosphate is present in tubulin, rather than being present in a highly phosphory‐ lated contaminant. A similar conclusion was reached by Lagnado *et al.* (79) who used a system of brain cortical slices.

These data suggest, therefore, that preparations of tubulin are differently phosphorylated according to the methods used for labelling and purification. Eipper (75) has reached the same conclusions having observed that *in vivo* and *in vitro* phosphorylated tubulin differ markedly (gel chromatography migration, number of labelled peptides).

However, Murray and Froscio (68) were unable to find any labelled neurotubulin after incubation of rat brain slices in the presence of ^{32}P orthophosphate. Very recently Haimo *et al.*(85) have isolated high molecular weight material (HMW) containing most of the ATPase activity of the preparation and which co‐purify with *in vitro* assembled microtubules. When ^{32}P is injected into brains of one day old chicks and tubulin purified by the assembly procedure, only this HMW material is phosphorylated and never the tubulin. The results of both Murray and Froscio (68) and Haimo *et al.* (85) agree with those obtained by Rubin and Filner (86) with microtubules of flagellae and with the *in vitro* data reported in this work.

POLYMERIZATION OF TUBULIN AND PHOSPHORYLATION REACTIONS

The results reported above strongly suggest that tubulin is not a good substrate for the "associated" protein kinase but that minor constituents always co‐purified with tubulin are labelled with a very high specific activity. The next question is to know if these phosphorylated constituents play a role in the poly‐ merization process. To answer this question, neurotubulin was prepared by the aggregation‐disaggregation procedure of Shelanski *et al.* (49) and its polymerization was followed in the conditions described by these authors (49). The results showed that poly‐ merization of this tubulin preparation was unaffected by the pre‐ sence of ATP and cyclic AMP.

This conclusion is strengthened by a further experiment where polymerization of disassembled tubulin was performed in the presence of the muscle thermostable inhibitor (76) of protein kinase. Under these conditions protein-kinase activity and phosphorylation were completely abolished whereas polymerization and probably microtubule formation were unaffected. Thus phosphorylation does not appear to be necessary for the polymerization process.

However, further experiments have shown that the phosphorylated minor constituents copolymerize with tubulin. Tubulin was allowed to polymerize in a medium containing $^{32}P-\gamma-ATP$ GTP 10^{-3} M in presence or absence of 5 x 10^{-6} M cyclic AMP. Protein bound ^{32}P was measured and polymerization was simultaneously monitored as described by Shelanski et al. (49). At the end of the polymerization process, reconstituted microtubules were sedimented and analyzed by ultracentrifugation on a very dense sucrose gradient (50 - 70 %) (Figure 9). Under these conditions ^{32}P sediments with very heavy structures probably microtubules. However, the gel electrophoresis profile showed that tubulin chains were not labelled with ^{32}P (Figure 7). Thus the ^{32}P minor constituents copolymerize with tubulin during the polymerization process. Inhibition of tubulin polymerization may be obtained after addition of either colchicine or Ca^2 to the medium. Under these conditions, no ^{32}P labelled heavy material was found after sucrose gradient centrifugation (51). Labelled reconstitued microtubules were also disrupted by exposure at 4°. Under these conditions, the microtubules dissociate to the 6 S subunit whereas ^{32}P radioactivity has a sedimentation coefficient higher than 6 S, as shown by the ^{32}P/protein ratio illustrated in Figure 10. (82)

CONCLUSIONS

The physiological significance of the phosphorylation reactions catalyzed by the protein-kinase associated with tubulin remains unclear. However, our experiments show that tubulin is not a substrate for this enzyme in vitro, when tubulin is prepared under conditions allowing the maintenance of a native structure which is also necessary for in vitro polymerization to microtubules. However purified tubulin contains phosphorus(18, 75) covalently bound to serine residues, the stoichiometry varying from one preparation to another (0.3 to 0.8 mole/mole of tubulin). Phosphorylation reactions of tubulin could therefore be present in vivo although only two of four authors have been able to show in vivo ^{32}P labelling of this molecule. Failure to demonstrate in vitro phosphorylation of the native tubulin molecule could thus mean that the reactive serine residues are already fully phosphorylated and that this reaction is not readily reversed suggesting that it has no regulatory significance. Our results show that in vitro only minor unknown components present in the tubulin preparation are phosphorylated. Their significance is unknown; it seems that the phosphorylation of these components is not necessary for the polymerization of tubulin into

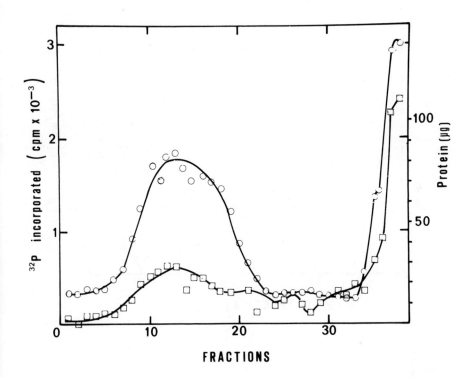

Figure 9. *Ultracentrifugation on sucrose gradients (50-70%) of a microtubule preparation polymerized and phosphorylated in conditions of Figure 6. Centrifugation was performed at 24°C immediately after polymerization in a Spinco SW 50-1 rotor at 50 000 rpm for 45 minutes. Aliquots of each fraction of the gradients were used for protein determination (□——□) and TCA precipitable radioactivity (O——O).*

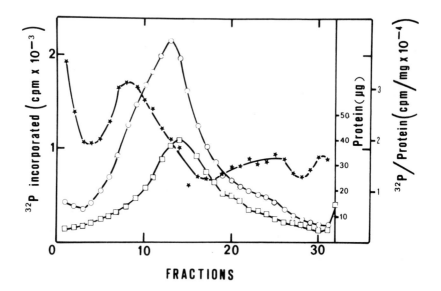

Figure 10. Ultracentrifugation on a sucrose gradient (5–20%) of a microtubule preparation, polymerized and phosphorylated under the same conditions as in Figure 6 and then depolymerized at 4°C for 30 minutes. The dissociated tubulin was visualized by protein determination (□——□); ^{32}P TCA precipitable radioactivity (O——O) was determined and ^{32}P/protein ratio (*——*) was calculted.

microtubules but that they co-polymerize with tubulin.

Thus the conclusions deduced from the inhibitory effect of colchicine upon hormone or cyclic AMP dependent secretion should be considered with great caution. It is probable that cyclic AMP does not act on secretion by a direct activation of the process of assembly into microtubules from tubulin subunits. Tubulin might be the basic structural subunit of these organelles but not the only molecule belonging to this structure. Other molecules or enzymes such as transphosphorylase, protein-kinase, dynein or other ATPases might form part of the structure of these organelles. Cyclic AMP action and the phosphorylation reactions may take place at the level of these or other constituents whose activity would be important for the biological activity of microtubules. Another possibility is that cyclic AMP acts on a system other than microtubules but which requires assembled microtubules to produce the final physiological response.

REFERENCES

(1) OLMSTED, J.B., BORISY, G.G. (1973b), Annual Review of Biochemistry, Vol. 42 (E.E. Snell Ed.) 507, Annual Review Inc.

(2) TILNEY, L.G., PORTER, K.R. (1967). J. Cell Biol., 34, 327

(3) GOODMAN, D.B.P., RASMUSSEN, H., DI BELLA, F., GUTHROW, C.E. (1970) Proc. Nat. Acad. Sci. 67, 652

(4) WEISENBERG, R.C., BORISY, G.G., TAYLOR, E.W. (1968). Biochemistry, 7, 4466

(5) FINE, R.E. (1971) Nature New Biol., 233, 283

(6) OLMSTED, J.B., WITMAN, G.B., CARLSON, K., ROSENBAUM, J.L. (1971), Proc. Nat. Acad. Sci. 68, 2273

(7) BRYAN, Y., (1974), Fed. Proc. 33, 152

(8) FEIT, H., SLUSAREK, L., SHELANSKI, M. (1971) Proc. Nat. Acad. Sci., 68, 2028

(9) EIPPER, B. (1972) Proc. Nat. Acad. Sci. 69, 2283

(10) SHELANSKI, M.L., TAYLOR, E.W. (1967) J. Cell. Biol. 34, 549

(11) SHELANSKI, M.L., TAYLOR, E.W. (1968) J. Cell. Biol. 38, 304

(12) RENAUD, F.L., ROWE, A.J., GIBBONS, I.R. (1968) J. Cell
      Biol. 36, 79

(13) STEPHENS, R.E. (1968) J. Mol. Biol. 32, 277

(14) WITMAN, G.B., CARLSON, K., BERLINER, J., ROSENBAUM, J.L.
      (1972) J. Cell Biol. 54, 507

(15) WILLIAMS, J.A., WOLFF, J. (1970) Proc. Nat. Acad. Sci.
      67, 1901

(16) RAPPAPORT, L., LETERRIER, J.F., NUNEZ, J. (1972) FEBS
      Letters, 26, 349

(17) JACOBS, M., BROWN, A.V.W., BROWN, G.L. (1972) FEBS Letters,
      24, 113

(18) EIPPER, B. (1974a), J. Biol. Chem. 249, 1398

(19) FALXA, M.L., GILL, T.J. (1969) Archiv. Biochem. Biophys.
      135, 194

(20) LUDUENA, R., WOODWARD, D. (1974) Conf. Biol. Cytoplasmic
      Microtubules - N. York Acad. Sci. Ed. in the press

(21) MARGOLIS, R.K., MARGOLIS, R.U., SHELANSKI, M.L. (1972)
      Biochem. Biophys. Res. Comm. 47, 432

(22) STEPHENS, R.E., RENAUD, F.L., GIBBONS, I.R. (1967) Science
      156, 1606

(23) BERRY, R.N., SHELANSKI, M. (1972), J. Mol. Biol., 71, 71

(24) WILSON, L., BAMBURG, J.R., MIZEL, S.B., GRISHAM, L.M. and
      CRESWELL, K.M. (1974) 33, 158

(25) MALAWISTA, S.E. (1965) J. Exp. Med. 122, 361

(26) INOUE, S. (1952) Exptl. Cell Res. 2, 305

(27) WILSON, L., FRIEDKIN, M. (1967) Biochemistry, 6, 3126

(28) BORISY, G.G., TAYLOR, E.W. (1967) J. Cell Biol. 34, 525

(29) WILSON, L. (1970) Biochemistry, 9, 4999

(30) VENTILLA, M., CANTOR, C.R., SHELANSKI, M.L. (1972) Bio-
      chemistry, 11, 1554

(31) PALMER, C.G., LIVENGOOD, D., WARREN, A.K., SIMPSON, P.J., JOHNSON, I.S. (1960) Exp. Cell Res. 20, 198

(32) CUTTS, J.H. (1961) Cancer Res. 21, 168

(33) MALAWISTA, S.E., BENSCH, K., SATO, H. (1968) Science 160, 770

(34) MALAWISTA, S.E., SATO, H., CREASEY, W.A., BENSCH, K.G. (1969) Fed. Proc. 28, 875

(35) WISNIEWSKI, H.M., SHELANSKI, M., TERRY, R.D. (1968) J. Cell Biol. 38, 224

(36) BENSCH, K.G., MALAWISTA, S.E. (1968) Nature, 218, 1176

(37) BENSCH, K.G., MALAWISTA, S.E. (1969) J. Cell Biol. 40, 95

(38) SCHOCHET, S.S., LAMPERT, P.W., EARLE, K.M. (1968), J. Neuropathol. 27, 645

(39) BRYAN, J., WILSON, L. (1971), Proc. Nat. Acad. Sci. 68, 1762

(40) BRYAN, J. (1972) Biochemistry, 11, 2611

(41) MARANTZ, R., VENTILLA, M., SHELANSKI, M.L. (1969) Science 165, 498

(42) WEISENBERG, R.C., TIMASHEFF, S.N. (1969), Biophys. Soc. Abst. 9, 174

(43) OLMSTED, J.B., CARLSON, K., KLEBE, R., RUDDLE, F., ROSENBAUM, J. (1970) Proc. Nat. Acad. Sci., 65, 129

(44) MARANTZ, R., SHELANSKI, M.L. (1970), J. Cell Biol. 44, 234

(45) WILSON, L., BRYAN, J., RUBY, A., MAZIA, D., (1970) Proc. Nat. Acad. Sci. 66, 807

(46) OWELLEN, R.J., OWENS, A.H., DONIGIAN, D.W. (1972) Biochem. Biophys. Res. Comm. 47, 685

(47) WEISENBERG, R.C. TIMASHEFF, S.N. (1970) Biochemistry, 9, 4110

(48) WEISENBERG, R.C. (1972) Science, 177, 1104

(49) SHELANSKI, M.L., GASKIN, F., CANTOR, C.R. (1973) Proc. Nat.
      Acad. Sci. 70, 765

(50) BORISY, G.G., OLMSTED, J.B., KLUGMAN, R.A. (1972) Proc. Nat.
      Acad. Sci. 69, 2890

(51) RAPPAPORT, L., LETERRIER, J.F., NUNEZ, J. (1974) Conf. Biol.
      Cytoplasmic Microtubules – N. York Acad. Sci. Ed. in press

(52) JEANRENAUD, B., PATZELT, Ch. (1974) Personal communication

(53) BHATTACHARYYA, B., WOLFF, J. (1974) Biochemistry, 13, 2364

(54) HINMAM, N.D., MORGAN, J.L., SEEDS, N.W., CANN, J. (1973)
      Biochem. Biophys. Res. Comm. 52, 752

(55) MORGAN, J.L., SEEDS, N.W. (1974) Conf. Biol. Cytoplasmic
      Microtubules – N. York Acad. Sci. Ed. in press

(56) OLMSTED, J.B., BORISY, G.G. (1973a) Biochemistry 12, 4282

(57) HAGA, T., ABE, T., KUROKAWA, M. (1974) FEBS Letters, 39,
      291

(58) OLMSTED, J.B., MARCUM, J.M., JOHNSON, K.A., MURPHY, D.B.,
      BORISY, G.G. (1974) Conf. Biol. Cytoplasmic Microtubules –
      N. York Acad. Sci. Ed. in press

(59) GASKIN, F., KRAMER, S.B., CANTOR, C.R., ADELSTEIN, R.,
      SHELANSKI, M.L. (1974) FEBS Letters, 40, 281

(60) KIRSCHNER, M.W., WILLIAMS, R.C., WEINGARTEN, M., GERHART,
      J.C. (1974) Proc. Nat. Acad. Sci. 71, 1159

(61) WEISENBERG, R.C., ROSENFELD, A., (1974) Conf. Biol. Cyto-
      plasmic Microtubules – N. York Acad. Sci. Ed. in press

(62) KIRSCHNER, M.W., WEINGARTEN, M. (1974) Conf. Biol. Cyto-
      plasmic Microtubules – N. York Acad. Sci. Ed. in press

(63) GIBBONS, I.R. (1963) Proc. Nat. Acad. Sci. 60, 1002

(64) GIBBONS, I.R., ROWE, A.J. (1965) Science, 149, 424

(65) SUMMERS, K.E., GIBBONS, I.R. (1973) J. Cell Biol. 58, 618

(66) BURNS, R.G., and POLLARD, T.D. (1974) FEBS Letters, 40, 274

(67)   LAGNADO, J.R., LYONS, C., WICKREMASINGHE, G. (1971) FEBS
       Letters, 15, 254

(68)   MURRAY, A.W., FROSCIO, M. (1971), Biochem. Biophys. Res.
       Comm. 44, 1089

(69)   SOIFER, D., LASZLO, A.H., SCOTTO, J.M. (1972) Biochim.
       Biophys. Acta 271, 182

(70)   SOIFER, D. (1974) Conf. Biol. Cytoplasmic Microtubules -
       N. York, Acad. Sci. Ed. in press

(71)   REDDINGTON, M., LAGNADO, J.R. (1973) FEBS Letters 30, 188

(72)   LETERRIER, J.F., RAPPAPORT, L., NUNEZ, J. (1974a) Molecular
       and Cellular Endocrinology, 1, 65

(73)   JACOKS, M., SMITH, H., and TAYLOR, E. (1974). J. Mol. Biol.
       89, 455

(74)   SUMMERS, K.E., GIBBONS, I.R. (1971) Proc. Nat. Acad. Sci.
       68, 3092

(75)   EIPPER, B. (1974b) J. Biol. Chem. 249, 1407

(76)   WALSH, D.A., ASHBY, C.D. (1973) Rec. Progr. Horm. Res. 29,
       (Acad. Press Ed.) 329

(77)   PIRAS, M.M., and PIRAS, R. (1974) Eur. J. Biochem. 47, 443

(78)   LAGNADO, J.R., LYONS, C.A., WELLER, M.G., PHILLIPSON, O.
       (1972) Biochem. J. 128, 95

(79)   LAGNADO, J.R., TAN, L.P., REDDINGTON, M. (1974) Conf. Biol.
       Cytoplasmic Microtubules - N. York Acad. Sci. Ed. in press

(80)   BEAVO, J.A., BECHTEL, P.J., and KREBS, E.G., (1974) Proc.
       Nat. Acad. Sci., 71, 3580

(81)   BORISY, G.G., OLMSTED, J.B., MARCUM, J.M., and ALLEN, G.
       (1974) Fed. Proc. 33, 167

(82)   LETERRIER, J.F., RAPPAPORT, L., NUNEZ, J. (1974b) FEBS
       Letters, 46, 285

(83)   QUINN, P.J., (1973) Biochem. J. 133, 273

(84)   EIPPER, B. (1974c) Conf. Biol. Cytoplasmic Microtubules -
       N. York Acad. Sci. Ed. in press

(85)   HAIMO, L., SLOBODA, R., BINDER, L., SNELL, W., DENTLER, W.,
       ROSENBAUM, J.L. (1974) Conf. Biol. Cytoplasmic Microtubules -
       N. York Acad. Sci. Ed. in press

(86)   RUBIN, R.W. and FILNER, P. (1973) J. Cell Biol. 56, 628

(87)   REIMANN, E.M., WALSH, D.A., KREBS, E.G. (1971) J. Biol.
       Chem. 246, 1986

(88)   WALTON, G.M., GARREN, L.D. (1970) Biochemistry, 9, 4223

(89)   MIYAMOTO, E., KUO, J.F., GREENGARD, P. (1969) J. Biol. Chem.
       244, 6395

PROSTAGLANDINS AND CYCLIC NUCLEOTIDES

C. Jacquemin

Laboratoire de Biochimie, Faculté des Sciences de
REINS, B.P. N° 347, 51062 Reims-Cédex, France

Contents

INTRODUCTION

Before discussing in detail the relationship between prostaglandins and cyclic nucleotides, it will be useful to briefly
summarise some properties of prostaglandins.

First of all their chemical structure : they are fatty acids
with twenty carbon atoms, atoms 8 to 12 constituting a pentagonal
cycle.

The discussion concerning the principles of nomenclature,
will be limited to "natural" prostaglandins since related compounds are considered their metabolites. The prostaglandins are
classified in series I, II and III according to the number of

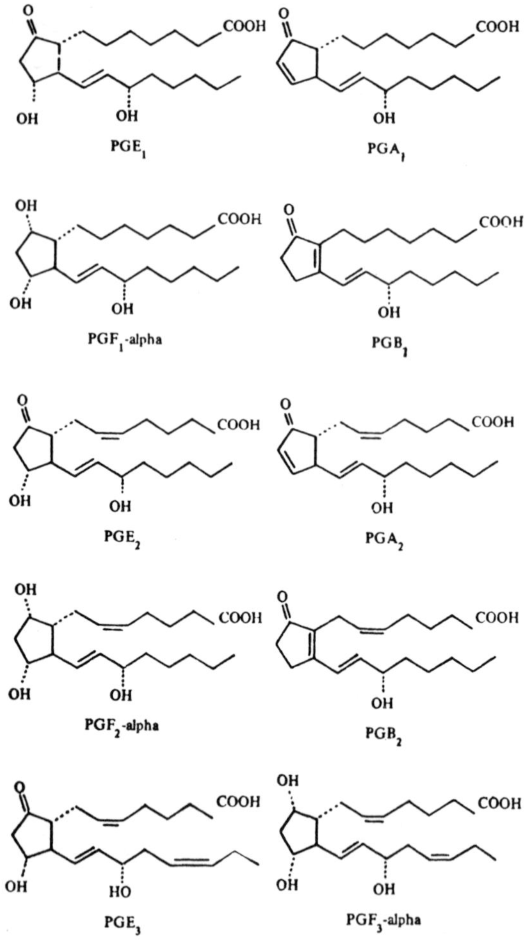

<u>FIGURE 1</u>. *Formula of naturally occurring prostaglandins.*

double bonds. The position of the substituents allows one to
distinguish the four types : A, B, E and Fα. The combination of
these two classifications furnishes twelve different prostaglandins
of which only ten are yet identified (Figure 1). Comparison between the biological properties of these compounds provides important differences among the four types, but only quantitative
differences exist within the series.

Prostaglandins are biologically synthesized from C_{20} polyunsaturated fatty acids : 8, 11, 14 eicosatrienoïc acid is the
precursor of series I, whilst 5, 8, 11, 14 eicosatetraenoïc acid
(arachidonic acid) and 5, 8, 11, 14, 17 eicosapentaenoïc acid are

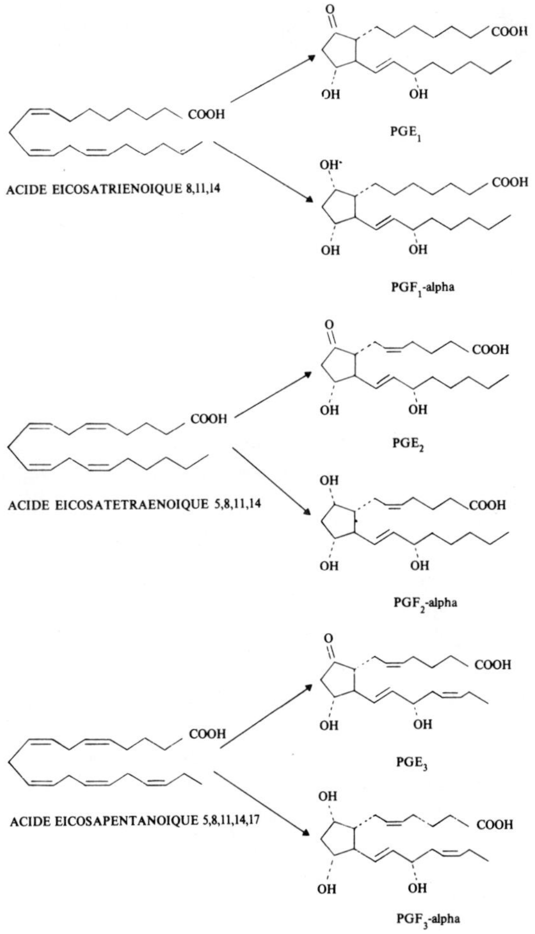

FIGURE 2. *Fatty acid precursors of primary prostaglandins.*

respectively the precursors of series II and III (Figure 2).

The extensive work which has lead to the elucidation of the following steps in prostaglandin biosynthesis (for a comprehensive review see (1)), will be outlined only.

Prostaglandin synthetase, a complex oxygenase, converts the fatty acid to a cyclic endoperoxide. This is converted by rearrangement to prostaglandin E and by reduction to prostaglandin F_α. Prostaglandin synthetase which has been incompletely purified, has a microsomal localization. In vitro we know that the addition of reduced glutathione and hydroquinone favours the synthesis of

PGE[1]at the expense of that of PGF_α. The mechanism operating in vivo, affecting the balance between prostaglandins E and F_α, is unknown.

Prostaglandins of the A series (PGA) are derived by dehydration of PGE, but this reaction is poorly understood.

The plasma enzyme, prostaglandin isomerase, converts PGA into PGB.

The subsequent metabolism of these compounds is based on four types of reactions :

β oxidation
ω oxidation
reduction of double bond in position 13
dehydrogenation of the hydroxyl group in position 15
  (Figure 3).

Generally, the different metabolites have less biological activity than the parent compounds. Therefore we can consider them as catabolites and that their formation leads to inactivation of prostaglandins.

What are the biological roles of prostaglandins ? Are they members of a new hormonal system or intracellular mediators ? It is impossible at present to effectively answer this question. The presence of prostaglandins has been established in most of the organs investigated,except the turkey erythrocyte (2). Their presence is the consequence of synthesis caused by various stimuli. Sometimes it is an artefact produced during processing of tissues when extracting prostaglandins (3, 4). In other cases it follows nervous, hormonal or pharmacological stimulations (5, 6, 7, 8).

There appear to be no storage pools of prostaglandins. The rapid accumulation of prostaglandins observed after stimulation results from synthesis in which the limiting factor is the low concentration of the precursors of prostaglandin synthesis e.g. free polyunsaturated fatty acids. These processus are probably mostly confined to the lipid fraction : cholesterol esters, tri-

---

[1]The abbreviations used are : PGE_1, prostaglandin E_1; PGE_2, prostaglandin E_2; PGE, either prostaglandin E_1 or prostaglandin E_2; $PGF_{1\alpha}$, prostaglandin $F_{1\alpha}$; $PGF_{2\alpha}$, prostaglandin $F_{2\alpha}$; PGF_α either prostaglandin $F_{1\alpha}$ or prostaglandin $F_{2\alpha}$; PGA, prostaglandins of the A series; PGB, prostaglandins of the B series; SC 19200, a dibenzoxazepine hydrazide derivative; PPP, polyphloretin phosphate; ACTH, adrenocorticotropic hormone; TSH, thyreostimulin; EFA, essential fatty acids; ADH, antidiuretic hormone; LH, luteotropin.

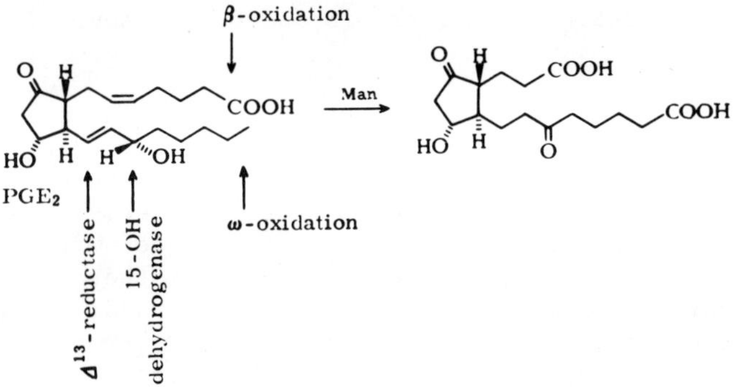

FIGURE 3. *Human urinary metabolism of* PGE_2.

glycerides and phospholipids. This suggests that the control of
esterase activity serves as a regulating factor in the synthesis
of prostaglandins (9, 10). This hypothesis is supported by the
fact that the addition of snake verom phospholipase to a homogenate of bovine seminal vesicles considerably augments the concentration of prostaglandins (3, 10).

Prostaglandin synthesis is sometimes accompanied by release
into the extracellular spaces and the circulation : in some cases
it is a normal phenomenon (e.g. contraction of the spleen induced
by catecholamines released from the splenic nerve fibers (11, 12)
and sometimes a pathologic phenomenon (e.g. medullary carcinoma of
the thyroid (13)).

Do the released prostaglandins play a biological role ? Many
possibilities can be considered.

The prostaglandins released might act as local hormones on the
cellular membranes increasing their resistance or modifying them
to adapt to new conditions created by the stimulus (14). In other
cases the prostaglandins released could act on cells of other
adjacent organs : e.g. PGF_α produced from the uterus might be transferred to the ovary and participate in luteolysis (14). However,
it does not seem a generality since, in laboratory animals, prostaglandins E and F_α are rapidly removed from the circulation by passage through the lung and the liver (11).

Hence, I think in our study of interactions between cyclic
nucleotides and prostaglandins, we must also consider the latter
as intracellular mediators biosynthesized in situ under the
action of certain stimuli, unlike hormones carried by the general
circulation.

When attempting to study this problem in a comprehensive
manner, determining both the concentration and rate of synthesis

of endogeneous prostaglandins, one is faced with several technical problems.

The first one is that of extraction. The tissues are extracted in ethanol; at pH 4.5 the extract is partitioned between water and ethyl acetate, and the organic phase is then reextracted at pH 8 by phosphate buffer. The pH of this aqueous phase is then adjusted to 4.5 and the prostaglandins reextracted with ethyl acetate (16) the crude extract being finally further purified by chromatography. With the method most commonly used, prostaglandins are eluted (in three fractions : A and B, E, F_α) from a silicic acid column with mixtures of benzene : ethyl acetate : methanol (17). The recoveries are determined by incorporation of labelled standards before extraction.

In place of bio-assays of prostaglandins, once widely employed, radioimmunological determinations which are more sensitive and reproducible are now commonly used (17). Cross reactivity exists, in particular between the prostaglandins of the same type belonging to different series (PGE_1 and PGE_2, $PGF_{1\alpha}$ and $PGF_{2\alpha}$,---) (Figure 4). However, practically speaking this is not too great a problem, because qualitative differences in biological activity exist between the different types. These methods are sufficiently sensitive to assay in the concentration range of 5 pg of prostaglandins A, E or F_α. Higher concentrations (µg) of prostaglandins E can be assayed spectrophotometrically after transformation to PGB in alkaline medium (18).

Finally there exist numerous thin layer chromatographic systems, separating prostaglandin mixtures either as to type or series (19). Gas chromatography is also used but less convenient to operate.

To finish this introduction we should also mention that in the study of prostaglandins one can also employ certain inhibitors. We can distinguish two categories of inhibitors : inhibitors of prostaglandin action and inhibitors of synthesis.

Among the inhibitors of prostaglandin action, some are structural analogues of prostaglandins. There is a complete series of such compounds synthesized by Fried et al. (21). The most representative is 7-oxa, 13-prostynoic acid which has been shown to be a competitive inhibitor of prostaglandin action.

In addition, different antagonists of prostaglandin action have been reported. SC-19220 appears to be a direct antagonist of prostaglandins (22). PPP, a heteregenous mixture of polyesters of phosphoric acid and phloretin, also antagonizes prostaglandin action. The low molecular weight component seems to be responsible for a direct blocking effect (23). The mechanism of action of these compounds is unknown.

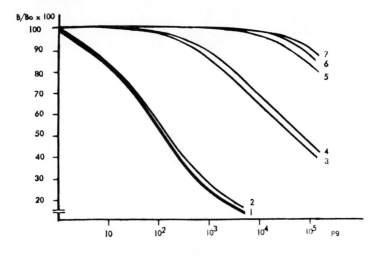

**Sensitivity
and specificity**

N°	Compounds		Cross reactivity for B/Bo = 0.5
1	Prostaglandin	$F_2\alpha$	100 %
2	Prostaglandin	$F_1\alpha$	100 %
3	Prostaglandin	E_1	0.25%
4	Prostaglandin	E_2	0.15%
5	Prostaglandin	A_1, A_2	< 0.1 %
6	Prostaglandin	B_1, B_2	< 0.1 %
7	15 Keto prostaglandin $F_2\alpha$		< 0.1 %

FIGURE 4. *Sensitivity and specificity of anti-PGF$_{2\alpha}$ antibody. Bo is the initial binding of labelled PGF$_{2\alpha}$ in the absence of any standard. Unpublished picture by courtesy of Dr. F. Dray, Institut Pasteur, Paris, France.*

Among the inhibitors of synthesis, one can distinguish between steric analogues of substrates of prostaglandin synthetase and other compounds.

The most effective steric analogues are linoleic acid (18 : 2ω6) (4), linolenic acid (18 : 3ω3); (4); 8 cis, 12 trans, 14 cis eicosatrienoïc acid (24), 5 cis, 8 cis, 12 trans, 14 cis eicosatetraenoïc acid (24) and 5, 8, 11, 14 eicosatetraynoïc acid (25).

The other substances which block prostaglandin biosynthesis belong to the family of non-steroïd-antiinflammatory agents. Aspirin and indomethacin are most widely used. Indomethacin is the strongest inhibitor of the two described and does not appear to act at any level other than prostaglandin synthetase (26, 27). Moreover it affects the synthesis of PGE and PGF_α identically. Aspirin however chiefly inhibits PGE synthesis (28).

Following this review covering the nomenclature of prostaglandins, biosynthesis, metabolism, biological roles and also the methodological principles for analysis, it is timely to discuss evidence for relationships between prostaglandins and cyclic nucleotides.

EFFECTS OF EXOGENOUS PROSTAGLANDINS ON ADENYLATE CYCLASE IN VARIOUS TISSUES

Many biological effects of prostaglandins are induced by the intermediate modification of adenylate cyclase activity. These modifications usually induce the accumulation of cAMP but this is not always so since we know of several examples of prostaglandins acting as antagonists of agents which stimulate adenylate cyclase.

Inhibition of the Cyclic AMP Formation

Historically these are the effects which were first described. Steinberg et al. in 1963 (29) showed that prostaglandins in vitro inhibited the lipolytic action of catecholamines in rat adipose tissue. Later prostaglandin blockade of other lipolytic agents such as ACTH, glucagon and theophylline on adipose tissue or isolated cells was also demonstrated (30, 31, 32, 33). To explain the PGE effect on phosphorylase activation, the hypothesis was postulated that the stimulation of cyclic-AMP accumulation was inhibited (30, 34). This hypothesis was supported by the fact that dibutyryl-c-AMP stimulated lipolysis was not affected by PGE, in isolated adipocytes of rat (30, 32), chick (33) and human (34). Generally it was reported that PGE_1 had no effect on the basal content of cyclic AMP in isolated adipocytes, but Shaw and Ramwell (35) found a two-fold increase in activity after PGE_1 (2.8 x 10^{-6}M). Contrarily, in intact adipose tissue PGE_1 increases the accumulation of cyclic AMP, this increase being attributed to the stimulation of adenylate cyclase of non-adipose cells. In the presence of stimulators of cyclic AMP accumulation (catecholamines, glucagon, ACTH, TSH with methylxanthine) PGE_1 has a strong inhibitory effect (32, 39, 37). This effect is related to the dose of PGE_1 (38).

Catecholamine stimulation of adenylate cyclase from adipocyte homogenates in the presence of theophylline has been found to be unaffected by PGE_1 (37, 39). Nevertheless this lack of PGE_1 action cannot be due to the absence of receptors because their existence has been demonstrated in this material (40, 41).

The antilipolytic actions of prostaglandins and their inhibitory effect on cyclic AMP accumulation were only observed with PGE_1 and PGE_2. Only structural analogues of the latter prostaglandins which possess other biological activity inhibit lipolysis (ω homo PGE_1), whereas the others ($\omega 7$ PGE_1, ω nor PGE_1, ω nor PGE_2, ω dinor PGE_2) have no action on theophylline stimulated lipolysis (42).

$PGF_{1\alpha}$ and β neither affect stimulated lipolysis (42), nor cyclic AMP accumulation (38), PGA_1 has less than 10 % of the antilipolytic activity of PGE_1 (43).

One suggestion for the biological role of the antilipolytic effect of prostaglandins E was proposed after the following observations.

Hormonal or neural stimulation of lipolysis is accompanied by the release of significant quantities of prostaglandins into the incubation media (8, 42). During a 2-hour period of adrenalin stimulation of lipolysis in fat pads, the quantity of PGE_1 and PGE_2 released ranged between 3 and 7 ng/g and 24 to 29 ng/g of tissue respectively (42, 44). Moreover dibutyryl-c-AMP stimulated PGE_2 accumulation by the rat fat cells (45). These results are compatible with the hypothesis of a negative feed-back system (8, 46) since polyunsaturated C_{20} fatty acids were among those released during lipolysis, which are limiting substrates of prostaglandin synthetase (Figure 5). Their conversion to prostaglandins, particularly PGE_1 and PGE_2 would inhibit adenylate cyclase and hence impede lipolysis.

However, experiments performed to verify this hypothesis have yielded conflicting results.

Christ and Nugteren (42) have compared dihomo-linolenic acid ($C_{20} : 3$) and arachidonic acid ($C_{20} : 4$) contents of triglycerides of epidydimal fat pads in normal rats and rats fed with diets poor in essential fatty acids (EFA). The content of $C_{20} : 3$ and $C_{20} : 4$ dropped from 0.1 % to 0 % and 1.7 % to 0.02 % respectively. These values in normal rats were compatible with the relative quantities of PGE_1 and PGE_2 secreted during lipolysis. The basal lipolysis was found to be higher in EFA deficient rats than in normal rats, but it was not inhibited by PGE_1. However, the stimulated lipolysis was found to be decreased by PGE_1 to the same extent in both groups of rats.

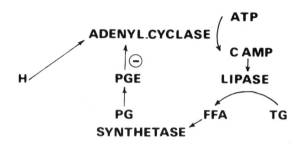

FIGURE 5. *A scheme representing the negative feedback of lipo-*
lysis by PGE in adipose tissue.

     Shaw et al. (35) performed a complementary experiment invol-
ving chronic treatment of rats with tetraynoïc acid, an inhibitor
of the conversion of arachidonate to prostaglandins (25). After
16 days of administration the basal concentration of cyclic AMP in
adipocytes increased by 200 % but was not further stimulated by
adrenalin in the presence of theophylline. The addition of PGE_2
decreased the cyclic AMP levels to an identical value in the control as well as the treated rats. Lipolysis was not measured in
this work but the PGE and PGFα compositions were determined. This
treatment resulted in a 50 % diminution of the content of PGFα but
the PGE content decreased by only 2 % which was curious since only
the latter have an inhibitory effect on cyclic AMP accumulation.

     However, the results of an experiment carried out by Iliano
and Cuatrecasas (47) supported the hypothesis of feedback. 7-oxa-
13-prostynoïc acid and SC 19220 which block prostaglandin action,
were found to increase adrenalin induced lipolysis in fat cells.
These compounds probably act by competitively suppressing lipolysis inhibition due to PGE. Moreover, indomethacin, an inhibitor
of endogeneous prostaglandin synthesis, was found to increase both
basal lipolysis and lipolysis stimulated by adrenalin, but aspirin
had no such effect. Indomethacin was reported to augment the basal
content of cyclic AMP by 200 % in 15 minutes. The accumulation of
cyclic AMP by adrenalin action,which was transient and shorter than
15 minutes,was also increased by the presence of indomethacin.

     These results are not in agreement with those of Fain et al.
(48). Using wide ranges of concentrations of indomethacin (5 to

50 µg/ml), these authors observed no effect on basal or stimulated lipolysis and cyclic AMP accumulation. The latter investigators are in agreement with Radzialowski and Novak (49) who found no effect of SC 19220 on adrenalin induced lipolysis. Nevertheless this compound was reported to suppress prostaglandin E_2 inhibition of induced lypolysis. Fain et al. (48) and Ho and Sutherland (50) postulated that the primary feedback regulator of lipolysis was not a prostaglandin. This conclusion was based both on their experimental results, and also on conflicting results in the literature which will be discussed later. Kuehl and Humes (40), using a binding system based on a poorly defined membrane preparation from fat cells, found that SC 19220 did not compete with PGE_1 which raised doubts as to the mechanism of its antiprostaglandin activity. Substances such as acetylcholine or histamine which possess no lipolytic activity on adipose tissue have been reported to stimulate the release of prostaglandins (8).

It is not absolutely certain that triglycerides are the sole source of arachidonate in adipocytes. Dalton and Hope (45) think that phospholipids can also play a role in this. They justify this hypothesis by the high arachidonate content in phospholipids and by the existence of a phospholipase A activity, apparently cyclic AMP dependent, in the adipocytes (51).

Therefore it is not possible at present to draw firm conclusions about the physiological role of prostaglandins in adipose tissue. Little information is available on the mode of prostaglandin action and the mechanism of their modification of intracellular cyclic AMP concentration in adipocytes. It seems that this is an action on synthesis, because PGE_1 has not been found to affect the phosphodiesterase activity (32, 42, 52). It has been proposed that PGE can interfere with ATP binding to adenylate cyclase (53). However the problem still remains unsolved, due to the failure to demonstrate an effect of PGE on cell free preparations of adenylate cyclase derived from adipose tissue (37, 39).

Absence of Action on Cyclic AMP Formation

In contrast to adipose tissue, where we see PGE antagonism of lipolytic hormones linked with the inhibition of synthesis and accumulation of cyclic AMP, there are other examples of hormone-prostaglandin interactions in which cyclic AMP has not been implicated. For example PGE_1 does not appear to affect either the basal, or adrenalin stimulated accumulation of cyclic AMP in the absence of caffein in turkey erythrocytes (2), although PGE_1 acts synergistically with adrenalin on the Ca^{2+} efflux. It should also be noted that endogenous prostaglandin synthesis is neglible in these cells.

Another example is furnished by the toad bladder where PGE_1
was reported to inhibit the effect of antidiuretic hormone (ADH)
on the osmotic water flux, without affecting cyclic AMP accumulation (54, 55). It seems that in this tissue the prostaglandins
are not implicated in a negative feedback system, since indomethacin, an inhibitor of prostaglandin synthesis, did not affect the
basal water flux, its stimulation by ADH, or the accumulation of
cyclic AMP resulting from ADH treatment (56).

Stimulation of Cyclic AMP Formation

Exogeneous prostaglandins particularly PGE_1 and PGE_2 have been
shown to stimulate cyclic AMP accumulation in many different tissues,
this phenomenon was first described by Butcher and Baird (36). It
would be fastidious to make a complete list, but it is more rewarding
to discuss examples where other parameters have been studied :
specially endogeneous prostaglandin biosynthesis during hormonal
stimulation of adenylate cyclase.

As a starting point for this discussion, let us consider
relative potencies of different prostaglandins when activating adenylate cyclase systems. When we determine the accumulation of cyclic
AMP or its formation from ^{14}C-adenine in intact cells, it is evident
that PGE_1 and PGE_2 are the most active on numerous types of tissues
(57). Dose-related responses are obtained with blood platelets (58)
mouse and rat ovary (59, 60), dog thyroid slices (61, 62), bovine
thyroid cells (62), fibroblasts (63), rat uterus (64, 65) and thymocytes (66).

However, results assaying adenylate cyclase activity ($\alpha^{32}P$-
ATP) in homogenates have shown that different prostaglandins (E, A,
Fα) often stimulate the enzyme activity equally in different
tissues and this effect has not increased with dose (61, 67, 68).
At the same time other authors have found a proportional stimulation by PGE_1 or E_2 of adenylate cyclase in thyroid homogenates
(69), in the 1000 g pellet of mammary gland homogenates (70) and
in corpus luteum homogenates (71).

Why differencies in response observed varied with the nature
of the material utilized (intact or non intact cells) has not been
explained in a satisfactory manner as yet.

During the last two years, the action of prostaglandin E on
adenylate cyclase has also been studied in the purified membrane
fractions, and even in this system differencies can be shown from
results obtained with intact tissue. The addition of GTP or
other nucleotide triphosphates to the incubation media as indicated

by Rodbell et al. (72) can be shown to have significant effects in membrane systems. Such addition for example was found necessary for hepatic membranes as reported by Sweat and Wincek (73), bovine thyroid membranes by Kowalski et al. (74), and for human thyroid membranes by Sato et al. (75). According to Wolff and Cook (76) however the addition of GTP was not necessary but amplified the response of bovine thyroid membranes to PGE_1. Finally Mashiter et al. (69) obtained a dose related response to PGE_1 using dose concentrations between 10^{-8} and 10^{-4}M with the same material, and without addition of nucleotide triphosphate. An explanation of the role of GTP was proposed by Kowalski et al. (74). These investigators obtained a response to PGE_2 when α ^{32}P-ATP was replaced by α ^{32}P-AMP-P-NP. Since the latter was not a substrate for ATPase, they considered that GTP could protect α ^{32}P-ATP from hydrolysis, maintaining concentrations for adenylate cyclase. This explanation is not absolutely convincing because addition of GTP is not indispensable to obtain stimulation by TSH with α ^{32}P-ATP. On the other hand, with human platelet membranes and AMP-PNP as the substrate, GTP appears to be essential for PGE_1 stimulation of adenylate cyclase (77).

Studies with membrane preparations have yielded further information concerning the mode of prostaglandin action. Receptors with high affinity for prostaglandin E were characterized in membrane preparations of liver (78), stomach (79), thyroid (80) luteal cells (81), and isolated rat thymocytes (82). These receptors showed binding characteristics similar to those described for adipocyte membrane fractions (40, 41). The exclusive localization of these receptors in preparations containing adenylate cyclase activity of the cell, argue in favour of prostaglandin E action on synthesis of cyclic AMP. These receptors show an affinity of the same magnitude for PGE_1 and PGE_2. The unique character of this type of receptor was confirmed by the absence of additivity of maximal doses of PGE_1 and PGE_2 on the synthesis of ^{14}C-cyclic AMP from ^{14}C-adenine by mouse ovary (59).

BIOLOGICAL SIGNIFICANCE OF CYCLIC AMP FORMATION INDUCED BY
PROSTAGLANDINS IN TARGET ORGANS OF HORMONES

It is now appropriate to examine the biological significance of prostaglandin induced stimulation of adenylate cyclase. Firstly many studies have been made comparing the action of prostaglandins with hormones normally found to stimulate the tissue in question. The results obtained by many groups in different or similar organs have frequently been contradictory.

Interaction between Prostaglandins and Hormones

LH has an additive effect with a maximal dose of PGE_2 on the adenylate cyclase of bovine corpus luteum(71). The action of the same agonists at maximal doses is only partially additive on rat ovary (60). The action of PGE_1 in the presence or absence of GTP is not additive with that of glucagon on adenylate cyclase of rat liver membranes (73). The lack of additivity of supramaximal doses of adrenaline and PGE_1 has also been described for the accumulation of ^{14}C-cyclic AMP by the rat myometrium (65) and on the stimulation of adenylate cyclase of a 600 g pellet of mammary gland homogenate (70). Finally, in the thyroid the additivity of submaximal doses of TSH and PGE_1 (or PGE_2) was studied by Burke with ovine cell-free adenylate cyclase (68), Sato et al. on cyclic AMP accumulation in dog slices (62) and on ^{14}C-cyclic AMP synthesis by isolated bovine cells (62). However, they observed no effect, or even an antagonistic action of a submaximal dose of one of the effectors in presence of maximal dose of the other one. This last phenomenon has not been confirmed by Mashiter et al. (69), when additive effects of PGE_1 and TSH were reported for the accumulation of cyclic AMP in dog thyroid slices.

The discrepancies which we face in the results of these experiments prevent one from drawing conclusions as to the possible existence of one or two distinct adenylate cyclase activities.

Effect of Prostaglandins Inhibitors on the Hormonal Stimulation

Another experimental approach which has not yielded any more conclusive results has been to use prostaglandin antagonists.

PPP was not found to inhibit PGE_1 stimulated adenylate cyclase of the ovary (83). However, this compound was reported to inhibit PGE_2 or TSH stimulation of adenylate cyclase in isolated thyroid cells (84). 7-oxa, 13-prostynoïc acid, which appears to be a true antagonist of prostaglandins, pharmacodynamically, yields equally contradictory results. According to Kuehl et al. (59), this acid competitively inhibited PGE_1 and LH stimulated accumulation of ^{14}C-cyclic-AMP, but Lamprecht et al. did not confirm this finding with the rat ovary, where 7-oxa, 13-prostynoïc acid failed to inhibit the action of PGE_2 and LH (60). Sato et al. (62) using isolated bovine thyroid cells or dog thyroid slices, like Kuehl et al. (69) observed competitive inhibition of cyclic AMP accumulation stimulated by TSH or PGE_2. Similar results were obtained with bovine thyroid homogenates by Kowalski et al. (74). Using the thyroid membrane system of Kowalski et al. (74), where adenylate cyclase did not respond to PGE_2 in the absence of GTP, 7-oxa, 13-prostynoïc acid inhibited only when PGE_2 was active. It did not affect TSH stimulation which occurred in the absence of GTP.

The result of Vesin and Harbon (65) that neither polyphloretin phosphate, nor 7-oxa, 13-prostynoïc acid inhibited PGE$_1$ induced stimulation of adenylate cyclase of the myometrium, whereas these substances were shown to totally inhibit contraction induced by prostaglandins, further adds to the confusion.

These contradictory results are very important because they throw doubt upon the hypothesis suggested by Kuehl et al. (59) and Burke et al. (62) in which prostaglandin E would be an obligatory intermediate in the normal stimulation of adenylate cyclase (Figure 6). This hypothesis implies that hormonal stimulation of adenylate cyclase is accompanied by new synthesis of prostaglandins E.

Hormonal Stimulation of Endogenous Prostaglandin Biosynthesis

Relationship with Cyclic AMP Synthesis

This last step has been demonstrated in the thyroid following stimulation by TSH (85, 86, 87) and in the ovary with stimulation by LH (57) or human chorionic gonadotrophin (88). The prostaglandin concentration was determined by radioimmunoassay. The elevation in concentration which we have observed resulted from new synthesis because it was inhibited by indomethacin.

Finally, the hypothesis of Vogt et al. (9), in which the control of a phospholipase A activity would be a regulating factor of prostaglandin biosynthesis, was demonstrated for the first time in porcine thyroid homogenates by Haye et al. (87). This TSH responsive system was found to be capable of synthesizing mainly PGE$_2$ and PGF$_2\alpha$ from ^{14}C-phosphatidylinositol emulsified in the incubation medium. This biosynthesis was inhibited by the addition of indomethacin. Moreover in the presence the latter, we observed, preferential accumulation in the medium of ^{14}C-arachidonate under the action of TSH. This effect of TSH on phospholipase A activity was not mediated by cyclic AMP (88).

More decisive experiments to find the role of new synthesis of endogenous prostaglandins, occurring with hormonal stimulation of adenylate cyclase, necessitated the use of prostaglandin synthetase inhibitors.

Kuehl et al. (59) were the first to perform this experiment and observed that fluoroindomethacin, inhibiting arachidonate stimulated ^{14}C-cyclic AMP accumulation, had no effect on LH stimulation of this in mouse ovary and bovine luteal cells. They concluded that the action of LH was to provoke depletion of prostaglandin stores.

LH ⟶ PGE ⟶ C_AMP   (KUEHL)

TSH ⟶ PGE ⟶ C_AMP   (BURKE)

FIGURE 6.   Hypothesis of the obligatory participation of PGE in adenylate cyclase activation.

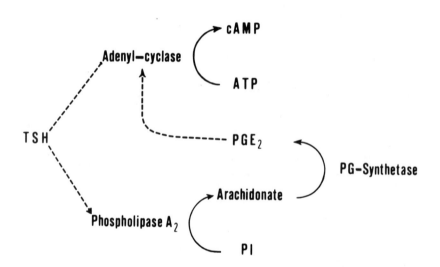

FIGURE 7.   A scheme showing the participation of a phospholipase A₂ activity in the synthesis of prostaglandins and the adenylate cyclase stimulation by TSH in the thyroid.   This illustration is reproduced from reference (87).

Similar results obtained by Lamprecht et al. (60) were not interpreted in this way and were considered to be "presumptive evidence against the idea that PGE$_2$ is an obligatory mediator of LH action on the ovary".

The action of indomethacin has been tested on cyclic AMP accumulation stimulated by TSH in pig (87) and of dog thyroid slices (69) and on adenylate cyclase stimulation by TSH with bovine thyroid membranes (90). In none of these cases could the biosynthesis of endogenous prostaglandins be considered to constitute a compulsory requirement for adenylate cyclase stimulation.

A diagram summarizing the concept of Haye et al. (87) for the relations between prostaglandin biosynthesis and cyclic AMP in the thyroid is shown in Figure 7.

Additional results of Kuehl (57) on the mouse ovary and of Burke et al. (91, 92) on the mouse thyroid have complicated the situation and shown that this diagram does not account for all the experimental facts. Dibutyryl cyclic AMP stimulated the biosynthesis of prostaglandins in vitro during long incubation intervals : this effect being impaired by prostaglandin synthetase inhibitors. This process would then appear to be similar to the one shown for adipose tissue except that it is a positive feedback system. The physiological significance of this device has been discussed by Butcher (93).

Kuehl (94) has combined his findings with those of Behrman and Armstrong (95) showing that LH stimulated activity of cholesterol esterase in the rat ovary provoked a depletion of cholesterol esters rich in arachidonate (96). A scheme was then proposed, in which the elevation of cyclic AMP content under the action of LH would stimulate protein kinases phosphorylating steroidogenesis enzymes and cholesterol esterase (Figure 8). The action of the latter enzyme would provide on the one hand cholesterol which would act as a substrate for steroidogenesis and on the other arachidonate which would be converted to PGE$_2$ prolonging the stimulation of adenylate cyclase.

Haye et al. (89) have shown that TSH, via the cyclic AMP accumulation it provoked in the thyroid, stimulated subsequent hydrolysis of triglycerides. This hydrolysis released amongst other fatty acids arachidonate, the precursor to PGE$_2$. These results have allowed us to complete the scheme described before (Figure 9). Participation of the cyclic AMP dependent protein kinase is postulated but has not yet been demonstrated.

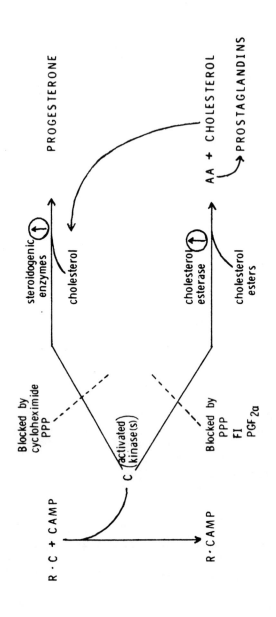

FIGURE 8.   *A scheme representing actions in the LH responsive cell, subsequent to cyclic AMP. This illustration is reproduced from reference (94).*

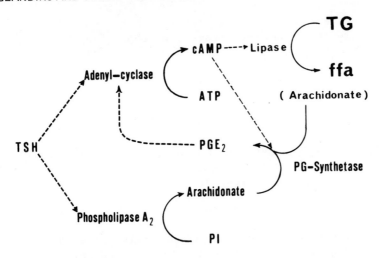

FIGURE 9. A scheme reproducing Figure 7 augmented to take into account the prostaglandin pool subsequent to cyclic AMP. This illustration is reproduced from reference (89).

Thus at present we can identify two pools of prostaglandins in the thyroid : one, which appears to be independent of cyclic AMP is formed by arachidonate released from phosphatidylinositol following stimulation of a phospholipase A (para cyclic AMP pool of PG). The other, subsequent to stimulation of cyclic AMP accumulation, results from the activation of triglyceride lipolysis by this cyclic nucleotide (post cyclic AMP pool of PG).

Moreover preliminary results (89) seem to show that cyclic AMP activates prostaglandin synthetase and increases conversion of arachidonate to prostaglandins.

PROSTAGLANDINS AS CONNECTING FACTORS BETWEEN CYCLIC AMP AND
CYCLIC GMP SYSTEMS : A TENTATIVE EXPLANATION

The above schemes do not assign prostaglandins Fα any role even though both prostaglandin E and Fα synthesis is stimulated by LH in the ovary (57) and by TSH in the thyroid (85, 86, 87). An extremely ingenious hypothesis was proposed by Kuehl (94) for the possible function of PGFα. The PGFα was thought to be associated with concentration changes in cyclic-GMP whereas PGE would be associated with those of cyclic AMP (Figure 10).

Evidence in favour of this conception is as follows.

Firstly, antagonism between cyclic-AMP and GMP appears to be valid and can be supported by Goldberg et al. (97) in their hypothesis illustrated by the oriental concept of opposite forces : Yin Yang. There are now several examples of systems in which cyclic GMP plays the role of second messenger to a first messenger such as acetylcholine, oxytocin, serotonin and calcitonin (97).

The nature of interaction between this new second messenger and cyclic AMP is an important problem to examine.

Is the production of the two nucleotides independent? Do cyclic AMP and cyclic GMP interact only on their intracellular targets ? This concept was supported by the results of Goldberg et al., where cyclic GMP in low doses partially antagonized the stimulation of a muscle protein kinase by cyclic AMP (97) and results of Kram and Tomkins on the reversion of cyclic GMP of "pleiotypic effects" of cyclic AMP on fibroblast culture from the mouse (98).

One should also ask whether the stimulation of synthesis of one cyclic nucleotide necessarily leads to a decrease in concentration of the other cyclic nucleotide ?

The answer appears to vary with the nature of the tissue studied. Among different cases described, rat lung might be considered a typical example (99). Acetylcholine stimulated accumulation of cyclic GMP but not cyclic AMP. This effect was inhibited by atropine. Isoproterenol stimulated accumulation of cyclic AMP but not cyclic GMP. This effect was inhibited by propranolol. The simultaneous action of acetylcholine and isoproterenol appeared to depend on their respective concentrations since the regulation was reciprocal. A relative increase in acetylcholine concentration augmented cyclic GMP accumulation and reduced that of cyclic AMP. The situation was reversed when the relative concentration of isoproterenol was increased.

However, the same result does not appear to be true for the guinea pig lung where acetylcholine alone or bradykinin alone provoked not only the accumulation of cyclic GMP but also cyclic AMP (100).

What could be the mechanism when antagonistic action between
respective concentrations of cyclic AMP and cyclic GMP was induced
via muscarinic or β-adrenergic stimulation ? Arguments have been
proposed following a study of the stability of liver lysozomes
(101). Adrenergic agents and cyclic AMP inhibited, whereas cholinergic agents and cyclic GMP stimulated the release of enzymes
from rat liver lysozomes in vitro. Acetylcholine, however, which
did not act on adenylate cyclase, stimulated phosphodiesterase
and this effect was reproduced by exogenous cyclic GMP. On the
other hand, acetylcholine induced cyclic GMP accumulation in the
liver (102). The stimulation by cyclic GMP of liver phosphodies
terase hydrolysing cyclic AMP has been previously reported (103).

Perhaps this is not the only explanation of a reciprocal
relationship between cyclic GMP and cyclic AMP systems. To date
only two papers suggest that prostaglandins might be implicated.

The first one by Stoner et al. (100) has been mentioned
earlier and concerns the effects of acetylcholine and bradykinin
of cyclic GMP and cyclic AMP content of guinea pig lung slices.
In this system indomethacin was found to be without effect on
cyclic GMP accumulation, but inhibited the accumulation of cyclic
AMP.

The second, by Champion et al. (104) concerns the antagonistic
effects of acetylcholine and TSH stimulation on cyclic AMP accu-
multion in pig thyroid slices. Yamashita and Field have shown
that TSH and PGE_1 have no effect on thyroid cyclic GMP content,
while on the other hand acetylcholine, without affecting cyclic AMP
content, stimulated the accumulation of cyclic GMP (105). The
cyclic AMP accumulation stimulated by TSH was decreased by acetylcholine (Figure 11). This increase could not be detected in the
presence of indomethacin. Prostaglandins therefore appeared to be
involved in this phenomenon. It does not seem realistic that they
would be PGE for this stimulates adenylate cyclase. They could
however be PGFα. This hypothesis was supported by the detection
of PGFα in great amounts in tissues where the release of prostaglandins have been induced by acetylcholine (5) or by nervous stimulation (6). In pig thyroid slices, $PGF_2\alpha$, without any action on
basal cyclic AMP content was found to decrease the stimulation by
TSH (Figure 12) (104). The existence of specific receptors for
PGFα, distinct from PGE receptors, in ovine corpus luteum (106) and
the 400 % stimulation by $PGF_2\alpha$ of the cyclic GMP content of the
rat uterus (107), supported the results that we have reported.

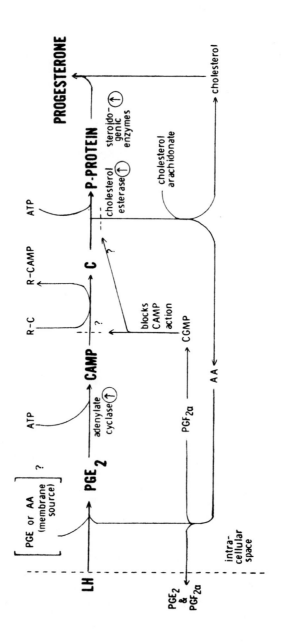

FIGURE 10.   *A hypothetical model representing the intracellular synthesis and disposition of prostaglandins in the LH-responsive cell. This illustration is reproduced from reference (94).*

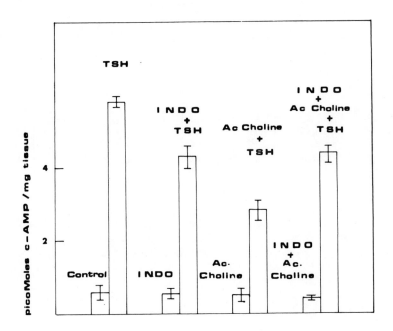

FIGURE 11.   Inhibition by indomethacin of the action of acetylcholine on the accumulation of cyclic AMP stimulated by TSH (20 mU/ml),
in pig thyroid slices.

Ac. choline = acetylcholine 5.5 x 10^{-5}M + eserine 3 x 10^{-4}M.

Indo.   = Indomethacin 10 μg/ml (during 30 minutes preincubation
              and 15 minutes incubation).

This illustration is reproduced from reference (104).

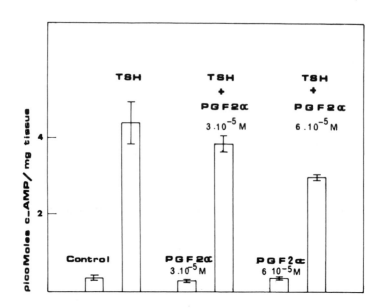

FIGURE 12. *Action of PGF$_2\alpha$ on the accumulation of cyclic AMP stimulated by TSH in pig thyroid slices (same general conditions as in Figure 11). This illustration is reproduced from reference (104).*

CONCLUSIONS

Many points remain speculative. The role of ions, particularly Ca^{2+}, has not been clearly established although they appear to have numerous effects.

According to Ramwell and Shaw hormonal stimulation produced a mobilization of membrane Ca^{2+}, increasing a phospholipase activity, which resulted in the formation of prostaglandins and an influx of Na^+ (108). The replacement of Ca^{2+} by Na^+ can remove the inhibition of adenylate cyclase in different tissues (109). Moreover, acetylcholine appeared to provoke an intracellular increase in Ca^{2+} (110, 111). In addition it has been shown that the presence of Ca^{2+} is necessary for accumulation of cyclic GMP under the action of acetylcholine (112).

The mechanism which permits control of the balance between PGE and PGFα biosynthesis is unknown. Its elucidation would be of great interest to enable one to gain a picture of the comprehensive role of prostaglandins in the regulation of intracellular cyclic nucleotide concentrations.

We know little about the mode of action of PGFα, but we can postulate that the relationship with guanylate cyclase may be symetrical with the one between PGE and adenylate cyclase.

We think that endogenous prostaglandins are components of a regulatory system in which their role is to adjust reciprocally the respective concentrations of cyclic AMP and cyclic GMP. This system of regulation does not constitute an obligatory building block in the cellular machinery and its participation can be of varying importance.

REFERENCES

(1)   SAMUELSSON, B. (1973) Prostaglandines, INSERM, Paris, 21

(2)   SHAW, J., GIBSON, W., JESSUP, S. and RAMWELL, P. (1971) Ann. N.Y. Acad. Sci., 180, 241

(3)   ELIASSON, R. (1959) Acta Physiol. Scand., 46, suppl. 158, 1

(4)   PACE-ASCIAK, C. and WOLFE, L.S. (1968) Biochim. Biophys. Acta, 152, 784

(5)   RAMWELL, P.W., SHAW, J.E. DOUGLAS, W.W. and POISNER, A.M. (1966) Nature (London) 210, 273

(6)   COCEANI, F., PACE-ASCIAK, C., VOLTA, F. and WOLFE, L.S. (1967) Amer. J. Physiol. 213, 1056

(7)   VOGT, W. and DISTELKÖTTER, B. (1967) Prostaglandins Proc.II Nobel Symp. S. Bergström and B. Samuelsson Eds., Almqvist and Wiksell, Stockholm, 237

(8)   SHAW, J.E. and RAMWELL, P.W. (1968) J. Biol. Chem., 243, 1498

(9)   VOGT, W.T., SUZUKI and BABILLI, S. (1966) Mem. Soc. Endocrinol. 14, 137

(10) KUNZE, H. and BOHN, R. (1969) Arch. Parmak. Exp. Path., 264, 263

(11) FERREIRA, S.H. and VANE, J.R. (1967) Nature, 216, 868

(12)   DAVIS, B.N., MORTON, E.W. and WITHRINGTON, P.G. (1968) Brit.
       J. Pharmacol. 32, 127

(13)   WILLIAMS, E.D., KARIM, S.M.M. and SANDLER, M. (1968) Lancet,
       1, 22

(14)   PIPER, P. and VANE, J. (1971) Ann. N.Y. Acad. Sci. 180, 363

(15)   FINDLAY, J.K., CERINI, M.E.D., CERINI, J.C., CHAMLEY, W.A.,
       HOOLEY, R.D., WILLIAMS, D.W., CUMMING, I.A., LEE, C.S. and
       O'SHEA, J.D. (1973) Prostaglandines, INSERM, Paris 235

(16)   SAMUELSSON, B. (1963) J. Biol. Chem. 238, 3229

(17)   JAFFE, B.M., BEHRMAN, H.R. and PARKER, C.W. (1973) J. Clin
       Invest. 52, 398

(18)   ANDERSON, N.H. (1969) J. Lipid. Res. 10, 320

(19)   GREEN, K. and SAMUELSSON, B (1964) J. Lipid. Res. 5, 117

(20)   RAMWELL, P.W. and DANIELS, E.G. (1969) Lipid Chromatographic
       Analysis, vol. 2, 313, G.V. Marinetti, Ed.; Marcel Dekker
       New York

(21)   FRIED, J., LIN, C., MEHRA, M., KAO, W. and DALVEN, P. (1971)
       Ann. N.Y. Acad. Sci., 180, 38

(22)   SANNER, J. (1971) Ann. N.Y. Acad. Sci., 180, 396

(23)   EAKINS, K. (1971) Ann. N.Y. Acad. Sci., 180, 386

(24)   NUGTEREN, D.H. (1970) Biochim. Biophys. Acta, 210, 171

(25)   DOWNING, D.T., AHERN, D.G. and BACHTA, M. (1970) Biochem.
       Biophys. Res. Comm., 40, 218

(26)   VANE, J.R. (1971) Nature New Biol., 231, 232

(27)   SMITH, W.L. and LANDS, W. (1971) J. Biol. Chem., 246, 6700

(28)   HORODNIAK, J.W., JULIUS, M., ZAREMBO, J.E. and BENDER, A.D.
       (1974) Biochim. Biophys. Res. Comm., 57, 539

(29)   STEINBERG, D., VAUGHAN, M., NESTEL, P. and BERGSTRÖM, S.
       (1963) Biochem. Pharmacol. 12, 764

(30)   STEINBERG, D., VAUGHAN, M., NESTEL, P., STRAND, O. and
       BERGSTRÖM, S. (1964) J. Clin. Invest. 43, 1533

(31) FAIN, J.N. (1968) Prostaglandin Symposium of the Worcester
      Foundation for Experimental Biology, 67, P.W. Ramwell and
      J.E. Shaw, Ed. Interscience Pub. New York

(32) HUMES, J.L., MANDEL, L.R. and KUEHL, Jr., J.A. (1968)
      Prostaglandin Symposium of the Worcester Foundation for
      Experimental Biology, 79, P.W. Ramwell and J.E. Shaw, Ed.
      Interscience Pub. New York

(33) LANDSLOW, D.R. (1971) Biochim. Biophys. Acta., 239, 33

(34) MOSKOWITZ, J. and FAIN, J.N. (1969) J. Clin. Invest. 48,
      1802

(35) SHAW, J.E. JESSUP, S.J. and RAMWELL, P.W. (1972) Adv. in
      Cyclic Nucleotides Res., Vol. 1

(36) BUTCHER, R.W. and BAIRD, C.E. (1968) J. Biol. Chem. 243,
      1713

(37) BUTCHER, R.W. and BAIRD, C.E. (1970) Proceedings of the
      Fourth International Congress on Pharmacol. R. Eigenmann
      Ed., volume 4, 42, Lippincott Philadelphia

(38) HITTELMAN, K.J. and BUTCHER, R.W. (1973) Biochim. Biophys.
      Acta, 316, 403

(39) VAUGHAN, M. and MURAD, F. (1969) Biochemistry, 8, 3092

(40) HUEHL, F.A., Jr., and HUMES, J.L. (1972) Proc. Natl. Acad.
      Sci., 69, 480

(41) GORMAN, R.R. and MILLER, O.V. (1973) Biochim. Biophys. Acta,
      323, 560

(42) CHRIST, E.J. and NUGTEREN, D.H. (1970 Biochim. Biophys. Acta
      218, 296

(43) BERGSTÖRM, S., CARLSON, L.A. and ORÖ, L. (1967) Life Sci.,
      6, 449

(44) JOUVENAZ, G.H., NUGTEREN, D.H., BERTHUIS, R.K. and VanDORP,
      D.A. (1970) Biochim. Biophys. Acta., 202, 231

(45) DALTON, C. and HOPE, W.C. (1974) Prostaglandins, 6, 227

(46) BERGSTRÖM, S. (1967) Science, 157, 382

(47) ILLIANO, G. and CUATRECASAS, P. (1971) Nature New Biol.,
      234, 72

(48) FAIN, J.N., PSYCHOYOS, S., CZERNIK, A.J. FROST, S. and
      CASH, W.D. (1973) Endocrinology, 93, 632

(49) RADZIALOWSKI, F.M. and NOVAK, L. (1971) Life Sci. (Part 1)
      10, 1261

(50) HO, R.J. and SUTHERLAND, E.W. (1971) J. Biol. Chem. 246,
      6822

(51) CHIAPPE de CINGOLANI, G.E., Van der BOSCH, H. and Van DEENEN,
      L.L.M. (1972) Biochim. Biophys. Acta, 260, 387

(52) MANGANIELLO, V. and VAUGHAN, M. (1973) J. Biol. Chem. 248,
      7164

(53) WESTERNMANN, E. and STOCK, K. (1970) Horm. Metab. Res. suppl.
      2, 47

(54) ORLOFF, J., HANDLER, J.S. and BERGSTRÖM, S. (1965) Nature,
      205, 397

(55) LIPSON, L., HYNIE, S. and SHARP, G. (1971) Ann. N.Y. Acad.
      Sci. 180, 261

(56) WONG, P.Y.D., BEDWANI, J.R. and CUTHBERT, A.W. (1972) Nature
      New Biol. 238, 27

(57) KUEHL, Jr. F.A., CIRILLO, V.J., HAM, E.A. and HUMES, J.L.,
      (1972) Advances in the biosciences, 9, 155

(58) MOSKOWITZ, J., HARWOOD, J.P., REID, W.D. and KRISHNA, G.
      (1971) Biochim. Biophys. Acta 230, 279

(59) KUEHL, F.A., Jr., HUMES, J.L., TARNOFF, J., CIRILLO, V.J.
      and HAM, E.A. (1970) Science, 169, 883

(60) LAMPRECHT, S.A., ZOR, U., TSAFRIRI, A. and LINDNER, H.R.
      (1973) J. Endocr., 57, 217

(61) FIELD, J., DEKKER, A., ZOR, U. and KANEKO, T. (1971) Ann.
      N.Y. Acad. Sci., 180, 278

(62) SATO, S., SZABO, M., KOWALSKI, K. and BURKE, G. (1972)
      Endocrinology, 90, 343

(63) MANGANIELLO, V. and VAUGHAN, M. (1972) Proc. Nat. Acad. Sci.
      U.S.A., 69, 269

(64) BHALLA, R.C., SANBORN, B.M. and KORENMAN, S.G. (1972) Proc. Nat. Acad. Sci. U.S.A., 69, 3761

(65) VESIN, M.F. and HARBON, S. (1974) Molecular Pharmacology, 10 457

(66) FRANKS, D.J., MacMANUS, J.P. and WHITFIELD, J.F. (1971) Biochim. Biophys. Res. Comm., 44, 1177

(67) MacLEOD, R.M. and LEHMEYER, J.E. (1970) Proc. Nat. Acad. Sci. U.S.A., 67, 1172

(68) BURKE, G. (1970) Amer. J. Physiol. 218, 1445

(69) MASHITER, K. MASHITER, G.D. and FIELD, J.B. (1974) Endocrinology 94, 370

(70) BÄR, H.P. (1973) Biochim. Biophys. Acta, 321, 397

(71) MARSH, J. (1971) Ann. N.Y. Acad. Sci., 180, 416

(72) RODBELL, M., BIRNBAUMER, L., POHL, S.L. and KRANS, H.M., (1971) J. Biol. Chem. 246, 1877

(73) SWEAT, F.W. and WINCEK, T.J. (1973) Biochem. Biophys. Res. Comm., 55, 522

(74) KOWALSKI, K., SATO, S. and BURKE, G. (1972) Prostaglandins 2, 441

(75) SATO, S., YAMADA, T., FURTHATA, R. and MAKIUCHI, M. (1974) Biochim. Biophys. Acta, 332, 166

(76) WOLFF, J. and COOK, G.H. (1973) J. Biol. Chem. 248, 350

(77) KRISHNA, G., HARWOOD, J.P., BARBER, A.J. and JAMIESON, G.A. (1972) J. Biol. Chem., 247, 2253

(78) SMIGEL, M. and FLEISCHER, S. (1973) Fed. Proc. 32, 454

(79) MILLER, O.V. and MAGEE, W.E. (1973) Advances in Biosciences, 9, 83

(80) MOORE, M.V. and WOLFF, J. (1973) J. Biol. Chem., 248, 5705

(81) RAO, C.V. (1974) Prostaglandins, 6, 533

(82) SCHAUMBURG, B.P. (1973) Biochim. Biophys. Acta., 326, 127

(83) KUEHL, F.A., Jr., HUMES, J.L., MANDEL, L.R., CIRILLO, V.J.,
      ZANETTI, M.E. and HAM, E.A. (1971) Biochim. Biophys. Res.
      Comm., 44, 1464

(84) SATO, S., KOWALSKI, K. and BURKE, G. (1972) Prostaglandin,
      1, 345

(85) YU, S.C., CHANG, L. and BURKE, G. (1972) J. Clin. Invest.,
      51, 1038

(86) BURKE, G. (1972) Prostaglandins, 2, 413

(87) HAYE, B., CHAMPION, S. and JACQUEMIN, C. (1973) FEBS
      Letters, 30 (3) 253

(88) LEMAIRE, W.J., YANG, N.S.T., BEHRMAN, H.R. and MARSCH, J.M.
      (1973) Prostaglandins, 3, 367

(89) HAYE, B., CHAMPION, S. and JACQUEMIN, C. (1974) FEBS
      Letters, 41, 89

(90) WOLFF, J. and MOORE, W.V. (1973) Biochem. Biophys. Res.
      Comm., 51, 34.

(91) BURKE, G. (1973) Prostaglandins, 3, 291

(92) BURKE, G., CHANG, L. and SZABO, M. (1973) Science, 180, 872

(93) BUTCHER, R.W. (1970) Advances in Biochemical and Psycho-
      pharmacology 3, 173. Greengard and Costa, Ed., Raven Press
      New York

(94) KUEHL, F.A. Jr. (1974) Prostaglandins, 5, 325

(95) BEHRMAN, H.R. and ARMSTRONG, D.T. (1969) Endocrinology, 85
      474

(96) MORIN, R.J. (1971) Lipids, 6, 815

(97) GOLDBERG, N.D., HADDOX, M.K., HARTLE, D.K. and HADDEN, J.W.
      (1973) Pharmacology and the future of the man Proc. 5th Int.
      Cgonr. Pharmacology San Francisco, 5, 146

(98) KRAM, R. and TOMKINS, G.M. (1973) Proc. Natl. Acad. Sci.
      U.S.A., 70, 1659

(99) KUD, J.F. and KUO, W.N. (1973) Biochem. Biophys. Res. Comm.,
      55, 660

(100) STONER, J., MANGANIELLO, V.C. and VAUGHAN, M. (1973) Proc.
      Natl. Acad. Sci. U.S.A., 70, 3830

(101)   IGNARRO, L.J., KRASSIKOFF, N. and SLYWKA, J. (1973) J.
        Pharmacol. Exp. Ther., 186, 86

(102)   ILLIANO, G., TELL, G.P.E., SIEGEL, M.I. and CUATRECASAS,
        P. (1973) Proc. Natl. Acad. Sci. U.S.A., 70, 2443

(103)   BEAVO, J.A., HARDMAN, J.G. and SUTHERLAND, E.W. (1971) J.
        Biol. Chem., 246, 3841

(104)   CHAMPION, S., HAYE, B., and JACQUEMIN, C. (1974) FEBS
        Letters, 46, 289

(105)   YAMASHITA, K. and FIELD, J.B. (1972) J. Biol. Chem., 247,
        7062

(106)   POWELL, W.S., HAMMARSTRÖM, S. and SAMUELSSON, B. (1974)
        Eur. J. Biochem., 41, 103

(107)   KUEHL, F.A., HAM, E.A., ZANETTI, M.E., SANFORD, C.H., NICOL,
        F.E. and GOLDBERG, N.D. (1974) Proc. Natl. Acad. Sci.
        U.S.A., 71, 1866

(108)   RAMWELL, P.W. and SHAW, J.E. (1970) Rec. Progr. Horm. Res.,
        26, 139

(109)   BÄR, H.P. and HECHTER, O. (1969) Biochem. Biophys. Res.
        Comm., 35, 681

(110)   SHANES, A.M. and BIANCHI, P. (1960) J. Gen. Physiol., 43,
        481

(111)   DURBIN, R.P. and JENKINSON, D.H. (1961) J. Physiol., 157,
        90

(112)   SCHULTZ, G., HARDMAN, J.G., SCHULTZ, K., BAIRD, C.E. and
        SUTHERLAND, E.W. (1973) Proc. Natl. Acad. Sci. U.S.A., 70
        3889

RE-EXAMINATION OF THE ROLE OF CYCLIC AMP IN THE ACTIONS OF GLUCAGON AND EPINEPHRINE

J. H. Exton and A. D. Cherrington

Department of Physiology
Vanderbilt University School of Medicine
Nashville, Tennessee   U. S. A.   37232

List of Contents

I.   INTRODUCTION

The classic investigations of Sutherland and coworkers into the actions of glucagon and epinephrine on hepatic glycogenolysis led to the discovery of cyclic AMP and largely formed the basis for the second messenger hypothesis of hormone action.   Figure 1 shows an early schematic representation of this hypothesis published by Sutherland and Robison in 1966.   It is interesting to note that in addition to the adenylate cyclase system, the figure depicts a generalized scheme with a plasma membrane receptor X and an

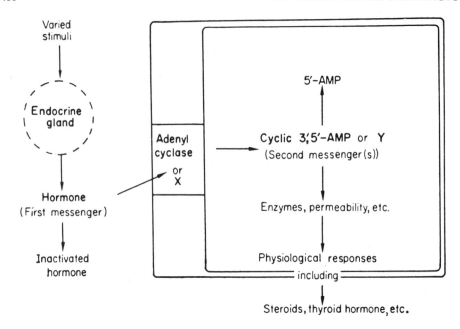

FIG. 1.   Schematic representation of the second messenger concept.   From Sutherland & Robison (6).

intracellular second messenger Y.   Thus, the authors recognized the possible existence of alternative mechanisms for hormones acting through cyclic AMP.

There is a multiplicity of data supporting the view that the hepatic actions of glucagon are entirely attributable to the intracellular accumulation of cyclic AMP (1).   The situation with epinephrine and other catecholamines, on the other hand, is less clear.   Although there is ample evidence that these agents can activate adenylate cyclase and raise cyclic AMP levels in liver (for reviews see References 2 and 3), recent observations by Sherline, Lynch and Glinsmann (4) and by Tolbert, Butcher and Fain (5) suggest that additional mechanism(s) may regulate hepatic metabolism.   This paper will present data obtained in recent experiments utilizing isolated perfused rat livers and isolated rat liver cells in which the role of cyclic AMP in the actions of glucagon and catecholamines on hepatic glycogen metabolism and gluconeogenesis was studied.   For more general reviews of glucagon and catecholamine action on liver, the reader is referred to References 1, 2, 3, 6, 7 and 8.

II. CYCLIC AMP AS THE MEDIATOR OF GLUCAGON ACTION IN LIVER

Table I lists the various hepatic effects of glucagon reported in the literature. Since pharmacological doses of the hormone were used in the majority of these studies, it is uncertain which of the actions (apart from those on glycogen metabolism and gluconeogenesis) occur under physiological conditions. In all instances tested the actions of glucagon could be mimicked by exogenous cyclic AMP, suggesting that most, if not all of the effects of this hormone are mediated by the nucleotide.

As illustrated in Figures 2 and 3, glucagon caused a very rapid rise in the levels of cyclic AMP in perfused livers and in isolated hepatocytes. An increase was detectable within 10 to 20 sec and a peak level was observed within 2 to 3 min. Thereafter the nucleotide concentration declined. In the experiments with perfused livers (Fig. 2) the subsequent fall in cAMP was less marked than in hepatocytes, since the glucagon dose was maintained by constant infusion.

TIME COURSE OF CYCLIC AMP RESPONSE TO GLUCAGON

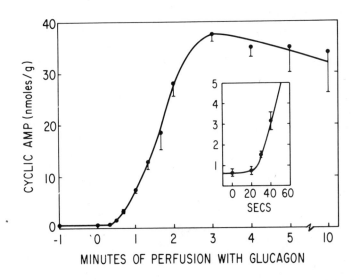

FIG. 2. Livers were perfused with a maximally effective concentration of glucagon (1.5 x 10^{-8} M) after a 20 min preliminary perfusion. Data are from Exton et al. (9).

TABLE I

Reported Effects of Glucagon on Liver

Process	Changes	Evidence for involvement of cyclic AMP
Glycogenolysis Phosphorylase	Increase	Yes
Glycogen synthesis Glycogen synthetase	Decrease	Yes
Gluconeogenesis	Increase	Yes
Ureogenesis	Increase	Yes
Ketogenesis	Increase	Yes
Lipogenesis Acetyl-CoA carboxylase	Decrease	Yes
Lipolysis	Increase	Yes
Cholesterol synthesis HMG-CoA reductase	Decrease	Yes
Protein catabolism	Increase	?
Lysosomal enzyme release	Increase	?
Overall protein synthesis	Decrease	Yes
Amino acid uptake	Increase	Yes
Krebs Cycle	Increase	?
Transamination	Increase	?
Triglyceride synthesis	Decrease	?

TABLE I (continued)

Process	Changes	Evidence for involve-ment of cyclic AMP
Lipoprotein release	Decrease	Yes
K$^+$ release	Increase	Yes
Ca^{++} release	Increase	Yes
Induction of phosphoenol-pyruvate carboxykinase	Increase	Yes
Induction of tyrosine transaminase	Increase	Yes
"Induction" of ornithine decarboxylase	Increase	Yes
"Induction" of glucose 6-Pase	Increase	Yes
"Induction" of serine dehy-dratase	Increase	Yes
"Induction" of glucokinase	Decrease	Yes
"Induction" of glucose-6-P dehydrogenase	Decrease	Yes
Phosphorylation of f 1 histone	Increase	Yes
Phosphorylation of ribo-somal protein	Increase	Yes
Synthesis of nuclear acidic proteins	Increase	?
RNA synthesis	Increase	Yes

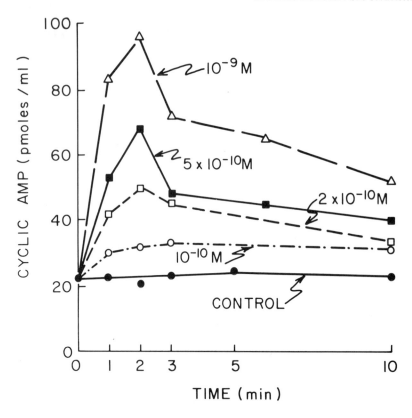

FIG. 3.   Isolated liver parenchymal cells prepared by a modification of the method of Berry and Friend (10) were incubated in
Krebs-Henseleit bicarbonate buffer containing 1.5% Difco gelatin
and the concentrations of glucagon shown. Cell suspensions were
fixed with $HClO_4$ at the times shown and cyclic AMP measured by
the method of Gilman (11) after purification using ion exchange
chromatography (Hardman and Sutherland, 12).   Values are means
of 3-6 determinations at each time point or glucagon concentration.

    The accumulation of cyclic AMP in the perfused liver and
isolated liver cells was related to the glucagon concentration in a
dose dependent manner (Figs. 3 and 4).   Infusion of glucagon into
the perfused liver at the rate of 1 pmole per min produced a hormone concentration of 1.5×10^{-10} M which significantly elevated
the cyclic AMP level (Fig. 4).   A similar dose was effective in
the isolated hepatocytes (Figs. 3 and 5).   Half maximal stimula-

tion of cyclic AMP accumulation was induced by 5×10^{-9} M glucagon in both systems and maximum accumulation was seen with 10^{-8} M hormone (Figs. 4 and 5).

Figure 6 shows the time courses of activation of glycogeno-lysis and lactate gluconeogenesis induced by glucagon in the perfused rat liver. It is seen that glycogenolysis (measured by glucose release) and gluconeogenesis (measured by the conver-sion of $[^{14}C]$ lactate to $[^{14}C]$ glucose) were activated almost con-currently. There was also an increase in lactate uptake which occurred pari passu with the activation of gluconeogenesis. The changes in carbohydrate metabolism were evident after 1 min, i. e. , about 40 sec after the rise in cyclic AMP and were maximal at about 4 min.

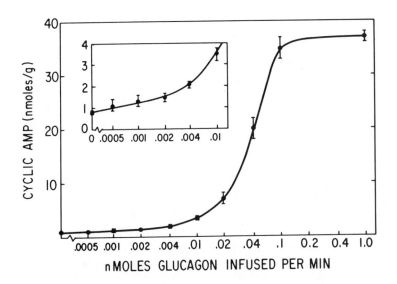

FIG. 4.   Dose response curve for the effect of glucagon on cyclic AMP levels in the perfused liver.   Levels were measured in tissue samples rapidly frozen 4 min after the start of glucagon infusion. Data are from Exton et al. (9).

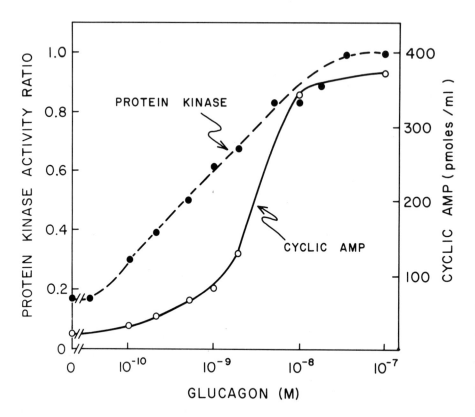

FIG. 5.   Dose response curves for the effects of glucagon on
cyclic AMP levels and protein kinase activity ratio in isolated
hepatocytes.   Cyclic AMP levels were measured at 3 min as
described in the legend to Fig. 3.   The protein kinase activity
ratio was determined at 5 min by the method of Corbin and
Reimann (13).   Values are from one representative experiment.
Similar findings have been obtained in at least four other experiments.

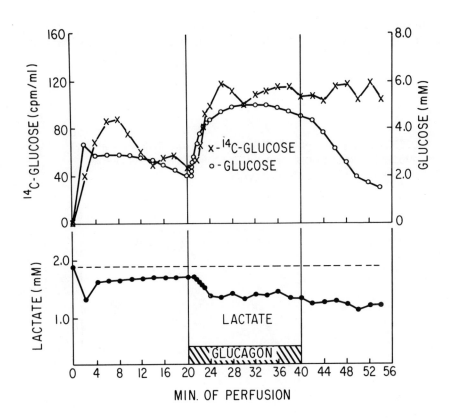

FIG. 6.   Time courses of glucagon activation of glycogenolysis and lactate gluconeogenesis in the perfused rat liver.   Glucagon was infused during the period shown to give a concentration of 10^{-8} M.   Data are from Exton and Park (14).

Figure 7 shows the dose response curves for the effects of glucagon on glycogenolysis and lactate gluconeogenesis in the perfused liver. Changes in cyclic AMP are also plotted for comparison. Activation of both glycogen mobilization and gluconeogenesis occurred with 2×10^{-10} M glucagon and was maximal at 10^{-9} M glucagon. The figures show that although only a 3- to 4-fold rise in cyclic AMP was necessary to fully activate glycogen breakdown and gluconeogenesis, glucagon was capable of increasing intracellular cyclic AMP 60- to 80-fold (Fig. 4). Very similar dose

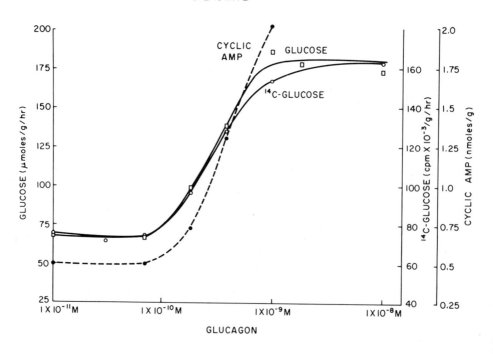

DOSE RESPONSE CURVES FOR GLUCAGON ON CYCLIC AMP, GLUCOSE PRODUCTION AND ^{14}C-GLUCOSE SYNTHESIS FROM ^{14}C-LACTATE

FIG. 7. Livers from fed rats were perfused for 1 hour with 10 mM [^{14}C] lactate and concentrations of glucagon shown. At the end of perfusion, livers were frozen and assayed for cyclic AMP (Exton et al. 9). Glucose release and [^{14}C] glucose synthesis were calculated as described by Exton and Park (15).

response curves for the actions of glucagon on glycogenolysis and gluconeogenesis were obtained in experiments with isolated hepatocytes (data not shown).

Glucagon concentrations in human portal blood are reported to be between 5×10^{-11} M and 4×10^{-10} M (16) while those in canine pancreaticoduodenal venous blood vary between 2×10^{-10} M and 2×10^{-9} M (17, 18). If similar levels occur in rat portal blood, it would seem that the perfused rat liver and isolated rat hepatocytes are capable of responding to physiological levels of glucagon.

The work of Krebs and associates (for review see Reference 19) has led to the hypothesis that the action of cyclic AMP on cellular processes in eukaryotes frequently, if not always, involves a cyclic AMP-dependent protein kinase which phosphorylates certain enzymes and other cellular proteins thereby altering their activity. This hypothesis is discussed in detail by Corbin in another section of this volume. Several workers have shown the existence of cyclic AMP-dependent protein kinases in rat liver (20-22). Evidence that activation of protein kinase is involved in the actions of glucagon on glycogenolysis and gluconeogenesis is presented in Figure 5. This shows the changes in the protein kinase activity ratio (which is the ratio of the kinase activity assayed in the absence of cyclic AMP to that assayed in the presence of saturating cyclic AMP) in hepatocytes incubated for 5 min with different concentrations of glucagon. With 10^{-10} M glucagon which produced a 50% increase in cyclic AMP there was a significant activation of protein kinase. Half-maximal activation occurred with glucagon concentrations ranging from 5×10^{-10} M to 10^{-9} M. Such levels of the hormone raised cyclic AMP 3- to 4-fold and maximally activated glycogenolysis and gluconeogenesis as in the perfused liver (Fig. 7). In another series of experiments using hepatocytes, the time course of protein kinase activation in response to various glucagon concentrations closely paralleled the changes in cyclic AMP (data not shown).

In summary, our findings strongly support the view that cyclic AMP is the mediator of glucagon action on glycogenolysis and gluconeogenesis in rat liver and that activation of a protein kinase is involved. No evidence of an alternative mechanism of glucagon action on the parameters measured was obtained. While all of glucagon's actions seem attributable to intracellular accumulation of cyclic AMP, modulation of the system by some as yet undefined factor remains possible.

III.   STUDIES ON THE ROLE OF CYCLIC AMP IN THE HEPATIC
       ACTIONS OF CATECHOLAMINES USING THE ISOLATED
       PERFUSED RAT LIVER

As stated in the Introduction, several workers have obtained
evidence that the cyclic AMP second messenger system might not
be the only means by which catecholamines act on the liver. Our
studies concerning hepatic effects of epinephrine and other adrenergic agents support this view. Figure 8 shows the changes in
cyclic AMP levels induced by maximally effective doses of glucagon and epinephrine in the perfused liver. Epinephrine was
strikingly less effective than glucagon in raising cyclic AMP
(Fig. 8). In response to the catecholamine, cyclic AMP rose
rapidly to a peak value 3-fold greater than basal at 30 sec.[1] and
thereafter declined to a value twice basal (Fig. 9).

Based on the facts that a maximally effective dose of epinephrine could not sustain a greater than 2-fold elevation in cyclic
AMP (Fig. 9) and that a 3- to 4-fold increase in the nucleotide
concentration was necessary to fully activate glycogenolysis and
gluconeogenesis (Fig. 7) one would predict that this agent would
be less effective than glucagon in stimulating these parameters.
Furthermore, since the two hormones produced the same time
course of cyclic AMP accumulation during the first 30 sec. (Fig.
9), one would also predict that they would induce glycogenolysis
equally rapidly. However, as shown in Fig. 10, with maximally
effective doses of the two hormones, epinephrine, in fact, produced a more rapid activation of glycogenolysis than glucagon and
sustained a greater maximal rate of glucose production.

Fig 11 depicts data from experiments in which livers from
fed rats were perfused with maximally effective concentrations
of epinephrine, glucagon and exogenous cyclic AMP. Again,
epinephrine was more effective than glucagon in stimulating glycogenolysis. In addition, it acted more quickly and was more
potent than exogenous cyclic AMP which produced changes almost
identical to those seen with glucagon. These data suggest that
epinephrine acts on glycogenolysis through some mechanism(s) in
addition to the adenylate cyclase-cyclic AMP system.

---

1.   In these experiments, zero time refers to the time at which
     the hormones reached the liver.

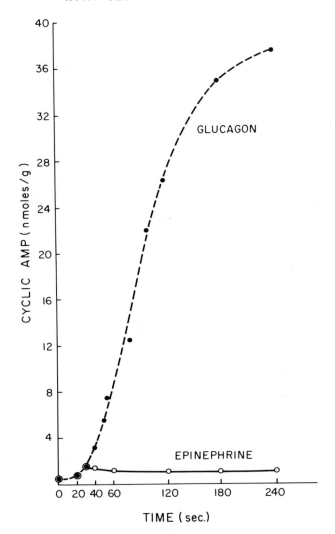

FIG. 8.   Livers were perfused with 10^{-7} M glucagon and 2 x 10^{-6} M epinephrine and cyclic AMP measured in frozen samples as described by Exton et al. (9).   Values are means of 4-6 determinations at each time point.

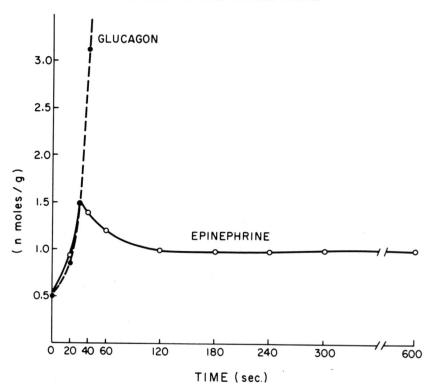

TIME COURSE OF CYCLIC AMP INCREASE WITH
GLUCAGON AND EPINEPHRINE

FIG. 9.   Data of Figure 8 plotted using an expanded ordinate scale.

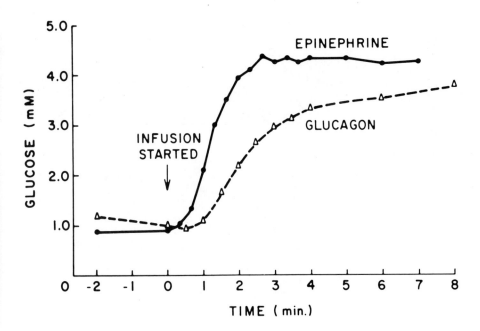

FIG. 10.   Time courses of glycogenolysis induced by maximally effective infusions of epinephrine (2×10^{-6} M) and glucagon (10^{-7} M) in perfused livers from fed rats.   The ordinate shows the concentration of glucose in the medium leaving the liver.   Data are the same experiments as in Fig. 8.

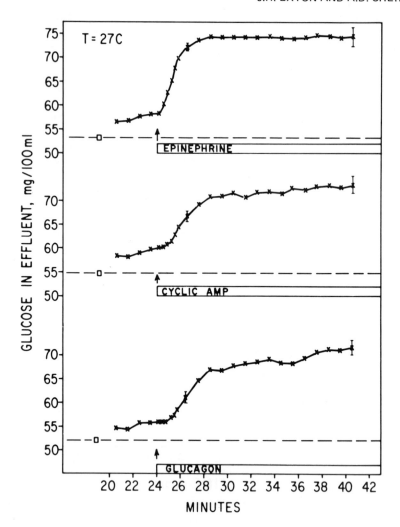

FIG. 11.   Time courses of glucose release induced by maximally
effective doses of epinephrine, cyclic AMP and glucagon.   Livers
from fed rats were perfused at 27° and infusions of 10^{-6} M epinephrine, 10^{-4} M cyclic AMP, and 5×10^{-8} M glucagon were commenced at 24 min.   Data are from Williams et al. (23).

Sutherland and Rall (2) first raised the possibility that some
adrenergic receptors might be related to adenylate cyclase.   It is
now believed that the adrenergic β-receptor is probably an integral component of the adenylate cyclase system in those tissues

where β-receptors occur, and that β-adrenergic effects result from
an increase in intracellular cyclic AMP (3, 24). Activation of α -
receptors, on the other hand, either does not change the level of
cyclic AMP or decreases it (3).

There has been considerable controversy regarding the nature
of the adrenergic receptors in rat liver, in contrast to the situation
in cat, dog and rabbit liver where the receptors are predominantly
of the β-type (7, 25). Sherline et al. using the perfused rat liver
(4) have obtained evidence that catecholamines act on glycogenolysis via two mechanisms, one involving β-receptors and cyclic AMP
and another involving α-receptors. In addition, Tolbert, Butcher
and Fain (5) and Tolbert and Fain (26) have reported that the stimulation of gluconeogenesis by epinephrine in isolated rat liver cells
is apparently unrelated to the rise in cyclic AMP induced by this
agent. The possibility that the additional mechanism might involve
activation of α-adrenergic receptors was supported by our finding
(Fig. 12) that the α-adrenergic antagonist phentolamine largely
abolished the glycogenolytic action of epinephrine in the perfused
liver without diminishing the release of cyclic AMP, a sensitive
index of the intracellular accumulation of the nucleotide (27). It
would seem in fact that glycogenolysis induced by epinephrine in
these experiments was largely due to activation of α-receptors
since the β-receptor antagonist propranolol produced little inhibition of glucose release.

Further evidence for α-receptor mediation of glycogenolysis
in rat liver was obtained in perfusion experiments using phenylephrine (an α-adrenergic agonist), and isoproterenol (a β-adrenergic
agonist). As illustrated in Fig. 13 (upper panel), epinephrine
which exhibits both α- and β-adrenergic activity was a much more
effective glycogenolytic agent than either phenylephrine or isoproterenol. The dose response curves for cyclic AMP release (Fig.
13, lower panel) did not correspond to those for glycogen mobilization. Epinephrine and isoproterenol promoted the accumulation
and efflux of cyclic AMP at concentrations between 10^{-7} M and 10^{-6}
M whereas phenylephrine produced a significant increment in cyclic
AMP production only at 2×10^{-5} M or higher concentrations. [2]

---

2. In these experiments the tissue levels of cyclic AMP were also
measured and changes in this parameter paralleled changes in cyclic
AMP efflux, i. e., the changes in nucleotide efflux induced by the
catecholamines were not due to effects in the efflux process per se.

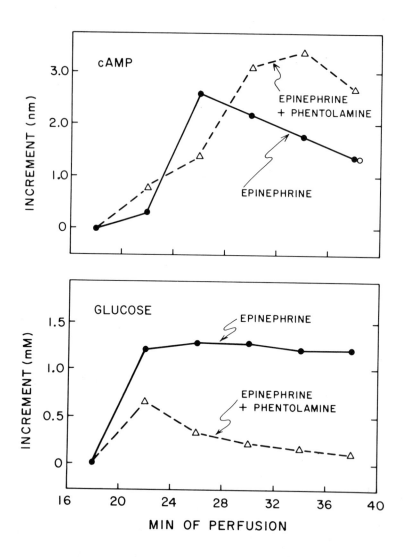

FIG. 12.   Effects of phentolamine on epinephrine-induced release
of glucose and cyclic AMP.   Livers were perfused for 20 min without additions.   Infusion of agents was then commenced to produce
final concentrations in the influent medium of 5×10^{-8} M epinephrine $\pm 5 \times 10^{-6}$ M phentolamine.   Glucose and cyclic AMP were
measured in sequential samples of effluent medium collected during
the 4 min prior to infusion and during five 4-min intervals after
infusion.   Mean values from 2 experiments are plotted.

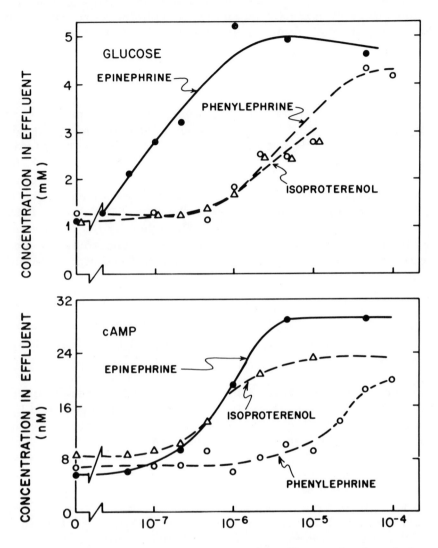

FIG. 13. Dose-response curves for the effects of epinephrine, isoproterenol and phenylephrine on the release of glucose and cyclic AMP from the perfused liver. Experiments were carried out as described in Fig. 12. Values plotted are mean values for cyclic AMP and glucose in the effluent medium collected during the period 8-20 min after commencement of catecholamine infusions. For a given concentration of catecholamine, at least 2 perfusions were carried out.

Comparison of the upper and lower panels of Figure 13 reveals that low doses of epinephrine and phenylephrine were capable of inducing substantial glycogenolysis without apparently increasing cyclic AMP efflux and that low levels of isoproterenol promoted significant efflux of cyclic AMP without activating glycogen breakdown. [3]

In preliminary series of experiments using the perfused rat liver (28), it was found that the glycogenolytic action of phenylephrine at doses which do not raise cyclic AMP was due both to activation of phosphorylase and inactivation of glycogen synthetase. It was also found that low levels of phenylephrine stimulated glucose synthesis from lactate, i. e. , an α-adrenergic mechanism exists for the activation of gluconeogenesis by catecholamines. All these actions of phenylephrine were abolished by the α-adrenergic antagonist phentolamine (28). The actions of phentolamine were specific since the agent was inactive by itself and did not inhibit the actions of glucagon or exogenous cyclic AMP.

IV. STUDIES ON THE ROLE OF CYCLIC AMP IN CATECHOL-
     AMINE ACTIONS USING ISOLATED LIVER PARENCHYMAL
     CELLS

Since it seemed possible that some of the apparently anomalous results obtained using the perfused liver might be explained by the presence of non-parenchymal cells which make up about 30% of the liver, it was decided to reexamine certain questions using isolated hepatic parenchymal cells. Figure 14 (lower panel) shows that in such cells epinephrine was once again more effective than phenylephrine or isoproterenol in inducing glycogenolysis. The findings regarding gluconeogenesis (upper panel) were different in that isoproterenol and epinephrine were about equally effective in stimulating this parameter. As was found for glycogenolysis,

---

3. The discrepancy between the effects of isoproterenol on cyclic AMP accumulation and glycogenolysis has been noted previously (9). It has been suggested that it is due to the formation of an inhibitory metabolite which affects phosphorylase activation, but evidence for this is lacking.

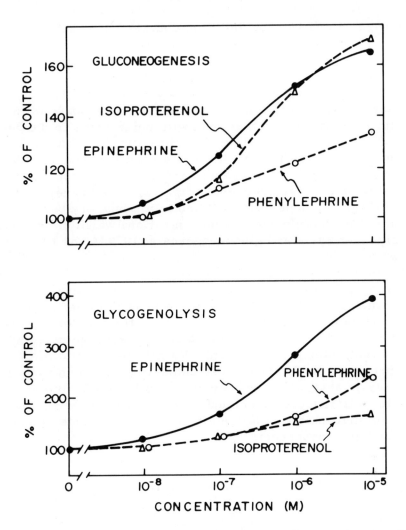

FIG. 14. Dose response curves for the effects of epinephrine, isoproterenol and phenylephrine on glycogenolysis and gluconeogenesis in isolated liver cells. Liver cells prepared from fed rats were incubated for 30 min with 5 mM [U-^{14}C] lactate. Glucose release was used as a measure of gluconeogenesis. The results are plotted as percentages of values obtained in the absence of added catecholamines. Values are means from 3 experiments in which all 4 concentrations of the 3 agents were tested.

phenylephrine was less potent than epinephrine.

Figure 15 and 16 show the time courses of the effects of different concentrations of epinephrine, isoproterenol and phenylephrine on cyclic AMP levels in the isolated parenchymal cells. Figure 15 (top panel) shows control data for incubations with saline in which cyclic AMP levels were steady for at least 10 min. With isoproterenol (Fig. 15, lower panel) there was a biphasic increase in cyclic AMP similar to that seen with epinephrine in the perfused liver. The minimally effective dose was 10^{-7} M. Maximally effective doses (10^{-6} M to 10^{-5} M) induced a peak increase of 2-fold. The pattern of cyclic AMP changes induced by epinephrine resembled that seen with isoproterenol (Fig. 16, lower panel). Phenylephrine (Fig. 16, upper panel) failed to produce any change in the level of the nucleotide even at concentrations which clearly stimulated glycogenolysis and gluconeogenesis (10^{-6} M and 10^{-5} M).

Norepinephrine was about as effective as epinephrine in activating glycogenolysis and gluconeogenesis and in promoting cyclic AMP accumulation in the cells. The effects of either agent on glycogenolysis and gluconeogenesis were greatly inhibited by the ⍺-adrenergic blockers phentolamine and phenoxybenzamine and by dihydroergotamine. These agents did not alter cyclic AMP levels in the presence or absence of catecholamines. In contrast, the β-adrenergic antagonist propranolol significantly inhibited the rise in cyclic AMP induced by epinephrine or norepinephrine, but produced minimal inhibition of the effects of these agents on glycogenolysis and gluconeogenesis.

V. A DUAL MECHANISM FOR CATECHOLAMINE ACTIONS IN LIVER

The findings with adrenergic agents reported herein are in essential agreement with those published by Sherline et al. (4) who studied the effects of different catecholamines and adrenergic antagonists on glucose output, phosphorylase activation and cyclic AMP levels in the perfused rat liver. They also support some of the findings of Tolbert et al. (5) who examined the effects of these agents on gluconeogenesis and cyclic AMP levels in isolated rat liver cells. In summary, these data indicate that in rat liver, the physiological catecholamines epinephrine and norepinephrine activate glycogenolysis and gluconeogenesis by more than one means. One mechanism involves interaction with β-adrenergic

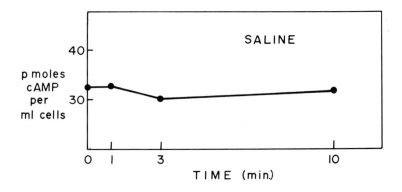

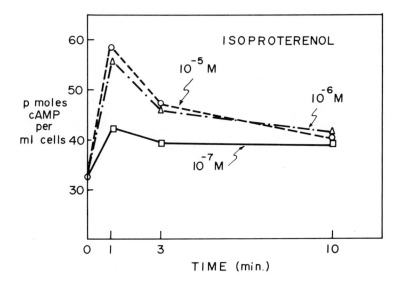

FIG. 15.   Time courses for the effects of saline and isoproterenol
on cyclic AMP levels in isolated liver cells.   Conditions were as
for Fig. 3.   Values from one experiment are given.   Similar results
were found in four other experiments.

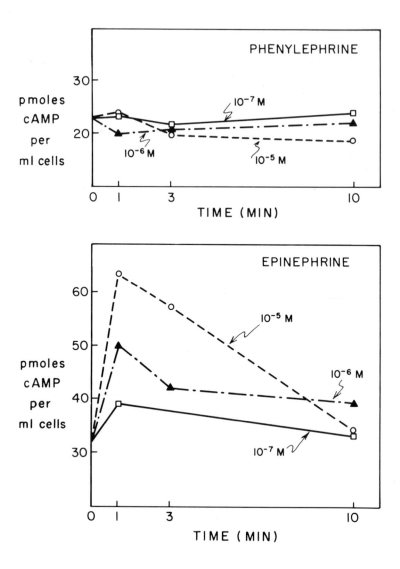

FIG. 16.   Time courses for the effects of phenylephrine and
epinephrine on cyclic AMP levels in liver cells.   Conditions were
as for Fig. 3.   Values from one experiment are given.   Similar
results were found in four other experiments.

receptors and consequent intracellular accumulation of cyclic
AMP leading to activation of phosphorylase, inactivation of glycogen synthetase and stimulation of some step(s) in the gluconeogenic pathway. Another mechanism involves interaction with α -
adrenergic receptors leading to changes in the activities of the
enzymes of glycogen metabolism and gluconeogenesis without an
overall increase in intracellular cyclic AMP.

The proposal that both α - and β-adrenergic receptors occur
in rat liver would explain the inability of previous investigators to
classify these receptors (see Reference 7). Our findings and those
of Sherline et al. (4) and Tolbert et al. (5) indicate that the effects
of epinephrine on glycogenolysis in rat liver are due predominantly
to activation of α-receptors. In other species, e. g. , dog, cat and
rabbit, β-receptors are apparently the major mediators of catecholamine-induced glycogenolysis (29-33). [4] The situation regarding
man is uncertain (25).

The mechanism of activation of hepatic glycogenolysis and
gluconeogenesis by α-receptor agonists is unknown. Preliminary
observations indicate the involvement of both phosphorylase activation and glycogen synthetase inactivation. The role of protein
kinase(s) is presently under investigation as is the role of two
possible second messengers.

The existence of alternative mechanisms for the control of
hepatic glucose production is probably of survival value. This
process plays a major role in increasing the supply of fuel to the
muscles and other organs during a "fight or flight" situation.
There exists a multiplicity of ways in which an animal can increase
glucose production when survival is at stake. These may include

---

4. In this respect, it is interesting to note that in their classic
studies on the mechanism of action of epinephrine on hepatic glycogenolysis, Sutherland and coworkers employed liver slices and
homogenates from dog, cat and rabbit, but not from rat. Sutherland apparently chose these species since they would provide large
amounts of tissue. It is interesting to speculate to what extent this
decision increased the probability of discovering cyclic AMP as a
second messenger for catecholamine action.

release of catecholamines not only from the adrenal medulla but also from nerve endings within the liver, increased glucagon release and diminished insulin secretion in response to sympa- thetic activation or other factors (34, 35), increased supply of gluconeogenic precursors (lactate, glycerol and alanine) to the liver (36) and the slower "permissive" effects of glucocorticoids on catecholamine and glucagon action on hepatic glycogenolysis and gluconeogenesis (37).

ACKNOWLEDGEMENTS

We thank Debbie Donahoo and Susan Jones for their very competent and capable assistance. Some of the initial studies in this project were carried out by J. H. Brown, H. W. Brooks, Jr., J. S. Dudney, A. S. Edgar and M. A. Whiting as part of the Physiology Practical Course in the Vanderbilt University School of Medicine. Support was received from U. S. Public Health Service Program Grant 5 P01 AM-07462 and Diabetes-Endocrino- logy Center Grant 1 P17-17026 from the National Institutes of Health.

REFERENCES

1. Exton, J. H., Robison, G. A., and Sutherland, E. W. (1971) In Handbook of Physiology. Endocrinology I (Eds. Freinkel, N. and Steiner, D.) pp. 425-436, American Physiological Society, Washington, D. C.

2. Sutherland, E. W., and Rall, T. W. (1960) Pharmacol. Rev., 12, 265.

3. Robison, G. A., Butcher, R. W., and Sutherland, E. W. (1971) Cyclic AMP. Academic Press, New York.

4. Sherline, P., Lynch, A., and Glinsmann, W. H. (1972) Endocrinology 91, 680.

5. Tolbert, M. E. M., Butcher, F. R., and Fain, J. N. (1973) J. Biol. Chem, 248, 5686.

6. Sutherland, E. W., and Robison, G. A. (1966) Pharmacol. Rev., 18, 145.

7. Hornbrook, K. R. (1970) Fed. Proc. , 29, 1381.

8. Park, C. R. , and Exton, J. H. (1972) In Glucagon: Molecular Physiology, Clinical and Therapeutic Implications (Eds. Lefebvre, P. J. and Unger, R. H.) pp. 77-108, Pergamon Press, New York.

9. Exton, J. H. , Robison, G. A. , Sutherland, E. W. , and Park, C. R. (1971) J. Biol. Chem. , 246, 6166.

10. Berry, M. N. , and Friend, D. S. (1969) J. Cell Biol. 43, 506.

11. Gilman, A. G. (1970) Proc. Nat. Acad. Sci. , 67, 305.

12. Hardman, J. G. , and Sutherland, E. W. (1969) J. Biol. Chem. 244, 6366.

13. Corbin, J. D. , and Reimann, E. M. (1975) In Methods in Enzymology (Eds. , Colowick, S. P. , and Kaplan, N. O.) Vol. 38, p. 287, Academic Press, New York.

14. Exton, J. H , and Park, C. R. (1968) J. Biol. Chem. 243, 4189.

15. Exton, J. H. , and Park, C. R. (1967) J. Biol. Chem. , 242, 2622.

16. Blackard, W. G. , Nelson, N. C. , and Andrews, S. S. (1974): Diabetes 23, 199.

17. Buchanan, K. D. , Vance, J. E. , Dinstl, K. , and Williams, R. H. (1969) Diabetes 18, 11.

18. Ohneda, A. , Aguilar-Parada, E. , Eisentraut, A. M. , and Unger, R. H. (1969) Diabetes 18, 1.

19. Krebs, E. G. (1972) Curr. Topics Cell. Regulation 5, 99.

20. Langan, T. (1968) Science, 162, 579.

21. Chen, L. J. , and Walsh, D. A. (1971) Biochemistry 10, 3614.

22. Kumon, A., Nishiyama, K., Yamamura, H., and Nishizuka, Y. (1972) J. Biol. Chem. 247, 3726.

23. Williams, T. F., Exton, J. H., Friedmann, N., and Park, C. R. (1971): Effects of insulin and adenosine 3', 5'-monophosphate on K^+ flux and glucose output in perfused rat liver. Am. J. Physiol. 221, 1645.

24. Robison, G. A., Butcher, R. W., and Sutherland, E. W. (1967) Ann. N. Y. Acad. Sci., 13, 703.

25. Jenkinson, D. H. (1973) Brit. Med. Bull. 29, 142.

26. Tolbert, M. E. M., and Fain, J. N. (1974) J. Biol. Chem., 249, 1162.

27. Exton, J. H., Lewis, S. B., Ho, R. J., Robison, G. A., and Park, C. R. (1971) Ann. N. Y. Acad. Sci., 185, 85.

28. Exton, J. H., and Harper, S. C. (1975) Adv. Cyclic Nucleotide Res., 5, 519.

29. Sutherland, E. W., and Cori, C. F. (1951) J. Biol. Chem. 188, 531.

30. Rall, T. W., Sutherland, E. W., and Berthet, J. (1957) J. Biol. Chem. 224, 463.

31. Ellis, S., and Beckett, S. B. (1963) J. Pharm. Exp. Therap. 142, 318.

32. Muhlbachova, E., Chan, P. S., and Ellis, S. (1972) J. Pharmacol. Exp. Therap., 182, 370.

33. Newton, N. E., and Hornbrook, K. R. (1972) J. Pharmacol. Exp. Therap. 181, 479.

34. Porte, D., Jr., and Bagdade, J. D. (1970) Ann. Rev. Med. 21, 219.

35. Marliss, E. G., Girardier, T., Seydoux, J., Wollheim, C. B., Kanazawa, Y., Orci, L., Renold, A. E., and Porte, D., Jr. (1973) J. Clin. Invest. 52, 1246.

36. Exton, J. H. , Mallette, L. E. , Jefferson, L. S. , Wong, E. H. A. , Friedmann, N. , Miller, T. B. , Jr. , and Park, C. R.   (1971) Rec. Prog. Horm. Res. ,   26, 411.

37. Exton, J. H. , Friedmann, N. , Wong, E. H. A. , Brineaux, J. P. , Corbin, J. D. , and Park, C. R.   (1972) J. Biol. Chem.   247, 3579.

THE ROLE OF CYCLIC AMP IN THE REGULATION OF GLYCOGEN METABOLISM

Georges Van den Berghe[1]

International Institute of Cellular
  and Molecular Pathology
Université de Louvain
75, Avenue Hippocrate, B-1200 Brussels, Belgium

Contents

INTRODUCTION

The study of glycogen metabolism has probably contributed more than the investigation of any other system to the knowledge of the biological role of cAMP. The cyclic nucleotide was discovered in 1956 as a heat-stable factor mediating the action of epinephrine and glucagon on the activation of liver phosphorylase (see (1) for a review). It was the further study of phosphorylase kinase that resulted in the recognition of a cAMP dependent protein kinase (2). This finding provided a unifying concept of the mechanism of action of the cyclic nucleotide (see (3) for a review).

---

[1] "Bevoegdverklaard Navorser" of the "Nationaal Fonds voor Weten-
schappelijk Onderzoek".

This lecture will be restricted to glycogen metabolism in skeletal muscle, heart and liver and will be divided in three parts. First, a brief outline of the pathway of glycogen metabolism will be given. The second part will be devoted to a more detailed review of the properties of the two rate-limiting enzymes, glycogen phosphorylase and glycogen synthetase and of the characteristics of their active and inactive forms. Finally, the role of cAMP in the interconversion of the two forms of phosphorylase and synthetase will be described. The discussion will be focussed mainly on physiological mechanisms. Attention will also be paid to additional controls, which besides the cyclic nucleotide, regulate the activity of both enzymes.

THE PATHWAY OF GLYCOGEN METABOLISM

Glycogen is found in almost all tissues but particularly in liver and muscle. The pathway of glucose to glycogen conversion and glycogenolysis is summarized in Figure 1. Glycogen synthesis from glucose occurs in muscle by the successive action of hexokinase {1}, phosphoglucomutase {2}, UDPG-pyrophosphorylase {3}, glycogen synthetase {4} and branching enzyme {5}. In the liver of certain species, glucose can also be phosphorylated by a specific glucokinase. The degradation of glycogen involves the coordinated operation of phosphorylase {6} and amylo-1,6-glucosidase {7}; glucose 1-phosphate formed by phosphorolysis is converted to glucose 6-phosphate by phosphoglucomutase {2}.. In muscle, glycogen provides a fuel reserve for ATP generation during contraction : glucose 6-phosphate is further degraded to lactate. In the liver, the presence of glucose 6-phosphatase {8} allows the polysaccharide to maintain blood glucose during the initial period of fasting.

Each pathway includes two irreversible steps : those catalyzed by hexo(gluco)kinase and by glycogen synthetase for the synthesis; by phosphorylase and, in the liver, glucose 6-phosphatase for the degradation. It is well established that phosphorylase and synthetase constitute the rate-limiting steps of each pathway. Both enzymes are subjected to a very complex regulation and exist in an active and an inactive form. As recently discussed by Hue and Hers (4), there is no need to postulate other controls than the concentration of substrate for the activity of glucokinase and glucose 6-phosphatase in the liver.

THE TWO FORMS OF GLYCOGEN PHOSPHORYLASE AND SYNTHETASE

General Properties and Nomenclature

Glycogen phosphorylase and glycogen synthetase belong to a group of enzymes whose activity can be modified by an enzyme-cata-

lyzed chemical modification (for reviews, see (5, 6)). For both
enzymes, the modification consists in the co-valent binding or in
the cleavage of an esterified phosphate group. The incorporation
of phosphate into phosphorylase results in the appearance of the
active form, whereas the phosphorylation of synthetase provides
the inactive form. The terms <u>active</u> and <u>inactive</u> refer to the
catalytic activity of the enzyme in physiological conditions.
This activity is related primarily to the affinity of the enzyme
for its substrates.The active forms of phosphorylase and synthetase have a lower Km for Pi and UDPG respectively than their
inactive counterparts. Modifications of the Vmax can also be
observed. The exact determination of the <u>in vivo</u> activity of the
active and inactive forms is, in principle, difficult to perform
since the kinetic parameters are influenced by a series of metabolites that modulate the enzymatic activity, often by allosteric

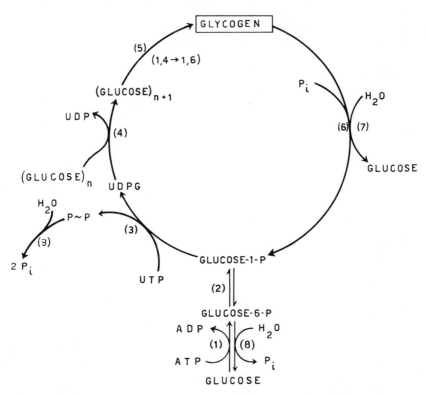

FIGURE 1. The pathway of liver glycogen metabolism

(1) Glucokinase   (6) Phosphorylase
(2) Phosphoglucomutase   (7) Amylo-1, 6-glucosidase
(3) UDPG-pyrophosphorylase   (8) Glucose 6-phosphatase
(4) Glycogen synthetase   (9) Inorganic pyrophosphatase
(5) Branching enzyme

control. The differentiation of the active and inactive forms is,
however, facilitated by the property that led to their discovery,
namely their different degree of stimulation by a single effector.
In muscle, active phosphorylase is independent of AMP for activity
whereas the inactive form is completely dependent on the nucleotide
(7); the active form of synthetase is largely active in the absence of glucose 6-phosphate, in contrast with the inactive form
which is nearly completely dependent on glucose 6-phosphate (8, 9).
It will become clear later that because of the complex conditions
that vary from tissue to tissue, the good correlation which exists
in muscle between the change in dependency towards the effector
and the modification of the physiological activity due to the
interconversion is not necessarily valid for other tissues.

   Cori and Green (10) have called the active form of phosphorylase, phosphorylase a and the inactive form, phosphorylase b.
The active form of glycogen synthetase is often called I (glucose
6-phosphate independent) and the inactive form D (glucose 6-phos-
phate dependent) (9). This operational nomenclature is, however,
misleading for the liver, since, in the ionic conditions prevailing
in the cell one form is nearly fully active and the other one
completely inactive, whereas neither form is significantly influenced by glucose 6-phosphate (11,12). The a and b terminology will
thus be used for the active (a) and inactive (b) form of glycogen
synthetase.

Glycogen Phosphorylase

Muscle. Muscle phosphorylase was the first enzyme shown to exist
in two interconvertible forms. Since this pioneering discovery of
Cori and his coworkers, the regulation of phosphorylase has become
probably the most thoroughly studied metabolic control system in
higher animals. Recent reviews of the subject have been published
(13, 14, 15).

   Muscle phosphorylase b is a dimeric molecule composed of two
subunits, each of molecular weight 92,500 (16). The monomer contains different sites, all affecting the activity of the enzyme
(Figure 2). The catalytic site binds the three substrates, glycogen,
Pi and glucose 1-phosphate and some inhibitors like glucose. The
nucleotide binding site is the site of allosteric control : binding
of AMP stimulates the inactive form of the enzyme mainly by decreasing the Km for Pi and glycogen. As said before, the b enzyme
from muscle is completely dependent on AMP for activity. Full
activity can be obtained and the half-maximal stimulation in the
presence of a physiological concentration of Pi is reached with
64 µM AMP (17). Binding of ATP or glucose 6-phosphate (probably
at a separate site) inhibits the b form by decreasing the
affinity for the substrates and AMP. The pyridoxal 5'-phosphate
binding site binds this cofactor which is indispensable to the

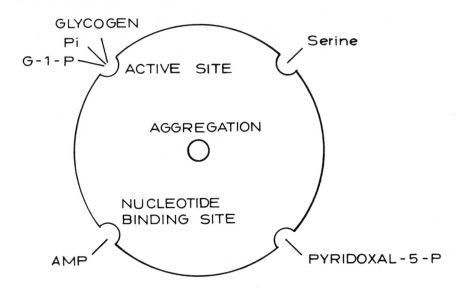

FIGURE 2.   *Schematic representation of the enzyme sites on the phosphorylase monomer*

activity of the enzyme. Probably several sites are involved in the aggregation of the monomers to a dimeric or in certain conditions a tetrameric molecule. Finally, phosphorylation of a specific seryl residue by ATP-Mg^{++} in a reaction catalyzed by phosphorylase kinase (164) converts inactive, dephosphorylated phosphorylase b into active phosphorylase a. Phosphorylase a is converted back to b by phosphorylase phosphatase (7). The stoichiometry of the interconversion was initially thought to occur according to the equation shown in Figure 3, but recent work has shown that in living muscle, phosphorylase a is probably also dimeric (18).

The activity of muscle phosphorylase is thus controlled by a multiplicity of factors. In resting muscle, in aerobic conditions, phosphorylase is in the b form and probably completely inactive although the concentration of the activator AMP is around 0.15 mM which is above the Ka of the b form for the nucleotide. The concentrations of the inhibitors ATP (8 mM) and glucose 6-phosphate (0.1 mM) result, however, in a Km for Pi of 20 mM. Since the concentration of Pi is only 3 mM in these circumstances, the activity of phosphorylase b must be very low (19). Phosphorylase a has a Km for Pi around 3 mM (20), is not dependent on AMP for activity (7, 17) and is not sensitive to the inhibitory effects of ATP and glucose 6-phosphate (19). It will thus promote glycogenolysis at a high rate. The conversion of phosphorylase b into

a by a complex mechanism, involving cAMP besides other factors,
thus plays a very important role in the regulation of the activity of phosphorylase. It should be noted, however, that the
multiple sites on the phosphorylase monomer allow regulation of
the activity of the b enzyme apart from any interconversion.
This has been documented mainly in two conditions :

(1) anaerobiosis : In the perfused rat heart, anoxia produces a
faster glycogenolysis than glucagon but less conversion of phosphorylase b to a. This has been explained by the decreased level
of the inhibitor ATP and the 3-4 fold increases of the substrate
Pi and of the activator AMP of phosphorylase b (21).

(2) Muscle phosphorylase kinase deficiency : In skeletal muscle of
I-strain mice, phosphorylase kinase as well as phosphorylase a can
hardly be detected (22). Nevertheless the animals produce glucose
6-phosphate and lactate during muscle contraction resulting from
exercize (52) or electrical stimulation (23). To our knowledge the
levels of AMP have however not been measured in these conditions.

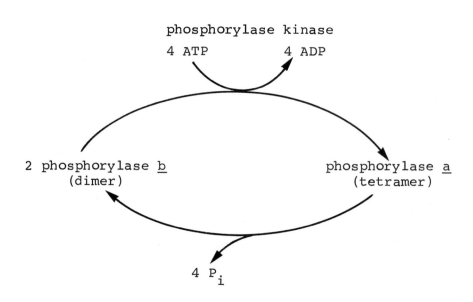

FIGURE 3. The interconversion of the action (a) and inactive (b)
           forms of muscle phosphorylase

<u>Liver</u>. The existence and properties of the two interconvertible forms of glycogen phosphorylase in the liver were originally established by Sutherland and his coworkers (for a review, see (24)). Many of the properties of liver phosphorylase are similar to those of the muscle enzyme.

An important difference between both enzymes is the effect of AMP. Inactive liver phosphorylase, in contrast to muscle phosphorylase <u>b</u> is not completely inactive when assayed in the absence of AMP. Therefore the correct measurement of the active form requires the addition of 0.5 mM caffeine to the assay in order to completely inhibit the <u>b</u> form (25). The dephosphorylated form of liver phosphorylase can also not be stimulated to full activity by the addition of AMP. The extent of the stimulation is very dependent on the composition and on the direction of the assay (Stalmans, unpublished results) and may also vary from species to species (26, 27). A Ka for AMP of 1 mM has been found for the rabbit liver enzyme (Stalmans, unpublished). It is difficult to evaluate the physiological significance of this effect since there is no certainty about the physiological concentrations of AMP in the liver. Faupel *et al*. (28) measured values as low as 30 nmol/g, 2-3 seconds after death of anesthetized rats and, by extrapolation at 0 time, calculated a basal value of 15 nmol/g. In this laboratory, values of 100-200 nmol/g have been observed, similar to those reported by Start and Newsholme (29).

There are, however, indications that similarly to the muscle enzyme, the activity of liver phosphorylase can be regulated not only by interconversion of the <u>b</u> and <u>a</u> enzyme, but also by various effectors that influence one or both forms. The increased rate of glycogenolysis observed in the perfused liver during anoxia, that was apparently not related to phosphorylase activation (30) might be explained by a stimulation of phosphorylase <u>b</u> by AMP. It has been hypothesized that the rise in blood glucose which is observed after the administration of glucagon to patients with glycogen storage disease due to the deficiency of liver phosphorylase kinase, might be the result of the stimulation of phosphorylase <u>b</u> by AMP provided by the degradation of cAMP (31).

Glycogen Synthetase

Glycogen synthetase was discovered by Leloir and his coworkers. The enzyme was first described in the liver (32) and subsequently in muscle (33). The existence of two interconvertible forms of the enzyme was shown by Larner in muscle (8) and in liver (34, 35). Glycogen synthetase has been the subject of a large amount of experimental work in recent years, which has been reviewed in detail (36, 37, 38).

Muscle. The physicochemical properties of glycogen synthetase are not yet known to the same extent as those of phosphorylase. The enzyme has been shown to be composed of subunits with molecular weight around 90,000 (39). These authors have proposed that these subunits are made of six smaller subunits of molecular weight around 15,000, each of which could be phosphorylated. From electron microscopic studies in conditions that would minimize the aggregation of the enzyme, it has been tentatively assumed that the enzyme is a tetramer and that the stoichiometry of the interconversion would be as shown in Figure 4 (40). As said before, the active (a) form is independent of glucose 6-phosphate for activity, whereas the inactive (b) form is dependent on the phosphate ester. Glucose 6-phosphate greatly increases the Vmax of the b enzyme and decreases the Km for UDPG of both forms.

The physiological inactivity of the b form of muscle glycogen synthetase is related mainly to its high Ka for glucose 6-phosphate (around 0.6 mM according to Leloir et al. (32) which is raised even further by various metabolites : a "physiological mixture", of ATP, ADP, creatine-P, Pi and MgCl$_2$ strongly inhibits the enzyme (41). As shown in Figure 5, the concentrations of glucose 6-phosphate during tetanic shock can rise to a level which is sufficient to stimulate the enzyme apart from any interconversion. This mechanism can contribute to the resynthesis of glycogen during the recovery period (42). Synthetase a has a much lower Ka for glucose 6-phosphate (5 µM according to Thomas et al. (43)), a slightly lower Km for UDPG than the b form and is less inhibited by the physiological mixture described (Figure 5). In the muscle cell, this inhibition is almost completely overcome because the concentration of glucose 6-phosphate is always much higher than the Ka of synthetase a for this effector. Synthetase a will thus promote glycogen synthesis at a high rate.

Liver. Glycogen synthetase b has been purified about 2,000-fold from rat liver (44). A subunit molecular weight of 85,000 was obtained and the enzyme could be a trimer. When measured at high levels of UDPG, the inactive (b) form of the enzyme is entirely dependent on glucose 6-phosphate, whereas the active (a) form is independent of this effector (34, 35). As said before, in the presence of physiological concentrations of UDPG (0.25 mM) and of Pi (5 mM) (11) or of a more complete physiological mixture (12) the b form is virtually inactive and cannot be stimulated to an appreciable extent by glucose 6-phosphate. In these conditions, the a form is largely active. In contrast with the muscle enzyme, the activity of liver glycogen synthetase will thus not be affected by the fluctuations of the glucose 6-phosphate level (Figure 6).

The inactivity of liver glycogen synthetase b is related to its high Km for UDPG and its inhibition by Pi and ATP. The a form

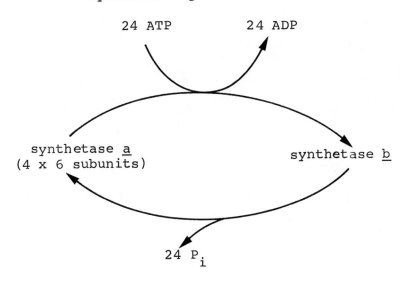

FIGURE 4. The interconversion of the active (a) forms and inactive
(b) forms of muscle synthetase

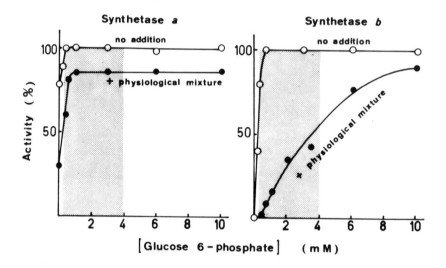

<u>FIGURE 5</u>.   *The effect of glucose 6-phosphate concentration on*
                 the activity of muscle glycogen synthetase <u>a</u> and <u>b</u>,
                 in the absence or in the presence of a "physiological
                 mixture" containing 10 mM P_i, 7.3 mM ADP plus ATP,
                 14 mM creatine-P, and 11 mM $MgCl_2$. (UDPG) was 0.4 mM
                 and pH 6.6. The concentration of glucose-6-P in
                 resting muscle is 0.3 mM; the shaded area indicates
                 the range observed in the muscle during tetanic sti-
                 mulation (Piras and Staneloni,1969). After Piras <u>et</u>
                 <u>al</u>. (41).

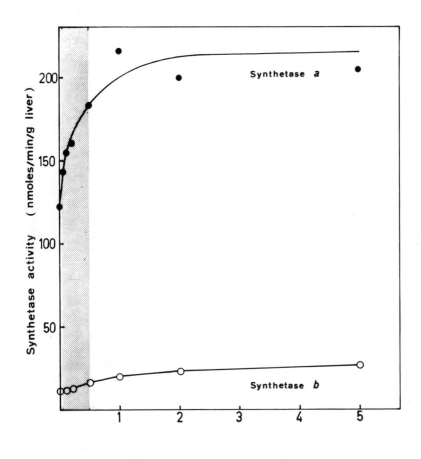

[Glucose 6 – phosphate] (mM)

FIGURE 6. *The effect of glucose 6-phosphate concentration on the activity of glycogen synthetase a and b in a liver extract in the presence of a physiological mixture containing 5 mM P_i, 3 mM ATP, and 3 mM Mg acetate. (UDPG) was 0.25 mM and pH 7.4. The shaded area indicates the in vivo range of liver glucose 6-phosphate concentration, the highest values being observed after the administration of glucagon. After De Wulf et al. (12).*

has a lower Km for UDPG and is also stimulated by Pi. The exact Km values in physiological conditions are difficult to determine as many factors, besides species differences, play a role in the kinetics of the reaction.

THE REGULATION OF THE INTERCONVERSION OF THE TWO FORMS

OF GLYCOGEN PHOSPHORYLASE AND SYNTHETASE

The role of cAMP in the regulation of glycogen metabolism is due to its stimulatory effect on the kinases that catalyse the incorporation of phosphate from ATP in the rate-limiting inter-convertible enzymes. This stimulation results in the simultaneous activation of phosphorylase and inactivation of synthetase (Figure 7). The obvious advantage of this mechanism is that synthesis and degradation of glycogen do not occur simultaneously at an important rate. The activation of phosphorylase by cAMP involves two enzymes : protein kinase (phosphorylase kinase kinase) and phosphorylase kinase, whereas the inactivation of synthetase requires only synthetase kinase. It has been shown, at least in muscle, that the same protein kinase acts as phosphorylase kinase kinase and as synthetase kinase (45).

The action of the kinases is antagonized by phosphorylase phosphatase, phosphorylase kinase phosphatase and synthetase phosphatase. Some important features of the regulation of these phosphatases will also be reviewed. The level of active phosphorylase and of active synthetase is thus the result of a balance between the antagonistic effects of the kinases and the phosphatases. An increase of the concentration of cAMP, by stimulating the kinases will obviously promote the degradation of glycogen. The possibility that a decrease of the concentration of the nucleotide, leaving the action of the phosphatases unopposed, may play a role in the synthesis of glycogen will also be discussed.

The Role of Cyclic AMP in the Degradation of Glycogen

The mechanism whereby cAMP promotes the activation of phosphorylase has been very thoroughly worked out, especially in muscle, and composes a complex sequence of events (Figure 7).

It involves 1) stimulation of adenylate cyclase by hormones and production of cAMP from ATP; 2) dissociation of protein kinase by cAMP and 3) activation of phosphorylase kinase by the catalytic subunit of protein kinase. The two first steps have been covered in great detail in other sections of this volume and will be reviewed only briefly here. More attention will be focussed on phosphorylase kinase and on the phosphatases.

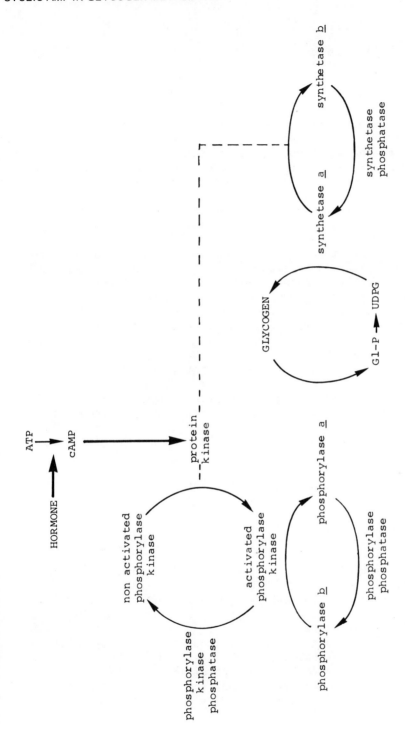

FIGURE 7. The regulation of the interconversion of glycogen phosphorylase and glycogen synthetase

Stimulation of adenylate cyclase

Muscle. The main hormones that stimulate the degradation of glycogen in mammalian skeletal muscle are the catecholamines. Of
these, only epinephrine is likely to have a physiological significance (46). Glucagon has no effect on adenylate cyclase in
skeletal muscle, but increases the activity of the enzyme in the
heart (47). This effect is, however, pharmacological, as the
concentration of the hormone required is far above its concentration in peripheral blood. The stimulation of adenylate
cyclase from cardiac tissue by thyroid hormone (48, 49) and by
histamine (50) may play a role in hyperthyroid and anaphylactic
states respectively. Prostaglandins of the E series have also
been reported to increase the concentration of cAMP in diaphragm
(51).

There is now ample evidence that the hormones that increase
the activity of phosphorylase in muscle act by way of cAMP (for
a review, see (1)). With very low doses of isoproterenol, however,
it has been shown that phosphorylase a could be formed in rabbit
gracilis muscle prior to or even without measurable change in
cAMP content or phosphorylase b kinase activation (53). The
significance of these findings is difficult to interpret. As will
be discussed later, the resting concentration of cAMP is more than
one order of magnitude above the Km of protein kinase. Small
variations of the concentration of free cAMP might not be measurable against the large background of cyclic nucleotide bound to
cell structures or proteins. The activation of phosphorylase on
the other hand, would be a more sensitive index by virtue of the
amplification mechanism provided by the sequence described in
Figure 7.

An important observation is that adenylate cyclase in skeletal
muscle (54, 55) and in cardiac muscle (56, 57, 58) is not
exclusively located in the plasma membrane (sarcolemma) but also
in the sarcoplasmic reticulum.

Liver. Glucagon constitutes the major physiological stimulus of
glycogenolysis in the liver. The minimal concentration of the
hormone required to stimulate adenylate cyclase in vitro (59)
or provoke an elevation of the level of cAMP in the perfused rat
liver (60) is around 2×10^{-10} M. This value is close to the basal
concentration of glucagon in portal blood (61, 62). Although the
concentrations of the catecholamines required to elevate the
hepatic level of cAMP (60) are not obtained in peripheral blood,
even during insulin hypoglycemia (63), the possibility exists that
such concentrations are reached locally at sympathetic nerve

endings in the hepatic tissue. A stimulation of liver glycogenolysis by secretin (64) and prostaglandin E_1 (65) has been reported but
not found by others (60). Vasopressin has also been shown to provoke degradation of glycogen in the perfused rat liver (66). When
tested on liver adenylate cyclase these hormones have given conflicting results. Whereas Pohl et al.(59) found no effect of
secretin and vasopressin, a stimulation by secretin was reported
by Thompson et al. (67) and by prostaglandin E_1 by Sweat and
Wincek (68). The preparation used for the adenylate cyclase assay
may play a role in these discrepancies.

Dissociation of protein kinase

A protein kinase, stimulated by cAMP, was discovered as a
contaminant of phosphorylase kinase purified from muscle (2) and
subsequently identified in liver (69) and in numerous tissues (70).
The mode of action of cAMP on protein kinase has been worked out
in great detail by E.G. Krebs and his coworkers in muscle (for a
review, see (3)) and an identical mechanism has been found by other
groups in various tissues (71, 72, 73).

The mechanism of the stimulation of protein kinase by cAMP is
unusual since it involves the binding of the cyclic nucleotide to
a regulatory subunit (R) of the enzyme, which promotes the dissociation of the inactive holoenzyme (R.C.) into a regulatory
subunit-cAMP complex and an active catalytic subunit (C) according
to the equation shown in Figure 8. The D and I nomenclature is
also used by certain authors, as the inactive holoenzyme is dependent on cAMP for activity, whereas the catalytic subunit does not
require the cyclic nucleotide (74, 75). As said before, evidence
has been obtained, at least in muscle, that protein kinase is
identical to phosphorylase kinase kinase and synthetase kinase.
The conclusion is based on the observation that synthetase kinase
catalyses the phosphorylation of synthetase, casein and phosphorylase kinase (165, 76) and on the co-purification of the enzyme
activities (45). The physicochemical properties of the purified
protein kinases from rat liver and rabbit skeletal muscle are close
(77). A functional similarity of the liver and muscle enzymes is
also apparent from the finding that C and R subunits from both
tissues are interchangeable (78) and that protein kinase from rat
liver phosphorylates rabbit muscle phosphorylase b kinase and
glycogen synthetase (79).

A heat stable protein inhibitor of the catalytic unit of protein kinase has been described in muscle as well as in other
tissues (80). Its physiological importance as modulator of the
activity of protein kinase is presently unknown.

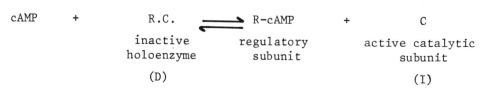

$$cAMP \quad + \quad \underset{\substack{\text{inactive} \\ \text{holoenzyme}}}{R.C.} \quad \rightleftharpoons \quad \underset{\substack{\text{regulatory} \\ \text{subunit}}}{R-cAMP} \quad + \quad \underset{\substack{\text{active catalytic} \\ \text{subunit}}}{C}$$

$$(D) \qquad\qquad\qquad\qquad\qquad\qquad (I)$$

FIGURE 8. The mechanism of action of cAMP on protein kinase

Phosphorylase kinase

Muscle. The discovery in muscle extracts of this enzyme that catalyses the conversion of phosphorylase b to phosphorylase a in the
presence of ATP-Mg^{++} is due to Fischer and Krebs (81). Phosphorylase kinase is a large molecule with a molecule weight greater than
1,000,000 and constitutes about 1 % of the soluble protein of
rabbit skeletal muscle (82). The enzyme has been shown to exist
in two forms : an activated and a non-activated form (83) that
are interconvertible by phosphorylation in the presence of ATP-Mg^{++}
(82) and by dephosphorylation (84).

The inactivity of the dephosphorylated form of the enzyme is
related primarily to its low affinity for the substrate phosphorylase b. Active phosphorylase kinase has a much higher affinity
for phosphorylase b (164). Inactive phosphorylase kinase has very
little activity at pH 6.8 but displays appreciable activity at
higher pH values, whereas active phosphorylase kinase is active
over a wide pH range. The ratio of activity at pH 6.8 to that at
pH 8.2 is used to measure the degree of activation of the enzyme:
a low ratio indicates that the enzyme is in the inactive form,
whereas an increased ratio indicates activation (85).

In muscle, the activity of phosphorylase kinase is subjected
to an important control mechanism, which does not involve interconversion of the enzyme. This mechanism was suggested by the
finding that electrical stimulation of muscle contraction was
accompanied by activation of phosphorylase and glycogenolysis,
but neither by an increase of the concentration of cAMP nor an
activation of phosphorylase kinase (86). The knowledge that the
intracellular Ca^{++} concentration controls muscle contraction led
to the study of the effect of Ca^{++} on the glycogenolytic mechanism.
Phosphorylase kinase has been shown to be Ca^{++} dependent (87).
Special precautions (Ca^{++} free solutions, Ca^{++} chelators) are
needed to demonstrate this metal requirement since the concentra-

tion of Ca^{++} required for half-maximal stimulation is in the range of 1×10^{-7} M to 3×10^{-6} M. The calcium effect results from a decrease of the Km of the enzyme for its substrate phosphorylase b. The activated form of phosphorylase kinase is more sensitive to Ca^{++} than the dephosphorylated form (88). Since the concentration of Ca^{++} in the sarcoplasm of resting muscle is in the order of 10^{-7} M and increases up to 10^{-6}-10^{-5} M during contraction (89), the conversion of phosphorylase b to phosphorylase a which is observed in response to nerve stimulation can be explained by the stimulation of non-activated phosphorylase kinase by Ca^{++} released from the sarcoplasmic reticulum.

Recent research has shown that the control of muscle phosphorylase kinase by Ca^{++} might also be influenced by cAMP. Entman et al. (56, 57) have found that epinephrine and glucagon stimulate the accumulation of Ca^{++} in a microsomal fraction of dog myocardium, thought to represent sarcoplasmic reticulum and that this effect could be mimicked by cAMP. Kirchberger et al. (90) have shown that protein kinase was involved in this process. Finally, Sulakhe and Drummond (92) have demonstrated that plasma membranes from rat skeletal muscle, phosphorylated by cAMP-dependent protein kinase accumulated more Ca^{++} than control membranes. cAMP could thus, by stimulating the phosphorylation of membranes, increase the amount of calcium available for delivery to the contractile proteins and to phosphorylase kinase and reinforce the coupling of glycogenolysis to muscle contraction.

Still additional factors have been shown to influence the activity of non-activated phosphorylase kinase : glycogen (1 %) is stimulatory whereas glucose (50 mM) and glucose 6-phosphate (10 mM) cause some inhibition (166). Recent studies have shown that phosphorylase kinase contains three different types of subunits, A, B and C. During the activation process peptide B is the first phosphoryl acceptor, peptide A can eventually also be phosphorylated but subunit C is not susceptible to phosphorylation (92, 93, 94).

Liver. Phosphorylase kinase has not been studied as extensively in liver as in muscle. The enzyme has been purified 75-fold from dog liver by Riley (95, 96) who found evidence of two interconvertible forms : activation as well as phosphorylation of the enzyme could be achieved by ATP-Mg^{++} and both processes were stimulated by cAMP. It appears that this preparation, like muscle phosphorylase kinase, could be contaminated by protein kinase (97). The characteristic effects of pH and Ca^{++} on the activity of muscle phosphorylase kinase have not been found with the liver enzyme, although the latter finding might be due to the failure to completely deplete liver tissue of Ca^{++}.

Phosphorylase_phosphatase

Muscle. Recently, phosphorylase phosphatase from rabbit muscle has
been purified 6,000-fold; due to aggregation phenomena, molecular
weights ranging from 30,000 to 120,000 or higher were observed (98).
As discussed by these authors, the potential activity of phosphorylase phosphatase is about a thousand-fold less than the potential
activity of phosphorylase kinase, so that the control of the amount
of phosphorylase a could be exerted easily by the kinase alone.
Modulation of the activity of the phosphatase however appears
possible. A marked inhibition by AMP has been described which
results from the binding of AMP to the substrate phosphorylase a
rather than from a direct effect on phosphorylase phosphatase (99).
This inhibition could contribute to maintain phosphorylase in the
active form in anaerobic conditions.

Stimulation of phosphorylase phosphatase by glucose (167, 100,
101), glucose 6-phosphate and glycogen (102, 103) has been demonstrated. The effect of glucose is devoid of physiological significance in muscle, since there is no free glucose in this tissue.
The Ka for glucose 6-phosphate was evaluated at 3 mM, which is in
the range of the concentrations of the hexose phosphate observed
in muscle (42). The prolonged increase of the concentration of
glucose 6-phosphate which is observed after a 20 s tetanic shock
may thus explain the decline of the level of phosphorylase a which
is observed after 10 s.

Interconvertible active and inactive forms of phosphorylase
phosphatase have been described in adrenal cortex (104), skeletal
muscle (105) and liver (106). cAMP has been reported to stimulate the inactivation of the enzyme in adrenal cortex and muscle
but not in liver. The physiological significance of these findings
is still unclear.

Liver. Like the muscle enzyme, liver phosphorylase phosphatase is
inhibited by AMP (107). The enzyme is also markedly stimulated by
glucose (108). This stimulation has been shown to be secondary to
the binding of the hexose to phosphorylase a, rendering this enzyme
a better substrate for its specific phosphatase (109). The Ka for
glucose is 3-7 mM in the absence of AMP and reaches 33 mM in the
presence of 10^{-4} M AMP (110). Physiological variations of the
hepatic glucose concentration, which is normally 5 to 10 mM could
thus profoundly affect the activity of phosphorylase phosphatase
and consequently the amount of phosphorylase a. The important
implications of the amount of phosphorylase a for the regulation
of glycogen synthesis will be discussed later.

Phosphorylase kinase phosphatase

Recent research suggests that phosphorylase kinase phosphatase is a protein phosphatase of broad specificity. In muscle, Zieve and Glinsmann (111) have shown that phosphorylase kinase phosphatase also functions as synthetase phosphatase. The latter enzyme was purified over 1,000-fold by Kato and Bishop (112) and shown to be similar to the histone phosphatase described in liver by Meisler and Langan (113). The synthetase phosphatase from bovine heart has also been reported to dephosphorylate phosphorylase a (114). In liver, the identity of synthetase phosphatase and phosphorylase phosphatase has been proposed (115). The possibility thus exists that the inactivation of glycogen phosphorylase and the activation of glycogen synthetase are catalyzed by a single enzyme, providing another mechanism to avoid simultaneous degradation and synthesis of glycogen.

Regulatory effects on these various enzymic activities have been reported. The activity of muscle phosphorylase kinase phosphatase might be controlled by the state of phosphorylation of the A subunits of phosphorylase kinase. Complete phosphorylation of this subunit promotes a rapid inactivation of phosphorylase kinase that might act as a shutdown process (116). Glycogen synthetase phosphatase has been shown to be inhibited by glycogen (117) and ATP (118, 119). The regulation of this enzyme will be considered in more detail in the next section.

The Role of Cyclic AMP in the Synthesis of Glycogen

Whereas there is considerable evidence that the hormones that stimulate the degradation of glycogen in muscle and liver act by increasing the concentration of cAMP, the question whether the major stimuli of glycogen synthesis, insulin, glucose and corticosteroids act through a lowering of the concentration of the cyclic nucleotide is more difficult to answer. Insulin is the principal effector of glycogen synthesis in muscle. In the liver, glucose and corticosteroids play a predominant role and the action of insulin on glycogenesis has been a subject of controversy. Each tissue will be considered separately.

Muscle. Insulin increases the proportion of the active form of glycogen synthetase in muscle in vitro (8) as well as in vivo (120).

The hypothesis that insulin activates muscle synthetase by decreasing the concentration of cAMP was not supported by experimental evidence. The administration of insulin at a dose of 2-4 U/kg in vivo produces a paradoxical rise of cAMP in rat skeletal muscle (120). This effect might however have been

caused by catacholamine release. In vitro, a previous incubation
of the isolated rat diaphragm with insulin reduces the increase of
cAMP in response to epinephrine, but insulin alone has no effect
(121).   Insulin in concentrations varying from 1 milliunit per ml
to 10 units per ml did not alter either basal or epinephrine
stimulated adenylate cyclase activity in plasma membranes from
rabbit skeletal muscle (122).

It has therefore been proposed that insulin induces a stable
change of the protein (synthetase) kinase. Indeed, a greater proportion of the enzyme has been found in the cAMP-dependent (or
R.C.) form after administration of insulin in vivo (74, 123) or
after the incubation of rat diaphragm with insulin (75).

The finding by Soderling et al.(124) that in the fat pad
treated with epinephrine, insulin decreases the concentration of
cAMP and the ratio of cAMP-independent protein kinase (C) to total
protein kinase (RC + C) in a parallel fashion is, however, not in
favour of alterations of protein kinase that are independent of
changes in the concentrations of the cyclic nucleotide. The effect
of insulin on muscle glycogen synthetase might thus be due to a
small undetectable change of the concentration of cAMP. Recently
it has been reported that insulin stimulates phosphodiesterase
activity localized at the external surface of small, intact frog
skeletal muscles (125).

Liver.

a) Glucose. It has been known for a long time that the hypergly-
caemia resulting from food intake causes deposition of glycogen in
the liver (126, 127). The mechanism of this effect has been studied
in recent years by Hers and associates (128, 129, 130). The intravenous administration of a load of glucose to mice provokes within
a few minutes an up to 40-fold increase of the rate of glucose to
glycogen conversion that parallels the increase of the amount of
synthetase a (150). The elevation of blood glucose also causes an
immediate partial or complete inactivation of phosphorylase in
the liver of the intact animal (149, 132) and in the isolated perfused liver (133, 134).

These observations have prompted the investigation of the
effect of a glucose load on the hepatic concentration of cAMP (135).
As shown in Table 1, a small but statistically significant decrease
of the concentration of cAMP together with a very large increase of
the amount of synthetase a was observed in the liver of intact fed
mice shortly after the administration of a large glucose load. It
is very difficult to evaluate if this slight decrease of the concentration of the cyclic nucleotide is sufficient to explain the
very large activation of glycogen synthetase. Even the lowest concentration of cAMP observed is several fold above the Ka values of

protein kinase for the cyclic nucleotide (3). In crude liver
extracts, half-maximal stimulation of both synthetase kinase (131)
and the complete activation system of phosphorylase (136) is
obtained with cAMP concentrations in the range of 2 x 10^{-7} to
1 x 10^{-8} M. To explain how the nucleotide can control the activity
of protein kinase, compartmentalization has been invoked (137).
However, recent experiments by Beavo et al. (138) have shown that
when the effect of cAMP is studied in the presence of physiological
concentrations of protein kinase, instead of in the usual conditions
where there is a large excess of ligand over enzyme, much higher
concentrations of cAMP are required to activate the kinase.
Identical conclusions have been reached by theoretical studies
(see Swillens, this volume) that have shown furthermore that the
Ka is dimensionless in the case of an enzyme which is activated by
dissociation. Experiments with the perfused rat liver (133, 134)
have shown that a decrease of the concentration of cAMP is not
required in order to observe the activation of glycogen synthetase
after a glucose load.

TABLE 1

EXPERIMENTAL GROUPS	cAMP nmol/g liver	Glycogen Synthetase a mU/g liver
Control (15)	0.83 + 0.03	11 + 1
6 min after glucose (1 mg/g) (8)	0.67 + 0.05	154 + 25
10 min after glucose (5 mg/g) (8)	0.63 + 0.04	223 + 8
3 h after prednisolone (1 mg/20 g) (13)	0.63 + 0.03	189 + 16

Influence of a glucose load and of prednisolone treatment on the
level of cAMP and on the activity of glycogen synthetase a in
mouse liver.

Values shown are means + the standard error of the means with the
number of determinations in parentheses (from Van den Berghe et
al.(135)).

Further investigations in this laboratory have provided the following mechanism to explain the activation of liver glycogen synthetase by glucose.

1° Glucose provokes the inactivation of phosphorylase a by a stimulation of phosphorylase phosphatase (108).

2° Phosphorylase a inhibits synthetase phosphatase by a protein-protein interaction (25). The activation of glycogen synthetase can proceed only when and if the level of phosphorylase a has been reduced below a threshold value equal to approximately 10% of the total amount of phosphorylase. This mechanism has been demonstrated by sequential studies in vitro (109) that have shown that the activation of synthetase is always preceded by a latency, which is the time required for phosphorylase a to be inactivated by its phosphatase.

The sequence described is difficult to elicit in fasted and diabetic animals. The increased concentration of cAMP which has been demonstrated in the liver of fasted rats (139) and mice (Van den Berghe, unpublished observations) and of insulin deficient rats (137) may explain this finding. The hepatic concentration of cAMP is, however, not significantly increased in insulin deficient mice (Van den Berghe, see this volume). The glucose effect on liver glycogen synthetase is not mediated by insulin since a rise of blood glucose is followed by glycogen synthesis in fasted depancreatized (140) fasted alloxan diabetic (141, 142, 143) or anti-insulin treated animals (129) and in the perfused liver.

b) Glucocorticoids. The administration of glucocorticoids induces an important deposition of glycogen in the liver (144). In normally fed mice the level of the polysaccharide can go up as high as 12 %. The effect is seen in fed as well as in fasted animals and is therefore not only the consequence of a stimulation of gluconeogenesis. It appears not to be insulin-dependent since it can also be observed in diabetic animals (145, 146).

The glucocorticoids require about 3 hours to stimulate liver glycogen synthesis but the effect can be observed in some animals after 30 minutes. Hornbrook et al. (147) were the first to report that the administration of hydrocortisone to adrenalectomized rats increases the amount of glycogen synthetase which is less dependent upon glucose 6-phosphate. De Wulf and Hers (148) demonstrated that in normal mice treated with prednisolone, the amount of glycogen synthetase a was markedly increased and that the rate of glycogen synthesis in vivo strongly correlated with the enzymic activity measured in vitro. A slight inactivation of glycogen phosphorylase has also been observed in the liver of mice treated with glucocorticoids (149, 143).

These observations led to the investigation of the effect of glucocorticoids on the hepatic level of cAMP. As shown in Table 1 a small decrease of the concentration of the cyclic nucleotide can be observed after the administration of prednisolone. This slight decrease of the concentration of cAMP is similar to the one observed after the administration of a glucose load and, for the same reasons, did not appear sufficient to explain the very large activation of glycogen synthetase. The study of the enzyme inter-conversions in the in vitro system described above showed two modifications :

1° The activity of phosphorylase phosphatase is increased in the liver filtrate of mice treated with prednisolone, resulting in a faster disappearance of phosphorylase a, allowing the activation of synthetase to occur earlier (108).

2° The activation of synthetase proceeds without latency, indicating that synthetase phosphatase is much less inhibited by phosphorylase a. Preliminary experiments indicate that this decreased inhibition is due to the formation in the liver of a protein factor, which, possibly by binding to phosphorylase a, prevents this enzyme from inhibiting synthetase phosphatase (130).

c) Insulin. Insulin is a much less potent stimulator of liver glycogen synthesis than glucose. The indications that insulin plays a role in the regulation of the accumulation of hepatic glycogen can be summarized as follows : 1° diabetic rats treated or not with glucose can rapidly accumulate glycogen in their liver but this synthesis levels off at a low concentration of about 3 %, while treatment with insulin allows normal levels of glycogen to be obtained (142). 2° in normal mice, insulin with glucose is more effective than glucose alone for the stimulation of glycogen synthesis since it allows the glucose effect to be obtained at a lower level of blood glucose (150). It should be noted that it has proven very difficult to show an effect of insulin on liver glycogen synthesis in vitro. Madison (151) has summarized the available evidence in favour of this effect.

It has been proposed, mainly from experiments with the per-fused rat liver, that the direct inhibitory effect of insulin on the production of glucose is, at least partly, due to a decrease of the formation of cAMP (for reviews see Exton et al.(151, 152), Park et al. (153)). In recent years, several studies have been performed to try to determine if the stimulatory action of insulin on liver glycogen synthesis might also be related to a decrease of the concentration of cAMP. This would result in a diminished sti-mulation of synthetase (protein) kinase, allowing the activation of glycogen synthetase to proceed.

In normal mice _in vivo_, a partial activation of liver glycogen synthetase, associated with a decrease of the concentration of cAMP, has been occasionally observed a few minutes after the injection of insulin (Figure 9A). This finding is, however, poorly reproducible (Figure 9B). In the normal isolated perfused rat liver, Miller and Larner (145) recently demonstrated that insulin could partially activate glycogen synthetase not only when infused simultaneously with glucagon, but also under basal conditions. Table 2 gives a summary of their results. The effect of insulin in livers perfused with glucagon was observed without as well as with simultaneous infusion of glucose to the control and insulin treated livers, to equalize their glucose outputs with those of the livers perfused with the hyperglycemic hormone. In these experiments the activation of glycogen synthetase was associated with a decrease of the concentration of cAMP and of the cAMP-independent form of synthetase (protein) kinase. The effect of insulin on the basal level of synthetase was associated with a similar decrease of the independent synthetase (protein) kinase but there were no changes of the concentration of the cyclic nucleotide. It should be noticed, however, that the effect of insulin on glycogen synthetase in the perfused liver seems to require well-defined experimental conditions and is of short duration. In cultured fetal rat liver insulin activates glycogen synthetase (156). Measurement of cAMP was not performed in these experiments.

TABLE II

EXPERIMENTAL CONDITIONS	GLUCOSE INFUSION	Sy I (%)	cAMP nmol/g liver	Sykinase I (%)
glucagon	0	14 + 2	0.68 + 0.06	
glucagon + insulin	0	21 + 3	0.42 + 0.03	
control	+	70 + 2	0.45 + 0.03	26.8 + 4.5
glucagon	0	25 + 1	0.67 + 0.07	42.5 + 3.3
glucagon + insulin	+	41 + 3	0.47 + 0.04	30.1 + 5.9
control 6'	0	29 + 2	0.37 + 0.02	46 + 2
insulin 6'	0	38 + 2	0.35 + 0.03	36 + 3
control 15'	0	31 + 3	0.30 + 0.02	53 + 2
insulin 15'	0	41 + 3	0.28 + 0.01	40 + 5

Effects of glucagon and insulin on the levels of active synthetase (Sy I), cAMP and cAMP-dependent protein kinase (sykinase I) in the isolated perfused liver of normal rats. The final concentration of glucagon was 3 x 10^{-10} M and of insulin 4 x 10^{-8}M. Glucose, when utilized, was perfused so as to equalize the glucose accumulation with that observed with glucagon alone. (Modified from Miller and Larner (162)).

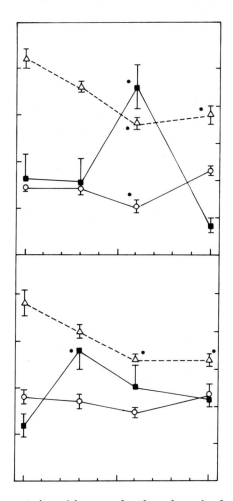

FIGURE 9. Effect of insulin on the levels of glucose, cAMP and synthetase a in the liver of normal mice.
Insulin was administered intravenously at a dose of 1 U/kg body weight to unanaesthetized mice that were killed by decapitation at the times indicated. The livers were quick-frozen according to Wollenberger et al. (154). cAMP was determined as described by Van den Berghe et al. (135) and synthetase a according to De Wulf et al. (155). There were 7 animals per group in experiment A and 3-5 animals per group in experiment B. Vertical bars represent ± the standard error of the mean and p < 0.05 in comparison with zero time is indicated by an asterisk (Van den Berghe, unpublished experiments).

In diabetic animals, glycogen synthetase is mostly in its inactive form, despite a high level of blood glucose. This might be explained by the higher level of cAMP in the rat (137), or hypothetically, by an increased concentration of the proportion of free cAMP in the mouse. In recently diabetic rats (157, 158, 130), dogs (132) or mice (Figure 10), insulin provokes a rapid activation of glycogen synthetase. Activation of the enzyme occurs, however, prior to or without a decrease of the concentration of cAMP. In chronically diabetic animals, the administrtion of insulin elicits an activation of glycogen synthetase only after about one hour (159, 160) without change of the concentration of cAMP (161).

Considered as a whole, the experimental data available make it difficult to conclude that the activation of glycogen synthetase, which can be observed after the administration of insulin, is mediated by a decrease of the concentration of cAMP. The mechanism of action of insulin on the synthesis of glycogen in the liver can thus not yet be considered as clarified.

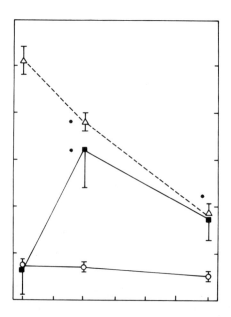

FIGURE 10. Effect of insulin on the levels of glucose, cAMP and synthetase a in the liver of diabetic mice.
Insulin was administered intraperitoneally at a dose of 1 U/kg to unanaesthetized mice that had received alloxan (70 mg/kg) 48 hours before. There were 10 animals per group. Experimental procedures and expression of the results are the same as for Figure 9 (Van den Berghe, unpublished results).

REFERENCES

(1) ROBISON, G.A., BUTCHER, R.W. and SUTHERLAND, E.W. (1971) Cyclic AMP, Academic Press, New York and London

(2) WALSH, D.A., PERKINS, J.P. and KREBS, E.G. (1968), J. Biol Chem. 243, 3763

(3) WALSH, D.A. and KREBS, E.G. (1973) in "The Enzymes" (Boyer, P.D., ed.) 3rd Edition, 8, 555, Academic Press, New York and London

(4) HUE, L. and HERS, H.G. (1974) Biochem. Biophys. Res. Commun. 58, 540

(5) HOLZER, H. (1969), Advanc. Enzymol. 32, 297

(6) SEGAL, H.L. (1973), Science, 180, 25

(7) CORI, G.T. and CORI, C.F. (1945) J. Biol. Chem., 158, 321

(8) VILLAR-PALASI, C. and LARNER, J. (1960) Biochim. Biophys. Acta, 39, 171

(9) ROSSELL-PEREZ, M., VILLAR-PALASI, C. and LARNER, J. (1962), Biochemistry, 1, 763

(10) CORI, G.T. and GREEN, A.A. (1943), J. Biol. Chem., 151, 31

(11) MERSMANN, H.J. and SEGAL, H.L. (1967) Proc. Natl. Acad. Sci. USA, 58, 1688

(12) DE WULF, H., STALMANS, W. and HERS, H.G. (1968) Eur. J. Biochem. 6, 545

(13) FISCHER, E.H., POCKER, A. and SAARI, J.C. (1970) "Essays in Biochemistry" (P.N. Campbell and F. Dickens, eds.) 6, 23, Academic Press, New York and London

(14) FISCHER, E.H., HEILMEYER, L.M.G. Jr. and HASCHKE, R.H. (1971) Curr. Top. Cell. Reg. 4, 211

(15) GRAVES, D.J. and WANG, J.H. (1972) in "The Enzymes" (Boyer, P.D., ed.) 3rd Edition, 7, 435, Academic Press, New York and London

(16) SEERY, V.L., FISCHER, E.H. and TELLER, D.C. (1970) Biochemistry, 9, 3591

(17)   HELMREICH, E. and CORI, C.F. (1964) Proc. Natl. Acad. Sci.
       USA, 51, 131

(18)   METZGER, B.E., GLASER, L. and HELMREICH, E. (1968) Bio-
       chemistry, 7, 2021

(19)   MORGAN, H.E. and PARMEGGIANI, A (1964b) J. Biol. Chem., 239,
       2440

(20)   BROWN, D.H. and CORI, C.F. (1961) in "The Enzymes", (Boyer,
       P.D., Lardy, H. and Myrback, K., eds.) 2nd Edition, 5, 207,
       Academic Press, New York and London

(21)   MORGAN, H.E. and PARMEGGIANI, A (1964a) J. Biol. Chem., 239,
       2435

(22)   LYON, J.B. Jr. and PORTER, J. (1962), Biochim. Biophys. Acta,
       58, 248

(23)   DANFORTH, W.H. and LYON, J.B. Jr. (1964) J. Biol. Chem.,
       239, 4047

(24)   SUTHERLAND, E.W. and RALL, T.W. (1960) Pharmacol. Rev., 12,
       265

(25)   STALMANS, W., DE WULF, H. and HERS, H.G. (1971) Eur. J.
       Biochem. 18, 582

(26)   WOSILAIT, W.D. and SUTHERLAND, E.W. (1956) J. Biol. Chem.
       218, 469

(27)   APPLEMAN, M.M., KREBS, E.G. and FISCHER, E.H. (1966),
       Biochemistry, 5, 2101

(28)   FAUPEL, R.P., SEITZ, H.J., TARNOWSKI, W., THIEMANN, V. and
       WEISS, C. (1972) Arch. Biochem. Biophys. 148, 509

(29)   START, C., and NEWSHOLME, E.A. (1968) Biochem. J., 107, 411

(30)   LEVINE, R.A. (1965) Am. J. Physiol., 208, 317

(31)   KOSTER, J.F., FERNANDES, J., SLEE, R.G., VAN BERKEL, T.J.C.
       and HULSMANN, W.C. (1973) Biochem. Biophys. Res. Commun.,
       53, 282

(32)   LELOIR, L.F. and CARDINI, C.E. (1957) J. Am. Chem. Soc.,
       79, 6340

(33)   LELOIR, L.F., OLAVARRIA, J.M., GOLDEMBERG, S.H. and
       CARMINATTI, H. (1959) Arch. Biochem. Biophys., 81, 508

(34)   HIZUKURI, S. and LARNER, J. (1963) Biochim. Biophys. Acta,
       73, 525

(35)   HIZUKURI, S. and LARNER, J. (1964) Biochemistry, 3, 1783

(36)   RYMAN, B.E. and WHELAN, W.J. (1971) Advan. Enzymol. 34, 285

(37)   LARNER, J. and VILLAR-PALASI, C. (1971) Curr. Top. Cell.
       Regul., 3, 195

(38)   STALMANS, W. and HERS, H.G. (1973) in "The Enzymes" (Boyer,
       P.D., ed.) 3rd. Edition, 9, 309, Academic Press, New York
       and London

(39)   SMITH, C.H., BROWN, N.E. and LARNER, J. (1971) Biochim.
       Biophys. Acta, 242, 81

(40)   REBHUN, L.I., SMITH, C. and LARNER, J. (1973) Mol. Cell
       Biochem. 1, 55

(41)   PIRAS, R., Rothman, L.B. and CABIB, E. (1968) Biochemistry,
       7, 56

(42)   PIRAS, R. and STANELONI, R (1969) Biochemistry, 8, 2153

(43)   THOMAS, J.A., SCHLENDER, K.K. and LARNER, J. (1973) Biochim.
       Biophys. Acta, 293, 84

(44)   LIN, D.C. and SEGAL, H.L. (1973) J. Biol. Chem., 248, 7007

(45)   SODERLING, T.R., HICKENBOTTOM, J.P., REIMANN, E.M., HUNKELER,
       F.L., WALSH, D.A. and KREBS, E.G. (1970) J. Biol. Chem.,
       245, 6317

(46)   BOWMAN, W.C. and NOTT, M.W. (1969) Pharmacol. Rev., 21, 27

(47)   MURAD, F. and VAUGHAN, M. (1969) Biochem. Pharmacol., 18,
       1053

(48)   LEVEY, G.S. and EPSTEIN, S.E. (1968) Biochem. Biophys. Res.
       Commun., 33, 990

(49)   LEVEY, G.S. and EPSTEIN, S.E. (1969) J. Clin. Invest., 48,
       1663

(50)   KLEIN, I. and LEVEY, G.S. (1971) J. Clin. Invest., 50, 1012

(51)   BUTCHER, R.W. and BAIRD, C.E. (1968), J. Biol. Chem., 243,
       1713

(52)   LYON, J.B., Jr. and PORTER, J. (1963), J. Biol. Chem., 238, 1

(53)   STULL, J.T. and MAYER, S.E. (1971) J. Biol. Chem., 246, 5716

(54)   RABINOWITZ, M., DESALLES, L., MEISLER, J. and LORAND, L.
       (1965) Biochim. Biophys. Acta, 97, 29

(55)   SERAYDARIAN, K. and MOMMAERTS, W.F.H.M. (1965) J. Cell Biol.
       26, 641

(56)   ENTMAN, M.L., LEVEY, G.S. and EPSTEIN, S.E. (1969a) Biochem.
       Biophys. Res. Commun. 35, 728

(57)   ENTMAN, M.L., LEVEY, G.S. and EPSTEIN, S.E. (1969b) Circ.
       Res., 25, 429

(58)   KATZ, A.M., TADA, M., REPKE, D.I., IORIO, J.A.M. and
       KIRCHBERGER, M.A. (1974) J. Mol. Cell Cardiol. 6, 73

(59)   POHL, S.L., BIRNBAUMER, L. and RODBELL, M. (1971) J. Biol.
       Chem., 246, 184

(60)   EXTON, J.H., ROBISON, G.A., SUTHERLAND, E.W. and PARK, C.R.
       (1971a), J. Biol. Chem., 246, 6166

(61)   OHNEDA, A., AGUILAR-PARADA, E., EISENTRAUT, A.M. and UNGER,
       R.H. (1969), Diabetes, 18, 1

(62)   BUCHANAN, K.D., VANCE, J.E., DINSTL, K. and WILLIAMS, R.H.
       (1969), Diabetes, 18, 11

(63)   GOLDFIEN, A., ZILELI, M.S., Despointes, R.H. and BETHUNE,
       J.E. (1958) Endocrinology, 62, 749

(64)   LEVINE, R.A., Pesch. L.A., KLATSKIN, G. and GIARMAN, N.J.
       (1964) J. Clin. Invest., 43, 797

(65)   CURNOW, R.T. and NUTTALL, F.Q. (1972) J. Biol. Chem., 247,
       1892

(66)   HEMS, D.A., and WHITTON, P.D. (1973) Biochem. J., 136, 705

(67)   THOMPSON, W.J., WILLIAMS, R.H. and LITTLE, S.A. (1973)
       Biochim. Biophys. Acta, 302, 329

(68)   SWEAT, F.W. and WINCEK, T.J. (1973) Biochem. Biophys. Res.
       Commun., 55, 52

(69)   LANGAN, T.A. (1968) Science, 162, 579

(70)   KUO, J.F. and GREENGARD; P. (1969) Proc. Natl. Acad. Sci.
       USA, 64, 1349

(71)   GILL, G.N. and GARREN, L.D. (1970) Biochem. Biophys. Res.
       Commun., 39, 335

(72)   KUMON, A., YAMAMURA, H. and NISHIZUKA, Y. (1970) Biochem.
       Biophys. Res. Commun., 41, 1290

(73)   TAO, M., SALAS, M.L. and LIPMANN, F. (1970) Proc. Natl.
       Acad. Sci. USA, 67, 408

(74)   VILLAR-PALASI, C. and WENGER, J.I. (1967) Fed. Proc., 26,
       563

(75)   SHEN, L.C., VILLAR-PALASI, C. and LARNER, J. (1970) Physiol.
       Chem. Physics, 2, 536

(76)   VILLAR-PALASI, C., LARNER, J. and SHEN, L.C. (1971) Ann.
       N.Y. Acad. Sci., 185, 74

(77)   CHEN, L.J. and WALSH, D.A. (1971) Biochemistry, 10, 3614

(78)   YAMAMURA, H., KUMON, A. and NISHIZUKA, Y. (1971) J. Biol.
       Chem., 246, 1544

(79)   YAMAMURA, H., NISHIYAMA, K., SHIMOMURA, R. and NISHIZUKA,
       Y. (1973), Biochemistry

(80)   WALSH, D.A., ASHBY, C.D., GONZALEZ, C., CALKINS, D.,
       FISCHER, E.H. and KREBS, E.G. (1971) J. Biol. Chem., 246,
       1977

(81)   FISCHER, E.H. and KREBS, E.G. (1955) J. Biol. Chem., 216,
       121

(82)   DELANGE, R.J., KEMP, R.G., RILEY, W.D., COOPER, R.A. and
       KREBS, E.G. (1968) J. Biol. Chem., 243, 2200

(83)   KREBS, E.G., GRAVES, D.J. and FISCHER, E.H. (1959) J. Biol.
       Chem., 234, 2867

(84)   RILEY, W.D., DELANGE, R.J. BRATVOLD, G.E. and KREBS, E.G.
       (1968) J. Biol. Chem. 243, 2209

(85)   POSNER, J.B., STERN, R. and KREBS, E.G. (1965) J. Biol.
       Chem., 240, 982

(86) DRUMMOND, G.I., HARWOOD, J.P. and POWELL, C.A. (1969) J.
      Biol. Chem., 244, 4235

(87) OZAWA, E., HOSOI, K. and EBASHI, S. (1967) J. Biochem., 61,
      531

(88) BROSTROM, C.O., HUNKELER, F.L. and KREBS, E.G. (1971) J.
      Biol. Chem., 246, 1961

(89) EBASHI, S. and ENDO, M. (1968) Progr. Biophys. Mol. Biol.,
      18, 125

(90) KIRCHBERGER, M.A., TADA, M., REPKE, D.I. and KATZ, A.M.
      (1972) J. Mol. Cell. Cardiol., 4, 673

(91) SULAKHE, P.V. and DRUMMOND, G.I. (1974), Arch. Biochem.
      Biophys., 161, 448

(92) HAYAKAWA, T., PERKINS, J., WALSH, D.A. and KREBS, E.G.
      (1973a), Biochemistry, 12, 567

(93) HAYAKAWA, T., PERKINS, J. and KREBS, E.G. (1973b) Bio-
      chemistry, 12, 574

(94) COHEN, P. (1973), Eur. J. Biochem., 34, 1

(95) RILEY, G.A. (1963) Fed. Proc., 22, 258

(96) RILEY, G.A. (1969) Pharmacologist, 11, 253

(97) WAHBA, W.W. and RILEY, G.A. (1969) Pharmacologist, 11, 253

(98) GRATECOS, D., DETWILER, T. and FISCHER, E.H. (1974) in
      "Metabolic Intern-conversion of Enzymes 1973" (E.H.
      Fischer, E.G. Krebs, H. Neurat and E.R. Stadtman, eds.) 43,
      Springer Verlag, Berlin, Heidelberg and New York

(99) NOLAN, C., NOVOA, W.B., KREBS, E.G. and FISCHER, E.H. (1964)
      Biochemistry, 3, 542

(100) DE BARSY, Th., STALMANS, W., LALOUX, M., DE WULF, H. and HERS,
      H.G. (1972) Biochem. Biophys. Res. Commun., 46, 183

(101) BAILEY, J.M. and WHELAN, W.J. (1972) Biochem. Biophys. Res.
      Commun., 46, 191

(102) BOT, G. and DOSA, I (1971) Acta Biochim. Biophys. Acad. Sci.
      Hung., 6, 73

(103) MARTENSEN, T.M., BROTHERTON, J.E. and GRAVES, D.J. (1973) J. Biol. Chem., 248, 8329

(104) MERLEVEDE, W. and RILEY, G.A. (1966) J. Biol. Chem., 241, 3517

(105) CHELALA, C.A., and TORRES, H.N. (1970) Biochim. Biophys. Acta, 198, 504

(106) MERLEVEDE, W., GORIS, J. and DE BRANDT, C. (1969) Eur. J. Biochem., 11, 499

(107) SUTHERLAND, E.W. (1951) Ann. N.Y. Acad. Sci., 54, 693

(108) STALMANS, W., DE WULF, H., LEDERER, B. and HERS, H.G. (1970) Eur. J. Biochem., 15, 9

(109) STALMANS, W., DE WULF, H., HUE, L. and HERS, H.G. (1974a) Eur. J. Biochem., 41, 127

(110) STALMANS, W., LALOUX, M. and HAS, H.G. (1974b), Eur. J. Biochem., 49, 415

(111) ZIEVE, F.J. and GLINSMANN, W.H. (1975) Biochem. Biophys. Res. Commun., 50, 872

(112) KATO, K. and BISHOP, J.S. (1972) J. Biol. Chem., 247, 7420

(113) MEISLER, M.H. and LANGAN, T.A. (1969) J. Biol. Chem., 244, 4961

(114) NAKAI, C. and THOMAS, J.A. (1973) Biochem. Biophys. Res. Commun., 52, 530

(115) KILLILEA, S.D., BRANDT, H., LEE, E.Y.C. and WHELAN, W.J. (1974) Fed. Proc., 33, 1431

(116) COHEN, P. and ANTONIW, J.F. (1973) FEBS Letters, 34, 43

(117) VILLAR-PALASI, C., GOLDBERG, N.D., BISHOP, J.S., NUTTALL, F.Q. and LARNER, J. (1969) FEBS Symp., 19, 149

(118) GILBOE, D.P. and NUTTALL, F.Q. (1972) Biochem. Biophys. Res. Commun., 48, 898

(119) GILBOE, D.P. and NUTTALL, F.Q. (1974) Biochim. Biophys. Acta, 338, 57

(120)   GOLDBERG, N.D., VILLAR-PALASI, C., SASKO, H. and LARNER,
        J. (1967) Biochim. Biophys. Acta, 148, 665

(121)   CRAIG, J.W., RALL, T.W. and LARNER, J. (1969) Biochim.
        Biophys. Acta 177, 213

(122)   SEVERSON, D.L., DRUMMOND, G.I. and SULAKHE, P.V. (1972) J.
        Biol. Chem., 247, 2949

(123)   LARNER, J. VILLAR-PALASI, C., GOLDBERG, N.D., BISHOP, J.S.
        HUIJING, F., WENGER, J.I., SASKO, H. and BROWN, N.B. (1968)
        in "Control of Glycogen Metabolism" (W.J. Whelan, ed.) 1,
        Academic Press, New York

(124)   SODERLING, T.R., CORBIN, J.D. and PARK, C.R. (1973) J.
        Biol. Chem., 248, 1822

(125)   WOO, Y.T. and MANERY, J.F. (1973) Arch. Biochem. Biophys.,
        154, 510

(126)   KURIYAMA, S. (1918) J. Biol. Chem., 33, 193

(127)   CORI, C.F. (1926) J. Biol. Chem., 70, 577

(128)   HERS, H.G., DE WULF, H. and STALMANS, W. (1970a) FEBS
        Letters, 12, 73

(129)   HERS, H.G., DE WULF, H., STALMANS, W. and VAN DEN BERGHE,
        G. (1970b), Advance Enzyme Regul. 8, 171

(130)   HERS, H.G., STALMANS, W., DE WULF, H., LALOUX, M. and HUE,
        L. (1974) in "Metabolic Interconversion of Enzymes 1973"
        (Fischer, E.H., Krebs, E.G., Neurath, H. and Stadtman,
        E.R., eds.), 89, Springer Verlag, Berlin, Heidelberg and
        New York

(131)   DE WULF, H. and HERS, H.G. (1968a) Eur. J. Biochem., 6, 552

(132)   BISHOP, J.S., GOLDBERG, N.D. and LARNER, J. (1971) Am. J.
        Physiol., 220, 499

(133)   BUSCHIAZZO, H., EXTON, J.H. and PARK, C.R. (1970) Proc.
        Natl. Acad. Sci. USA, 65, 383

(134)   GLINSMANN, W., PAUK, G. and HERN, E. (1970) Biochem.
        Biophys. Res. Commun., 39, 774

(135)   VAN DEN BERGHE, G., DE WULF, H. and HERS, H.G. (1970) Eur.
        J. Biochem., 16, 358

(136) VAN DE WERVE, G., VAN DEN BERGHE, G. and HERS, H.G. (1974)
       Eur. J. Biochem., 41, 97

(137) JEFFERSON, L.S., EXTON, J.H., BUTCHER, R.W., SUTHERLAND,
       E.W. and PARK, C.R. (1968) J. Biol. Chem., 243, 1031

(138) BEAVO, J.A., BECHTEL, P.J. and KREBS, E.G. (1974) Proc.
       Natl. Acad. Sci. USA, 71, 3580

(139) PAUK, G.L. and REDDY, W.J. (1971) Diabetes, 20, 129

(140) LONGLEY, R.W., BORTNICK, R.J. and ROE, J.M. (1957) Proc.
       Soc. Exptl. Biol. Med., 94, 108

(141) FRIEDMANN, B., GOODMAN, E.H. Jr. and WEINHOUSE, S. (1963)
       J. Biol. Chem., 238, 2899

(142) FRIEDMANN, B., GOODMAN, E.H. Jr. and WEINHOUSE, S. (1967)
       Endocrinology, 81, 486

(143) HORNBROOK, K.R. (1970) Diabetes, 19, 916

(144) LONG, C.N.H., KATZIN, B. and FRY, E.G. (1940) Endocrinology,
       26, 309

(145) MILLER, A.M. (1949) Proc. Soc. Exptl. Biol. Med. 72, 635

(146) TARNOWSKI, W., KITTLER, M. and HILZ, H. (1964) Biochem. Z.
       341, 45

(147) HORNBROOK, K.R., BURCH, H.B. and LOWRY, O.H. (1966) Mol.
       Pharmacol., 2, 10

(148) DE WULF, H. and HERS, H.G. (1967b) Eur. J. Biochem., 2, 57

(149) DE WULF, H. and HERS, H.G. (1968b) Eur. J. Biochem., 6, 558

(150) DE WULF, H. and HERS, H.G. (1967a) Eur. J. Biochem., 2, 50

(151) EXTON, J.H., LEWIS, S.B., HO, R.J., ROBISON, G.A. and PARK,
       C.R. (1971b) Ann. N.Y. Acad. Sci., 185, 85

(152) EXTON, J.H., LEWIS, S.B., HO, R.J. and PARK, C.R. (1972)
       Advan. Cyclic Nucl. Res., 1, 91

(153) PARK, C.R., LEWIS, S.B. and EXTON, J.H. (1972) Diabetes, 21,
       Suppl., 2, 439

(154)   WOLLENBERGER, A., RISTAU, O. and SCHOFFA, G. (1960) Arch.
        Gesamte Physiol. Menschen Tiere, 270, 399

(155)   DE WULF, H., STALMANS, W. and HERS, H.G. (1970) Eur. J.
        Biolchem., 15, 1

(156)   EISEN, H.J., GOLDFINE, I.D. and GLINSMANN, W.H. (1973)
        Proc. Natl. Acad. Sci. USA, 70, 3454

(157)   VILLAR-PALASI, C. (1969) Ann. N.Y. Acad. Sci., 166, 719

(158)   NICHOLS, W.K. and GOLDBERG, N.D. (1972) Biochim. Biophys.
        Acta, 279, 245

(159)   STEINER, C. and NEWSHOLME, E.A. (1968) Biochem. J., 107,
        411

(160)   STEINER, D.F. and KING, J. (1964) J. Biol. Chem., 239,
        1292

(161)   BISHOP, J.S., GOLDBERG, N.D. and LARNER, J. (1971) Am. J.
        Physiol., 220, 499

(162)   MILLER, T.B., Jr. and LARNER, J. (1973) J. Biol. Chem.,
        248, 3483

(163)   MADISON, L.L. (1969) Arch. Intern. Med., 123, 284

(164)   KREBS, E.G., LOVE, D.S., BRATVOLD, G.E., TRAYSER, K.A.,
        MEYER, W.L. and FISCHER, E.H. (1964) Biochemistry, 3, 1022

(165)   SCHLENDER, K.K., WEI, S.H. and VILLAR-PALASI, C. (1969),
        Biochim. Biophys. Acta, 191, 272

CYCLIC AMP AND PYRUVATE DEHYDROGENASE

H. G. Coore

Department of Biochemistry
University of Birmingham
Birmingham B15 2TT, U.K.

Contents

Introduction

The mammalian enzyme pyruvate dehydrogenase (PDH) catalyses a
coordinated series of reactions summarized as:-

$$CH_3\text{--}CO\text{--}COOH + CoA\text{--}SH + NAD \longrightarrow CH_3\text{--}\underset{O}{\overset{}{C}}\text{--}S\text{--}CoA + CO_2 + NADH + H^+$$

The enzyme is situated within the inner mitochondrial membrane. It
has been suggested that pyruvate dehydrogenase is rate limiting for
the utilization of pyruvate for fatty acid synthesis by adipose
tissue (1). Earlier work (2) indicated that in muscle the availability of fatty acids for oxidation could restrict pyruvate
utilization by inhibiting PDH. One mechanism for this inhibition

533

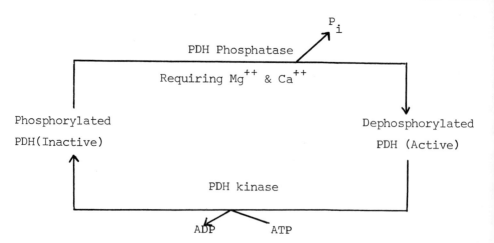

Fig. 1 <u>Activation-inactivation cycle of mammalian pyruvate dehydrogenase</u>

suggested by the above authors was an increase in the ratios of NADH/NAD and acetyl CoA/CoASH within mitochondria. This would appear to be simply product inhibition. In 1969 Linn <u>et al.</u>, (3) reported the discovery that the activity of PDH from kidney could be regulated by a phosphorylation/dephosphorylation cycle shown in Fig. 1. The phenomenon was shown to apply also to the enzyme from heart, liver, brain and adipose tissue (4,5,6,7,8). It was subsequently demonstrated that phosphorylation (by a kinase tightly bound to the multi-enzyme complex) and dephosphorylation (by a weakly associated phosphatase) were confined to serine residues in certain sub-units of the complex. These subunits catalysed the first decarboxylating step of the reaction series (9). If one defines percentage activation of PDH as the initial activity of a given enzyme preparation divided by the activity exhibited after complete dephosphorylation and multiplied by 100 then for tissues so far examined the percentage activation of extracted PDH varies between 15-70%. One imagines that in the living cell the activity of the enzyme complex is poised by the relative activities of its kinase and phosphatase. Pyruvate dehydrogenase therefore appeared to fall into the same category as glycogen phosphorylase, phosphorylase b kinase, glycogen synthetase and triglyceride lipase. In these enzymes phosphorylation of certain serine residues by the γ-phosphate group of ATP leads to a profound change in enzymic activity. This resemblance was reinforced when it appeared that hormonal treatments of adipose tissue altered the degree of phosphorylation and hence activity of PDH extracted from the tissue (1, 7). In the cases of phosphorylase b kinase, glycogen synthetase and triglyceride lipase it is generally accepted that phosphorylation is effected by cAMP activated protein kinase (10). It is the purpose of this survey to assess whether an analogous mechanism is involved in the hormonal

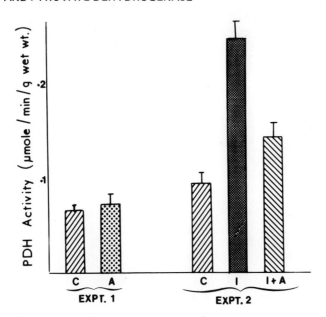

Fig. 2 <u>Effect of insulin with and without adrenalin on PDH activity of rat epididymal fat pads</u>
Following 30 min preincubation in Krebs bicarbonate containing fructose (2 mg/ml) fat pads from fed rats were incubated for a further 30 min with indicated hormones in fresh medium. C = controls, no addition: A = adrenalin present at 1 µg/ml: I = insulin present at 1 mU/ml: I + A = insulin (1 mU/ml) and adrenalin (1 µg/ml) present. Four observations were made for each group. Based on data of Coore <u>et al</u>. (1).

effects on the phosphorylation state of PDH with particular reference to adipose tissue. Essential details of methods are indicated in text or in legends to figures or tables. For other details of methods reference may be made to the original papers quoted.

Effects of Hormones on Adipose Tissue PDH
    Fig. 2 drawn from the data of Coore <u>et al</u>. (1) shows the effects of adrenalin and insulin separately or together on the apparent activity of PDH from extracted adipose tissue after incubation for 30 min <u>in vitro</u>. The mode of extraction of the enzyme (from freeze-clamped tissue using a medium containing EDTA) was designed to preserve the phosphorylation state of the enzyme. It appeared from this work and from that of Weiss <u>et al</u>., (8, 11), that insulin treatment did not alter the total amount of PDH present in the tissue but only diminished the degree of phosphorylation of the complex and hence increased its activity. Sica and Cuatrecasas (12) asserted on the contrary that the insulin effect was mainly to increase the total amount of PDH. However, these authors relied on the endogenous PDH

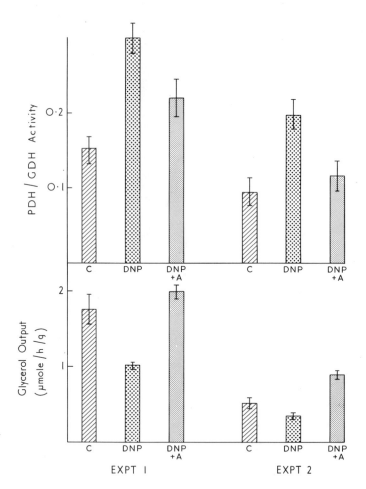

Fig. 3 Effect of adrenalin and dinitrophenol on PDH activity and
glycerol output of rat epididymal fat pads

Fat pads were preincubated in Krebs bicarbonate containing fructose
(2 mg/ml) for 30 min. Some pads were then exposed to adrenalin
(1 µg/ml) for 5 min after which these pads were transferred to
fresh media containing dinitrophenol (2 mM) and adrenalin (1 µg/ml)
for a further 20 min incubation. Other pads were exposed to DNP
only during this incubation, with no previous exposure to adrenalin.
Control pads were treated similarly except that they were not exposed
to either agent. Fructose (2 mg/ml) was present throughout.
Glycerol was measured in the medium, PDH and glutamate dehydrogenase
were measured in extracts of fat pads as described by Coore et al.(1)
C = controls: DNP = dinitrophenol present at 2 mM; DNP + A =
dinitrophenol (2 mM) and adrenalin (1 µg/ml) present. There were
four observations in each group. Glutamate dehydrogenase activity
(GDH) was used as an index of extraction recovery as explained by
Coore et al. (1).

phosphatase to achieve dephosphorylation and thus furnish an estimate of the potential activity of the enzyme. The use of exogenous
phosphatase (11) would appear a more reliable method by eliminating
ambiguity between an apparent increase in the PDH complex itself and
an increase in the activity of the associated phosphatase. We shall
assume in the subsequent discussion that all the effects observed
over short periods (30 min) are due to changes in rates of phospho-
phorylation or dephosphorylation while bearing in mind that the
constancy of the potential PDH activity has not always been demonstrated in papers reporting activity of PDH extracted from tissues.
As shown in Fig. 2 adrenalin did not by itself alter the activity
of PDH but blocked activation by insulin. Again, Sica and
Cuatrecasas (12) disagreed, reporting considerable activation of
adipose tissue PDH following in vitro incubation with adrenalin or
dibutyryl cyclic AMP. However, Taylor et al. (13) showed that when
adipose tissue is incubated for prolonged periods (> 60 min) in
the absence of substrate and the presence of adrenalin (conditions
similar to those in the experiments of Sica and Cuatrecasas) there
is a large fall in the ATP concentration of the tissue. Similar
findings had been reported earlier (14, 15). This ATP depletion
presumably diminishes the activity of pyruvate dehydrogenase kinase
(by lowering the intra-mitochondrial ATP/ADP ratio - see later).
In fact, Taylor et al. (13) showed that uncoupling agents, dinitrophenol and oligomycin in the incubation medium of adipose tissue
also activated PDH. Briefer incubations of adipose tissue in the
presence of glucose and adrenalin led to smaller but still significant falls in ATP content (14). It is likely therefore, that in the
absence of a large fall in the tissue ATP/ADP ratio the effect of
adrenalin is to diminish the activity of adipose tissue PDH.
Actually, under certain conditions adrenalin treatment can reduce
the activation of PDH due to exposure of adipose tissue to dinitrophenol (Fig. 3). It may be noted that both the papers of Taylor
et al. (13) and Halperin & Denton (14) showed no change of tissue
ATP content due to insulin. These effects of insulin and adrenalin
are reflected in observations on rates of fatty acid synthesis from
glucose and pyruvate output of adipose tissue. The stimulation by
insulin of fatty acid synthesis is of course well recognized. The
observations that adrenalin added to the incubation medium of adipose tissue diminished the rate of fatty acid synthesis from glucose
in the presence of insulin (16) and increased the output of lactate
and pyruvate (17) are obviously consistent with reduction in the
activity of PDH. Fig. 4 again drawn from data in the paper by Coore
et al. (1) shows that ACTH and dibutyryl cyclic AMP, like adrenalin,
antagonized the activation of PDH due to insulin treatment of adipose
tissue. If glycerol output from incubated fat pads is taken as an
index of lipolysis (due to low activity of glycerokinase) it would
further appear that there is an inverse correlation between rate of
lipolysis and activation of PDH. Fig. 5 based on data from Martin
et al. (18) indicates that other anti-lipolytic treatments - exposure
to ouabain and to K^+-free incubation medium led to activation of

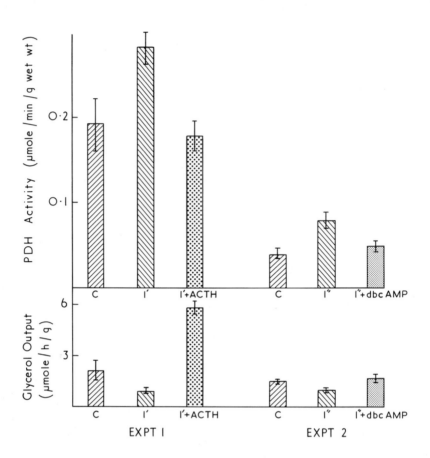

Fig. 4 <u>Effect of insulin with and without adrenocorticotrophic</u>
<u>hormone or dibutyryl cyclic AMP on PDH activity and glycerol output</u>
<u>of rat epididymal fat pads</u>
Procedure as in legend for Fig. 2 and data also from Coore <u>et al</u> (1).
C = controls, no additions: I' = insulin present at 1.25 mU/ml:
I" = insulin present at 5 mU/ml: ACTH = adrenocorticotrophic
hormone present at 2 μg/ml: dbcAMP = dibutyryl cyclic AMP present
at 1 mM. Four observations were made for each group.

adipose tissue PDH. ATP content of the tissue was not significantly
affected by these treatments. If one further assumes that lipolysis
in adipose tissue is regulated by cyclic AMP concentration in the
cells (19) then one might suppose that the phosphorylation of PDH
(and its inactivation) is directly regulated by cyclic AMP. PDH
would then be analogous in its regulation to glycogen synthetase.

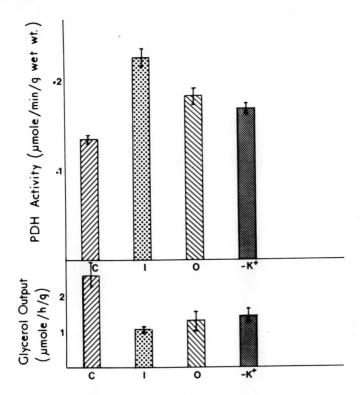

Fig. 5 Effects of insulin, ouabain and K^+ free medium on PDH acti-
vity and glycerol output of rat epididymal fat pads
Based on data of Martin et al. (18). Procedure as in legend for
Fig. 2. Other details given in above reference.
C = controls: I = insulin present at 2 mU/ml: 0 = ouabain present
at 300 μM: $-K^+$ = k^+ free medium for incubation.
There were eight observations in each group.

There are however many observations that cannot easily be reconciled
with this view.

Failure in Inverse Correlation of Lipolysis Rate with PDH Activity
of Adipose Tissue
        Table 1 lists data from which it can be seen that at the given
concentrations prostaglandin E_1 and 5-methyl-pyrazole-3 carboxylate
were as effective as insulin in reducing the rate of lipolysis in
incubated adipose tissue but were without significant effect on
pyruvate dehydrogenase. In contrast to these results Taylor et al.
(13) were unable to find concentrations of these two substances which
were anti-lipolytic and yet did not activate pyruvate dehydrogenase.
Taylor et al.noted occasional inconsistencies between different

batches of rats in the relative effectiveness of agents which stimulated PDH and suggested that such differences might underlie the conflict of data. Weiss et al. (11) found that prostaglandin E_1 stimulated adipose tissue PDH only if the tissue was from fasted-refed
rats. The data could be summarized by saying that, compared to any
given control situation, a reduction in lipolysis rate (and by implication a fall in intra-cellular cyclic AMP concentration) is a
contributary but not sufficient condition for activation of adipose
tissue PDH. It would be desirable to have actual measurements of
cyclic AMP and PDH in adipose tissue in the same experiments but I
am unaware of such studies. In other tissues there is also a need
for such correlative studies. Patzelt et al. (20) could find no
effect of insulin or glucagon on % activation of PDH in perfused
liver though an increase in % activation followed injection of

Agent	Effect on pyruvate dehydrogenase activity compared to controls	Effect on glycerol output from fat pads	Reference
Prostaglandin E_1 (1 µg/ml)	− 21%	− 60% *	1
Insulin (1.25 mU/ml)	+ 46% *	− 56% *	1
Prostaglandin E_1 (10 µg/ml)	+ 17%	− 51% *	18
Insulin (2 mU/ml)	+ 55% *	− 51% *	18
5-Methyl pyrazole-3 -carboxylate (10 µM)	0%	− 30%*	18
Insulin (2 mU/ml)	+ 64% *	− 30%*	18

Table 1: Effects of insulin, prostaglandin E_1 and 5-methyl
pyrazole-3-carboxylate on PDH activity and glycerol
output of rat epididymal fat pads

*significantly different from appropriate control at $p < 0.05$.

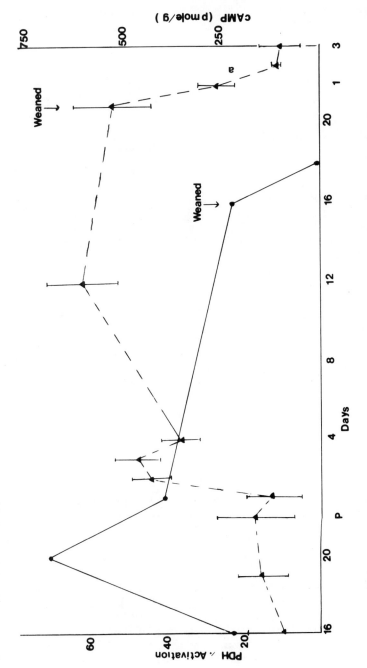

Fig. 6   Percentage activation of PDH and cyclic AMP content of rat mammary tissue during pregnancy
lactation and weaning
Based on data of Coore & Field (24) and Sapag-Hagar & Greenbaum (23)

● — ● — ●   cAMP concentration;   ▲ — ▲ — ▲   PDH % activation (explained in text)
Horizontal axis: days of pregnancy 16, 20;   P = parturition;   days of lactation 4,8,12,16,20;
days of weaning after full term 1,3.

insulin into the intact animal (21). However, insulin had little
effect on cyclic AMP concentration in perfused liver from normal
rats (22). In the case of rat mammary tissue Sapag-Hagar &
Greenbaum (23) have published data on cyclic AMP concentration
during pregnancy and lactation. Fig. 6 compares their data with
that of Coore & Field (24) on % activation of PDH over the same
period. Unfortunately the data are sparse and the picture is not
clear in that during early lactation an increase of % activation of
PDH accompanied the fall in cyclic AMP while during weaning both
parameters fell together.

Attempts to Demonstrate Direct Effects of cyclic AMP on the PDH Complex

A report by wieland & Siess (25) that cyclic AMP promoted
phosphorylation of the PDH phosphatase and that its activity was
thereby increased has not been confirmed (26) and in any case this
would not be the expected direction of effect. Activation of the
PDH kinase by cyclic AMP analogous to the activation of protein
kinase has been looked for but not found (27,28). Regulation of PDH
kinase by means of a dissociable regulator unit binding cyclic AMP
would therefore seem unlikely. The only reservation that one might
make for experiments with purified PDH is that extraction of PDH
from mitochondria is always incomplete and it is just possible that
such a regulator unit might be left behind. The possibility that
cyosolic cyclic AMP might act on isolated mitochondria to influence
in some way the activity of PDH has also been investigated (1).
The experiments involved exposure of adipocyte mitochondria to incubation media with and without ATP alone or plus diluted cytosol
or protein kinase. Cyclic AMP was without effect on the activity
of PDH extracted from mitochondria thus treated though extra-
mitochondrial ATP caused a reduction in activity of the enzyme.

Possible Roles for cyclic AMP in Pyruvate Dehydrogenase Regulation

The experiments reviewed above lead to an apparent paradox.
According to current belief insulin, adrenalin and ACTH act at the
plasma membrane of the fat cell to alter the internal concentration
of cyclic AMP and thereby influence intracellular processes and yet
in this instance we are unable to detect any intervention by cyclic
AMP in the process itself. There are at least three possible explanations.
(a) Cytosolic cyclic AMP concentration is irrelevant to PDH control.
This seems unlikely in view of the data quoted at the beginning of
this article and would involve accepting a failure of the "second
messenger hypothesis". Although Weiss et al. (11) state that the
effect of insulin on adipose tissue PDH from normally fed rats is
dependent on stimulation of membrane transport of metabolizable
sugar this was not the case for adipose tissue from fasted-refed
rats nor in the experiments of Coore et al. (1) and Jungas (7).
In any case adrenalin does not diminish the effect of insulin on

	Experimentally controlled factors	Tissues	Effect: Increase (+) or decrease (−) in % activation of PDH	Refs.
EXTRA-CELLULAR FACTORS	Insulin	Adipose tissue	+	1, 7
	Adrenalin, ACTH	Adipose tissue	−	1, 7
	Free fatty acid and aceto-acetate	Liver, heart, kidney, adipose tissue	−	13, 20
	Pyruvate or metabolizable sugar	Adipose tissue, liver	+	13, 20
EXTRA-MITOCHONDRIAL FACTORS	Pyruvate	Adipose tissue, liver mitochondria	+	18, 36
	ADP	liver mitochondria	+	36
	ATP	Adipose tissue, liver mitochondria	−	1, 33
	Palmitoyl-1 (−) carnitine	liver mitochondria	−	36
	3-hydroxy-butyrate	liver mitochondria	−	36
INTRA-MITOCHONDRIAL FACTORS	Diminished ATP/ADP ratio	Adipose tissue, liver mitochondria	+	18, 33
	Depleted Ca^{++}	Adipose tissue, liver mitochondria	−	33, 37

Table 2 : Some factors affecting PDH activation.

Addition to Incubation Medium	Glycerol output μmole/h/g wet wt.	Ratio of activities PDH to glutamate dehydrogenase	Effect of insulin on PDH compared to appropriate control
Control: no addition	1.27 ± .04	0.056 ± .003	
	*	*	
Insulin (10 mU/ml)	0.74 ± .05	0.097 ± .009	+ 73%
4-Pentenoic Acid (0.4 mM)	1.08 ± .03	0.076 ± .01	
	*	*	
4-Pentenoic Acid (0.4 mM) + Insulin (10 mU/ml)	0.74 ± .04	0.127 ± .007	+ 67%

Table 3:   Effects of insulin and 4-Pentenoic acid on PDH activity and glycerol output of incubated rat epididymal fat pads

After 30 min pre-incubation in Krebs bicarbonate containing fructose (10 mM) fat pads were incubated for a further 30 min in the same medium with additions as indicated. Glycerol was measured in the incubation medium and enzyme activities in extracts of freeze-clamped fat pads. The extraction medium was 100 mM phosphate containing EDTA (2 mM), pH 7. Means and standard errors are based on four observations. The use of glutamate dehydrogenase as an index of extraction recovery is explained by Coore et al. (1).

*p< 0.01 for differences of means.

membrane transport (14) and hence antagonistic effects of the two hormones on PDH cannot originate there.
(b) Cyclic AMP acts in concert with another "second messenger" e.g. Ca^{++} (29) or cyclic GMP. The role of Ca^{++} will be referred to again below. Relatively little attention has been devoted to the possible role of cyclic GMP though Illiano et al. (30) have shown it to increase transiently in fat cells exposed to insulin. Hucho et al. (27) and Cooper et al. (28) did not find any effects of cyclic GMP on purified PDH kinase. According to Illiano et al. (30) carbachol and acetyl choline were as effective as insulin in increasing fat cell cyclic GMP concentration. In a few preliminary experiments I did not find any influence of these agents on adipose tissue PDH. It might be interesting however to test the effect of a combination

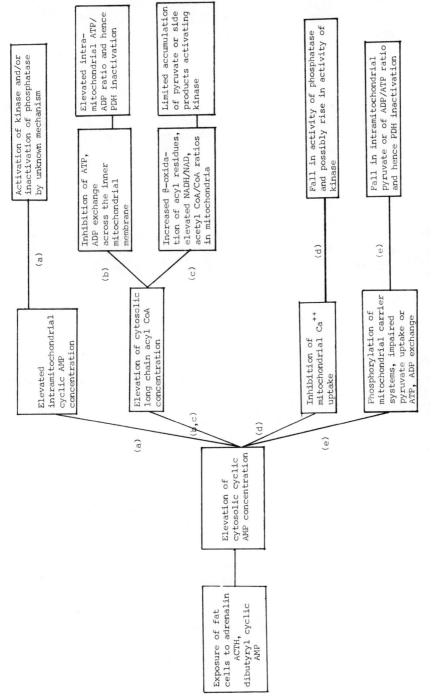

Fig. 7 Hypothetical mechanisms of effects of hormones on PDH of adipose tissue
Note. "Kinase" and "phosphate" refer to the specific enzymes associated with
the PDH complex.

of agents which affect cyclic AMP and cyclic GMP independently.
(c) Cyclic AMP influences the concentration of some other cytosolic
or mitochondrial factor which in turn alters the relative activities
of PDH kinase and/or PDH phosphatase. Table 2 lists some factors
which have been shown by various workers to affect these activities
by acting on the intact cell ("extra cellular factors"), the isolated
mitochondria ("extra-mitochondrial factors") or extracted PDH
("intra-mitochondrial factors"). An increase of intra-mitochondrial
pyruvate or ADP is supposed to act by inhibiting the PDH kinase and
a fall in intra-mitochondrial ATP is supposed to act by freeing
bound Mg^{++} required for the activity of PDH phosphatase (4, 27).
Depletion of Ca^{++} may act by weakening the binding of PDH phosphatase to the complex (31, 32). Inhibition of PDH kinase by Ca^{++} in
the range 10^{-8} - 10^{-5}M has also been noted (28). Fig. 7 sets out
hypothetical schemes whereby cytosolic cyclic AMP would influence
these factors in adipocytes. Possibility (a) has been discussed
above. Possibility (b) has been advanced by Wieland & Portenhauser
(33). This has the merit of explaining the effects of insulin and
adrenalin on adipose tissue PDH in terms of changes in tissue concentrations of long-chain acyl-CoA (see (17)) and also the effects
of fatty acids on liver, heart and kidney PDH extensively studied
by Wieland and co-workers (33). However, it remains to be demonstrated that in the conditions prevailing in the adipocyte reported
cytosolic concentrations of long-chain acyl-CoA would in fact have
the postulated effect on mitochondrial ATP/ADP levels. This scheme
may not fully explain the effect of insulin. The experimental results of Table 3 show that 4-pentenoic acid, which inhibits fatty
acid utilization possibly by sequestering CoA (34) did not prevent
insulin from further activating adipose tissue PDH.

Possibility (c) has been suggested by Cooper et al. (28). It
appears that low concentrations of pyruvate ($<$100 µM) or acetoin
(a possible side product of PDH catalysis) may activate PDH kinase.
Higher concentrations of pyruvate, as mentioned earlier, inhibit
PDH kinase. Possibility (d) is raised by the work of Borle (35).
Possibility (e) has up to now no published experimental support.

In general, as can be seen further resolution of the problem
requires methods for determination of metabolite and ion content of
mitochondria in situ or removed from tissues with a minimum of dis-
turbance - a formidable technical challenge.

Financial support from the Wellcome Trust is gratefully
acknowledged.

REFERENCES

1. Coore, H.G., Denton, R.M., Martin, B.R. & Randle, P.J. (1971)
    Biochem. J. 124, 115

2. Garland, P.B. & Randle, P.J. (1964) Biochem. J. 91, 6C

3. Linn, Tracy C., Pettit, Flora H. & Reed, L.J. (1969) Proc. Natl.
    Acad. Sci. U.S. 62, 234

4. Linn, Tracy C., Pettit, Flora H., Hucho, F. & Reed, L.J. (1969)
    Proc. Natl. Acad. Sci. U.S. 64, 227

5. Wieland, O. & von Jagow-Westermann, B. (1969) FEBS Lett. 3, 271

6. Siess, E., Wittmann, J. & Wieland, O. (1971) Hoppe-Seyler's Z.
    Physiol. Chem. 352, 447

7. Jungas, R.L. (1971) Metabolism 20, 43

8. Weiss, L., Loffler, G., Schirmann, A. & Wieland, O. (1971)
    FEBS Lett. 15, 229

9. Roche, T.E. & Reed, L.J. (1972) Biochem. Biophys. Res. Commun.
    48, 840

10. Robison, G.A., Butcher, R.W. & Sutherland, E.W. (1971) Cyclic AMP.
    Academic Press, New York and London

11. Weiss, L., Loffler, G. & Wieland, O.H. (1974) Hoppe-Seyler's Z.
    Physiol. Chem. 355, 363

12. Sica, V. & Cuatrecasas, P. (1973) Biochemistry 12, 2282

13. Taylor, S.I., Mukkerjee, C. & Jungas, R.L. (1973) J. Biol. Chem.
    248, 73

14. Halperin, M.L. & Denton, R.M. (1969) Biochem. J. 113, 207

15. Bihler, I. & Jeanrenand, B. (1970) Biochim. Biophys. Acta
    202, 496

16. Denton, R.M. & Randle, P.J. (1967) Biochem. J. 104, 423

17. Denton, R.M. & Halperin, M.L. (1968) Biochem. J. 110, 27

18. Martin, B.R., Denton, R.M., Pask, H.T. & Randle, P.J. (1972)
    Biochem. J. 129, 763

19. Butcher, R.W. (1970) in Adipose Tissue:Regulation and metabolic
    functions, (Ed. by Jeanrenand, B. & Hepp, D) p.5 London,
    Academic Press.

20. Patzelt, C., Loffler, G. & Wieland, O.H. (1973) Eur. J. Biochem.
    33, 117

21. Wieland, O.H., Patzelt, C. & Loffler, G. (1972) Eur. J. Biochem.
    26, 426

22. Park, C.R., Lewis, S.B. & Exton, J.H. (1972) In Insulin Action.
    (Ed. by I.B. Fritz) p.509, Academic Press, New York & London

23. Sapag-Hagar & Greenbaum, A.L. (1973) Biochem. Biophys. Res.
    Commun. 53, 982

24. Coore, H.G. & Field, Barbara. (1974) Biochem. J. 142, 87

25. Wieland, O. & Siess, E. (1970) Proc. Natl. Acad. Sci. U.S.
    65, 947

26. Hucho, F. (1974) Eur. J. Biochem. 46, 499

27. Hucho, F., Randall, D.D., Roche, T.E., Burgett, M.W., Pellery,
    J.W. & Reed, L.J. (1972) Arch. Biochem. Biophys. 151, 328

28. Cooper, R.H., Randle, P.J. & Denton, R.M. (1974) Biochem. J.
    143, 625

29. Rasmussen, H. (1970) Science 170, 404

30. Illiano, G., Tell, G.P.E., Siegel, M.I. & Cuatrecasas, P.
    Proc. Natl. Acad. Sci. U.S. 70, 2443

31. Denton, R.M., Randle. P.J. & Martin, B.R. (1972) Biochem. J.
    128, 161

32. Pettit, Flora H., Roche, T.E. & Reed, L.J. (1972) Biochem.
    Biophys. Res. Commun. 49, 563

33. Wieland, O.H. & Portenhauser, R. (1974) Eur. J. Biochem. 45, 577

34. Loken, S.C. & Fain, J.N. (1971) Am. J. Physiol. 221, 1126

35. Borle, A. (1973) Fed. Proc. 32, 1944

36. Portenhauser, R. & Wieland, O. (1972) Eur. J. Biochem. 31, 308

37. Severson, D.L., Denton, R.M., Pask, H.T. & Randle, P.J. (1974)
    Biochem. J. 140, 225

CYCLIC AMP AND PROTEIN SYNTHESIS

J.E. Loeb

Institut de Recherches Scientifiques sur le Cancer
B.P. N° 8, 94-Villejuif (France)

Contents

Introduction
Suppression of enzyme induction
References

INTRODUCTION

In contrast to the consistent stimulation of lipolysis and glycogenolysis in most tissues, the effects of cyclic AMP (cAMP) on protein synthesis are tissue dependent.

Table I below lists some examples where the influence of various effectors on protein synthesis is mediated via cAMP. The suggested level(s) of regulation is also indicated. (More complete discussion of the literature can be found in the excellent review by Wicks (1).)

It appears that cAMP usually induces the synthesis of only selected proteins and that there are only a few general effects, either positive or negative. In tissues responding with a general increase in protein synthesis (anterior pituitary, thyroid) this stimulation may be explained as the sum of an increase in specific proteins. In adipose tissue, the general decrease of protein synthesis, following cAMP or epinephrine administration, is attributed to ATP depletion secondary to the cAMP mediated lipolysis.

549

TABLE I

TISSUE	EFFECTOR	EFFECT	SITE OF ACTION
Adrenal cortex (2)	ACTH* dBcAMP*	Enzyme induction for steroid bio-synthesis	Translation
Gonads (3)	LH	Enzyme induction for steroid bio-synthesis	Translation
Anterior pituitary (4)	dB cAMP	General increase in protein synthesis	Translation
Thyroid (5)	TSH	Increase of protein synthesis	Translation?
Adipose tissue (6)	dB cAMP	General inhibition of protein synthesis	?
Neural tissue (7, 8)	dB cAMP Epinephrine adrenalin	Induction of tyrosine hydroxylase	?
Melanocytes (9) melanoma	MSH	Induction of tyro-sinase	?
Fibroblasts (10, 11)	PGE_1 dB cAMP	Induction of phospho-diesterase	Translation?

dBcAMP : dibutyryl cyclic AMP
ACTH   : adrenocorticotropic hormone
LH   : luteinizing hormone
TSM   : thyrotropic stimulating hormone
MSH   : melanocyte stimulating hormone

Caution must be exercised when distinguishing a true increase in protein content from a mere activation of the existing enzyme templates. This may be most accurately assessed by immunochemical quantitation of the enzyme antigen, though with all the requisite precautions. However, this necessitates a prior purification of the enzyme to homogeneity with a view to preparing specific antibodies. Inhibition by antimetabolites is an argument very often used suggesting effect of cAMP on protein synthesis, but the antibiotics used for this purpose have been reported to exert side effects that might secondarily result in the decreased activity (12). On the other hand, inhibitors with known mechanism of action (actinomycin, cycloheximide) are useful in elucidating the possible step(s) of protein synthesis susceptible to cAMP.

Furthermore, it should be noted that enzymes induced by cAMP also respond to other hormones and stimuli (see the section on the liver). Late effects on enzyme induction may most easily be explained as an indirect consequence of differentiation or maturation of the tissue stimulated by cAMP.

The increase in the rate of protein synthesis following cAMP administration varies with tissues and the nature of the protein(s) in question, although this is generally lower than that caused by the steroids. It is important to bear in mind that the circadian rhythms may provoke unsuspected variations. However, these may be minimized by including a control with each determination, and by conducting experiments at times when the rate of synthesis is lowest. Indeed, the cAMP content of the tissues may itself exhibit diurnal variations (13) leading to secondary retroactive adjustments in parameters under study.

Most of the studies on cAMP and protein synthesis had been conducted in the liver which responds well to hormones, where extensive biochemical information is available, and where cAMP exerts primarily a selective and not a general influence on protein synthesis. After administration of glucagon a small decrease (20 to 30 %) in total amino acid incorporation is however observed (14), although the proportion of active polysomes, remains unchanged (15). At the same time, cAMP increases the rate of degradation of proteins and stimulates the transport of selected amino acids. Thus the effects of cAMP on total protein synthesis in liver appear to be indirect.

In the intact rat liver, serine dehydrase (16), tyrosine transaminase (17), phosphoenol-pyruvate carboxykinase (18, 19) and ornithine decarboxylase (20) are induced, by both glucagon and dbcAMP, and in liver cells in culture (hepatoma cells or hepatoblasts) by dbcAMP or other derivatives of cAMP. It is not known

whether the microsomal enzymes of detoxification, like arylhydro-
carbon benzoapyrene hydroxylase, which are induced by their substrates and by steroids (31), are responsive to cAMP.

SUPPRESSION OR ENZYME INDUCTION

In rat liver glucagon or dbcAMP can also prevent the induction of a number of enzymes : the ability of glucose infusion to
elevate glucokinase activity (which is sensitive to inhibition by
cycloheximide) is also suppressed by glucagon, epinephrine, or
dbcAMP (22). Furthermore, the induction of glucose-6-phosphate
dehydrogenase and fatty acid synthetase, in response to feeding,
is suppressed by glucagon and dbcAMP (23, 24). These results
suggest that cAMP normally exerts both positive and negative
effects on the synthesis of specific proteins in the liver. The
enzymes induced by cAMP are primarily associated with catabolic
reactions and glucose synthesis. In contrast to this, at the same
time, enzymes subject to negative effects by cAMP are involved in
glucose utilization and lipogenesis (1).

Some more precise examples on the mode of action of cAMP in
the regulation of specific hepatic enzyme synthesis are given below,
taken from Wicks et al. (25). As already mentioned, the synthesis
of these enzymes can also be induced by other hormones such as
steroids and insulin, though possibly via different mechanisms.
Other effectors, such as amino acids, are also active though after
prolonged fasting and there may again be mediation by cAMP.

Figure 1, taken from Wicks et al. (26), shows the temporal
change in rat liver of carbokinase and transaminase activities and
glycogen content, following administration of dbcAMP.

It is evident that glycogen depletion (through activation of
phosphorylase) follows a doubling of liver tyrosine transaminase
and PEP carboxykinase within 2-3 hours after cAMP treatment.

This increase in activity is a consequence of a net synthesis
of these enzymes as evidenced by immunoprecipitation of carboxykinase protein (26). The effects are similar in intact animal and
in cultured hepatoma cells.

Liver PEP carboxykinase, like tyrosine transaminase, can be
induced by steroids, such as dexamethasone, but it is very unlikely
that the effects of the corticoid are mediated by cAMP. Thus,
corticoids and cAMP exert antagonistic effects on glycogen synthesis; PEP carboxykinase is not induced by corticoids in organ
culture under conditions where tyrosine transaminase is extremely

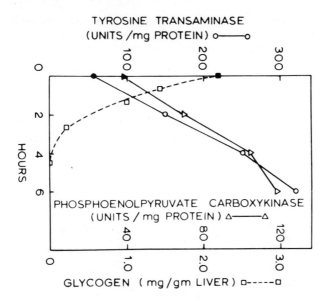

<u>FIGURE 1</u>. *Male rats, 100–125 g previously fed a low protein diet*
were injected intraperitoneally every 90 minutes with 2 mg dbcAMP
and 2 mg theophylline. At the intervals indicated the rats were
killed by decapitation and their livers removed.
Standard erros were less than 5 %.

▫ ‒ ‒ ‒▫	*Glycogen*
Δ ——— Δ	*PEP carboxykinase*
O ——— O	*tyrosine transaminase*

responsive, but both enzymes are sensitive to dbcAMP. The effects
of dexamethasone and dbcAMP are additive. Further differences are
evident by the fact that progesterone, which competes with glucocorticoids for binding to cytoplasmic receptor proteins, and inhibits the induction of transaminase and carboxykinase by dexamethasone, does not inhibit the induction of these enzymes by dbcAMP.
Insulin can also induce tyrosine transaminase but has no effect on
carboxykinase under conditions in which the two enzymes are
induced by dbcAMP (26).

Cyclic AMP influences the synthesis of tyrosine transaminase
and PEP carboxykinase in a very transient manner. After removal
of dbcAMP from the medium, in the case of cultured hepatoma cells,
the rate of synthesis returns abruptly to the basal state (25).

The rapid but transient nature of this influence of cAMP on both
enzymes suggests action at a post-transcriptional step. Experiments with actinomycin D also favour this possibility. It is
evident from Figure 2, taken from Wicks and McKibbin (27) that
actinomycin D does not block the early response to dbcAMP although
the response to dexamethasone is antagonized by this antibiotic.
In contrast, the regulation of synthesis of some proteins in the
liver by cAMP, serine dehydratase in particular, is perhaps effected
at a transcriptional level as indicated by the kinetics of induction
and its inhibition by actinomycin D (28).

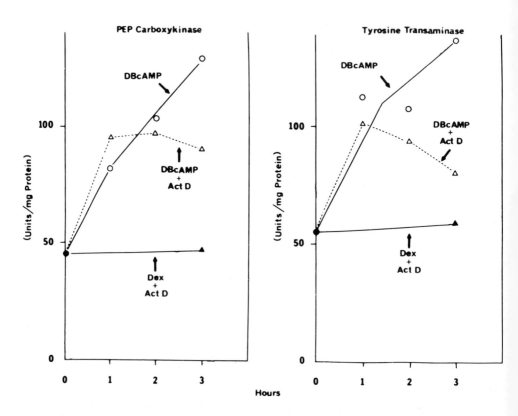

FIGURE 2. Effects of actinomycin D on the early response of transaminase and carboxykinase to dbcAMP and dexamethasone. Confluent
H35 cultures were placed in medium free of serum 16 hours before
additions.   Actinomycin D was added at 0.1 uM and dbcAMP at 0.5
mM. Incubation was continued for the intervals indicated and the
cells were harvested, lysed, and enzyme assays performed.
O control cultures :
    O———O dbcAMP added to control cultures,
    Δ----Δ dbcAMP and actinomycin D added to control cultures
Δ dexamethasone and actinomycin D added to control cultures.

What is the molecular mechanism of action of cyclic AMP ? It seems well established that the effects of cAMP in eukaryotes are mediated through the activation of a protein kinase which is able to phosphorylate a number of proteins (29). On the other hand, no kinase activity has actually been demonstrated in bacteria and cAMP is seen to act at the transcriptional level promoting the binding of the cap protein to the promotor region.

By assessing the relative efficiency of a series of P-substituted analogues of cAMP on induction of tyrosine transaminase, and on activation of protein kinase in vitro (Figure 3), Wicks et al. (25) have recently provided evidence that cAMP dependent protein phosphorylation may be involved in enzyme induction. There is a significant degree of correlation between the two parameters.

Which phosphorylated substrates may participate in the regulation of synthesis of specific proteins by cAMP ?

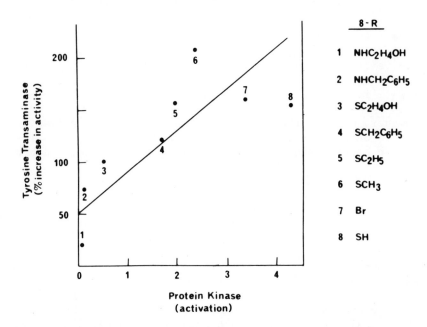

FIGURE 3. Correlation of effects of 8-substituted cAMP analogues on tyrosine transaminase induction in H35 cells and protein kinase activation in vitro. Confluent H35 cultures were placed in serum-free medium 16 hours prior to addition of analogues. The analogues were all added at 0.5 mM. Five hours later, cells were harvested, lysed, and enzyme assays performed. Correlation coefficient is 0.80 with a P value of 0.02. The numbers refer to the substituent in the 8 positions (8-H = cyclic AMP) of each analogue.

At the transcriptional level, in the nucleus, the phosphoproteins such as histones and non-histone chromatin proteins (NHP)
are generally believed to exert negative and positive control,
respectively.

- Histones are very good substrates for cAMP-dependent protein
kinase, they are phosphorylated in vivo but only phosphorylation
of histone f 1 is stimulated in vivo by cAMP (30). This phosphorylation can be responsible for the induction of serine dehydratase
although the mechanism is not known.

- Non-histone chromatin proteins are phosphorylated in vitro
by cAMP-independent protein kinases (31). But Johnson and Allfrey
(32) observed that the phosphorylation of 2 NHP was doubled after
administration of glucagon. Although in Escherichia coli a factor
of RNA polymerase can be phosphorylated in vitro by cAMP-dependent
protein kinase (33) as yet there is no evidence for this in
eukaryotes.

Nucleolar proteins are phosphorylated in vitro by a cAMP-
independent kinase (34, 35) while in vivo, the mechanism of their
phosphorylation is not yet known. There can also be a regulation
in nuclei at the posttranscriptional level (splitting of giant-RNA
by specific nucleases) or phosphorylation of proteins from nuclear
mRNP (36). Proteins of nuclear membranes can also be phosphorylated.

However, most of the effects of cAMP on protein synthesis are
believed to be at the translational level, not only in the liver
but also in other tissues such as the adrenals, gonads, and hypophysis.

At the translational level the specific mechanisms of regulation of protein synthesis are very poorly understood. But this
should not impair the search for phosphoproteins among the proteins that might intervene in the machinery for protein synthesis.

Phosphoproteins appear to form a part of ribosomal constituents as evidenced by ^{32}P administration in rat liver (37-38),
rabbit reticulocytes (39) rat sarcoma cells (40), bovine anterior
hypophysis gland (41), and mouse mammary gland (42). Phosphorylated ribosomal proteins have even been found in the plant Lemna
minor (43). Rat liver ribosomes, purified by magnesium precipitation, contain 0.5 µg phosphorus per mg protein (37), which
implies approximately 10 phosphate groups per ribosome but not
necessarily 10 different phosphoproteins, since some phosphorylated proteins may contain more than one phosphate group.

The range of ribosomal proteins is extensive. Among the phosphoproteins found in the ribosomes, some form the structural

elements of the subunits, but others may play an active role in
translation. The proteins of the mRNP could also be considered
as associated ribosomal proteins in a wider sense. The presence
of two phosphoproteins in purified mRNP has been shown by two
different groups : in ascites cells by Egly et al., 1972 (44),
and in duck reticulocytes by Grander et al., 1973 (46). It is not
yet known if cAMP has an influence on the phosphorylation of the
proteins of the mRNP, although at least two of them can be phosphorylated in vitro by a cAMP-dependent protein kinase (M. Pierre,
unpublished).

Phosphorylation of ribosomal proteins is perhaps not restricted
to eucaryotes. However, except for the work of Kuo and Greengard
(46), the attempt to demonstrate protein kinases and phosphoproteins
in E. Coli has been fruitless, although a recent publication (47)
indicates that, after phage T7 infection in E. Coli, a protein
kinase is induced and the phosphorylation of some ribosomal proteins in vivo is observed.

In rat liver, the phosphorus of ribosomal proteins was mostly
found on structural ribosomal proteins. After extraction at high
ionic strength, 80 % of alkalinelabile ^{32}P remained attached to
ribosomal particles (48).

Among the proteins extracted at high ionic strength and which
remained at the top of the gradient (Figure 4), three or four
radioactive components were detected in the subsequent one dimensional gel electrophoresis.

These components may be ribosome-associated factors or proteins from bound mRNP which are at least partially dissociated
from the mRNA at high ionic strength. It should be noted that
electrophoresis was performed at pH 4.5 and that acidic proteins
do not migrate at this pH. As some radioactivity remained in the
slot, electrophoresis performed at basic pH could indicate the
presence of more phosphoproteins.

Phosphoproteins resisting extraction at high ionic strength
were mainly localized on the small subunit (Figure 4).

Most of the labelling was in band M which seems to be composed of two components; bi-dimensional electrophoresis should
elucidate this point. A slower migrating band L was always
visible. Three or four weakly labelled bands were also observed
in the large subunit. Those corresponding to band M may be a
contamination from the small subunit. The preferential in vivo
phosphorylation in the small subunit of ribosomes of rat liver
is comparable to the results of Kabat (39) who found one major
labelled protein in the small subunit from reticulocytes after

dissociation with EDTA. M band is probably identical to the protein II of Kabat although they are derived from different tissues. Bitte and Kabat 1972 (40) described the same patterns of _in vivo_ phosphorylation in reticulocytes and sarcomas.

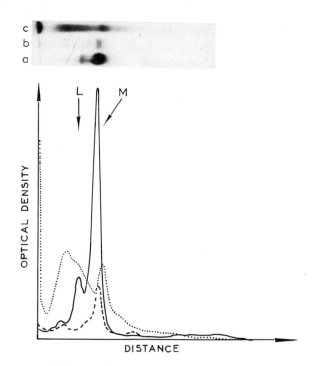

FIGURE 4. _Autoradiographic patterns of proteins from ribosomal subunits and supernatant, under the conditions described in the text. Densitometry of the autoradiograms (a,————) small subunit (b,......) large subunit (c,........) supernatant. Pierre et al. (48)._

In the plant _Lemna minor_, Trewawas (43) also found one ribosomal protein, located on the small subunit, and heavily labelled _in vivo_.

More recently, Wool (49) and Stahl and Bielka (50) observed that, after ^{32}P injection in rat liver, the radioactivity was mainly localized on the small subunit; after two dimensional electrophoresis they found a major radioactive spot (M6 according to Wool's nomenclature and S9 according to Stahl and Bielka's).

In rat liver, if the same proteins from free and bound polysomes are labelled X (Figure 5), M is more strongly labelled in boun polyribosomes, whereas L is predominantly labelled in free polysomes

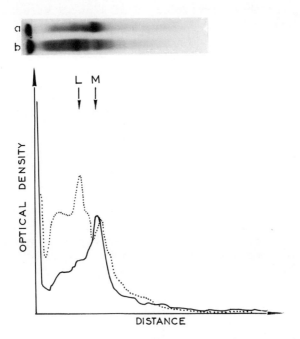

FIGURE 5. *Autoradiographic patterns of proteins from bound and free polysomes densitometry of the autoradiograms (a,————) bound polysomes (b,......) free polysomes. Pierre et al. (48).*

Ribosomal proteins from different tissues are also phosphorylated in vitro by a cAMP-dependent protein kinase (37, 51, 52).

In rat liver, with the 80 S polysomes as substrate in bidimensional electrophoresis, ten proteins appear phosphorylated (53, 54); under these conditions the similar proteins from reticulocyte polysomes are also found phosphorylated. More proteins are phosphorylated (52) if one takes the subunits as substrate instead of the 80 S polysomes.

In yeast, at least 8 ribosomal proteins can be phosphorylated by a muscle protein kinase (Pierre and Loeb, unpublished data).

In vitro studies should be interpreted with caution, since the artificial conditions may expose sites inaccessible in vivo. The meaning of soluble cytoplasmic kinase is questionable. This may represent more or less tightly bound protein kinases or multienzyme complexes that are dislocated during tissue homogenization.

However, the cell contains kinases that are not cAMP dependent. In vitro GTP-dependent phosphorylation is also accomplished by a cAMP-independent protein kinase (55, 56).

In vivo, the phosphorylation of at least 2 structural ribosomal proteins appears to be stimulated by cAMP.

In rat liver an increase of 200 % to 300 % in ^{32}P labelling of phosphoproteins is observed after glucagon injection (57). In vivo stimulation of phosphorylation by cAMP has also been found in anterior pituitary, mammary gland and reticulocytes (58). It seems that cAMP increases the turnover of the phosphate groups and not the quantity of phosphate (58, 59).

The turnover of phosphate in ribosomal proteins was much higher than that of the ribosomal proteins themselves (60). Ribosomal proteins should thus be dephosphorylated on the ribosome by a phosphatase. It has been shown by different authors that in the cytoplasm of different eucaryotic tissues, one can find at least two different types of phosphoprotein phosphatases capable of releasing phosphorus from phosphoproteins. The muscle glycogen synthetase phosphatase (61) can dephosphorylate ribosomal proteins in situ (on the ribosomes).

Incubation of ribosomes with muscle protein phosphatase showed disappearance of label (Table II).

TABLE II. Dephosphorylation of phosphorylated ribosomes by a muscle phosphatase

Phosphorylated ribosomes (specific radioactivity of 35,200 cpm per mg RNA) were incubated in assay medium described in (65) with rabbit muscle phosphatase (600 μg per ml; specific activity of 0.13 nanomoles of ^{32}P phosphate liberated/min/mg ptein and the radioactivity of the extracted ribosomal proteins was counted.

	Control	Incubation time	
		5 min	30 min
	CPM/mg protein		
Specific radioactivity of protein extracted from ribosomes (cpm per mg)	45860	10650	9200
per cent control	100	23	20

Taken from Perlès and Loeb (64).

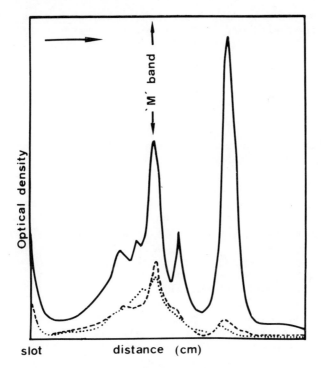

FIGURE 6. *Dephosphorylation of phosphorylated ribosomes by a muscle protein phosphatase.* ——— *control;* ········ *assay 5 min;* ------- *assay 30 min; Perlès and Loeb (64).*

However, when ribosomal proteins extracted with acetic acid were electrophoresed at pH 4.5 in 6 M urea and, subsequently autoradiographed, the different ribosomal proteins were not dephosphorylated at the same rate (Figure 6). The labelling in most of the bands of the autoradioelectrophoregram disappeared almost completely after 5 minutes of incubation, whereas a band in the middle of the electrophoregram retained an appreciable part of its radioactivity even after 30 minutes of incubation. The position of this band corresponds to the M band which exhibits the heaviest labelling in vivo.

Physiological regulation of phosphoprotein phosphatase activity by cAMP (62) and by insulin (63) has been described. That these may also modulate the ribosomal phosphoprotein phosphatase activity is an attractive possibility.

At the present time there is no direct evidence for a change in ribosome function following phosphorylation.

Experiments comparing some properties of in vitro phosphorylated ribosomes with native ribosomes (66) have failed to show
significant differences but this is not very surprising if one
remembers that cAMP induces a specific increase in synthesis of
only some proteins. Experiments with either pure or at least
enriched fractions of messengers for these proteins may afford
some elucidation or an eventual reason for the phosphorylation of
ribosomal proteins.

Since in vivo phosphorylation was essentially observed in the
small subunit, to which initiation factors and mRNA appear to bind,
it is tempting to postulate that phosphorylation is required for
the initiation of eucaryotic protein synthesis. Perhaps the phosphorylation of proteins of the small subunit may locally modify
the structure of the ribosome, and render it recognizable by a
specific signal(s) on the messenger, or modify the binding of the
initiation factors.

It should be remembered that these studies have been conducted with ribosomes artificially phosphorylated in vitro. It
may be more interesting to compare "native" ribosomes with ribosomes dephosphorylated by a phosphatase. Such experiments must be
conducted with purified factors, otherwise the presence of protein
kinase and phosphatase in the crude extract may give erroneous
results.

Krebs (67) has proposed a set of criteria which should be
satisfied when determining whether a particular effect of cAMP is
mediated by protein phosphorylation. Thus, one should affirm
that : 1) the cell-type involved contains a cAMP-dependent protein-
kinase, 2) protein substrate exists which bears a functional
relationship to the cAMP mediated process, 3) phosphorylation of
the substrate alters its function in vitro, 4) protein substrate
is modified in vivo in response to cAMP, 5) a phosphoprotein
phosphatase exists to reverse the process.

As regards the ribosomal proteins criteria 1, 4 and 5 appear
well satisfied. Criterion 1, however, is only partially satisfied,
since the potential protein substrate exists but it is not yet
proved that phosphorylation of ribosomal or associated proteins is
related to the cAMP mediated induction of synthesis of specific
proteins. The criterion 3, for the moment, remains unsatisfied.
Further work is required to elucidate possible relationships
between ribosomal protein phosphorylation and regulation of protein synthesis.

REFERENCES

(1) WICKS, W.D. (1974) Advances in cyclic nucleotide research. Editors P. Greengard, A. Robison, Raven Press, 3, 335

(2) GARREN, L.D., NEY, R.L., DAVIS, W.W. (1965), Proc. Nat. Acad. Sci. USA, 53, 1443

(3) HERMIER, C., COMBARNOUS, JUTISZ (1971), Biochim. Biophys. Acta, 244, 625

(4) LABRIE, F., BERAUD, G., GAUTHIER, M., LEMAY, A. (1971), J. Biol. Chem., 246, 1902

(5) DUMONT, J.E. (1971) Vitamins and Hormones, 29, 287

(6) JARETT, L. STEINER, A.L., SMITH, R.M. and KIPNIS, D.M. (1972) Endocrinology, 90, 1277

(7) WAYMIRE, J.C., WEINER, N. and PRASAD, K.N. (1972) Proc. Nat. Acad. Sci. USA, 69, 2241

(8) GUIDOTTI, A. and COSTA, E. (1973), Science, 179, 902

(9) WONG, G. and PAWELEK, J. (1973), Nature New Biology, 241, 213

(10) MANGANIELLO, V., VAUGHAN, M. (1972) Proc. Nat. Acad. Sci. USA 69, 269

(11) D'ARMIENTO, M., JOHNSON, G.S. and PASTAN, I. (1972) Proc. Nat. Acad. Sci. USA, 69, 459

(12) MANCHESTER, K.L. (1970), In Mammalian Protein Metabolism, Ed. H.N. Munro, 229, Academic Press

(13) MARKS, F. and GRIMM, W. (1972) Nature New Biol., 240, 178

(14) AYUSO, M.-PARRILLA, M. and PARRILLA, R. (1973) Bioch. Biophys. Res. Comm., 52, 582

(15) SELLERS, A., BLOKHAM, D.P., MUNDAY, K.A. and AKHTAR, M. (1974) 138, 335

(16) JOST, J.P., KHAIRALLAH, E.A. and PITOT, H.C. (1968), J. Biol. Chem., 243, 5057

(17) WICKS, W.D. (1969) J. Biol. Chem., 244, 3941

(18) YEUNG, D., OLIVER, I.T. (1968), Biochemistry, 7, 3231

(19) WICKS, W.D., KENNEY, F.T. and LEE, K.L. (1969), J. Biol. Chem., 244, 6008

(20) BECK, W.T., BELLANTONE, R.A. and CANELLAKIS, E.S. (1972) Biochem. Biophys. Res. Commun., 48, 1649

(21) NEBERT, D.W. and GELBOIN, H.V. (1969) Arch. Biochem. Biophys. 134, 76

(22) URETA, T., RADOJKOVIC and NIEMEYER, H. (1970), J. Biol. Chem., 245, 4819

(23) RUDACK, D., DAVIE, B. and HOLTEN, D. (1971) J. Biol. Chem., 246, 7823

(24) LAKSHMANAN, M.R., NEPOKROEFF, C.M. and PORTER, J.W. Proc. Nat. Acad. Sci. USA, 69, 3516

(25) WICKS, W.D., BARNETT, C.A. and McKIBBIN, J.B. (1974) Fed. Proceed., 33, 1105

(26) WICKS, W.D., LEWIS, W. and McKIBBIN, J.B. Biochim. Biophys. Acta, 246, 177

(27) WICKS, W.D. and McKIBBIN, J.B. (1972) Biochim. Biophys. Res. Commun., 48, 205

(28) JOST, J.P., HSIE, A., HUGHES and RYAN, L. (1970) J. Biol. Chem. 245, 351

(29) KUO, J.F. and GREENGARD, P. (1969) Proc. Nat. Acad. Sci. USA, 64, 1349

(30) LANGAN, T.A. (1969), Proc. Nat. Acad. Sci. USA, 64, 1276

(31) DASTUGUE, B., TICHONICKY, L. and KRUH, (1974) Biochimie, 56, 491

(32) JOHNSON, E.M. and ALLFREY, V.G. (1972) Arch. Biochem. Biophys. 152, 786

(33) MARTELO, D.J., WOO, S.L., REIMANN, E.M. and DAVIE, E.W. (1970) Biochem., 9, 6807

(34) GRUMMT, I. and GRUMMT, E. (1974), FEBS Letters, 39, 129

(35) OLSON, M.O., ORRICK, L.R., JONES, C. and BUSCH, H. (1974), J. Biol. Chem., 249, 2823

(36) GALLINARO—MATRINGE, H. and JACOB, M. (1973) FEBS Letters, 36, 105

(37) LOEB, J.E. and BLAT, C. (1970) FEBS Letters, 10, 105

(38) CORREZE, C., PINEL, P. and NUNEZ, J. (1972), FEBS Letters, 23, 87

(39) KABAT, D. (1970), Biochemistry, 9, 4160

(40) BITTE, L. and KABAT, D. (1972) J. Biol. Chem. 247, 5345

(41) BARDEN, N. and LABRIE, F., (1973), Biochemistry, 12, 3096

(42) MAJMUNDER, G.C. and TURKINGTON, R.W. (1972), J. Biol. Chem. 247, 7207

(43) TREWAVAS, A., (1973) Plant. Physiol., 51, 760

(44) EGLY, J., JOHNSON, B.C., STRICKLER, C., MANDEL, P. and KEMPF, J., (1972) FEBS Letters, 22, 181

(45) GRANDER, E.S., STEWART, A.C., MOREL, C.M. and SCHERBER, K. (1973), Eur. J. Biochem., 38, 443

(46) KUO, J.F., GREENGARD, P. (1969), J. Biol. Chem., 244, 3417

(47) RAHMSDORF, H.J., PAI, S.H., PONTA, H., HERRLICH, P. ROSKOSKI, R., Jr., SCHWEIGER, M., and STUDIER, F.W. (1974), Proc. Nat. Acad., Sci., USA, 71, 586

(48) PIERRE, M. CREUZET, C., and JOEB, J.E. (1974) FEBS Letters, 45, 88

(49) WOOL, I.G. (1974) (personal communication)

(50) STAHL, G., and BIELKA, H. (1974), (personal communication)

(51) WALTON, G.M., GILL, G.N., ABRASS, I.B. and GARREN, L.D. (1971) Proc. Nat. Acad. Sci. USA, 68, 886

(52) EIL, C. and WOOL, I.G. (1973) J. Biol. Chem., 248, 5122

(53) DELAUNAY, J., LOEB, J.E., PIERRE, M. and SCHAPIRA, G. (1973), Biochim. Biophys. Acta, 312, 147

(54) STAHL, G., WELFLE, M. and BIELKA, H. (1972) FEBS Letters, 26, 233

(55) TRAUGH, J.A., MUMBY, M. and TRAUT, R.A. (1973) Proc. Nat. Acad. Sci. USA, 70, 373

(56) VENTEMIGLIA, F.A. and WOOL, I.C. (1974) Proc. Nat. Acad. Sci., USA, 71, 350

(57) BLAT, C. and LOEB, J.E. (1971) FEBS Letters, 18, 124

(58) CANTHON, M.L., BITTE, L.F., KRYSTOSEK, A. and KABAT, D., (1974) J. Biol. Chem., 249, 275

(59) ZAHLTEN, R.N., HOCHBERG, A.A., STRATMAN, F.W. and LARDY, M.A. (1972), Proc. Nat. Acad. Sci. USA, 69, 800

(60) KABAT, D. (1972) J. Biol. Chem., 247, 5338

(61) KATO, K. and BISHOP, J.S. (1972) J. Biol. Chem., 247, 7420

(62) CHELALA, C.A., and TORRES, H.P. (1969) Biochim. Biophys. Acta, 178, 423

(63) BISHOP, J.S. (1970), Biochim. Biophys. Acta, 208, 208

(64) PERLES, B. and LOEB, J.E. (1974) Biochimie, 56, 1007

(65) MEISLER, M.H. and LANGAN, T.A. (1969) J. Biol. Chem. 244, 4961

(66) EIL, C. and WOOL, I.G. (1973) J. Biol. Chem., 248, 5130

(67) KREBS, E.G. (1973) In Endocrinology, Proceedings of the 4th International Congress. Excerpta Medica, Amsterdam, 17

CYCLIC AMP AND THE CONTROL OF LIPOLYSIS IN FAT CELLS
OF THE RAT

K.D. Hepp, R. Renner, and H.U. Häring

Institut für Diabetesforschung, 8 München 4o

Kölner Platz 1, W.-Germany

Contents

Introduction

The isolated fat cell has become a widely used
model for studies on the control of lipolysis because
of its special sensitivity to lipolytic hormones as
well as to insulin, and because of the relatively
simple procedures involved in its preparation. Rat adipose tissue responds to a variety of hormones such as
the catecholamines, ACTH, TSH, LH, glucagon and secretin but it is questionable as to whether it can be regarded as a physiological target for all of them. In
vitro however, all were found to raise the levels of
cAMP in intact cells, and stimulate the adenylate cyclase system in membrane preparations. In view of the
similarity of dose response curves of lipolytic hormones when cAMP levels and lipolysis (glycerol and FA-
release) are compared, the lipolytic effect of cAMP or
its derivatives, and the effect of cAMP upon interconversion of the hormone sensitive lipase, cAMP is currently considered to be the key factor in the control
of lipolysis. Fig. 1 depicts the mechanisms involved in
the activation of the interconvertible triglyceride
lipase in adipose tissue under the influence of a lipolytic hormone, with a causal chain of events leading
from receptor binding to substrate release in the cell.

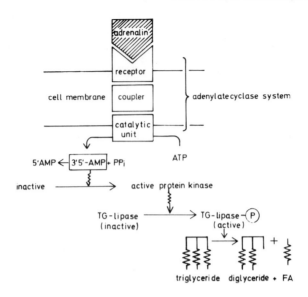

Fig. 1
Mechanism of action of lipolytic hormones. Rate-limiting
step is the activation of the adenylate cyclase system
in the plasma membrane of the fat cell, here operation-
ally defined as receptor, coupler, and catalytic unit
which obtains ATP/Mg from the interior of the cell. cAMP
binds to the regulatory subunit of the protein kinase,
the catalytic subunit is in turn released and catalyzes
the interconversion of the triglyceride lipase to its
phospho-form. The active form cleaves one fatty acid
from the triglyceride molecule which is further broken
down by di- and monoglyceride lipases which are not
rate limiting.

Insulin, so far the only known physiological antagonist, was found to modulate the metabolic effects of
the lipolytic hormones and to prevent the rise in cAMP
concentrations. This suggested that the nucleotide is
involved also in mediating the antilipolytic effect
of insulin. Insulin could thus act by interfering with
the effects of catabolic hormones upon formation of
cAMP, or by stimulation of cAMP catabolism, both resulting in the observed lowering of cAMP in the fat cell.

Although the central role of cAMP as a mediator
of lipolytic hormones seems to be well established,
this has not been accepted by all workers in the field.

Two pertinent problems are currently under debate: (1)
the lack of correlation between cAMP levels and rate
of lipolysis, and (2) the mechanism of action of
insulin.

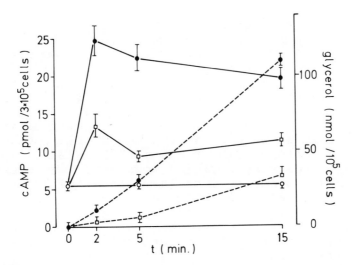

Fig. 2
Kinetics of cAMP and lipolysis in the isolated fat cell
under the influence of isoproterenol alone ($1o^{-6}M$)
● —— ● and with insulin (1oo μU/ml) □——□ Points represent the mean $\pm$ S.E.M. of 8 experiments. In contrast
to cAMP levels, glycerol release, after a lag period,
proceeds in a linear fashion without ● --- ● and with
insulin □---□ .The basal cAMP concentrations o-o indicate a steady state in the absence of hormones. Incubation medium: Tris-bicarbonate-albumin, pH 7.4.

Correlation of cyclic AMP Levels and Lipolysis

     Addition of a lipolytic hormone leads to a rapid
elevation of the overall cAMP concentration in the fat
cell of approximately fivefold from a basal steady
state of a mean of 1.7 p moles/$1o^5$ cells within 2 min,
depending on the incubation conditions (fig. 2). This
"burst" in cAMP formation is nonlinear and the initial
rate is about 1o times faster than the rate in "ghosts"
prepared from the same number of cells, as measured by
conversion of ^{32}P-ATP to ^{32}P-cAMP. Depending on the
number of cells and rate of agitation during incubation,
the level of cAMP falls or remains constant during

2o min of incubation. The fall was ascribed to feedback
inhibition of the adenylate cyclase, which could be due
to an unknown inhibitor (1), to adenosine (2,3) or free
fatty acids (G.A. Robison, this volume), all produced
in the course of lipolysis. Furthermore, cAMP itself
was found to activate the phosphodiesterase in the intact cell (M. Vaughan, this volume, and 4), and this
could also lead to the observed decrease in cAMP accumulation. In contrast to cAMP, the rate of lipolysis
proceeds in a linear fashion for as long as 6o min and
more, depending on the incubation conditions (5) (fig.
2). Addition of a β-blocker to a catecholamine-stimul-
ated system which is known to interfere with stimulation of the adenylate cyclase, leads to an immediate reduction of the rate of lipolysis at any point of incubation (5). This shows that at a point where lipolysis
continues in spite of almost basal cAMP levels, lipase
activation is fully reversible. Apparently the overall
levels of cAMP do not reflect the metabolically active
portion of the nucleotide which can also be shown in
the perfused liver, where glucagon leads to an enormous
"overshoot" of cAMP and where a better correlation is
observed between metabolic effects and cAMP released
from the liver than with the cAMP concentration in the
liver cell (J. Exton, this volume and 6). Thus compartmentation is quite likely to occur also in the fat cell
but it has not been possible to further characterize
the active pool of cAMP. Changes in the metabolically
active portion may be masked by a large background of
inert cAMP. In this light it would be unwise to postulate a correlation of cAMP levels and lipolysis, or to
deduce physiological mechanisms from levels measured at
a given point during incubation. As to the question of
the key role of cAMP and the validity of the scheme
presented in fig. 1, the data of Soderling (7) and Khoo
et al. (8) provide good evidence for an activation of
the lipolytic system as mediated by cAMP (7). On the
other hand, Lang et al. pointed out that lipolysis may
be stimulated without activation of the adenylate cyc-
lase-cAMP system (9). Thus at present, the exclusive
role of cAMP as a mediator of lipolysis is not fully
established.

Insulin Action: Adenylate Cyclase or Phosphodiesterase?

Insulin was found to inhibit the action of lipolytic hormones at concentrations below 1 µU/ml. In
lipocytes from fed rats the effect on basal lipolysis
is variable and the physiological importance lies in
the antagonism between the lipolytic hormones and

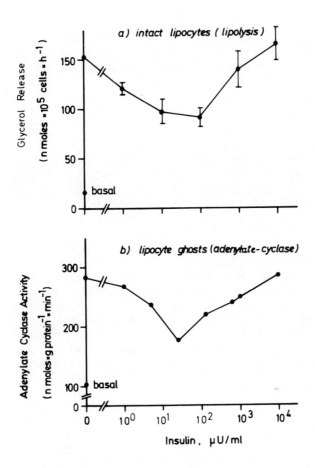

Fig. 3
Comparison of lipolysis in intact cells and adenylate cyclase activity in lipocyte "ghosts" in presence of norepinephrine (10^{-6} M) and various concentrations of insulin (from R. Renner et al. (19)).

insulin. Characteristically, the effect of insulin is poor in the presence of supramaximal concentrations of lipolytic hormone and a paradoxical bimodal effect is observed beginning at concentrations beyond the physiological range (approx. 2oo uU/ml) (fig. 3). Insulin can also antagonize the lipolytic effect of methylxanthines which are thought to act by blocking the phosphodiesterase. Unfortunately the many studies measuring lipolysis in intact lipocytes could provide no conclusive evidence regarding the mechanism of insulin action.

In view of the antilipolytic effect, a mediation of insulin action by cAMP levels seemed a good possibility and indeed, Butcher et al. (1o) found a decrease of cAMP concentrations in lipocytes under the influence of insulin. Although there are negative reports (11,12) this has now been confirmed by us (fig. 4) and several other groups (5,7,13,14) (fig. 2 and 4). Enzymes which could be involved in the observed lowering of cAMP in the cell are either the phosphodiesterase or the adenylate cyclase systems. Insulin could act through stimulation of a phosphodiesterase or modulation of the stimulatory effect of catabolic hormones on the adenylate cyclase, or both. Loten and Sneyd have reported that previous treatment of intact cells with insulin can lead to activation of a low K_M phosphodiesterase (15), a finding which has been confirmed in other laboratories (4,16). It is interesting to note that in no case was a direct effect of added insulin observed on phosphodiesterase in broken cell preparations, thus indicating that functions of the whole cell - such as for instance, intact energy metabolism - may be involved. Another finding was the stimulation of this unexpected low K_M activity by lipolytic hormones and cAMP, although again only in the intact cell (4). This raises the question whether the observed antagonism to the lipolytic hormones can be ascribed to the stimulation of phosphodiesterase activity. The activation of phosphodiesterase activity follows a dose response curve which is similar to that observed when glucose oxidation serves as a parameter, and no paradoxical reversal is found with high concentrations as in the case of lipolysis or cAMP levels (4).

On the other hand, a direct effect of insulin has been shown by us and others on adenylate cyclase activity in crude membranes or "ghosts" from fat cells (17,18). The effect upon the rate of cAMP formation is rapid (fig. 5) and was found only in presence of sub-

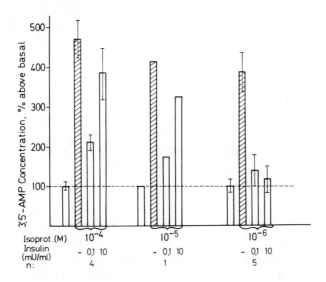

Fig. 4
Paradoxical effect of 1o mU/ml of insulin on cAMP
levels in isolated fat cells after 5 min of incubation.
At 10^{-6} M isoproterenol a bimodal effect was obtained
after 1o min of incubation (not shown in figure)

maximal concentrations of lipolytic hormone. A similar
paradoxical reversal with high concentrations can be
observed as in the case of lipolysis (fig. 4).

The effect of insulin is abolished by trypsin treatment of intact cells before preparation of ghosts
which is characteristic for the insulin receptor (19).
The effect of high concentrations of lipolytic hormone
cannot be inhibited and the dose response kinetics are
of a "pseudocompetitive" character (19). It is interesting that NSILA-S, a polypeptide which is believed
to be one of the somatomedins and which mimicks many
metabolic effects of insulin, can also inhibit the
adenylate cyclase system in ghosts (2o) and plasma
membrane preparations (unpublished results). Although
a number of negative reports have appeared (21-23)
insulin effects upon the adenylate cyclase have now
been found in neurospora (24) fibroblasts (25) and the
islets of Langerhans (26). In our hands, experiments
with purified plasma membranes gave inconsistent
results; although binding remains unimpaired, exten-

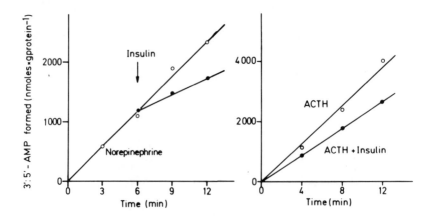

Fig. 5
Effect of insulin on adenylate cyclase activity in
lipocyte "ghosts". All samples contained norepinephrine (10^{-6} M) or ACTH (30 ng/ml) as indicated.
Insulin was added at a concentration of 50 µU/ml
at 6 min (left) or before starting the reaction
with the addition of "ghosts" (from (19)).

sive manipulation during preparation may have led to
a selective loss of responsiveness to insulin. In view
of similarities in dose-response kinetics of adenylate
cyclase activity in ghosts and cAMP levels and lipolysis in intact cells,we believe that the adenylate
cyclase system is an important control point in the
antagonism between insulin and lipolytic hormones.
Lack of correlation between cAMP concentrations and
lipolysis in the presence of insulin (27) could well
be explained on the basis of compartmentation as discussed above. However, insulin may yet have other
messengers such as cyclic GMP (28) or Ca^{++} (29), but
the evidence for this is still meagre.

REFERENCES

(1) HO, R.J. and SUTHERLAND, E.W., (1971), J. Biol. Chem. 246,
     6822

(2) FAIN, J.N., POINTER, R.H. and WARD, W.F., (1972), J. Biol.
     Chem. 247, 6866

(3) SCHWABE, U., EBERT, R. and ERBLER, H.C. (1973), Naunyn-
     Schiedeberg's Arch. Pharmacol. 276, 133

(4) ZINMAN, B. and HOLLENBERG, C., (1974), J. Biol. Chem. 249,
     2182

(5) MANGANIELLO, V.C., MURAD, F. and VAUGHAN, M., (1971) J. Biol.
     Chem. 246, 2195

(6) EXTON, J.H., ROBISON, G.A., SUTHERLAND, E.W., and PARK, C.R.,
     (1971) J. Biol. Chem., 246, 6166

(7) SODERLING, T.R., CORBIN, J.D. and PARK, C.R., (1973) J. Biol.
     Chem. 248, 1822

(8) KHOO, J.C., STEINBERG, D., THOMPSON, B., and MAYER, S.E.
     (1973), J. Biol. Chem. 248, 3823

(9) LANG, U. and SCHWYZER, R. (1972), FEBS letters 21, 91

(10) BUTCHER, R.W., BAIRD, C.E. and SUTHERLAND, E.W. (1968), J.
     Biol. Chem. 243, 1705

(11) FAIN, J.N. and ROSENBERG, L., (1972) Diabetes 21, 414

(12) JARRETT, L., STEINER, A.L., SMITH, R.M. and KIPNIS, D.M.,
     Endocrinology 90, 1277

(13) DESAI, K.S., LI, K.C. and ANGEL, A., (1973) J. Lipid Res.
     14, 647

(14) KONO, T. and BARHAM, F.W., (1973) J. Biol. Chem. 248, 7417

(15) LOTEN, E.G. and SNEYD, J.G.T., (1970) Biochem. J. 120, 187

(16) VAUGHAN, M. (1972) in Insulin Action. I.B. Fritz ed.,
     Academic Press, New York, 297

(17) HEPP, K.D. and RENNER R. (1972), FEBS letters 20, 191

(18)   ILLIANO, G. and CUATRECASAS, P. (1972), Science 175, 906

(19)   RENNER, R., KEMMLER, W. and HEPP, K.D., (1974) Eur. J.
       Biochem., 49, 129

(20)   RENNER, R., HEPP, K.D., HUMBEL, R.E. and FROESCH, (1973)
       Horm. Metab. Res. 5, 56

(21)   RODBELL, M. (1967), Biochem. J. 105, 2

(22)   VAUGHAN, M. and MURAD, F. (1969), Biochemistry 8, 3092

(23)   COMBRET, Y. and LAUDAT, P. (1972), FEBS letters 21, 45

(24)   FLAWIA, M.M. and TORRES, H.N. (1973), J. Biol. Chem. 248,
       4517

(25)   DE ASUA, L.J. and SURIAN, E.S., FLAWIA, M.M. and TORRES,
       H.N., (1973), Proc. Nat. Acad. Sci. USA, 70, 1388

(26)   KUO, W.N., HODGKINS, D.S. and KUO, J.F. (1973), J. Biol.
       Chem. 248, 2705

(27)   SIDDLE, K. and HALES, C.N. (1974), Biochem. J. 142, 97

(28)   ILLIANO, G., TELL, G.P.E., SIEGEL, M.I. and CUATRECASAS, P.
       (1973), Proc. Nat. Acad. Sci. USA, 70, 2443

(29)   HOPE-GILL, H.F., KISSEBAH, A.H., TULLOCH, B.R., VYDELINGUM,
       N. and FRASER, T.R., (1973),Eighth Congress of the Internat.
       Diabetes Fdn. Brussels, July 1973.

STUDIES ON THE PERMISSIVE EFFECT OF THE THYROID ON FAT CELLS

G.A. Robison
R.G. Van Inwegen
W.J. Thompson
J.E. Stouffer

The University of Texas Medical School and
Baylor College of Medicine
Houston, Texas, 77025, USA

Fat cells from normal rats respond to a variety of hormones (including the catecholamines, glucagon and ACTH with an increase in the rate of lipolysis. Most of the available evidence is compatible with the hypothesis that this effect is mediated by cyclic AMP (1). Fat cells from hypothyroid rats are unresponsive to these hormones, which is to say that thyroid hormones exert a permissive effect for lipolysis. We have recently carried out a series of studies designed to elucidate the mechanism of this effect.

Fat cells from adipose tissue (epididymal fat pads) of normal rats respond to epinephrine and dibutyryl cyclic AMP as illustrated in Figure 1. In these experiments the amount of glycerol released after 30 minutes of incubation was taken as an index of the rate of lipolysis. The cell density was approximately 70,000 cells/ml.

Rats were made hypothyroid by placing them on an iodine-deficient diet containing 0.15 % PTU for at least two weeks (2). Fat cells prepared from the adipose tissue of these rats still

---

ACTH : *Adrenocorticotrophic hormone* T_3 : *triiodothyronine*
PDE : *phosphodiesterase*
PTU : *propylthiouracil*
MIX : *1-methyl-3-isobutylxanthine (SC2964)*

responded to dibutyryl cyclic AMP, albeit to a somewhat reduced
degree, but did not respond at all to any concentration of epinephrine (Figure 2). Similar results were obtained with glucagon
and isoproterenol, i.e. normal fat cells responded to these agents
whereas the cells from hypothyroid rats did not. These results
are basically similar to those reported by many other investigators
(e.g., see (3)).

Treatment with T_3 (750 µg/kg daily for five days) restored
the ability of adipocytes to respond to epinephrine (Figure 3).
The fact that these rats were still on the PTU-containing diet
indicates that PTU had no direct effect on the fat cells. This is
further evidenced by the results of experiments in which concentrations of PTU as high as 70 mM in vitro had no substantial effect
on the ability of the fat cells to respond to epinephrine (2).
Administration of T_3 (250 µg/kg) to normal rats increased the response to epinephrine above the control value, in agreement with
previous results (3, 4).

Sensitivity to epinephrine could be partially restored by
including either theophylline or MIX in the incubation medium
(Figure 4). The effect of these drugs was initially interpreted
as a result of their ability to inhibit phosphodiesterase activity
(6), although at this cell density other interpretations are certainly possible.

One alternate interpretation is suggested by the results
shown in Figure 5, from an important paper by Schwabe and Ebert
(7). At high cell densities (approximately 100,000 cells/ml,
similar to that employed in our experiments), isoproterenol had
a relatively small effect by itself on the level of cyclic AMP,
and this was greatly increased in the presence of theophylline.
This was similar to many previous observations (e.g. see (6, 8)),
and could easily be interpreted in terms of the expected syner-
gism between a stimulator of adenylate cyclase and an inhibitor of
PDE. At lower cell densities, however, isoproterenol produced
a relatively large effect by itself, almost as large as in the
presence of theophylline (Figure 5, right hand panel). Schwabe
and Ebert interpreted these findings to mean that an inhibitor of
lipolysis was being released from the fat cells and that it accumulated in the medium in proportion to the cell density. They
suggested that theophylline was acting not to inhibit PDE but
rather to antagonize the action of the proposed inhibitor. There
is now evidence that this inhibitor may be adenosine (9, 10, 11),
the actions of which generally are inhibited by methylxanthines.

Regardless of the mechanism by which these drugs partially
restored sensitivity to lipolytic hormones, we felt that our data
was consistent with an impaired ability of fat cells from hypothyroid rats to accumulate cyclic AMP. This was demonstrated

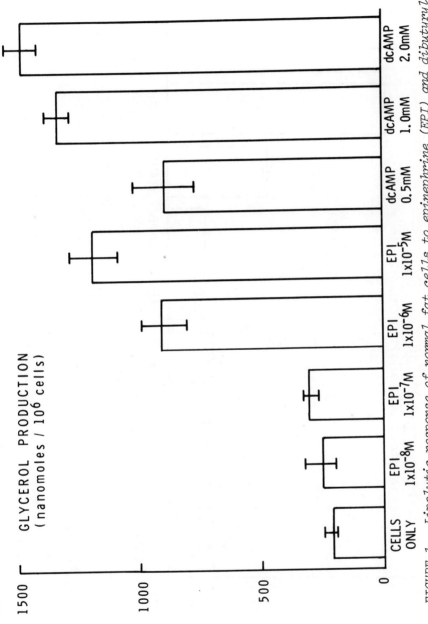

FIGURE 1. Lipolytic response of normal fat cells to epinephrine (EPI) and dibutyryl cyclic AMP (dcAMP). Cells were obtained from three male rats, and each bar represents the mean of 2 to 3 incubations, with the range indicated by a vertical line. From Armstrong et al. (2).

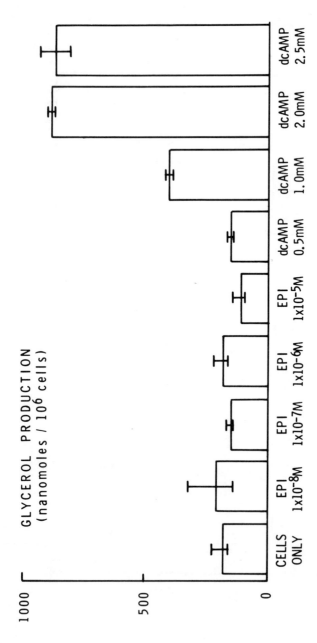

FIGURE 2. Lack of response to epinephrine of fat cells from hypothyroid rats. Cells were obtained from three male rats which had been fed a goitrogenic diet for 31 days. Each bar represents the mean of 2 to 3 incubations, with the range indicated by a vertical line. From Armstrong et al. (2).

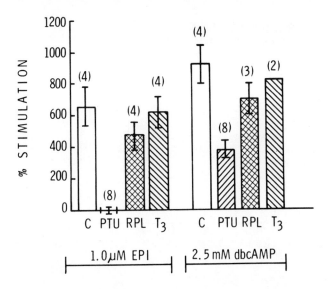

FIGURE 3. *Stimulation of lipolysis by epinephrine (EPI) and dibutyryl cyclic AMP (dbcAMP) in fat cells from control (c) and hypothyroid (PTU) rats, from hypothyroid rats after replacement therapy with 750 μg/kg of T3 daily for 5 days (RPL), and from control rats after the same treatment (T3). Each bar and vertical line represents the mean and standard error of the mean respectively. The numbers in parentheses refer to the number of separate cell preparations from which the data were pooled. From Van Inwegen et al. (5).*

directly by the experiments summarized in Table 1, showing that epinephrine produced a smaller rise in cyclic AMP in hypothyroid cells than it did in normal cells, either in the presence or absence of theophylline (2). These measurements were made at a higher cell density (approximately 250,000 cells/ml), and additional experiments at lower densities will be needed before they can be related quantitatively to our earlier measurements of lipolysis.

An interesting finding in these experiments was that basal levels of cyclic AMP were not lower in the cells from hypothyroid animals, and in fact, if anything, they tended to be higher than control values. This was not reflected when we measured protein kinase activity, using the procedure described by Corbin et al. (12). We found that protein kinase activity in the absence of added cyclic AMP was significantly lower in the hypothyroid cells than in controls, although activity was similar in the presence of a saturating concentration of cyclic AMP (Table 2). This result could be interpreted to mean that the concentration of cyclic AMP

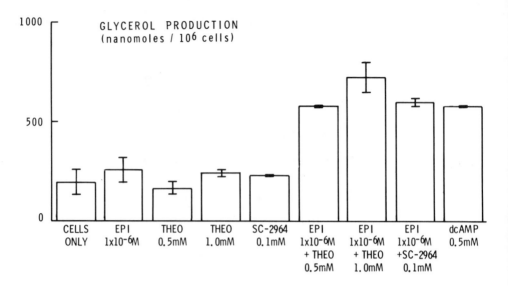

FIGURE 4. Effect of theophylline (THEO) and MIX (SC-2964) on the lipolytic response to epinephrine of fat cells from hypothyroid rats. Cells were obtained from three male rats which had been fed the goitrogenic diet for 27 days. Data plotted as in Figure 1 and 2. From Armstrong et al. (2).

in contact with the protein kinase was in fact lower in the hypo-thyroid than in normal cells, and our failure to detect this when we measured total cyclic AMP could be taken as evidence that cyclic AMP is compartmentalized in fat cells. Here again, however, cell density could have been a factor, since the protein kinase measurements were made using the lower cell density of about 70,000 cells/ml. Like many other investigators, we have not paid as much attention to cell density as we should have, in view of its apparent importance as a determinant of fat cell function.

It was nevertheless clear that fat cells from hypothyroid rats were less capable than normal fat cells of accumulating cyclic AMP in response to lipolytic hormones, and we sought to establish the reason for this. The first possibility to be tested was that the membrane adenylate cyclase might be defective. When we measured cyclase activity in membrane ghosts, however, using the procedure of Harwood et al. (13), we found that the response to isoproterenol was essentially similar regardless of whether the ghosts were obtained from normal or hypothyroid cells (Figure 6). In other experiments we found that stimulation by epinephrine, glucagon,

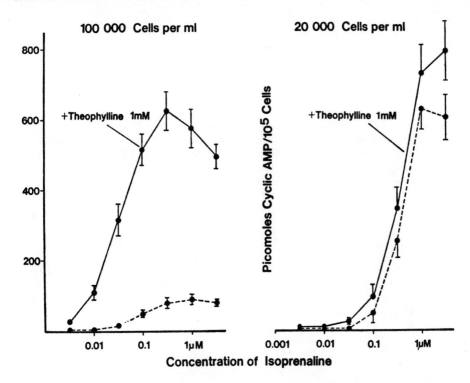

FIGURE 5. *Accumulation of cyclic AMP in rat fat cells at different cell densities. Cells were incubated for 4 minutes in the presence of increasing concentrations of isoproterenol (isoprenaline) with and without 1 mM theophylline. Each value represents the mean ± standard error of 5 experiments. From Schwabe and Ebert (7).*

or fluoride was also similar, both with respect to the concentrations needed for half-maximal activation and to the magnitude of the maximal effect obtained (on the order of 550 pmoles/min/mg protein in the case of fluoride). These findings do not support the earlier suggestion by Krishna et al. (14) that thyroid hormones might act by stimulating the synthesis of adenylate cyclase. We had previously found that thyroidectomy was without effect on the development or activity of the brain adenylate cyclase system (15).

We next examined phosphodiesterase activity after fractionation on a discontinuous sucrose gradient (16). We found that the activity of the particulate fraction, using cyclic AMP as the substrate, was significantly increased in hypothyroid cells, and that this could be restored or even reduced below normal by pretreatment of the animals with T_3 (5) as shown in Figure 7. The extrapolated

TABLE 1

CYCLIC AMP LEVELS IN FAT CELLS
FROM NORMAL AND HYPOTHYROID RATS

Cells were incubated at a density of 10^6 cells per 10 min, and cyclic AMP measured in purified extracts after perchloric acid fixation. Cyclic AMP is expressed as picomoles per flask ± standard deviation. Numbers in parentheses refer to the number of incubations per point, using aliquots from the same pool of cells for each group of rats.

Additions	Normal	Hypothyroid
None	6.1 ± 1.8 (4)	8.0 ± 2.0 (4)
Theophylline (1 mM)	35.0 ± 6.3 (3)	35.4 ± 5.0 (3)
Epinephrine (10^{-6} M)	37.3 ± 4.9 (3)	14.6 ± 3.0 (3)
Theophylline and epi	966 ± 125 (3)	74 ± 7.1 (3)

TABLE 2

PROTEIN KINASE IN FAT CELLS
FROM NORMAL AND HYPOTHYROID RATS

Homogenates were incubated in the presence and absence of cyclic AMP, using calf thymus histone as substrate. Activity expressed as picomoles of phosphate incorporated per min per mg. protein. Each value is the mean ± s.e. of three separate pooled cell preparations.

	− cyclic AMP	+ cyclic AMP	$\dfrac{+ \text{ cyclic AMP}}{- \text{ cyclic AMP}}$
Control	29 ± 1	128 ± 16	4.4
Hypothyroid	13 ± 3	134 ± 32	10.3

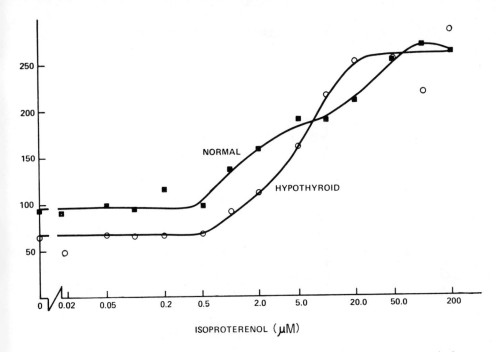

FIGURE 6. *Effect of isoproterenol on adenylate cyclase activity of fat cell ghosts. Ghosts were prepared from 4 normal and 4 hypothyroid rats. Activity expressed as picomoles of cyclic AMP produced per minute per mg protein. From Armstrong et al. (2).*

kinetic parameters for both the "high K_m" and "low K_m" cyclic AMP phosphodiesterases as well as cyclic GMP phosphodiesterase (which is almost totally soluble) are summarized in Table 3, from which it can be seen that the affinity of PDE for substrate does not appear to be affected by thyroid status. The most highly significant changes were in the specific activities of the "low K_m" cyclic AMP phosphodiesterase, which is predominantly present in the particulate fraction, and the soluble cyclic GMP phosphodiesterase (5).

By pretreating the rats with dexamethasone, we have in some experiments been able to restore cyclic GMP phosphodiesterase activity to normal without restoring the sensitivity of fat cells to lipolytic hormones. By contrast, the restoration of the particulate low K_m cyclic AMP phosphodiesterase has in all cases gone hand in hand with the restoration of the lipolytic response. We have suggested, therefore, that an important effect of T₃ on fat

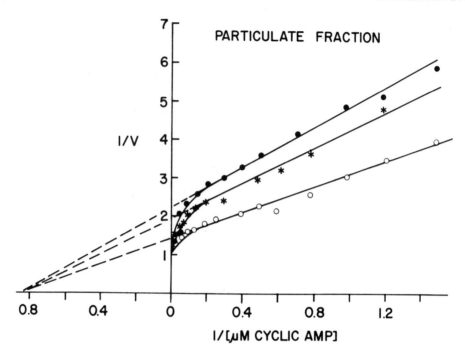

<u>FIGURE 7</u>. *Lineweaver-Burk plot of phosphodiesterase activity in particulate fractions of fat cell homogenates from control rats (asterisks), hypothyroid rats (open circles), and hypothyroid rats after T₃ treatment (closed circles). Activity expressed as nanomoles of cyclic AMP hydrolyzed per min per mg protein. From Van Inwegen et al. (5).*

cells is to somehow suppress the activity of the membrane-bound phosphodiesterase which has a high affinity for cyclic AMP. In the intact cell, this enzyme is presumably located in close proximity to adenylate cyclase. It seems possible or even likely that the increased activity of this enzyme seen in hypothyroid cells could account for the impaired ability of these cells to accumulate lipolytically significant amounts of cyclic AMP. Under these conditions, in other words, the cyclic AMP resulting from adenylate cyclase stimulation could be destroyed almost as rapidly as it is formed.

The mechanism by which T₃ produces this effect on phosphodiesterase is unknown, as is its relevance for other effect of T₃ in other types of cells. To date we have been able to produce the effect only by injecting T₃ into intact animals. Concentrations of the hormone in excess of 10^{-5}M have no effect when added to the enzyme <u>in vitro</u> (5), although higher concentrations may be inhibi-

TABLE 3. KINETIC PARAMETERS OF PHOSPHODIESTERASE ACTIVITIES

Cell Fraction	Kinetic Parameters	"Control"	"Hypothyroid"	"Hypo. + T_3"	"Hyperthyroid"
"Supernatant"	V_{max}hi A	1460 ± 318 (5)	2275 ± 443 (5)	2208 ± 403 (5)	1314 ± 283 (4)
	$K_m$hi A	49 ± 4 μM	49 ± 4 μM	49 ± 6 μM	37 ± 1 μM
	V_{max}lo A	300 ± 78 (5)	465 ± 100 (5)	322 ± 99 (4)	289 ± 67 (3)
	$K_m$lo A	2.2 ± 0.7 μM	2.2 ± 0.7 μM	2.4 ± 0.8 μM	2.9 ± 0.9 μM
	V_{max}G	723 ± 165 (4)	1051 ± 122 (4)	665 ± 63 (4)	613 ± 74 (4)
	K_mG	19 ± 6 μM	20 ± 5 μM	21 ± 6 μM	25 ± 4 μM
"Particulate"	V_{max}lo A	684 ± 60 (4)	1046 ± 110 (4)	556 ± 278 (3)	499 (2)
	$K_m$lo A	1.4 ± 0.4 μM	1.4 ± 0.4 μM	1.1 ± 0.2 μM	1.1 μM

Vm's are given in picomoles/min·mg protein ± S. E. Km's also given ± S. E.

V_{max}hi A	=	Maximum velocity (V_{max}) of cyclic AMP PDE extrapolated from the linear portion of the Lineweaver-Burk plots at high substrate concentrations.
K_m hi A	=	Michaelis-Menten constant (K_m) derived from the extrapolated lines deriving V_{max}hi A.
V_{max}lo A	=	V_{max} of cyclic AMP PDE determined as above except with low substrate concentrations.
$K_m$lo A	=	K_m derived from extrapolated lines determining V_{max}lo A
V_{max}G	=	V_{max} of cyclic GMP PDE
K_mG	=	K_m for cyclic GMP PDE
(N)	=	No. of separate cell preparations.

tory.(17). Such concentrations are of doubtful physiological significance, however.

In speculating about the mechanism of action of T_3, several
points could be raised. The first and most general point, emphasized in a recent essay by J.E. Rall (18), is that thyroid hormones appear to be unique among known hormones in that their
blood levels are not normally subject to large fluctuations. In
this respect T_3 resembles such plasma constituents as calcium and
hydrogen ions more than it resembles other hormones. This points
to the possibility of a mechanism of action fundamentally different
from other hormones, a possibility rendered even more likely by
the recognition that T_3 probably affects more different types of
cells than any other hormone. The presence of cytoplasmic
receptors for T_3 has raised the possibility of a mechanism of
action similar to that of steroid hormones (19), but this remains
to be substantiated.

The evidence that methylxanthines promote lipolysis by inhibiting the effect of adenosine (see discussion of Figure 5),
combined with our finding that methylxanthines can partially restore the response to lipolytic hormones of hypothyroid fat cells
(Figure 4), suggests the possibility that one component of the
action of T_3 on rat fat cells might be to reduce the sensitivity
of these cells to the inhibitory effect of adenosine. To state the
converse, it seems possible that hypothyroid cells seem less responsive to lipolytic hormones because they are more responsive to
the inhibitory influence of adenosine. It is interesting to note
in this regard that human fat cells, in apparent contrast to rat
fat cells, do not seem to be affected by adenosine, even at high
concentrations, either in terms of cyclic AMP accumulation or
lipolysis (T.W. Burns, P.E. Langley and G.A. Robison,unpublished
observations). In line with this, adenosine deaminase has no
effect on human fat cells, again in apparent contrast to rat fat
cells (20). Thus, even if T_3 does alter the sensitivity of rat
fat cells to adenosine, and this is a possibility which is
currently being investigated, it could hardly explain the effect
of T_3 on human fat cells.

Another difference between human and rat fat cells is that
human cells possess adrenergic alpha receptors, which are
inhibitory (21). Here it is especially interesting to note that
Rosenquist (22) has shown that fat cells from hypothyroid patients
are more sensitive to alpha adrenergic inhibition than normal human
fat cells, and he has suggested on this basis that T_3 may act by
reducing the sensitivity of fat cells to α-adrenergic agonists.

But just as it seems clear that T_3 could not affect human fat
cells by altering their sensitivity to adenosine, so also does it

seem clear that it could not affect rat fat cells by altering their sensitivity to α-adrenergic agonists. But might not the inhibition of rat fat cells by adenosine and the inhibition of human fat cells by α-adrenergic agonists have something in common which <u>could</u> be affected by thyroid hormones ? One of the aims of our current research is to answer this question.

REFERENCES

(1) ROBISON, G.A., BUTCHER, R.W. and SUTHERLAND, E.W. (1971) "Cyclic AMP", Acedemic Press, New York

(2) ARMSTRONG, K.G., STOUFFER, J.E., VAN INWEGEN, R.G., THOMPSON, W.J. and ROBISON, G.A. (1974) J. Biol. Chem. <u>249</u>, 4226

(3) FISHER, J.N. and BALL, E.G. (1967) Biochemistry <u>6</u>, 637

(4) GOODMAN, H.M. and REAY, G.A. (1966) Amer. J. Physiol. <u>210</u>, 1053

(5) VAN INWEGEN, R.G., ROBISION, G.A., THOMPSON, W.J., ARMSTRONG, K.J. and STOUFFER, J.E. (1975) J. Biol. Chem. <u>250</u>, in press

(6) BEAVO, J.A., ROGERS, N.L., CROFFORD, O.B., BAIRD, C.E., HARDMAN, S.G., SUTHERLAND, E.W. and NEWMAN, E.V. (1971) Ann. N.Y. Acad. Sci. <u>185</u>, 129

(7) SCHWABE, U. and EBERT, R. (1972) Naunyn-Schmied. Arch. Pharmacol. <u>274</u>, 287

(8) BUTCHER, R.W., BAIRD, C.E. and SUTHERLAND, E.W. (1968) J. Biol. Chem. <u>243</u>, 1705

(9) EBERT, R. and SCHWABE, U. (1972) Naunyn-Schmied. Arch. Pharmacol. <u>278</u>, 247

(10) FAIN, J.N. (1973) Molec. Pharmacol. <u>9</u>, 595

(11) SCHWABE, U., SCHÖNHÖFER, P.S. and EBERT, R. (1974) Europ. J. Biochem. <u>46</u>, 537

(12) CORBIN, J.D., SODERLING, T.R. and PARK, C.R. (1973) J. Biol. Chem. <u>243</u>, 1813

(13) HARWOOD, J.P., LÖW, H., and RODBELL, M. (1973) J. Biol. Chem. <u>248</u>, 6239

(14) KRISHNA, G., HYNIE, S. and BRODIES, B.B. (1968) Proc. Nat. Acad.-Sci. 59, 884

(15) SCHMIDT, M.J. and ROBISON, G.A. (1972) J. Neurochem. 19, 937

(16) THOMPSON, W.J., LITTLE, S.A. and WILLIAMS, R.H. (1973) Biochemistry 12, 1889

(17) MANDEL, L.R. and KUEHL, F.A. (1967) Biochem. Biophys. Res. Commun. 28, 13

(18) RALL, J.E. (1974) Perspectives Biol. Med. 17, 218

(19) STERLING, K., SALDANHA, V.F., BRENNER, M.A. and MILCH, P.O. (1974) Nature 250, 661

(20) SCHWABE, U. and EBERT, R. (1972) Naunyn-Schmied. Arch. Pharmacol. 274, 287

(21) ROBINSON, G.A., LANGLEY, P.E. and BURNS, T.W. (1972) Biochem. Pahrmacol. 21, 589

(22) ROSENOUIST, U. (1972) Acta Med. Scand. 192, 353

CYCLIC NUCLEOTIDES, CALCIUM AND ION TRANSPORT

Michael J. Berridge and William T. Prince

A.R.C. Unit of Invertebrate Chemistry and Physiology
Department of Zoology, Downing Street, Cambridge
England, CB2 3EJ

CONTENTS

INTRODUCTION

Fluid transport across epithelia plays an important role not only in osmoregulation, but also in digestion. In many cases, the rate of fluid movement is carefully regulated by hormonal or nervous stimuli. Although the nature of the hormones and nerves responsible for this regulation have been characterized, not much is known about how these various stimuli bring about the very large changes in fluid flow which are seen during stimulation of such epithelia as the pancreas or mammalian salivary gland. One reason for our ignorance about how epithelia are controlled stems from the fact that we still know very little about how ions and water are transported across most epithelia. In order to unravel the control mechanisms within epithelial cells, it is first necessary to understand the basic features of the transport mechanisms. Such essential information has been difficult to obtain for most vertebrate epithelia because of their structural complexity. Such problems are greatly reduced in various insect epithelia such as the salivary glands of adult blowflies. These insect salivary glands not only have a relatively simple structure (1) but they are particularly amenable to _in vitro_ studies which have provided

591

insights into both the mechanism and the control of secretion.

Both cyclic AMP and calcium have been implicated in the control of a number of transporting epithelia including toad bladder,
pancreas and mammalian salivary gland (2). In order to fully
appreciate the role of these second messengers during cell activation it is desirable to study them at work in their normal cellular environment. These insect salivary glands provide a unique
opportunity for studying how cyclic AMP and calcium act in the
intact cell because it is possible to continuously monitor their
intracellular effects by making appropriate rate and potential
recordings.

II. THE MECHANISM OF FLUID SECRETION

The salivary gland of the adult blowfly consists of a long
thin tube composed of a layer of uniform secretory cells. During
stimulation with 5-hydroxytryptamine (5-HT) the gland rapidly
secretes fluid which exudes from the open end of the gland (3).
Since the techniques used for studying the secretory activity of
this salivary gland have been described in several previous publications (4,5,6) they will not be dealt with in detail. Fluid
secretion is studied by setting the gland up in a drop of saline
maintained under liquid paraffin; the rate of fluid secretion is
estimated by measuring the volume of saliva which escapes from the
open end of the gland. Various electrical parameters are monitored
by setting the gland up in a perfusion chamber which contains three
parallel baths. The two outer baths contain saline and are insu-
lated from each other by liquid paraffin contained in the central
bath. A salivary gland is set up such that the closed end lies
in one saline bath whereas the open end lies in the opposite bath.
Calomel electrodes connected to these two saline baths record
transepithelial potentials and microelectrodes are used to make
intracellular and resistance measurements.

Earlier studies established that after applying low concentrations of 5-HT (5×10^{-9}M) to isolated glands the rate of secretion
increased from 2 to 37 nl/min with a half time of approximately 30
seconds (3). This rapid stimulation of secretion could be mimicked
by cyclic AMP (1×10^{-2}M). Since theophylline (1×10^{-2}M) was capable
of stimulating secretion and was also capable of potentiating the
action of both 5-HT and cyclic AMP,it seemed likely that the action
of 5-HT was mediated by cyclic AMP. However, detailed studies on
the mechanism of secretion have revealed that exogenous cyclic AMP
is not capable of mimicking all the effects of 5-HT. For example,
exogenous cyclic AMP cannot reproduce the potential responses recorded during the action of 5-HT(4,7). At rest, the lumen is 15-30 mV
positive with respect to the bathing medium.(Earlier measurements of
the transepithelial potential made across the paraffin gap were much
lower than those recorded subsequently by inserting a microelectrode

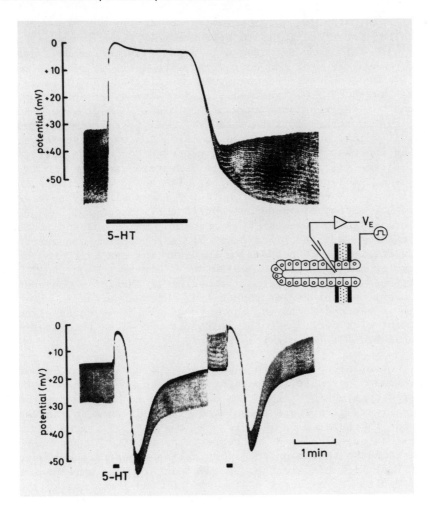

Fig. 1. Transepithelial potential responses of an isolated salivary gland during long (top) or short (bottom) treatment with 10^{-8} M 5-HT. The potential was recorded by a microelectrode inserted in the lumen close to the liquid paraffin gap (stippled area in inset). Changes in the resistance across the membrane can be determined by the potential deflections produced by passing regular current pulses (0.11 µA) across the gland. Note that during the action of 5-HT the height of these deflections is greatly reduced indicating a large decrease in resistance. In the bottom trace, the direction of the current pulses was reversed in between the two 5-HT treatments which demonstrates that the transepithelial resistance behaves linearly because the potential deflections remained the same size (Taken from reference 6).

directly into the lumen). During the action of 5-HT the transepithelial potential falls to approximately 0 mV within 3-5 secs
(Fig. 1). This sudden increase in negativity is rapidly restored
after removal of 5-HT and during recovery there is often a marked
positive undershoot. The magnitude of this undershoot is related
to the length of 5-HT treatment; it is large after short applications but is greatly reduced after long treatment with 5-HT
(Fig. 1). Contrary to this effect of 5-HT, cyclic AMP causes the
transepithelial potential to go positive instead of negative. A
similar increase in positivity is recorded during the action of
theophylline (7). These potential measurements seemed to indicate
that 5-HT had two effects. Firstly, it caused an increase in
potassium transport which accounts for the positivity observed
during the action of exogenous cyclic AMP. Secondly, 5-HT seemed
to increase anion movement by a mechanism which was independent of
cyclic AMP. This inability of cyclic AMP to stimulate anion transport sufficiently to produce an increase in negativity may explain
why cyclic AMP is a poor stimulant of fluid secretion under
conditions where chloride in the medium is partially replaced with
the impermeant anion isethionate (5). When chloride in the bathing
medium is reduced to 50 mM, the rate of fluid secretion after
treatment with cyclic AMP (5 nl/min) is much less than that
produced by 5-HT (21 nl/min) (Fig. 2).

The ability of 5-HT to accelerate the movement of both cations
and anions apparently independently of each other can be further
revealed by studying the action of 5-HT in a chloride-free medium.
When salivary glands are stimulated with 5-HT in a saline where
chloride is replaced by isethionate, the potential goes positive
instead of negative. The increase in positivity is probably due
to an increase in cation transport taking place in the absence of
a parallel flow of chloride. The potential rapidly returns to the
level typical of a normal 5-HT response when isethionate is
replaced with chloride. Therefore, although anion transport had
been switched on, it was not expressed because isethionate was
unable to permeate the cell membrane. These results suggested
that the active transport of potassium may be the prime mover
during fluid secretion. Physiological observations which show
that fluid secretion can be maintained in salines containing very
low potassium concentrations further indicate that potassium is
transported uphill. On the other hand, chloride movement appears
to be passive. Resistance measurements indicate that there is a
sudden decrease in transepithelial resistance immediately after
the application of 5-HT (Fig. 1) (6). The change in membrane
permeability, which seems to be specific for chloride, occurs
simultaneously across both the basal and apical membranes. On the
basis of such electrical measurements, a model has been developed
which adequately accounts for all the changes in potential observed
during the action of 5-HT (6). 5-HT stimulates fluid secretion by
increasing the active transport of potassium which provides the

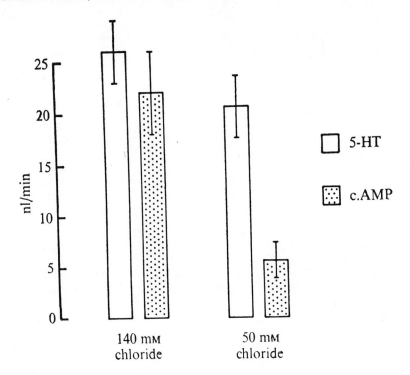

Fig. 2. The effect of 5-HT (10^{-8} M) and cyclic AMP (10^{-2} M) on
the rate of fluid secretion by isolated salivary glands maintained
in solutions containing either 140 or 50 mM chloride (Taken from
reference 5).

driving force for a parallel flow of both chloride and water. This
passive movement of chloride is facilitated by the large increases
in chloride permeability which occur across both surfaces of the
cell. This understanding of the basic features of the secretory
mechanism has provided a powerful tool for studying the intracellular signals responsible for regulating the changes in ion
transport induced by 5-HT.

III. THE ROLE OF CYCLIC AMP AND CALCIUM

As mentioned earlier, there is reason to believe that cyclic
AMP may function as a second messenger during the action of 5-HT.
Cyclic AMP by itself is capable of stimulating secretion and during

the action of 5-HT there is an increase in the intracellular level
of cyclic AMP (3,8).   The effect of cyclic AMP on potential seems
to suggest that it may stimulate cation transport.   The fact that
5-HT causes the potential to go positive in chloride-free media is
also consistent with the notion that cyclic AMP stimulates cation
transport.   However, this evidence is somewhat indirect and it is
still not clear whether or not cyclic AMP acts directly on the
potassium pump.   The possibility exists that cyclic AMP may stimulate potassium transport indirectly and this aspect will be discussed further in Section IV.

The stimulatory effect of 5-HT on chloride permeability seems
to be regulated by calcium.   If salivary glands are stimulated with
5-HT in a calcium-free saline, there is a normal increase in fluid

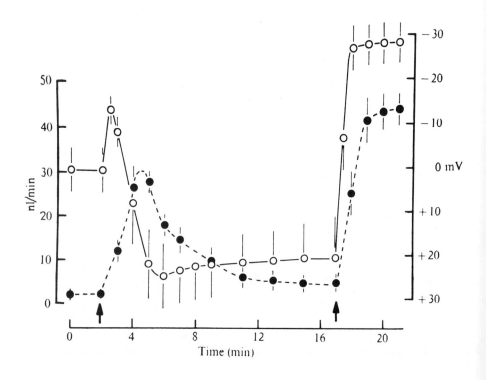

Fig. 3.   Changes in transepithelial potential (o) and rate of fluid
secretion (●) of isolated salivary glands when stimulated with
10^{-8} M 5-HT (first arrow) in a calcium-free saline (5 mM EGTA).
At the second arrow calcium was re-admitted and both the potential
and secretory response returned to normal (Taken from reference 5).

secretion and the potential goes negative in the usual way (Fig.
3) (5). However, these normal responses are not maintained and
first the potential goes rapidly positive and, sometime later,
the rate of fluid secretion falls to a low level. When calcium is
readmitted, both the potential and secretory rate return to normal
(Fig. 3). The temporary independence of external calcium is
achieved by the mobilization and utilization of an internal pool
of calcium, but once this pool is depleted the gland becomes dependent upon external calcium. Calcium is apparently responsible
for mediating the increase in chloride permeability because when
glands are stimulated in a calcium-free medium there is no change
in resistance (Fig. 4) except during the brief negative phase when
the glands may be running on their internal supplies of calcium.

The importance of calcium in the control of fluid secretion
has emerged from studies using either the calcium ionophore
A 23187 or elevated potassium to stimulate fluid secretion. The
calcium ionophore A 23187 is capable of stimulating fluid secretion
(Fig. 5) by a mechanism which is apparently independent of an
increase in the intracellular level of cyclic AMP (9). Similarly,
salines containing elevated potassium concentrations can stimulate
fluid secretion with no significant increase in the intracellular
level of cyclic AMP (10). However the stimulatory effects of
A 23187 and high potassium are both dependent upon external calcium.
However, like 5-HT, A 23187 can induce a temporary elevation in
fluid secretion in a calcium-free saline (Fig. 5) (2) indicating
that this ionophore enters the gland and can stimulate the release
of stored calcium. A 23187 can also stimulate the release of
granules from blood platelets in the absence of external calcium
(1) again suggesting that it may act by altering the distribution
of stored calcium. These results with A 23187 and high potassium
seem to indicate that an increase in the intracellular level of
calcium may be directly responsible for stimulating fluid secretion
without the mediation of cyclic AMP. These observations have high-
lighted our ignorance concerning the role of cyclic AMP in the
control of fluid secretion during a normal response to 5-HT.
One possibility is that cyclic AMP functions in a feedback loop
which is responsible for regulating the transfer of calcium
between the cytoplasm and various intracellular reservoirs.

IV. INTERACTIONS BETWEEN CYCLIC AMP AND CALCIUM

There is considerable evidence from other cell systems
to indicate that cyclic AMP may play an important role in
adjusting the intracellular level of calcium (2). In some systems,
such as in heart and smooth muscle, which are bidirectional in
character, cyclic AMP acts to lower the intracellular level of
calcium by stimulating the mechanisms responsible for removing

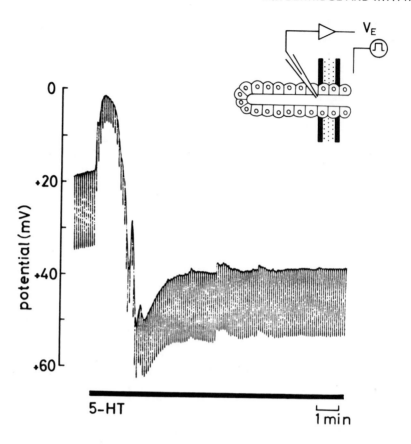

<u>Fig. 4.</u> Changes in transepithelial potential and resistance during
stimulation of a salivary gland with 10^{-8} M 5-HT in a calcium-free
medium. The inset illustrates the arrangement of the recording
electrode which was similar to that described for figure 1. Note
the temporary early negative phase and decrease in resistance after
which the potential goes much more positive and the potential deflections (an indication of the resistance) are similar to those
observed before the application of 5-HT (Taken from reference 6).

calcium from the cell. In monodirectional systems (eg. β-cells,
liver), however, cyclic AMP may act to augment the calcium signal.
Borle (12) has recently demonstrated that cyclic AMP can stimulate
the release of calcium from isolated liver mitochondria. In the
case of these insect salivary glands there is evidence that cyclic
AMP may also act to mobilize the internal reservoirs of calcium.
Earlier it was described how salivary glands were able to respond

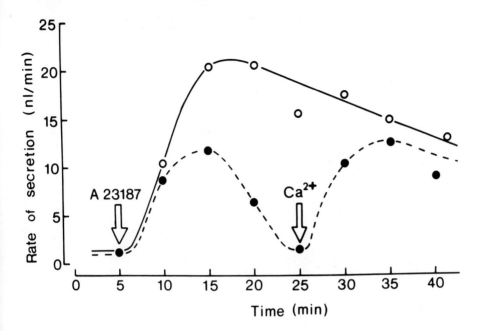

Fig. 5. The effect of the calcium ionophore A 23187 (2×10^{-5}M) on the rate of fluid secretion by isolated salivary glands. One group was treated in the presence of 2×10^{-4} M calcium (o—o) whereas the second group was in a calcium-free saline (•---•) containing 1 mM EGTA. Calcium was readmitted to this latter group as indicated.

normally to 5-HT for a short period in the absence of external calcium (Fig. 3). This temporary independence of external calcium seems to depend upon the mobilization of internal reservoirs which occurs during stimulation with either 5-HT or cyclic AMP (5). Other experiments have shown that there is little mobilization of internal calcium in the absence of stimulation (13). The fact that both 5-HT and exogenous cyclic AMP can markedly enhance the efflux of calcium from prelabelled glands, seems to indicate that cyclic AMP is responsible for mobilizing this internal calcium (8).

Various drugs known to alter calcium metabolism have been tested in an attempt to find out more about the role of intracellular calcium in cell activation. Local anaesthetics such as procaine and tetracaine are thought to act by inhibiting calcium influx into cells and can thus be used to determine the contribution of internal and external calcium to cell activation. Studies with procaine suggest that there may be a mobilization of

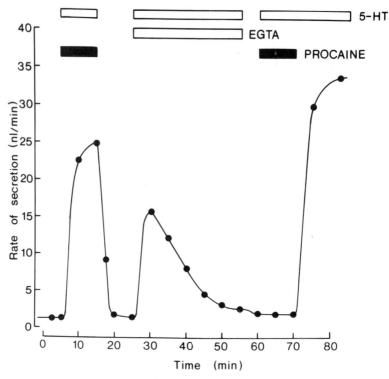

Fig. 6.   The effect of procaine (10^{-3} M) on fluid secretion stimulated with 5-HT (10^{-8} M).   When first tested procaine had little
inhibitory effect but after being stimulated in calcium-free
medium (5 mM EGTA), which deplete the internal reservoirs of
calcium, procaine was able to fully inhibit the stimulatory
effect of 5-HT.   Note the very rapid recovery to normal high
rates of secretion when procaine was removed.

internal calcium during normal cell activation.   In normal cells,
procaine causes little inhibition.   However, after the cells have
been depleted of calcium by being stimulated in EGTA, procaine
completely inhibits the stimulatory effect of 5-HT (Fig. 6).

The inability of procaine to inhibit the action of 5-HT in
normal cells suggests that intracellular calcium might be utilized as part of the signal which initiates secretion.   This
contribution of internal calcium is apparently not sufficient
to maintain secretion by itself because when salivary glands are
treated with tetracaine, which is a more potent drug than procaine,
there is a complete and immediate cessation of secretion.   The

complete inhibition seen with tetracaine may indicate that external calcium is of primary importance during the stimulation of salivary glands. This conclusion must be accepted with caution because it depends on the assumption that the main action of tetracaine is to prevent the influx of calcium. Tetracaine may inhibit the action of calcium directly which would effectively mask any contribution of calcium from the intracellular reservoirs. An interesting feature of this tetracaine inhibition is that it can be overcome either by raising the concentration of 5-HT or by the addition of exogenous cyclic AMP (14). If the concentration of 5-HT is increased from 10^{-8} M to 10^{-5} M, the amount of tetracaine necessary to inhibit secretion is increased almost tenfold (Fig. 7). The protective action of 5-HT can also be demonstrated electrically (Fig. 8). At 10^{-8} M to 10^{-5} M, the amount of tetracaine necessary to inhibit secretion is increased almost tenfold (Fig.7). The protective action of 5-HT can also be demonstrated electrically (Fig. 8). At 10^{-8} M 5-HT, tetracaine (10^{-3} M) caused the potential to go positive and the resistance increased as might be expected if tetracaine acts by blocking either the influx or action of calcium. However, this same concentration of tetracaine had a much smaller effect on potential and resistance when the glands were stimulated with 10^{-5} M 5-HT (Fig. 8). When the glands are treated with such an excess of 5-HT, the intracellular cyclic AMP level is elevated considerably above that normally associated with salivary gland stimulation (14). Therefore, it appears as if excess cyclic AMP is able to overcome the inhibition imposed by tetracaine and this protective action of cyclic AMP could be explained through its proposed role as a regulator of internal calcium homeostasis.

These studies on the control of fluid secretion by isolated salivary glands have emphasized the central importance of calcium in the control of ion transport. Calcium certainly seems to have a direct effect on chloride movement through its ability to increase the chloride permeability of both the basal and apical membranes. The action of cyclic AMP is not so clear cut. On the basis of available information it is difficult to decide whether the ability of cyclic AMP to stimulate potassium transport, and hence fluid secretion, is a direct effect or whether it occurs indirectly through its ability to release calcium from various intracellular reservoirs. This ability of cyclic AMP to alter internal calcium homeostasis is of considerable interest in that it may prove to be of central importance in the control of a wide range of different cell types (2).

V. COMPARISON WITH MAMMALIAN SYSTEMS

It is of interest to compare some of the features which are beginning to emerge from these studies on insect salivary glands

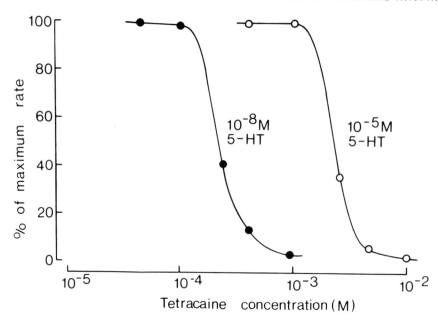

Fig. 7. The ability of excess 5-HT to overcome the inhibitory effect of tetracaine. The rates of secretion have been expressed as percentage of the rate obtained with a control dose of 5-HT $(1 \times 10^{-8}$ M) which gives a maximal response.

with what is known about the control of secretory events in various mammalian systems. The mammalian salivary gland receives a dual innervation. Fluid secretion is under cholinergic control whereas adrenergic nerves regulate the release of enzyme. The way in which acetylcholine stimulates fluid secretion is not fully understood but there are suggestions that, like the insect salivary gland, calcium may be involved (15,16). This idea is substantiated by the observation that the calcium ionophore A 23187 stimulates a large release of potassium which is a characteristic feature of salivary gland activation during cholinergic stimulation (17). There is no evidence that cyclic AMP plays any role in stimulating fluid secretion during cholinergic stimulation but Schultz et al. (18) have noted a large increase in the level of cyclic GMP during the action of methacholine. However, cyclic AMP has been implicated in the release of enzymes induced during adrenergic stimulation (19,20). The control of enzyme release is complicated by the obser- vation that there is always a small but significant activation of fluid secretion during adrenergic stimulation. On the basis of the

feedback relationships uncovered in the insect salivary gland, it
might be worthwhile to consider the possibility that cyclic AMP may
cause a release of intracellular calcium which could switch on fluid
secretion (Fig. 9). Salivary glands possess an enormous intracellular store of calcium (21). Selinger et al. (22) have isolated
a microsomal preparation from rat parotid and sub-maxillary glands
which displays energy-dependent calcium accumulation. This microsomal preparation also possesses a very specific cyclic AMP binding
site so it is conceivable that cyclic AMP may release calcium from
this intracellular reservoir to induce a small increase in fluid
secretion by the same mechanism as that used during cholinergic
stimulation. Such a view is strengthened by the observations that
adrenergic stimulation induces very similar secretory potentials
(24) and losses of potassium (25) as occur during cholinergic
stimulation.

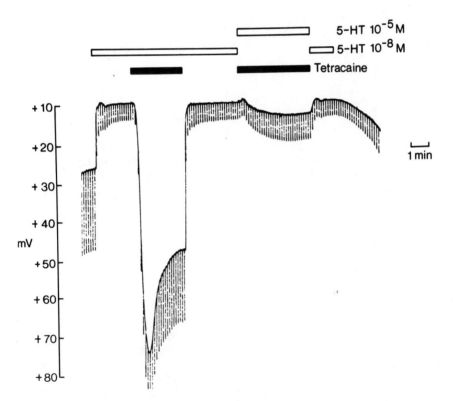

Fig. 8. The protective action of excess 5-HT in the inhibitory
action of tetracaine (1 x 10^{-3} M). Application of tetracaine during
stimulation with 10^{-8} M 5-HT caused the potential to go positive
and the resistance increased markedly. This effect of tetracaine
was greatly reduced during stimulation with 10^{-5} M 5-HT.

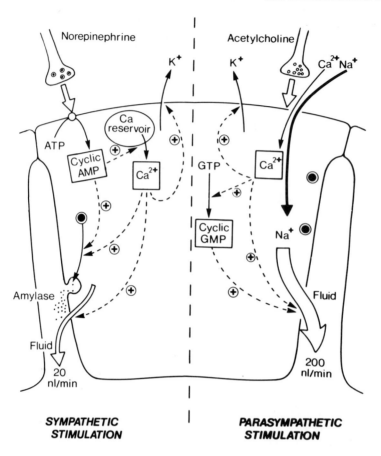

Fig. 9. A summary of some of the current speculations concerning
the role of second messengers in the control of fluid and enzyme
secretion by the mammalian salivary gland. See text for further
details (Taken from reference 2).

        During liver activation with glucagon or epinephrine there
is a loss of potassium with a resulting membrane hyperpolarization
which is remarkably similar to that just described in the mammalian
salivary gland (25). Potassium efflux and hyperpolarization of the
membrane is not a direct effect of the catabolic hormones because
these membrane events can be mimicked by either cyclic AMP or cyclic
GMP (26,27). These cyclic nucleotides may have a direct effect on
membrane permeability, or they may act indirectly by releasing calcium (Fig. 10). There is some evidence for the latter possibility

because Borle (12) has found that cyclic AMP can stimulate the
release of calcium from isolated liver mitochondria.   Such mobilization of calcium from the mitochondria may account for the increased efflux of calcium which occurs during the action of glucagon
or cyclic AMP (28,29).   The increase in calcium efflux preceeds
the efflux of potassium suggesting that the two events may be related especially since calcium is known to increase potassium
permeability in red blood cells (30,31) and in nerve cells (32).

     Control of insulin secretion represents another example
where cyclic AMP may act through an effect on calcium metabolism.
The ability of glucose to stimulate the release of insulin is
apparently mediated by calcium.   Glucose seems to have a direct
effect on the permeability of the plasma membrane which results in

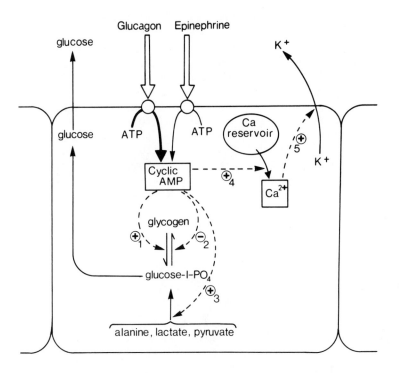

Fig. 10.   The role of intracellular second messengers in regulating liver function.   The effect of cyclic AMP on carbohydrate
metabolism is well-established.   Cyclic AMP may also act on
intracellular reservoirs (4) to release calcium which, in turn,
may account for the efflux of potassium (5) which is associated
with the action of glucagon or epinephrine (Taken from Reference 2).

an influx of calcium (33) and characteristic changes in membrane
potential (34,35). Although cyclic AMP has no role to play in this
stimulatory effect of glucose, it does seem to mediate the action
of glucagon on insulin release. However, cyclic AMP is effective
only when operating in the presence of a certain critical level of
glucose. For example, glucagon does not stimulate insulin release
in the presence of 3.3 mM glucose but becomes an effective stimulus
when the glucose level is elevated to 16.5 mM (36). These studies
seem to indicate that cyclic AMP can potentiate the effect of
glucose. One possible explanation is that cyclic AMP may sensitize
β-cells to glucose by modulating calcium homeostasis. A clue to the
internal action of cyclic AMP was provided by Brisson et al. (37)
and by Brisson and Malaisse (38) who showed that theophylline increased the efflux of calcium from prelabelled β-cells. It would
be of interest to know whether glucagon, or cyclic AMP, was capable
of causing a similar efflux of calcium.

VI. CONCLUSION

Studies on the role of intracellular second messengers in the
control of insect salivary glands have stressed the central importance of calcium in the control of cellular activity. Cyclic AMP
also plays an important role but its exact function within the cell
is still unclear. There are strong indications that it may regulate intracellular calcium homeostasis. In particular, there is
evidence that cyclic AMP may promote the release of calcium from
intracellular reservoirs. There are indications in the control
mechanisms found in several mammalian systems (salivary glands,
liver and β-cells) to suggest that this action of cyclic AMP on
calcium homeostasis may be of general significance.

REFERENCES

1. Oschman, J.L. and Berridge, M.J. (1970) Tissue and Cell 2, 281
2. Berridge, M.J. (1975) Advances in Cyclic Nucleotide Research
    Vol.6, Raven Press, N.Y. pp.1
3. Berridge, M.J. (1970) J. exp. Biol. 53, 171
4. Berridge, M.J. and Prince, W.T. (1972) Advances in Cyclic
    Nucleotide Research Vol.1, Raven Press, N.Y. pp.137
5. Prince, W.T. and Berridge, M.J. (1973) J. exp. Biol. 58,
    367
6. Berridge, M.J., Lindley, B.D. and Prince, W.T. (1975) J.Physiol.
    244, 549
7. Berridge, M.J. and Prince, W.T. (1972) J. exp. Biol. 56, 139
8. Prince, W.T., Berridge, M.J. and Rasmussen, H. (1972) Proc.Natl.
    Acad.Sci.U.S.A. 69, 553
9. Prince, W.T., Rasmussen, H. and Berridge, M.J. (1973) Bioch.
    Biophys. Acta 329, 98

10. Berridge, M.J., Lindley, B.D. and Prince, W.T.(1975) J. exp. Biol. 62, 629

11. Feinman, R.D. and Detwiler, T.C. (1974) Nature 249, 172

12. Borle, A.B. (1974) J. Membrane Biology 16, 221

13. Berridge, M.J., Lindley, B.D. and Prince, W.T. (1974) In: Alfred Benzon Sympsoium VII. Secretory Mechanisms of Exocrine Glands. pp.2101-2109, Munksgaard, Copenhagen.

14. Berridge, M.J. and Prince, W.T. (1975) J. Cyclic Nucleotide Res. 1, 169.

15. Petersen, O.H. (1970) J. Physiol. 210, 205

16. Schneyer, L.H., Young, J.A. and Schneyer, C.A. (1972) Physiol. Rev. 52, 720

17. Selinger, Z., Eimerl, S. and Schramm, M. (1974) Proc. Natl. Acad. Sci. U.S.A. 71, 128

18. Schultz, G., Hardman, J.G., Schultz, K., Baird, C.E. and Sutherland, E.W. (1973) Proc. Natl. Acad. Sci. U.S.A. 70, 3889

19. Bdolah, A. and Schramm, M. (1965) Biochem. biophys. Res. Commun. 18, 452

20. Guidotti, A., Weiss, B. and Costa, E. (1972). Mol. Pharm. 8, 521

21. Feinstein, H. and Schramm, M. (1970) European Journal of Biochemistry 13, 158

22. Selinger, Z., Naim, E. and Lasser, M. (1970) Bioch. Biophys. Acta. 203, 326

23. Salomon, Y. and Schramm, M. (1970) Bioch. Biophys. Res. Commun. 38, 106

24. Creed, K.E. and Wilson, J.A.F. (1969) Australian Journal of Experimental Biology and Medical Science 47, 135

25. Petersen, O.H. (1970) In: Electrophysiology of Epithelial Cells, pp.207-221. Schattauer Verlag, Stuttgart.

26. Friedmann, N., Somlyo, A.V. and Somlyo, A. (1971) Science 171, 400

27. Friedmann, N. and Dambach, G. (1973) Bioch. Biophys. Acta 307, 399

28. Friedmann, N. and Park, C.R. (1968) Proc. Natl. Acad. Sci. U.S.A. 61, 504

29. Friedmann, N. (1972) Bioch. Biophys. Acta 274, 214

30. Gárdos, G. (1958) Bioch. Biophys. Acta 30, 653

31. Romero, P.J. and Whittam, R. (1971) J. Physiol. 214, 481

32. Meech, R.W. (1974) J. Physiol. 237, 259

33. Malaisse-Lagae, F. and Malaisse, W.J. (1971) Endocrinology 88, 72

34. Dean, P.M. and Matthews, E.K. (1970) J. Physiol. 210, 255

35. Dean, P.M. and Matthews, E.K. (1970) J. Physiol. 210, 265

36. Hales, C.N. and Milner, R.D.G. (1968) J. Physiol. 199, 177

37. Brisson, G.R., Malaisse-Lagae, F. and Malaisse, W.J. (1972) J. Clin. Invest. 51, 232

38. Brisson, G.R. and Malaisse, W.J. (1973) Metabolism 22, 455

INSULIN SECRETION - THE ROLE AND MODE OF ACTION OF CYCLIC AMP

W. MONTAGUE
Department of Chemical Pathology and
Diabetic Department
King's College Hospital Medical School
Denmark Hill
London SE5 8RX

I.C.GREEN and S.L.HOWELL
Biochemistry Group
School of Biological Sciences
University of Sussex
Brighton BN1 9QG
Sussex
England

CONTENTS

E THE ROLE OF CYCLIC AMP IN THE REGULATION OF INSULIN SECRETION
        (a) Short Term Regulation
        (b) Long Term Regulation

F MODE OF ACTION OF CYCLIC AMP IN REGULATING INSULIN SECRETION
        (a) Cyclic AMP as a modulator of islet cell metabolism
        (b) Cyclic AMP and microtubules
        (c) Cyclic AMP and calcium
        (d) Membranes
        (e) Speculation on the mechanism of action of cyclic AMP

G CONCLUSIONS

H ACKNOWLEDGEMENTS

I REFERENCES

INTRODUCTION

There is much evidence to suggest that intracellular levels of
cyclic AMP in endocrine cells may play an important role in determining rates of hormone release, and that many secretagogues influence cyclic AMP levels, and hence rates of secretion, by interaction with receptors which are related to adenylate cyclase, or by
inhibition of phosphodiesterase.   A mechanism of this type seems
to operate during activation of secretion by physiological agents
in, for instance, the anterior pituitary (1) and thyroid (2).   A
widely accepted model for the regulation of hormone secretion is
shown in Fig. 1, and it is the purpose of this paper to determine
how far this model is applicable to the regulation of insulin secretion by the B cells of mammalian islets of Langerhans.

Studies on the biochemical basis of the regulation of insulin
secretion have been greatly facilitated in the past 10 years by the
availability of techniques for the isolation from pancreatic tissue
of large numbers of metabolically active and functionally and structurally intact islets of Langerhans (3,4).   An islet isolated in
this way represents a heterogeneous cell population composed typically of 70-80% B cells, responsible for the synthesis, storage and
secretion of insulin and 20-30% of A cells most of which are concerned with the synthesis, storage and secretion of glucagon.   Homogenates or extracts of isolated islets are generally assumed to
reflect the characteristics of the predominating B cells, an assumption which has also been made in this paper.

THE PROCESS OF INSULIN SECRETION

The release of insulin from the B cell is a rapid process occurring within seconds of the addition of a stimulus such as glu-

cose (5). Whilst glucose also has dramatic effects in stimulating rates of insulin biosynthesis by B cells in isolated islets (6) this newly synthesised insulin is not available for secretion for periods up to 1 hour after its synthesis (7). In general, therefore, insulin released from the B cell, at least during the first hour of stimulation, comes from the cytoplasmic pool of insulin storage granules and it is the number of these granules released at any given time which determines the rate of secretion. There appears to be no good evidence for a pathway of secretion in normal cells which by-passes the granule stage, and the secretory mechanisms which we shall consider in this article relate to the process of insulin secretion by the extrusion of granule contents. The final extrusion occurs by fusion of the granule membrane and the plasma membrane of the cell with the release of the granule contents into the extracellular space and is termed exocytosis or emiocytosis (8). The movement of storage granules from the cytoplasmic pool, where they are present in large numbers, approximately 13,000 per cell in the mouse (9), to the plasma membrane for release has been termed margination (8). A role for microtubules in transporting granules from the cytoplasmic storage pool to the plasma membrane was proposed by Lacy, Howell, Young and Fink (10) on the basis of morphological studies and of evidence of the inhibition of insulin secretion by colchicine, a specific inhibitor of microtubule function. These observations have been confirmed and extended by Malaisse, Malaisse-Lagae, Walker and Lacy (11) and current concepts of the role of microtubules in the process of insulin secretion have been reviewed by Lacy and Malaisse (12).

In addition to the involvement of microtubules, two other factors have so far been identified as essential for insulin secretion to occur by this mechanism: the presence of adequate intracellular concentrations of ATP (13) and the availability of extracellular calcium (14). ATP is required for the final secretory process itself, presumably for the movement of granules through the cytoplasm and/or in the final membrane fusion involved in granule extrusion. The requirement for calcium, which like that for ATP is shared with many other secretory cell types, appears to be specific for the secretory process itself since insulin biosynthesis and granule formation are relatively unaffected by the absence of extracellular calcium (15).

COMPONENTS OF THE CYCLIC AMP SYSTEM IN ISLETS OF LANGERHANS

All the components of the cyclic AMP system depicted in Fig. 1 have been demonstrated in islets of Langerhans. Their characteristics have been investigated in detail and are described in this section. The interaction of secretagogues with the components of the B cell cyclic AMP system are described in the next section.

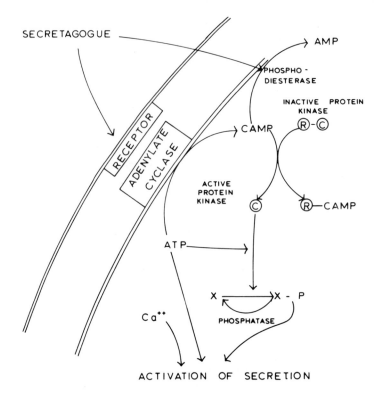

<u>Fig. 1</u> Model for the regulation of hormone secretion

Adenylate Cyclase

Cytochemical localisation of adenylate cyclase in islets of
Langerhans has shown the enzyme to be distributed apparently uni-
formly in the plasma membrane of both A and B cells, no activity
being found in any other organelle (16).

Two separate assay procedures have been used in studies of
islet adenylate cyclase: (1) Broken cell systems in which homogenates or subcellular fractions of islets are incubated in the
presence of radioactively labelled ATP and the labelled cyclic AMP
formed is then separated chromatographically.   (2) Surviving cell
techniques, in which intact islets are preincubated with [14]C-
adenosine or ^{3}H-adenine to label ATP within the cell, and after

further incubation of the tissue in the presence of a secretory stimulus cyclic AMP formed from this pool of ATP is separated and its radioactivity determined.

Using these techniques the properties of islet cell adenylate cyclase have been investigated in mouse (17,18) and rat islets (19-22) and hamster (23) and human islet cell tumours (24). In general the characteristics of the enzyme are similar in these different species. It is predominantly particulate, 80-90% being sedimented with a force of 10,000g x 10 min. The Km for ATP lies in the range $1 - 4 \times 10^{-4}$M and the pH optimum is approximately 7.6.

In common with all other mammalian adenylate cyclase systems islet cell adenylate cyclase in broken cell preparations is markedly stimulated by 10 mM sodium fluoride. The mechanism of this effect of fluoride is not known but it seems unlikely to play an important role in the physiological regulation of islet cell adenylate cyclase activity. As is the case in other tissues, nucleotides apparently play a role in the modulation of adenylate cyclase activity in islets of Langerhans. Thus, GTP or CTP increase both basal and hormone stimulated levels of adenylate cyclase activity (19, 20, 25).

Phosphodiesterase

Cyclic AMP phosphodiesterase activity has been investigated in islet cell tumours (23, 26, 27) and in islets isolated from guinea pigs (28) and mice (17, 29, 30). Subcellular distribution studies have indicated that both soluble and particulate activities exist, although the majority (70%) of the activity appears to be soluble. The pH optimum of the activity is in the range 8.0 to 8.7. Detailed electrophoretic and kinetic studies of the enzyme in islet cells has given evidence of distinct forms, one activity with a Km in the range 2-10μM and one or more with Km's in the range 30-500μM. Since the concentration of cyclic AMP in islets lies in the μMolar range, studies have largely been confined to the low Km phosphodiesterase activity.

Protein Kinase Activity

Protein kinase activity has been demonstrated in islets isolated from rat (31-33), guinea pig (34), mouse (35) and cod (35) and in an islet cell tumour (27).

Two approaches have been made to the study of islet cell protein kinase activity. In the first the enzyme has been partially purified from islet cells and its characteristics investigated using histone as an exogenous phosphate acceptor and in the second

approach protein kinase activity in subcellular fractions of islet
cells has been investigated using the endogenous substrates present
in the same fractions.   Subcellular distribution studies have
shown that most of the enzyme is soluble, the major portion of the
activity being recovered in the post-microsomal supernatant although significant activity was also demonstrated in granule and
microsomal fractions.   The general characteristics of the soluble
enzyme with histone as a substrate are very similar to those of
protein kinases extracted from other mammalian tissues.   Thus the
islet enzyme was activated by cyclic AMP with an intrinsic association constant for cyclic AMP of $1.15 \times 10^{-8}M$ (34).

The mechanism by which cyclic AMP stimulates islet cell protein
kinase activity appears to be similar to that for this enzyme isolated from heart, adrenal cortex and skeletal muscle (36-38).
Thus, protein kinase in islet cells consists of two subunits, one
of molecular weight 90,000 which binds cyclic AMP (receptor subunit)
and the other of molecular weight 75,000 which possesses protein
kinase activity (catalytic subunit).   In the presence of cyclic
AMP the receptor subunit binds the nucleotide and dissociates from
the catalytic subunit which then exhibits maximal kinase activity
(34).

Phosphoprotein Phosphatase Activity

Phosphoprotein phosphatase activity has been demonstrated in
islets of Langerhans (32, 33, 35).   Studies on the time course of
phosphorylation and dephosphorylation of islet cell proteins by
endogenous protein kinase and phosphoprotein phosphatase suggest
that both activities play an important role in regulating the level
of phosphorylation of islet proteins.

INTERACTION OF SECRETAGOGUES WITH COMPONENTS OF THE B CELL CYCLIC AMP SYSTEM

The major problem in trying to relate the model as depicted
in Fig. 1 to the process of insulin secretion concerns the wide variety of agents that affect the process.   These include metabolites
such as glucose, mannose, leucine and arginine; peptide hormones
such as glucagon, ACTH, pancreozymin and secretin; prostaglandins,
catecholamines and pharmacological agents such as methylxanthines,
imidazole and sulphonylureas.   In this section an attempt has
been made to summarise the current information concerning the effects of these agents on the various components of the cyclic AMP
system in the B cell with a view to determining the role of cyclic
AMP in mediating the effects of each agent on the release process.

Glucose

Since glucose is the major physiological stimulus to insulin release in many species, it is a question of crucial importance to determine whether the effects of glucose on insulin secretion are mediated via direct short term activation of adenylate cyclase, as postulated by Cerasi, Effendic and Luft (39). Results of studies using broken cell preparations to measure adenylate cyclase activity have so far been unequivocal; in none of the five studies has an increase in the glucose concentration of the incubation medium in the physiologically important range of 2-20 mM had any effect on adenylate cyclase activity (17-20, 40). The results of two studies using intact cell preparations of rat islets for adenylate cyclase estimations have also shown no effect of glucose on cyclase activity at concentrations up to 300 mg% (21, 22) even though this concentration of glucose induced maximal rates of insulin secretion.

Effects of glucose on islet cell phosphodiesterase activity have been investigated and in none of the four studies was there any evidence of a change (27-30).

Effects of glucose on protein kinase activity have also been investigated. Montague and Howell (34) and Steiner (41) reported a lack of effect of glucose on cyclic AMP dependent protein kinase activity in extracts of rat islets, while in experiments in which protein kinase was assayed immediately after incubation of intact islets in the presence of high glucose concentration there was no change in protein kinase activity in conditions in which effects of phosphodiesterase inhibitors and stimulants of adenylate cyclase were readily detectable (31).

Thus, in none of the studies on the enzymes of the cyclic AMP system in islets has an effect of glucose in the physiologically important range up to 20mM been observed, even though this concentration of glucose induces almost maximal rates of insulin secretion. This general agreement contrasts with the disturbing anomalies in the data relating to the effects of variation of glucose concentration on cyclic AMP concentrations in islet cells. Kipnis (42) and Montague and Cook (43) found that 30 or 60 min incubation with 20mM glucose in a static incubation system did not alter cyclic AMP levels in rat islets. These results have been confirmed with mouse islets in a perifusion system in which observations were made from 0.5 to 60 min by Cooper, Ashcroft and Randle (44). Hellman, Idahl, Lernmark and Täljedal (45) also found that 20 mM glucose had no effect on the cyclic AMP content of mouse islets save a very small initial rise detectable by a freeze-stop perfusion technique only. However, Charles, Fanska, Schmid, Forsham and Grodsky (46) found significantly elevated levels of cyclic AMP 2 and 20 min after exposure of rat islets to glucose in a perifusion

system.   The reason for this difference in results has not yet
been determined.   Zawalich, Ferrendelli and Matschinsky (47) have
reported that raising the glucose concentration from 2.75mM to
27.5mM increased the concentration of cyclic AMP in rat islets at
1 and 2 minutes, although it returned to pre-stimulatory control
levels by 5 minutes and was still at this level at 20 minutes.   The
use of 27.5mM glucose to obtain this effect must question the physiological significance of these observations.

Grill and Cerasi (21) have also found that high concentrations
of glucose (>20mM) stimulate the accumulation of cyclic AMP as
measured in their system, although over this concentration range
glucose has no further effect on secretion, perhaps suggesting
that the effect was unrelated to the insulin releasing action of
glucose.

Changes in the concentration of cyclic AMP which have been observed in islet cells in response to glucose do not correlate
either quantitatively or temporally with the effect of glucose on
insulin release (45, 46) suggesting that glucose does not exert its
short term effects on secretion directly by increasing cyclic AMP
concentrations in the B cell.

Amino Acids

Interaction of amino acids with components of the cyclic AMP
system has been considered as a possible site of action of these
agents in stimulating insulin release (48,49).   However, none of
the amino acids investigated, including leucine and arginine, has
any stimulatory effect on islet adenylate cyclase (19,20,23).
Phosphodiesterase activity of islet cell extracts does not appear
in general to be affected by amino acids (19,29).   Montague and
Howell (31) could demonstrate no change in the protein kinase activity of islets which had been incubated with either leucine or arginine.   There is thus little evidence to date which suggests a role
for cyclic AMP in mediating the insulin secretory response to
amino acids.

Imidazole

Imidazole inhibits the release of insulin (50) and it has been
shown to stimulate islet cell phosphodiesterase activity (28,29)
suggesting that the effect on insulin release may be related to a
lowering of islet cell cyclic AMP by this agent.

Sulphonylureas

The hypoglycaemic sulphonylureas exert their major effects by

stimulating the release of insulin and the effects of these agents
on the components of the cyclic AMP system of isolated islets have
been extensively investigated.   Tolbutamide has been shown to increase islet cell adenylate cyclase activity (19,40) and inhibit
phosphodiesterase activity (23,26,28,30).   Glibenclamide has also
been shown to inhibit islet cell phosphodiesterase activity (28,29).
Protein kinase activity and cyclic AMP concentrations are increased
in islets incubated with tolbutamide or glibenclamide (31,51,52).
It thus seems likely that the mechanisms of action of the sulphonylureas may involve elevation of cyclic AMP levels as a result of activation of B cell adenylate cyclase, inhibition of phosphodiesterase or of both.

Methylxanthines

There is general agreement that the methylxanthines theophylline, caffeine and 3-isobutyl-1-methylxanthine, increase rates of
insulin release, by affecting components of the cyclic AMP system
in islets of Langerhans.   All three agents have been shown to inhibit islet cell cyclic nucleotide phosphodiesterase activity
(17,23,26,28-30).   The relative effectiveness of these agents as
inhibitors of phosphodiesterase activity parallels their order of
potency in increasing insulin secretion, intracellular cyclic AMP
concentrations, and islet cell protein kinase activity, 3-isobutyl-
1-methylxanthine having the most dramatic effect on all three parameters (31,43,44).

These results suggest that the effects of methylxanthines on
insulin release are related to an increased intracellular cyclic AMP
concentration, consequent upon phosphodiesterase inhibition.

Prostaglandins

Johnson, Fujimoto and Williams (53) demonstrated that PGE_1,
PGE_2 and $PGF_{2\alpha}$ stimulated insulin release in response to glucose
from isolated rat pancreatic islets.   Stimulatory effects of PGE_1
on insulin release in mouse (54) and dog (55) have also been reported.

Studies on rat islet cell adenylate cyclase have shown that
PGE_1, E_2, A_1 and $F_{1\alpha}$ increase its activity (19,20,53), the order of
potency paralleling the relative effectiveness of the various prostaglandins in stimulating insulin release.   The information available at present suggests that prostaglandins may stimulate insulin
release by activation of adenylate cyclase in the B cell, thereby
increasing intracellular cyclic AMP concentrations.

Hormones and Neurohumoral Agents

Peptide hormones which have been shown to stimulate rates of insulin secretion and to activate islet cell adenylate cyclase include glucagon (20,23,24), corticotropin (19), secretin (18,56) and pancreozymin (18). Furthermore, glucagon has been shown to increase islet cell cyclic AMP concentrations (43,57,58) and to increase protein kinase activity in islet cells (31).

The catecholamines, epinephrine and norepinephrine inhibit the release of insulin in response to almost all agents tested and this effect appears to be mediated through the cyclic AMP system of the B cell. Turtle and Kipnis (57) and Montague and Cook (43) demonstrated that epinephrine decreased the concentration of cyclic AMP in rat islets incubated in vitro. This effect of epinephrine on cyclic AMP levels appears to result from the inhibition of islet cell adenylate cyclase activity since Montague and Howell (31) and Kuo et al. (19) have reported an inhibitory effect of epinephrine on islet cell adenylate cyclase activity. Protein kinase activity has also been shown to be decreased in islets previously incubated with epinephrine (31). It seems likely that the inhibitory effects of catecholamines on insulin release are mediated through the cyclic AMP system of the pancreatic B cell.

THE ROLE OF CYCLIC AMP IN THE REGULATION OF INSULIN SECRETION

Short Term Regulation

The extensive studies of Malaisse on the secretory response of the B cell to a variety of secretagogues have led him to postulate the existence of two separate types of stimuli: 'primary' stimuli which will increase rates of secretion in the absence of other agents (e.g. glucose, mannose or leucine) and 'potentiators' which will stimulate secretion only in the presence of a 'primary' stimulus (59).

The weight of evidence available at present suggests that glucose and possibly other 'primary' stimuli do not exert their short term effects on insulin secretion via direct interaction with components of the cyclic AMP system in islet cells. However, the effects of many other agents, including 'potentiators', on insulin release appear to be directly attributable to their interaction either with adenylate cyclase or phosphodiesterase activities in B cells producing alteration of the B cell cyclic AMP levels.

An increase in the concentration of cyclic AMP such as occurs in the presence of peptide hormones, prostaglandins or phosphodiesterase inhibitors will not per se lead to an increased rate of insulin release unless a 'primary' stimulus such as glucose is

present at a stimulatory concentration (6mM or above. Fig. 2).
However, it will increase the effectiveness of a given stimulatory
concentration of glucose and also lower the threshold glucose concentration at which the response is observed; the cell becomes
sensitized to the effects of 'primary' stimuli (Fig.2). A decrease
in the concentration of cyclic AMP such as occurs in the presence
of epinephrine, norepinephrine or imidazole lowers the responsiveness of the B cell to a primary stimulus and increases the minimal
concentration at which glucose becomes effective (Fig. 2). Thus
the role of cyclic AMP in the short term regulation of rates of
insulin release would seem to be to modulate the sensitivity of

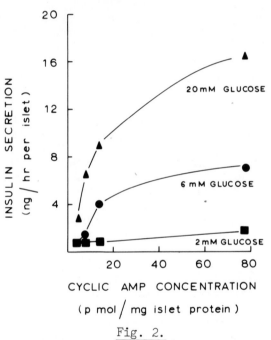

RELATIONSHIP BETWEEN CYCLIC
AMP CONCENTRATION AND INSULIN
SECRETORY RESPONSE TO
GLUCOSE

Fig. 2.

Rat islets of Langerhans were incubated in vitro for 1 hour in medium
containing 2, 6 or 20 mM glucose. Intracellular cyclic AMP concentrations were varied by the addition of epinephrine (to lower
cyclic AMP) or 3-isobutyl-1-methylxanthine (to increase cyclic AMP).
At the end of the incubation the insulin released into the medium
was measured by immunoassay and the cyclic AMP content of the islets was determined by a competitive binding assay. These procedures have been described in detail (61). The normal concentration of cyclic AMP in islets incubated in the presence of glucose alone was 8 pmol/mg islet protein.

the B cell to primary stimuli, in response to the Minute-by-Minute
changes in the levels of circulating hormones or to neuro-humoral
agents.

Long Term Regulation

There is some evidence that in addition to the acute alterations of rates of secretion there may exist in the B cell regulatory mechanisms responsible for longer term adaptations of the
secretory response to maintained changes in the physiological
status of the animal.   These longer term adaptations have been
identified in the case of pregnancy and diet, and the possible
role of cyclic AMP in achieving the observed changes has been considered in some detail.

Pregnancy.   The insulin secretory responses of B cells in
pregnancy are characterized by a lower threshold concentration
required for glucose stimulation and an increased response to a
given glucose stimulus (60) and these responses are comparable to
those achieved by short term incubation of islets from normal
rats in the presence of theophylline, a phosphodiesterase inhibitor (Fig. 3).   Green, Howell, Montague and Taylor (61) have
compared some components of the cyclic AMP system in islets from
pregnant rats with their non-pregnant littermates and observed
elevated adenylate cyclase activity and increased cyclic AMP
levels and cyclic AMP dependent protein kinase activity in islets
from pregnant rats.   Pair feeding experiments suggested that the
increased cyclase activity might be a result of the higher food
and particularly carbohydrate intake of the pregnant rats (62) although it is probable that hormonal influences, particularly of
placental lactogen, progesterone and oestriol may also be involved (63).

Dietary changes. Starvation has been recognized to have a profound effect on patterns of insulin secretion.   Thus starvation
of rats for 48 hours results in a drastic inhibition of the normal insulin secretory response to glucose (64 and Fig. 3), although
the responses to tolbutamide or theophylline remain relatively unimpaired (65).   The fact that the two agents which most readily
restore the normal response to glucose in islets from starved
rats were both phosphodiesterase inhibitors suggested that a defect
in the cyclic AMP system might be important.   In support of this
concept Howell, Green and Montague (66) showed that islets from
fasted rats had lower adenylate cyclase activity and reduced cyclic
AMP dependent protein kinase activity in comparison with their fed
controls.   Furthermore, adenylate cyclase activity and the insulin secretory response to glucose of isolated islets could be increased by prior loading of animals with glucose (2g/kg every hour)
for 4 hours by either intraperitoneal or intravenous route (66),

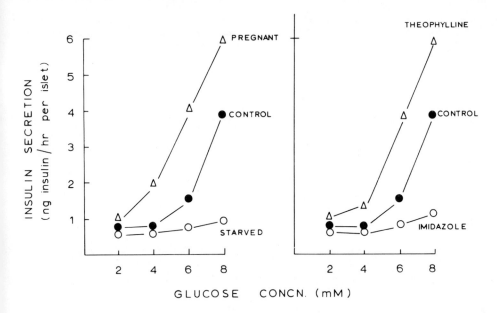

INSULIN SECRETION (ng insulin / hr per islet)

GLUCOSE CONCN. (mM)

Figure 3   Insulin Secretory Responses to Glucose

Islets of Langerhans isolated from 19-day pregnant, 2-day starved
or control female rats were incubated in vitro for 1 hour in medium containing various concentrations of glucose and the insulin
released into the medium was determined (left hand graph).   In a
separate series of experiments islets from fed control rats were
incubated in the presence or absence of theophylline (5mM) or imidazole (13mM) and various concentrations of glucose and rates of
insulin release determined (right hand graph)

suggesting a role for glucose in the long term regulation of islet
adenylate cyclase.   A direct effect of glucose on islet adenylate
cyclase activity was established by incubation of islets with 5.5
or 17 mM glucose for periods of up to 24 hours: a progressive
activation was achieved over a period of 2 - 7 hours and maintained through a 24-hour period (66).   Thus the longer term regulation of adenylate cyclase and cyclic AMP in islets by glucose
might be responsible for the altered secretory responses of islets
from fasted or glucose loaded rats.   Some support for this hypothesis derives from the observation that over a range of glucose
concentrations of 2-8 mM the secretory response of islets from
starved rats incubated in the presence of theophylline closely
resembles that of control rats to glucose alone (66).   Similarly,
insulin secretion from islets isolated from control rats and incubated with theophylline resembles the response of islets from glu-

cose-loaded rats incubated with glucose alone.   Finally, incubation of islets from control rats with imidazole, a stimulant of islet phosphodiesterase which would be expected to lower B cell cyclic AMP levels, results in a reduced response to 2-8 mM glucose resembling that seen in starvation (Fig. 3).

Thus with the proviso that these results refer to the physiologically important range of glucose concentrations (2-8 mM) and not necessarily to maximum rates of secretion, it seems that the effects of pregnancy, fasting and glucose loading on insulin secretion may be the result at least in part of alterations of B cell cyclic AMP levels, and that these changes are mediated by direct long term effects of glucose in regulating B cell adenylate cyclase activity.

MODE OF ACTION OF CYCLIC AMP IN REGULATING INSULIN SECRETION

The effects of cyclic AMP in many mammalian tissues appear to be related to the ability of the nucleotide to activate cyclic AMP-dependent protein kinases (67,68) and comparable enzyme activity has been demonstrated in the islets of Langerhans.   Incubation of intact islets with glucagon or methylxanthines, agents which raise cyclic AMP concentrations in islets of Langerhans and stimulate hormone release, has been shown to increase the protein kinase activity of islet homogenates where this is determined immediately after the incubation period, whereas diazoxide and epinephrine which lower cyclic AMP levels and inhibit insulin release, decreased protein kinase activity (31).   Thus, cyclic AMP may exert its effect on insulin secretion by increasing the activity of a cyclic AMP-dependent protein kinase in islets, thereby promoting the phosphorylation and altering the activity of one or more rate-determining components of the secretory mechanism.   The interplay between the activities of protein kinase and phosphoprotein phosphatase in regulating the state of phosphorylation of the components of the secretory process may provide a mechanism whereby the rate of secretion could be regulated on a minute to minute basis.   The characteristics of protein kinase substrates which may be important in the regulation of insulin secretion demand a rapid phosphorylation to initiate and dephosphorylation to terminate secretion after stimulation, and this will make the identification of proteins which are important in this respect even more difficult.   Cellular components which appear to play an essential role in secretion and which might be considered as possible substrates for the protein kinase are regulatory enzymes of glucose metabolism, protein components of the granule and plasma membranes, components of the microtubular/microfilamentous system, and calcium binding phosphoproteins.

Cyclic AMP as a Modulator of Islet Cell Metabolism

Since cyclic AMP potentiates glucose induced insulin release (69) and the effect of glucose on the release process may be related to glucose metabolism (70), the possibility exists that cyclic AMP might promote glucose metabolism by the B cell (69,71). However, the available biochemical data do not provide evidence to support the suggestion that cyclic AMP has any major effect on glucose metabolism in the B cell, apart from a role in the regulation of glycogenolysis, which is more likely to be important in the glycogen-rich B cell of the obese hyperglycaemic mouse than in normal animals (72).   Thus, glucagon has been shown to have no significant effect on glucose oxidation as measured by $^{14}CO_2$ production from ^{14}C-glucose by mouse islets (73).   Furthermore, neither glucagon nor dibutyryl cyclic AMP stimulated the respiration of isolated islets in the presence of 11 mM glucose (74). These observations do not rule out the possibility of more subtle changes in glucose metabolism by the B cell.   However, since theophylline and glucagon will stimulate insulin release in the presence of certain amino acids such as leucine in the total absence of glucose, it seems unlikely that the effects of cyclic AMP on insulin release can be accounted for solely on the basis of alterations in the metabolism of glucose by the B cell.

Cyclic AMP and Microtubules

Rasmussen (75) first suggested that microtubular protein (tubulin) might provide a substrate for cyclic AMP dependent protein kinase in nervous tissue and that this phosphorylation might provide the mechanism for the control of intracellular movements by cyclic AMP via the microtubular network.   The experimental basis for the hypothesis of the direct phosphorylation of tubulin or proteins closely associated with tubulin by protein kinase has subsequently been confirmed (76,77).   Recent studies have indicated that cyclic AMP may directly or indirectly affect insulin release by promoting the polymerisation of microtubules from subunits in islets of Langerhans (84).   A role for cyclic AMP in maintaining a pool of phosphorylated (activated) microtubule subunits ready for polymerisation or in maintaining microtubules in a state which would facilitate secretion would certainly provide a conceivable mechanism of action of this nucleotide in the regulation of insulin secretion.

Cyclic AMP and Calcium

Since both cyclic AMP and calcium play a role in regulating insulin secretion, it seems possible that there might be a direct

relationship between the two agents and this has been proposed as
a general mechanism of action of cyclic AMP by Rasmussen and Tenenhouse (78).   Malaisse and collaborators have undertaken a series
of studies designed to examine the role of calcium in insulin secretion by a study of the efflux and uptake of calcium-45 during
secretion from islets of Langerhans.   On the basis of these experiments Malaisse (59) has proposed that glucose inhibits the normal
outward flow of calcium from the B cell, causing an increase in the
intracellular calcium concentration which in turn triggers secretion possibly by interaction with the microtubular/microfilamentous
system.   Cyclic AMP did not appear to alter rates of calcium uptake or efflux, although possible effects on the intracellular distribution of calcium in islet cells were indicated by the observation that theophylline caused a dramatic increase in calcium efflux
from perifused islets in the absence of glucose when secretion was
not stimulated.   These observations have been interpreted as
showing that cyclic AMP may promote the intracellular translocation
of calcium within the B cell from an organelle bound 'vacuolar'
to a cytoplasmic pool of free ionized calcium, the increased concentration of which serves to activate the secretory process (59).
A model of this type requires the demonstration of calcium binding
sites within the B cell, and we have recently initiated a series of
studies which are designed to identify these sites and to investigate their characteristics.   Preliminary studies of calcium-45
accumulation by organelles present in homogenates of rat islets have
suggested the presence of multiple sites of accumulation within .
islet cells (79).   Mitochondria and endoplasmic reticulum (microsomes) both represent major sites of a rapid calcium accumulation
which is markedly stimulated by the addition of 1.25 mM ATP;   the
characteristics of uptake by these organelles resemble those already
reported for mitochondria and microsomes in other mammalian cell
types.   Insulin storage granules on the other hand, while containing high concentrations of calcium, do not appear to represent
a readily exchangeable pool which is subject to metabolic regulation
by nucleotides.

    Addition of cyclic AMP (10^{-6}-10^{-3} M)   to islet homogenates redu-
ces the calcium-45 accumulation by organelles by up to 60%   and preliminary subcellular fractionation studies suggest that this action
of cyclic AMP is exerted predominantly on the mitochondrial calcium
pool.   The effect may be similar in nature to that reported by
Borle (80) in experiments which showed that low concentrations of
cyclic AMP caused a dramatic efflux of calcium from preparations of
mitochondria isolated from kidney, heart and liver.   There is thus
direct experimental evidence from studies of calcium handling in
islets to support the suggestion of Malaisse (59) that one of the
effects of cyclic AMP in B cells may be to release calcium from an
organelle bound (mitochondrial) to a soluble calcium pool.

Further investigations are required to determine whether these effects are mediated through a cyclic AMP dependent protein kinase, and how the implied increase in cytosolic calcium concentration could serve to promote rates of insulin secretion.

Membranes

Interaction of insulin storage granules with the B cell plasma membrane is an essential component of the secretory process and it is possible that changes in the membrane proteins induced by phosphorylation could play a role in this interaction. Protein kinase activity has been demonstrated in membrane fractions from cod and mouse islets (35,81) and specific proteins in the membrane were shown to be readily phosphorylated and dephosphorylated, their phosphorylation being enhanced in the presence of cyclic AMP. Although formidable difficulties remain in the isolation and characterization of purified granule and plasma membrane fractions from mammalian islets, the results of these studies indicate that phosphorylation of membrane proteins in the B cell may form an essential component in the regulation of the secretory response.

Speculation on the Mechanism of Action of Cyclic AMP

Cyclic AMP and a primary stimulus both contribute to the regulation of the secretory process in the B cell, the effect of each one being dependent on the presence of an adequate concentration of the other and on adequate concentrations of ATP and calcium.

The reason why cyclic AMP is unable to stimulate release in the absence of a primary stimulus such as glucose is uncertain. The effects of phosphodiesterase inhibitors and adenylate cyclase activators on intracellular cyclic AMP concentrations are not dependent on glucose concentration. Thus 3-isobutyl-1-methylxanthine will increase cyclic AMP concentrations whether glucose is present at 2 mM or 20 mM (43,45) and similar results have been obtained with caffeine by Cooper et al. (44) and with theophylline by Charles et al. (46). Cholera toxin will also increase the concentration of cyclic AMP in islet cells independently of glucose concentration but will only potentiate the effect of glucose on insulin release (45). Thus glucose does not appear to be essential for the maintenance of B cell cyclic AMP levels.

It has been suggested (82) that glucose might simply be providing a source of energy for the secretory response since citrate or pyruvate, metabolites which by themselves did not alter secretion, were found to stimulate release from perifused minced pancreas pieces provided that theophylline was also present. It has

not been possible to confirm these results using isolated rat islets of Langerhans.   Thus, pyruvate or succinate had no effect on
insulin release in the presence or absence of 3-isobutyl-1-methyl-
xanthine and the effect of citrate on insulin release was not potentiated by 3-isobutyl-1-methylxanthine (83).

Thus glucose and other primary stimuli evidently have some specific role in the stimulation of secretion by cyclic AMP which is
unrelated merely to maintenance of cyclic AMP levels or of energy
supplies.   The simultaneous presence of a signal for secretion
appears to be necessary before a cyclic AMP-induced potentiation
effect can be observed.

Cyclic AMP might play its permissive role in the process by
maintaining a hypothetical pool of phosphorylated intermediates or
calcium at levels which would allow a satisfactory input into
the secretory mechanism.   If this pool falls below a critical
level then the secretory response to a primary stimulus cannot be
maintained and the threshold concentration required for secretion
to be initiated is increased.   Conversely, when the size of the
pool is increased the secretory response to a primary stimulus is
enhanced and the threshold is lowered.   The existence of such a
pool and the nature of the intermediates which might comprise it
remain a matter for further investigation.

CONCLUSIONS

The following general conclusions can be made concerning the
role and mode of action of cyclic AMP in insulin secretion.

1.   Islets of Langerhans possess all the enzymes involved in the
generation, hydrolysis and action of cyclic AMP which have been
observed in other mammalian cell types, and changes in the intracellular concentrations of cyclic AMP appear to play an important
role in regulating the rate of insulin release.

2.   Primary stimuli of insulin release such as glucose or leucine
at concentrations which affect release have no effect on the components of the cyclic AMP system in islet cells, so that the weight
of available evidence suggests that they do not exert their short
term effects on secretion directly through elevation of cyclic AMP
levels.   However, the effects of modifiers of secretion, which
require the presence of a critical concentration of primary stimulus
before they are effective, are directly attributable to their
effects on cyclic AMP levels.   These agents include glucagon,
corticotropin, secretin, pancreozymin, epinephrine, norepinephrine,
prostaglandins and acetylcholine which affect adenylate cyclase;
and sulphonylureas, imidazole and methylxanthines which affect
phosphodiesterase activity.

3.   Changes of cyclic AMP levels in islets may be produced in at least two ways: a.   Transient changes produced by short term alterations in B cell adenylate cyclase or phosphodiesterase activity. b.   Longer term adaptive changes which occur over a period of days in response to maintained changes in adenylate cyclase activity, these have been detected in starvation and in pregnancy.   Blood glucose concentrations, as well as hormonal influences, may have an important role in the long term modulation of adenylate cyclase activity under these conditions.

4.   The effects of alteration of cyclic AMP levels whether produced by short term regulatory or long term adaptive changes are similar.   An increase in cyclic AMP will potentiate the effect of a primary stimulus of secretion and lower the threshold concentration at which glucose becomes an effective secretagogue.   A decrease in cyclic AMP concentration will diminish and eventually abolish the secretory effect of a primary stimulus and increase the

Fig. 4

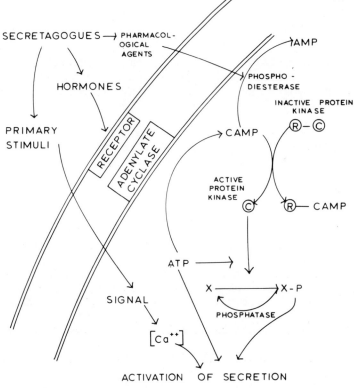

Hypothesis for the involvement of cyclic AMP in insulin secretion.

minimal concentration of glucose which is required to obtain an effect on secretion.

5.   The mode of action of cyclic AMP in regulating rates of secretion appears to be related to the ability of the nucleotide to increase cyclic AMP-dependent protein kinase activity.   This enzyme promotes the phosphorylation and possibly activity of rate determining components of the secretory mechanism.   Possible substrates for protein kinase in islet cells include granule and plasma membranes, microtubule protein (tubulin) and calcium binding proteins.

6.   The simple scheme proposed in Fig. 1 has to be modified to include additional regulatory factors, so that the rate of insulin release can be controlled by primary stimuli such as glucose or amino acids which do not exert their effects directly via cyclic AMP (Fig. 4).   Regulation of secretion by these agents is, however, still subject to modification by the prevailing cyclic AMP concentration in the B cell, and this in turn is regulated by short and long term changes in the hormonal and nutritional balance and physiological status of the animal.

ACKNOWLEDGEMENTS

Financial assistance from the Medical Research Council, British Diabetic Association, Hoechst Pharmaceuticals and King's College Hospital and Medical School Joint Research Committee is gratefully acknowledged. SLH is a CIBA fellow.

A more complete discussion of the topics presented in this article can be found in a review "Cyclic AMP and the Physiology of the islets of Langerhans", published in Vol.6 of Advances in Cyclic Nucleotide Research (Raven Press) 1975.

REFERENCES

(1) Steiner, A.L., Peake, G.T., Utiger, R.D., Karl, I.E. and Kipnis, D.M. (1970): Endocrinology, 86: 1354-1363.
(2) Dumont, J.E., Willems, C., Van Sande, J. and Neve, P. (1971): Annals of New York Academy of Science, 185: 291-316.
(3) Moskalewski, S. (1965): General and Comparative Endocrinology, 5: 342-353.
(4) Kostianovsky, M. and Lacy, P.E. (1966): Federation Proceedings, 25:377.
(5) Curry, D.L., Bennett, L.L. and Grodsky, G.M. (1968): Endocrinology, 83: 572-584.
(6) Howell, S.L. and Taylor, K.W. (1966): Biochimica et Biophysica Acta, 130: 519-521.
(7) Howell, S.L. and Taylor, K.W. (1967): Biochemical Journal, 102: 922-927.

(8) Lacy, P.E. (1961): American Journal of Medicine, 31: 851-859.
(9) Dean, P.M. (1973): Diabetologia, 9: 115-119.
(10) Lacy, P.E., Howell, S.L., Young, D.A. and Fink, C.J. (1968):
      Nature, 219: 1177-1179.
(11) Malaisse, W.J., Malaisse-Lagae, F., Walker, M.O. and Lacy,
      P.E. (1971): Diabetes, 20: 257-265.
(12) Lacy, P.E. and Malaisse, W.J. (1973): Recent Progress in
      Hormone Research, 29: 199-228.
(13) Coore, H.G. and Randle, P.J. (1964): Biochemical Journal,
      93: 66-78.
(14) Grodsky, G.M. and Bennett, L.L. (1966): Diabetes, 15:
      910-913.
(15) Steiner, D.F., Kemmler, W., Clark, J.L., Oyer, P.E. and Ru-
      benstein, A.H. (1972): Handbook of Physiology, Section
      7, Vol.1, edited by D.F.Steiner and N.Freinkel. Ameri-
      can Physiological Society, pp 175-198.
(16) Howell, S.L. and Whitfield, M. (1972): Journal of Histo-
      chemistry and Cytochemistry, 20: 873-879.
(17) Atkins, T. and Matty, A.J. (1971): Journal of Endocrin-
      ology, 51:67-78.
(18) Davis, B. and Lazarus, N.R. (1972): Biochemical Journal,
      129:373-379.
(19) Kuo, W., Hodgins, D.S. and Kuo, J.F. (1973): Journal of Bio-
      logical Chemistry, 248:2705-2711.
(20) Howell, S.L. and Montague, W. (1973): Biochimica et Bio-
      physica Acta, 320:44-52.
(21) Grill, V. and Cerasi, E. (1974): Journal of Biological
      Chemistry, 249:4196-4201.
(22) Miller, E.A., Wright, P.H. and Allen, D.O. (1972): Endocrin-
      ology, 91:1117-1119.
(23) Rosen, O.M., Hirsch, A.H. and Goren, E.N. (1971): Archives
      of Biochemistry and Biophysics, 146:660-663.
(24) Goldfine, I.D., Roth, J. and Birnbaumer, L. (1972): Journal
      of Biological Chemistry, 247:1211-1218.
(25) Johnson, D.G., Thompson, W.J. and Williams, R.H. (1974:
      Biochemistry, 13: 1920-1924.
(26) Goldfine, I.D., Perlman, R. and Roth, J. (1971): Nature,
      234:295-297.
(27) Schubart, U., Udem, L., Baum, S. and Rosen, O.M. (1973):
      Diabetes, 22, Suppl. 1:306.
(28) Sams, D.J. and Montague, W. (1972): Biochemical Journal,
      129:945-952.
(29) Ashcroft, S.J.H., Randle, P.J. and Taljedal, I.B. (1972):
      FEBS letters, 20:263-266.
(30) Bowen, V. and Lazarus, N.R. (1973): Diabetes, 22:738-743.
(31) Montague, W. and Howell, S.L. (1973): Biochemical Journal,
      134: 321-327.
(32) Dods, R.F. and Burdowski, A. (1973): Biochemical and Bio-
      physical Research Communications, 51:421-427.

(33) Müller, W.A. and Sharp, G.W.G. (1974): Diabetologia, 10:380.

(34) Montague, W. and Howell, S.L. (1972): Biochemical Journal, 129:551-560.

(35) Davis,B. and Lazarus, N.R.(1973): Excerpta Medica ICS,280,p7.

(36) Erlichman, J., Hirsch, A.H. and Rosen, O.M. (1971): Proceedings of the National Academy of Sciences, 68:731-735.

(37) Gill, G.N. and Garren, L.D. (1971): Proceedings of the National Academy of Sciences, 68:786-790.

(38) Reimann, E.M., Walsh, D.A. and Krebs, E.G. (1971): Journal of Biological Chemistry, 246:1986-1995.

(39) Cerasi, E., Effendic, S. and Luft, R. (1969): Lancet, 2: 301-302.

(40) Levey, C.S., Schmidt, W.M.T. and Mintz, D.H. (1972): Metabolism, 21:93-98.

(41) Steiner, D.F. (1972): Diabetes, 21, Suppl. 2:571.

(42) Kipnis, D.M. (1970): Acta Diabetologica Latina 7, Suppl. 1:314-337.

(43) Montague, W. and Cook, J.R. (1971): Biochemical Journal, 122:115-120.

(44) Cooper, R.H., Ashcroft, S.J.H. and Randle, P.J. (1973): Biochemical Journal, 134:599-605.

(45) Hellman, B., Idahl, L.A., Lernmark, A. and Täljedal, I.B. (1974): Proceedings of the National Academy of Sciences, 71 No.9, 3405-3409.

(46) Charles, M.A., Fanska, R., Schmid, F.G., Forsham, P.H. and Grodsky, G.M. (1973): Science, 179:569-571.

(47) Zawalich, W., Ferrendelli, J. and Matschinsky, F.M. (1973): Diabetes, 22: 331.

(48) Milner, R.D.G. (1970): Biochimica et Biophysica Acta, 192: 154-156.

(49) Effendic, S., Cerasi, E. and Luft, R. (1972): Journal of Clinical Endocrinology, 34:67-72.

(50) Malaisse, W.J., Malaisse-Lagae, F. and King, S. (1968): Diabetologia, 4:370-375.

(51) Charles, M.A., Lawecki, J. and Grodsky, G.M. (1973): Diabetes, 22: Suppl. 1:297.

(52) Sams, D.J. and Montague, W. (1974): Biochemical Society Transactions, 2:411-412.

(53) Johnson, D.G., Fujimoto, E.Y. and Williams, R.H. (1973): Diabetes, 22:658-663.

(54) Bressler, R., Vargas-Cordon, M. and Lebovitz, H.E. (1968): Diabetes, 17:617-624.

(55) Lefèbvre, P.J. and Luyckx, A.S. (1972): Diabetes, Suppl.1, 21:369.

(56) Thompson, W.J., Johnson, D.G. and Williams, R.H. (1973): Diabetes, 23, Suppl. 1:297.

(57) Turtle, J.R. and Kipnis, D.M. (1967): Biochemical and Biophysical Research Communications, 28:797-802.

(58) Selawry, H., Marcks, C., Fink, G., Lavine, R., Cresto, J. and Recant., L. (1973): Diabetes, 22, Suppl. 1:295.

(59) Malaisse, W.J., (1973): Diabetologia, 9:167-173.
(60) Green, I.C. and Taylor, K.W. (1972): Journal of Endocrinology, 54: 317-325.
(61) Green, I.C., Howell, S.L., Montague, W. and Taylor, K.W. (1973): Biochemical Journal, 134:481-487.
(62) Green, I.C. and Taylor, K.W. (1974): Journal of Endocrinology, 62:137-143.
(63) Costrini, N.V. and Kalkhoff, R.K. (1971): Journal of Clinical Investigation, 50:992-999.
(64) Malaisse, W.J., Malaisse-Lagae, F. and Wright, P.H. (1967): American Journal of Physiology, 213:843-848.
(65) Grey, N.J., Goldring, S. and Kipnis, D.M. (1970): Journal of Clinical Investigation, 49:881-889.
(66) Howell, S.L., Green, I.C. and Montague, W. (1973): Biochemical Journal, 136:343-349.
(67) Miyamoto, E., Kuo, J.F. and Greengard, P. (1969): Journal of Biological Chemistry, 244:6395-6402.
(68) Walsh, D.A. and Ashby, C.D. (1973): Recent Progress in Hormone Research, 29:329-359.
(69) Malaisse, W.J., Malaisse-Lagae, F. and Mayhew, D. (1967): Journal of Clinical Investigation, 46:1724-1734.
(70) Randle, P.J., Ashcroft, S.J.H. and Gill, J.R. (1968): Carbohydrate Metabolism and its Disorders, Vol.1, edited by F.Dickens, P.J., Randle and W.J.Whelan. Academic Press, London, pp. 427-447.
(71) Samols, E., Marri, G. and Marks, V. (1966): Diabetes, 15: 855-866.
(72) Idahl, D.A. and Hellman, B. (1971): Diabetologia, 7:139-142.
(73) Ashcroft, S.J.H., Hedeskov, C.J. and Randle, P.J. (1970): Biochemical Journal, 118:143-154.
(74) Hellerström, C. and Gunnarsson, R (1970): Acta Diabetologica Latina, 7, Suppl. 1:127-151.
(75) Rasmussen, H. (1970): Science, 170:404-412.
(76) Reddington, M. and Lagnado, J.R. (1973): FEBS Letters, 30: 188-194.
(77) Leterrier, J.P., Rappaport, L. and Nunez, J. (1974): Molecular and Cellular Endocrinology 1:65-75.
(78) Rasmussen, H. and Tenenhouse, A. (1968): Proceedings of the National Academy of Sciences, 59:1364-1370.
(79) Howell, S.L. and Montague, W. (1975): FEBS Letters 52, 48-52.
(80) Borle, A. (1974) J.Membrane Biol. 16, 221-236.
(81) Davis, B. and Lazarus, N.R. (1974): Biochemical Society Transactions, 2, No.3, 409-411.
(82) Burr, I.M., Balant, L., Stauffacher, W. and Renold, A.E. (1970): Journal of Clinical Investigation, 49:2097-2105.
(83) Green, I.C. and Taylor, K.W. Diabetologia (in press).
(84) Montague, W., Howell, S.L. and Green, I.C. Diabetologia (in press).

EFFECTS OF CYCLIC AMP ON B-CELL FUNCTION

Willy J. MALAISSE

Laboratory of Experimental Medicine
Brussels University
Brussels, Belgium

CONTENTS

INTRODUCTION

The role of adenosine-3',5'-cyclic monophosphate (cAMP) in the function of the pancreatic B-cell was recently and extensively reviewed (1). In order to avoid duplication, we will restrict the present contribution to a synoptic view of such a topic.

Two major aspects of cAMP involvement in B-cell physiology should be considered. The first of these, reviewed by Montague elsewhere in this volume, deals with the regulation of cAMP concentration in the B-cell and the concomitant changes in B-cell protein kinase activity. Recent investigations on the localization and regulation of both adenylate cyclase and phosphodiesterase activity in insular tissue, the influence of insulinotropic agents on cAMP accumulation and release in isolated islets, and the characterization of the insular protein kinase and phosphoprotein phosphatase systems have left some intriguing problems partially unsolved, such as the precise influence and mechanism of action of glucose upon cAMP level in the B-cell (2), the concomitant stimulation by cAMP of insular protein kinase and phosphoprotein phosphatase (3), and the nature of the endogenous proteins serving as a substrate for the latter enzymes.

With these queries in mind, we wish to concentrate on the second of the above-mentioned aspects, which deals with the influence and mode of action of cAMP upon physiological processes in the pancreatic B-cell.

THE INSULINOTROPIC ACTION OF cAMP

Any proposed mechanism for the action of cAMP in the B-cell should be able to account for the fact that cAMP provokes little if any release of insulin in the absence of glucose, but markedly enhances secretion evoked by either glucose, mannose, leucine or sulfonylurea (4, 5, 6, 7, 8). In other terms, cAMP does not initiate the secretory process, but potentiates the insulinotropic action of other secretagogues. Incidentally, the failure of cAMP to cause sustained stimulation of insulin release in the absence of glucose cannot be attributed to a shortage of such a permissive factor as ATP (1).

THE EFFECT OF cAMP ON INSULAR GLUCOSE METABOLISM

The enhancing effect of cAMP upon glucose-induced insulin release is dependent on the integrity of glucose metabolism in the B-cell (4). It is conceivable, therefore, that cAMP mediates its insulinotropic action through an alteration of glucose metabolism in the B-cell. However, as well as other authors, we have been unable, at least at high glucose concentration, to detect any effect of cAMP upon exogenous glucose uptake and metabolism in isolated islets (9, 10).

As a matter of fact, the only documented action of cAMP upon insular glucose metabolism is to stimulate glycogenolysis. Thus, cAMP indeed lowers the glycogen content of the islets (11). Moreover, even in the absence of exogenous glucose, cAMP stimulates insulin release in glycogen-enriched B-cells removed from rats rendered hyperglycemic for several hours prior to sacrifice. Under these experimental conditions, the insulinotropic effect of cAMP is not inhibited by mannoheptulose (4). It should be stressed that the glycogenolytic effect of cAMP, by mimicking the insulinotropic action of exogenous glucose, may lower the threshold value for the stimulant action of glucose upon the B-cell, but is unlikely to account for an enhancement of insulin release at high glucose concentrations (12).

THE EFFECT OF cAMP ON CALCIUM HANDLING BY ISOLATED ISLETS

Whereas glucose, leucine and sulfonylurea stimulate the net uptake of ^{45}calcium by isolated islets, cAMP only exerts such an effect at an intermediate glucose concentration (5.6 mM). At higher glucose levels, this glucose-like effect of cAMP is no more detectable. The insulinotropic action of the nucleotide, which is indeed most marked at these high glucose concentrations, cannot be attributed, therefore, solely to an imbalance between the influx and efflux of calcium across the plasma membrane of the B-cell (7).

The suggestion was made that cAMP provokes an intracellular translocation of calcium from an organelle-bound pool into the cytosol. Insulinotropic agents such as glucose or sulfonylurea, by inhibiting the outward transport of calcium, would allow the translocated load of calcium to remain intracellulary and, hence, cAMP to cause a sustained enhancement of insulin release. In support of such a concept, it was shown that (i) at low extracellular calcium concentration, cAMP partially restores the insulinotropic action of glucose or leucine ; (ii) cAMP provokes an increase in ^{45}calcium efflux from perifused islets ; and (iii) glucose minimizes the cAMP-induced increase in ^{45}calcium efflux (7, 13).

THE EFFECT OF cAMP ON PROINSULIN BIOSYNTHESIS

From recent work (9, 14), it appears that cAMP exerts two main effects on insular biosynthetic activity, namely a stimulation of ^{3}H-leucine incorporation into all insular peptides and a preferential stimulation of proinsulin synthesis. Both effects require the presence of glucose but fade out at high glucose concentrations. For instance, the preferential stimulation of proinsulin synthesis is most marked at low glucose (4.2 mM) or glyceraldehyde (5.0 mM) concentration, whilst failing to achieve statistical significance at a much higher glucose level (16.7 mM). Such a glucose-like effect represents a calcium-independent process. It is not due to enhanced uptake of glucose by the B-cell, but could correspond to the glycogenolytic effect of cAMP (9).

THE EFFECT OF cAMP ON THE B-CELL MICROTUBULAR-MICROFILAMENTOUS SYSTEM

No study of tubulin metabolism in isolated islets has as yet been completed. Only indirect information on the possible effect of cAMP on insular tubulin metabolism is available. The postmicrosomal supernatant of insular homogenates contains 80 per cent of the colchicine-binding proteins and colchicine may interfere with the cAMP-dependent phosphorylation of such endogenous pro-

teins (15). It is thus tempting to consider that cAMP could influence insulin release by interfering with the function of the
B-cell microtubular - microfilamentous system, a system which is
thought to participate in the dynamics of insulin secretion by
providing both the structural framework for the segregation of
β-granules and the motive force for their intracellular translocation and eventual release (16). However, a primary effect of cAMP
on such a translocator-releasing system is unlikely, since the alteration of the microtubular system by either colchicine or vincristine and that of the microfilamentous cell web by cytochalasin B do not differentially affect the respective insulinotropic
action of either glucose or cAMP (7, 17).

CONCLUSIONS

The present review underlines the fact that cAMP apparently
exerts a dual effect upon physiological processes in the pancreatic B-cell : a calcium-independent effect responsible for its glucose-like action and a calcium-translocating effect responsible
for its glucose-potentiating action. As a provocative and unifying
hypothesis, we wish to suggest that both the glucose-simulating
and glucose-potentiating actions of cAMP are secondary to altered
(de)phosphorylation of enzymes controlling glucose metabolism and
of membrane constituents involved in the subcellular distribution
of cations, respectively.

Acknowledgment
We wish to thank Mrs. B. Noël for secretarial help. The experimental work on which the present review is partially based was
supported in part by a grant from the Fonds de la Recherche Scientifique Médicale (Brussels, Belgium) and a grant-in-aid of Farb-
werke Hoechst A.G. (Frankfurt, Germany).

References[1]

1. Malaisse, W.J. Participation of the adenylate cyclase system.
   In O. Eichler, A. Farah, H. Herken and A.D. Welch : "Handbook
   of experimental Pharmacology", vol. XXXII/2 (A. Hasselblatt and
   F. von Bruchhausen, ed.), Springer Verlag, Berlin, in press,
   1975.
2. Hellman, B. The possible dependence of cyclic AMP on glucose
   metabolism in the pancreatic β-cells. Diabetologia 10, 368,
   1974 (abstract).
3. Müller, W.A. and Sharp, G.W.G. Cyclic AMP dependent protein
   kinase and phosphoprotein phosphatase in rat islets. Diabeto-

[1]The references were completed in September 1974.

logia 10, 380, 1974 (abstract).
4. Malaisse, W.J., Malaisse-Lagae, F. and Mayhew, D.   A possible
   role for the adenylcyclase system in insulin secretion.   J.
   Clin. Invest. 46, 1724-1734, 1967.
5. Malaisse, W., Malaisse-Lagae, F. and Mahy, M.   Effets du mannose sur la sécrétion d'insuline. Ann. Endocrin. (Paris) 30,
   595-597, 1969.
6. Malaisse, W.J., Brisson, G. and Malaisse-Lagae, F. The stimulus-secretion coupling of glucose-induced insulin release.   I.
   Interaction of epinephrine and alkaline earth cations. J. Lab.
   Clin. Med. 76, 895-902, 1970.
7. Brisson, G.R., Malaisse-Lagae, F. and Malaisse, W.J. The stimulus-secretion coupling of glucose-induced insulin release.
   VII. A proposed site of action for adenosine-3',5'-cyclic monophosphate. J. Clin. Invest. 51, 232-241, 1972.
8. Malaisse, W.J., Mahy, M., Brisson, G.R. and Malaisse-Lagae, F.
   The stimulus-secretion coupling of glucose-induced insulin release.   VIII. Combined effects of glucose and sulfonylureas.
   Europ. J. Clin. Invest. 2, 85-90, 1972.
9. Malaisse, W.J., Pipeleers, D.G. and Levy, J. The stimulus-secretion coupling of glucose-induced insulin release.   XVI. A
   glucose-like and calcium-independent effect of cyclic AMP.
   Biochim. Biophys. Acta 362, 121-128, 1974.
10. Ashcroft, S.J.H. and Randle, P.J. Metabolism and insulin secretion in isolated islets.   Acta diabet. lat. 6 (suppl. 1),
   538-553, 1969.
11. Hellman, B. and Idahl, L.-A. On the functional significance of
   the pancreatic β-cell glycogen. Wenner-Gren International Symposium Series 16, 253-261, 1970.
12. Malaisse, W.J. Insulin secretion : multifactorial regulation
   for a single process of release. The Minkowski Award Lecture.
   Diabetologia 9, 167-173, 1973.
13. Brisson, G.R. and Malaisse, W.J.   The stimulus-secretion coupling of glucose-induced insulin release.   XI. Effects of theophylline and epinephrine on ^{45}Ca efflux from perifused islets.
   Metabolism 22, 455-465, 1973.
14. Schatz, H., Maier, V., Hinz, M., Nierle, C. and Pfeiffer, E.F.
   Stimulation of H-3-leucine incorporation into the proinsulin
   and insulin fraction of isolated pancreatic mouse islets in the
   presence of glucagon, theophylline and cyclic AMP.   Diabetes
   22, 433-441, 1973.
15. Montague, W. and Howell, S.L. The mode of action of adenosine
   3':5'-cyclic monophosphate in mammalian islets of Langerhans.
   Preparation and properties of islet-cell protein phosphokinase.
   Biochem. J. 129, 551-560, 1972.
16. Malaisse, W.J., Malaisse-Lagae, F., Van Obberghen, E., Somers,
   G., Devis, G., Ravazzola, M. and Orci, L. Role of microtubules
   in the phasic pattern of insulin release. Ann. N.Y. Acad. Sci.,
   in press, 1975.

17. Malaisse, W.J., Hager, D.L. and Orci, L. The stimulus-secretion coupling of glucose-induced insulin release. IX. The participation of the beta cell web. Diabetes 21, 594-604, 1972.

ROLE OF CYCLIC NUCLEOTIDES IN THE ANTERIOR PITUITARY GLAND

B. L. Brown

Department of Nuclear Medicine
The Middlesex Hospital Medical School
Thorn Institute of Clinical Science
Mortimer Street
London W1N 8AA (United Kingdom)

Contents

Abbreviations

TSH = thyroid stimulating hormone (thyrotrophin);
LH = luteinising hormone; FSH = follicle stimulating hormone;
ACTH = Adrenocorticotrophic hormone; GH = growth hormone;
TRH = thyrotrophin releasing hormone;
GnRH (also LHRH) = Gonadotrophin releasing hormone;
CRF = corticotrophin releasing factor;
GHRH = growth hormone releasing hormone;
GHRIH (somatostatin) = growth hormone release inhibiting hormone;
PRF = prolactin releasing factor;
PIF = Prolactin inhibiting factor
TS = Triiodothyronine; T4 = Thyroxine

INTRODUCTION

It is now well established that a number of hormones synthesised in the hypothalamic area and carried to their adenohypophyseal site of action by a portal system, act to modulate the release of anterior pituitary hormones. Some of these hypothalamic regulating factors have now been characterised. The first to be demonstrated (1) was corticotrophin releasing factor (CRF); however, its structure is still not known. Thyrotrophin releasing hormone (TRH) was the first hypothalamic factor to be fully characterised, largely through the efforts of two groups led by Guillemin and Schally respectively (2,3) and shown to be a tripeptide (pyroglutamyl-histidyl-proline amide). The synthesis of TRH was closely followed by the identification and synthesis of gonadotrophin releasing hormone (GnRH), a decapeptide which stimulates the release of both LH and FSH.

The majority of studies on the mode of action of hypothalamic regulating hormones have employed TRH and GnRH and therefore much of the subsequent discussion will be concerned with this area. However, the existence of at least 7 hypothalamic regulating factors (some of which are inhibitory) has been reasonably well established (see Table 1) and some have been synthesised.

The secretion of ACTH, FSH and LH is known to be under positive control, whereas that of prolactin and growth hormone (and possibly TSH) results from a balance of the action of inhibitory and stimulatory hormones. The overall hypothalamic influence on GH and TSH is stimulatory, whereas prolactin is primarily under inhibitory control.

There have been, so far, two basic approaches to the investigation of the action of the hypothalamic regulating hormones and of other hormones acting on the anterior pituitary. They involve, on the one hand, the measurement of response parameters specific to particular cell type such as hormone secretion, and the incorporation of labelled amino acids into hormones, and, on the other, the measurement of non-specific effects, e.g. calcium movements, membrane potentials, cyclic AMP or cyclic GMP concentrations. However, due to the heterogeneity of cells in this tissue, special problems are involved in interpreting results concerning the latter non-specific effects. For example, since thyrotrophs comprise less than 5 per cent of the cells in a normal rat pituitary, observations of changes in these latter parameters in response to TRH stimulation could be insignificant when compared to the background effects arising in the other cells of the gland. Clearly, such studies would be more significant and

Table I

Cell Type	Hormone Secreted	Hypothalamic Factors Increasing Secretion	Hypothalamic Factors Inhibiting Secretion
Somatotroph	Growth Hormone (somatotrophin)	GHRH (?) TRH	GHRIH (Somatostatin)
Mammotroph	Prolactin	TRH (?) PRF	PIF Dopamine
Gonadotroph	LH FSH	GnRH (LH.RH)	
Corticotroph	ACTH	CRF	
Thyrotroph	TSH	TRH	(?) GHRIH

smaller changes more readily detected if they were conducted on
cell populations containing a high proportion of functioning
thyrotrophs. In practice, enriched populations can be obtained
either by selecting pituitaries from chronically physiologically
altered donors, (e.g. following thyroidectomy) or by preparing
cells from hormone-secreting tumours, (assuming that these cells
retain the relevant characteristics of normal cells). Alternatively, anterior pituitary cells prepared by enzymic dis-
aggregation may be fractionated by various physical and physicochemical techniques (4-7).

MECHANISM OF ACTION OF HYPOTHALAMIC REGULATORY HORMONES

Role of Calcium

Studies on other secretory processes (e.g. in the neuro-
hypophysis and adrenal medulla) have suggested that Ca^{++} may play
an essential role in stimulus-secretion coupling (8,9). For
example, it has been suggested that releasing factors might act
to alter the permeability of the cell membrane, leading to
increased uptake of calcium ions which, by a mechanism as yet
unknown, activates the release of the hormone by emiocytosis.
Poisner and Trifaro (10) suggested that Ca^{++} may serve to link
negatively charged groups at the surface of a secretory granule
and at the inner surface of the plasma membrane, thus bringing the
two membranes close together. Omission of Ca^{++} in vitro lowers
the amount of hormone released in response to releasing factors
and readdition restores the response. The removal of Ca^{++} also
inhibits the response to high potassium concentration, another
pituitary hormone secretogogue. It has been suggested that high
K^+ and hypothalamic regulating hormones may act through similar
mechanisms involving an increased permeability to Ca^{++}. However,
the fact that releasing factors can cause an additional increase
in the response of pituitaries treated with high K^+ militates
against, but does not rule out a similar mechanism.

Receptors for Hypothalamic Hormones

The binding of ^3H - TRH to plasma membranes prepared from
the pituitaries of various species has been reported (11-14), and
binding activity has been co-purified with the activity of adenylate cyclase (12). Hinkle and Tashjian (15,16) and Vale et al.
(17) reported that TRH was also bound by the prolactin and growth
hormone secreting cell line, GH_3. Since both TSH and prolactin
release are stimulated by TRH, it is reasonable to suppose that
both thyrotrophs and mammotrophs possess similar receptors. The

dissociation constant for (^3H)-TRH binding to GH_3 cells, TSH-secreting tumour cells and to bovine pituitary plasma membranes (15,14,11) is similar at approximately $1 - 2 \times 10^{-8}M$. The specificity of the receptors in GH_3 cells and TSH secreting tumour cells appears to be identical. Half maximal binding of TRH to GH_3 cells occurred at a higher TRH concentration (11nM) than the half maximal biological effect (2nM).

The binding of TRH was reported to be unaffected by other hypothalamic peptides, pituitary hormones or thyroid hormones (11), although the latter have been shown recently to alter the number of binding sites for TRH (18). The number of TRH binding sites was increased in hypothyroid rats as compared to the pituitaries of normal rats. Furthermore, one injection of L-thyroxine (60 ug) caused a drop in the number of sites within 6 hours, suggesting that the thyroid hormones may modulate the sensitivity of the anterior pituitary to TRH by controlling the availability of receptors.

The binding of LH-RH to rat pituitary cells (55) and to bovine cells and purified plasma membranes (19) has been reported. The rat cells possess two orders of binding site; one with a high affinity ($\sim 2 \times 10^{-9}M$) which corresponds well with the half-maximal effect of LHRH on both LH release and cyclic AMP accumulation (55,23). This binding site also possesses a specificity for LHRH analogues which relates well to the relative biological potencies of these analogues. The second binding site has a lower affinity ($2 \times 10^{-8}M$) but a higher capacity to bind LHRH. In a more recent study with isolated bovine pituitary cells binding reached a maximum in 1-minute at 37°C and was shown to be specific and saturable (19). In addition, it was reported that oestradiol treatment caused some alteration in the binding parameters.

Effect of Hypothalamic Hormones on Cyclic AMP Metabolism

a. Hypothalamic extracts

The addition of crude hypothalamic extracts to pituitary gland homogenates results in an increase in adenylate cyclase activity (20,21). These extracts had no effect on the adenylate cyclase of other tissues and extracts of cerebral cortex were inactive on the anterior pituitary. Hypothalamic extracts also caused significant increases in cyclic AMP concentrations in intact pituitaries in vitro (20, 21). Since these extracts contained a number of regulatory hormones, it is not possible to ascertain in which cell types the cyclic AMP concentration was increased. The rise in cyclic AMP concentrations with hypothalamic extract was not due to changes in phosphodiesterase activity and

was independent of Ca^{++} concentration. It has been suggested
that Ca^{++} acts at a site subsequent to changes in cyclic AMP
production.

b. Releasing Hormones

     Bowers (22) reported that synthetic TRH caused an
elevation in pituitary cyclic AMP concentration. This has also
been observed by Labrie et al. (23), a significant increase being
observed at 15 minutes of incubation. The rise in cyclic AMP is
small, amounting to a maximum of 50 per cent over control after
two hours of incubation with 10^{-6}M TRH. The small alterations of
cyclic AMP levels observed are not surprising in view of the
probability that only a small percentage of the cells (i.e. the
thyrotrophs and mammotrophs) would be stimulated. The addition
of TRH to cultures of GH_3 cells (a clonal strain of rat pituitary
cells) caused a significant increase in intracellular cyclic AMP
concentrations within 5 minutes. This effect of TRH was dose
dependent (16). Although the increase in cyclic AMP occurred
before the effect on prolactin release, in some experiments TRH
induced an increase in prolactin release from cells in which there
was no measurable change in cyclic AMP concentrations.

     Stimulation of cyclic AMP accumulation by LH-RH has also
been reported (24,25). Again, these changes are not thought to
be due to alterations in phosphodiesterase activity. A close
correlation between gonadotrophin release and changes in cyclic
AMP accumulation was reported by Borgeat et al. (24); the concentration of LHRH required for half-maximal stimulation of both
parameters being 1 x 10^{-10} -1 x 10^{-9}M. However, surprisingly,
the increases in cyclic AMP were delayed; no apparent changes
being observed until 120 minutes of incubation. These results
conflict with those of Kaneko et al. (25) who reported a rise in
cyclic AMP within 1 minute of stimulation with LHRH albeit at a
much higher dose ($\sim 10^{-6}$M). The minimally effective dose in this
study was 10^{-8}M. Rigler et al. (26) recently reported that,
although LH release was increased within the first 30 minutes of
incubation of pituitaries with LHRH, there was no change in cyclic
AMP levels at times shorter than 180 minutes. They concluded
that cyclic AMP did not appear to be an obligatory mediator for
the action of LHRH.

     Growth hormone - releasing hormone (GHRH) has also been
shown to lead to stimulation of cyclic AMP accumulation (27). In
this case, there was a rapid increase in cyclic AMP concentration
reaching a maximum at 5 minutes. However, Peake et al. (28)
reported that a partially purified GHRH preparation failed to
alter the activity of pituitary adenylate cyclase, or to increase

pituitary cyclic AMP concentrations.

Borgeat et al. (29) have recently reported that addition of EGTA to the incubation medium leads to inhibition of the LH-RH-induced rise in pituitary cyclic AMP concentrations, suggesting that Ca^{++} acts at an early site as well as at the late site, i.e. on hormone secretion itself. The effect of EGTA was reversed by the addition of Ca^{++}, the basal secretion of LH was enhanced in the absence of Ca^{++}. In the same study, it was shown that the GHRH-stimulation of cyclic AMP accumulation was not dependent on the presence of Ca^{++}.

c. Inhibiting Hormones

Somatostatin (growth hormone release inhibiting hormone) at a relatively high concentration of $10^{-6}M$ caused a rapid inhibition of prostaglandin E_2-induced accumulation of cyclic AMP in rat pituitary tissue (30), half maximal inhibition being seen after three minutes. A parallel inhibition of both GH and TSH secretion stimulated by PGE_2 was observed. It was suggested that somatostatin led to an almost complete inhibition of cyclic AMP production in the somatotrophs and thyrotrophs. Somatostatin lowered basal GH release in addition to that stimulated by theophylline, prostaglandins and cyclic AMP derivatives.

Prolactin release is predominantly controlled by a prolactin inhibiting factor (PIF) from the hypothalamus. Nicoll reported that when hypothalamic extract and theophylline were incubated with rat pituitaries in vitro, the effect of each on prolactin release was nullified by the other, possibly suggesting that elevation of cyclic AMP concentrations could overcome the inhibiting action of PIF (31). However, hypothalamic extract is as effective in inhibiting prolactin release in the presence as in the absence of theophylline suggesting that PIF and theophylline affect prolactin secretion by different mechanisms. As yet, there are no reports of cyclic AMP measurements in pituitaries exposed to PIF (or to dopamine, another inhibitor of prolactin release).

Effect of Theophylline, Exogenous Cyclic AMP and Prostaglandins

One of the first pieces of evidence suggesting a role for cyclic AMP as a mediator of the action of hypothalamic regulating hormones came from observations that theophylline could augment the release of growth hormone (32). Subsequently, it was shown that theophylline stimulated the release in vitro of TSH (33),

ACTH (34), LH (35) and prolactin (36,37). Theophylline was also
shown to act synergistically with hypothalamic hormones or
exogenous cyclic AMP on hormone release. Exogenous cyclic AMP, or
its derivatives stimulate the release of TSH (38,39), ACTH (34),
LH (35,40), FSH (41), GH (37,42,43) and prolactin (37). Prostaglandins E_1, E_2, and $F_{2\alpha}$ have been demonstrated to enhance growth
hormone release and synthesis (an effect that is potentiated by
theophylline), activation of adenylate cyclase and intracellular
cyclic AMP concentrations, (44,28). Prostaglandin E has been
observed to stimulate TSH secretion in vitro (45). However, there
appears to be no effect of the prostaglandins on LH (44,46) or
prolactin (44) release. The prostaglandin antagonist, 7 oxa-
prostanoic acid, inhibits both the release of TSH in response to
either TRH or high potassium concentration, and the release of ACTH
in response to high potassium (47). If this inhibition is
specific this may suggest a role for prostaglandins in hormone
secretion. It is possible that the action of prostaglandin in the
pituitary is mediated through the adenylate cyclase-cyclic AMP
system.

Cyclic AMP-Dependent Protein Kinase

Labrie and his co-workers have reported on the properties
and subcellular localisation of cyclic AMP-dependent protein kinase,
in the anterior pituitary (48,49). Perhaps one of the more
interesting aspects of this work was the finding that pure isolated
secretory granules were phosphorylated by a protein kinase present
on the granules. Cyclic AMP does not, however, stimulate this
activity. The proteins phosphorylated are reported to be structural
proteins of the granules (50). It has been suggested that phosphorylation of the plasma membrane and/or of the secretory granule
membrane could lead to an altered rate of membrane fusion-fusion
processes leading to emiocytosis. In addition, the occurrence of
a ribosome-associated protein kinase that is stimulated by cyclic
AMP could enhance protein synthesis at the translational level.
We have recently observed a dose and time-dependent increase in
protein kinase activity in resonse to hypothalamic extract and, in
preliminary work, to TRH in pituitaries from treated rats (51).
Kraicer (56) has recently reviewed the literature relevant to the
role of protein kinase in the pituitary and has suggested that
activation of a contractile microtubule system by protein kinase
may be involved in the release process. This is clearly an area
which is wide open to investigation.

Cyclic GMP

In contrast to the amount of evidence concerning a role for cyclic AMP in pituitary hormone release (which is by no means substantial) the evidence for a role for cyclic GMP is very sparse. Hypothalamic extract caused a fourfold increase in cyclic AMP and a two-fold increase in cyclic GMP. Incubation of pituitary tissue in the presence of aminophylline resulted in an up to tenfold rise in cyclic GMP concentration concomittant with a threefold increase in both cyclic AMP concentration and GH release. As mentioned earlier, no increase in intracellular cyclic AMP in the presence of GHRH was observed by Peake (28); instead an increase in cyclic GMP occurred. Exogenous cyclic GMP stimulated GH release; an effect that could be potentiated by aminophylline. In addition dibutyryl cyclic AMP caused an increase in intracellular cyclic GMP and in GH release (28).

Thus it is probably fair to say that at this juncture the role of cyclic AMP in pituitary hormone secretion is, at best, unclear. Many, if not all, of the effects mentioned in this section could be mediated by changes in the intracellular concentration of cyclic AMP.

TARGET GLAND HORMONE FEEDBACK

Target gland hormones act to modify the release of pituitary hormones. Taking the pituitary-thyroid axis as an example, it has been shown that there is a functionally competitive relationship between TRH and the thyroid hormones. TRH acts rapidly to stimulate TSH release whereas the thyroid hormones need several hours in vivo for expression of their inhibitory effects. Thyroxine also inhibits the stimulatory action of K^+ and theophylline. The accumulated evidence suggests that the thyroid hormones act at pituitary level by stimulating the production of a labile protein which blocks the action of the releasing hormone (52,53). Thus, actinomycin D prevents the blockade of TRH action by the thyroid hormones and cycloheximide can prevent and even reverse the effect of these hormones (52). Similarly, actinomycin D can block the effects of dexamethasone on ACTH release (54).

Very little is known concerning the involvement of cyclic AMP in this feedback control. It has been reported that thyroidectomy results in a rise in pituitary cyclic AMP content and that treatment with T3 in vivo returned this to normal values (22). In addition, prior treatment with T3 led to an inhibition of the rise in cyclic AMP caused by TRH. Wilber et al. reported that thyroxine inhibited TSH secretion even in situations where

presumably the intracellular concentrations of cyclic AMP were
high, i.e. in the presence of theophylline or dibutyryl cyclic AMP,
suggesting that the action of thyroxine was beyond the activation
of adenylate cyclase (39). Similarly, adrenalectomy and castration
have been shown to increase pituitary cyclic AMP concentrations.
Dexamethasone inhibited the effect of dibutyryl cyclic AMP-stimu-
lated ACTH release (34). Thus it is possible that steroid and
thyroid hormones affect not only the metabolism, but also the action
of the nucleotide. As noted earlier, the target gland hormones
may also affect the number of receptors on the cell for the regulating hormones. As redundancy in control systems is to be suspected, it is also possible that several mechanisms of inhibition
co-exist.

SUMMARY

     There is little doubt that hypothalamic hormones influence
the intracellular concentration of cyclic AMP in the anterior
pituitary. Indeed, the criteria for cyclic AMP mediation of
hormone action have been largely met. Hypothalamic extracts and,
in some reports, individual regulating hormones increase adenylate
cyclase activity and intracellular cyclic AMP concentrations,
exogenous cyclic AMP and its derivatives increase hormone release,
and phosphodiesterase inhibitors increase pituitary cyclic AMP
levels, stimulate hormone release and potentiate the action of
hypothalamic hormones. However, it is worth emphasising that
this simple view is not universally held. There are reports of
failure to demonstrate changes in intracellular cyclic AMP
accumulation in response to individual releasing hormones (e.g.
GHRH).   In addition, the reported LHRH-induced increase in LH
release preceding cyclic AMP changes mitigates against a necessary
role of cyclic AMP in hormone release. Some of this controversy
may well stem from the experimental conditions employed. The
adenohypophysis is an heterogeneous tissue and so the effects of a
releasing (or inhibiting) hormone on only one or two of the cell
types may be obscured by the background contributed by the other
cell types. The use of phosphodiesterase inhibitors may further
complicate the situation, particularly if some cells have a greater
basal adenylate cyclase activity. It is becoming clear that the
detailed elucidation of the role of cyclic AMP in the secretion
of individual pituitary hormones will have to await the preparation
of reasonably pure samples of the particular cell type. This is
likely to be particularly true in the case of the hypothalamic
hormones acting on cells which comprise only a small fraction of
the total cell number (e.g. TRH, CRF). The development of the
methodology for specific cell isolation will also be invaluable
in the investigation of the role of cyclic GMP which is currently
largely obscure.

Two principal hypothesis have been proposed for the mechanism of the hypothalamic hormones, one involving membrane depolarisation and Ca^{++} movements ("stimulus-secretion coupling") and the other involving the adenylate cyclase-cyclic AMP system. These two theories may be combined in a unitary hypothesis. One possibility is that cyclic AMP might act at the cell membrane or an intracellular organelles to bring about a change in the distribution of Ca^{++}. Protein kinase activated by cyclic AMP might be the mediator of this re-distribution of Ca^{++}. It is also possible that the protein kinase (with Ca^{++}) catalyses the phosphorylation of a protein, perhaps a contractile protein associated with the release process. Since K^+ ions also stimulate the release of pituitary hormones in the absence of changes in intracellular cyclic AMP, the redistribution of Ca^{++} may be all that is needed to trigger the release mechanism. Clearly, more detailed investigations will be necessary to determine the validity of this theory for the mechanism of action of releasing hormones, and also for the mechanism of action of hypothalamic inhibitors, (e.g. PIF, GHRIH). How the feedback control by hormones (e.g. thyroid hormones and steroid hormones) operate within this proposed scheme must also await further investigation.

REFERENCES

(1)   SAFRAN, M., SCHALLY, A.V., and BENFEY, B.G., (1955) Endocrinology, 57, 439

(2)   BURGUS, R., DUNN, T.F., DESIDERIO, D., and GUILLEMIN, R., (1969). Compt. Rend. Acad. Sci., 269, 1870

(3)   BØLER, J., ENZMANN, F., FOLKERS, K., BOWERS, C.Y., and SCHALLY, A.V. (1969). Biochem. Biophys. Res. Commun. 37, 705

(4)   HYMER, W.C., KRAICER, J., BENCOSME, S.A., and HASKILL, J.S., (1972), Proc. Soc. Exp. Biol. Med., 141, 966

(5)   HYMER, W.C., SNYDER, J., WILFINGER, W., SWANSON, N. and DAVIS, J. (1974), Endocrinology, 95, 107

(6)   LLOYD, R.V., and McSHAN, W.H. (1973), Endocrinology, 92, 1639

(7)   GARD, T.G., ATKINSON, D., BROWN, B.L., TAIT, J.F. and BARNES, G.D. (1975), J. Endocrinol. (in press)

(8)   DOUGLAS, W.W., and POISNER, A.M. (1964) J. Physiol. 172, 1

(9)   DOUGLAS, W.W., KANNO, T., and SAMPSON, S.R. (1967) J. Physiol., 191, 107

(10) POISNER, A.M., and TRIFARO, J.M. (1967). Mol. Pharmacol., 3, 561

(11) LABRIE, F., BARDEN, N., POIRIER, G., and DE LEAN, A. (1972) Proc. Nat. Acad. Sci. (USA), 69, 283

(12) POIRIER, G., LABRIE, F., BARDEN, N., and LEMAIRE, S. (1972), FEBS Letters, 20, 283

(13) GRANT, G., VALE, W., and GUILLEMIN, R. (1972) Biochem. Biophys. Res. Commun., 46, 28

(14) GRANT, G., VALE, W., and GUILLEMIN, R. (1973) Endocrinology 92, 1629

(15) HINKLE, P.M., and TASHJIAN, A.H. (Jr.) (1973). J. Biol. Chem. 248, 6180

(16) HINKLE, P.M., and TASHJIAN, A.H. (Jr.) (1974) Hormones and Cancer, 203, edited by McKerns, K.W., Academic Press Inc.

(17) VALE et al. (1973), Frontiers in Neuroendocrinology

(18) DE LEAN, A., BEAULIEU, D., and LABRIE, F. (1975). Proc. of the Seventh International Thyroid Conference, Boston. Excerpta Medica, Amsterdam

(19) ZOLMAN, J., and WARREN, J.C. (1975) Abstract. American Endocrine Society, New York

(20) ZOR, U., KANEKO, T., SCHNEIDER, H.P.G., McCANN, S.M., LOWE, I.P., BLOOM, G., BORLAND, B., and FIELD, J.B. (1969), Proc. Nat., Acad. Sci (USA), 63, 918

(21) STEINER, A.L., PEAKE, G.T., UTIGER, R.D., KARL, I.E., and KIPNIS, D.M. (1970) Endocrinology, 86, 1354

(22) BOWERS, C.Y., (1971) Ann. N.Y. Acad. Sci., 185, 263. Edited by Robison, G.A., Nahas, G.G., and Triner, L.

(23) LABRIE, F., BORGEAT, P., LEMAY, A., LEMAIRE, S., BARDEN, N., DROUIN, J., LEMAIRE, I., JOLICOEUR, P., and BELANGER, A. (1975). Advances in Cyclic Nucleotide Research, 5, 787. Edited by Drummond, G.I., Greengard, P., and Robison, G.A. Raven Press

(24) BORGEAT, P., CHAVANCY, G., DUPONT, A., LABRIE, F., ARIMURA, A., and SCHALLY, A.V. (1972) Proc. Nat. Acad. Sci (USA), 69, 2677

(25) KANEKO, T., SAITO, S., OKA, H., ODA, T., and YANAIHARA, N.
     (1973). Metabolism, 22, 77

(26) RIGLER, G.L., RATNER, A., SRIVASTAVA, L., and PEAKE, G.T.,
     (1975) Abstract. American Endocrine Society, New York.

(27) BORGEAT, P., POIRIER, G., CHAVANCY, G., DUPONT, A., and LABRIE,
     G.T. (1972) Hypothalamic Hypophysiotrophic Hormones.
     Excerpta Medica, Amsterdam, Int. Cong. Series N° 263, 174

(28) PEAKE, G.T. (1973) Frontiers in Neuroendocrinology, 173,
     edited by Ganong, W.F. and Martini, L.

(29) BORGEAT, P., GARNEAU, P., and LABRIE, F. (1975) Mol. and Cell.
     Endocrinology, 2, 117

(30) BELANGER, A., LABRIE, F., BORGEAT, P., SAVARY, M., COTE, J.,
     DROUIN, J., SCHALLY, A.V., COY, D.H., COY, E.J., IMMER, H.,
     SESTANJ. K., NELSON, V., and GOTZ, M. (1974). Mol. and Cell.
     Endocrinology, 1, 329

(31) NICOLL, C.S. (1971) Frontiers in Neuroendocrinology, 291.
     Edited by Martini, L. and Ganong, W.F., Oxford Univ. Press,
     London and New York

(32) SCHOFIELD, J.G. (1967) Biochem. J., 103, 331

(33) WILBERG, J.F., PEAKE, G.T., MARIZ, I., UTIGER, R.D., and
     DAUGHADAY, W.H. (1968), Clin. Res., 16, 277

(34) FLEISCHER, H., DONALD, R.A., and BUTCHER, R.W. (1969) Am. J.
     Physiol., 217, 1287

(35) RATNER, A., (1970) Life Sci. 9, 1221

(36) PARSONS, J.A., and NICOLL, C.S. (1970) Fed. Proc., 29, 377

(37) LEMAY, A., and LABRIE, F. (1972), FEBS Letters, 20, 7

(38) CEHOVIC, G. (1969), Compt. Rend. Acad. Sci., Ser. D. 268,
     2929

(39) WILBER, J.F., PEAKE, G.T. and UTIGER, R.D. (1969) Endocrino-
     logy, 84, 758

(40) LABRIE, F., PELLETIER, G., LEMAY, A., BORGEAT, P., BARDEN, N.,
     DUPONT, A., SAVARY, M., COTE, J., and BOUCHER, R. (1973)
     Karolinska Symposium on Research Methods in Reproductive
     Endocrinology, 301. Edited by Diczfalusy E.

(41) JUTISZ, M., and DE LA LLOSA, M.P., (1970) Endocrinology
     86, 761

(42) CEHOVIC, G., LEWIS, U.J., and VAN DER LAAN, W.P. (1970)
     Compt. Rend. Acad. Sci., Ser. D (Paris), 270, 3119

(43) LABRIE, F., BERAUD, G., GAUTHER, M., and LEMAY, A. (1971)
     J. Biol. Chem., 246, 1902

(44) MACLEOD, R.M., and LEHYMEYER, J.E. (1970). Proc. Nat. Acad.
     Sci. (USA), 67, 1172

(45) GUILLEMIN, R., BURGUS, R., and VALE, W. (1971) Vitamins and
     Hormones, 29

(46) ZOR, U., KANEKO, T., SCHNEIDER, H.P.G., McCANN, S.M., and
     FIELD, J.B. (1970), J. Biol. Chem., 245, 2883

(47) VALE, W., RIVIER C., and GUILLEMIN, R. (1971) Fed. Proc. Fed.
     Amer. Soc. Exp. Biol., 30, 363

(48) LABRIE, F., LEMAIRE, S., and COURTE, C. (1971) J. Biol. Chem.
     246, 7293

(49) LEMAIRE, S., PELLETIER, G., and LABRIE, F. (1971) J. Biol.
     Chem., 246, 7303

(50) LABRIE, F., LEMAIRE, S., POIRIER, G., PELLETIER, G., and
     BOUCHER, R. (1971) J. Biol. Chem., 246, 7311

(51) BARNES, G.D., and BROWN, B.L. Unpublished observations

(52) VALE, W., BURGUS, R., and GUILLEMIN, R. (1968), Neuroendo-
     crinology, 3, 34

(53) BOWERS, C.Y., LEE, K.L., and SCHALLY, A.V. (1968) Endocrino-
     logy, 82, 75

(54) ARIMURA, A., BOWERS, C.Y., SCHALLY, A.V., SAITO, M., and
     MILLER, M.C. (1969) Endocrinology, 85, 300

(55) GRANT, G., VALE, W., and RIVIER, J., (1973) Biochem. Biophys.
     Res. Commun., 50, 771

(56) KRAICER, J. (1975) in Ultrastructure in Biological Systems,
     7, 21, edited by Tixier-Vidal A., and Farquhar, M.G.

MECHANISM OF LH AND FSH ACTION ON THE TESTIS

Brian A. Cooke

Dept. of Biochemistry (Div. of Chem. Endocrino-

logy), Med. Fac., Erasmus University Rotterdam

CONTENTS

1. Introduction
2. Preparation of testis tissues and cells
3. Experimental models for the mechanisms of LH and FSH action
4. LH and FSH receptors
5. Cyclic AMP and testosterone production
6. Protein kinase
7. Protein and RNA synthesis
8. Summary and conclusions

1. INTRODUCTION

The testes fulfil a dual role analogous to that of the ovaries i.e. an endocrine function in the formation of steroid hormones and a germinal one in the production of spermatozoa. The seminiferous tubules are the site of spermatogenesis and they occupy approximately 85% of the gland volume. They are highly coiled (in the rat there are about 6 separate tubules) and are embedded in connective tissue containing the Leydig (interstitial) cells, the site of steroidogenesis. In contrast to the seminiferous tubules, the Leydig cells have an excellent blood supply. The whole testis is surrounded by a dense white inelastic capsule, the tunica albuginea.

It is generally accepted that the two trophic hormones follicle stimulating hormone (FSH) and luteinizing hormone (LH) secreted by the pituitary in

the male, control the endocrine and germinal function of
the testis although it is possible that other hormones
e.g. prolactin may also be involved. FSH (together with
the androgens) has an effect on spermatogenesis in the
seminiferous tubules whereas LH controls steroidogenesis
in the leydig cells. However, not only are the precise
mechanisms unknown, but until recently these actions of
the trophic hormones had not been studied at a cellular
and molecular level.

        Our knowledge of the sites and mode of action of
these trophic hormones is now expanding rapidly. It is
apparent that LH and FSH evoke specific responses in
specific cell types in the testis in terms of activation
of adenylate cyclase, cyclic AMP, testosterone and androgen binding protein production and activation of protein
kinase, RNA and protein synthesis. The following is a
review of these events and possible interpretation in
terms of mechanism of trophic hormone action especially
with regard to steroidogenesis.

2. PREPARATION OF TESTIS TISSUES AND CELLS

The cellular and molecular effects of trophic hormones
on the testis cannot be adequately understood unless the
specific tissue and cell types can be isolated. In the
rat the testis interstitial tissue and seminiferous
tubules can be obtained by wet dissection of the
decapsulated testis (1) and also by dissection of freeze
dried sections of the testis (2). The relative merits
and characterization of these separated tissues have been
investigated (3). It is particularly important to
determine the purity of the separated tissue fractions;
this can be achieved by using suitable enzyme markers
such as non-specific esterase and 3β-hydroxysteroid
dehydrogenase which are localized almost exclusively in
the interstitial tissue. Thus the contamination of the
seminiferous tubule fraction with this tissue can be
calculated (3). Unfortunately a suitable marker enzyme
for the seminiferous tubules is not available. The
interstitial tissue (and seminiferous tubules) obtained
by wet dissection do, however, show specific interactions
with trophic hormones and respond in terms of cyclic AMP
and testosterone when the trophic hormones are added in
vitro. The capacity of the interstitial tissue to form
testosterone (but not cyclic AMP) is, however, reduced
compared with the interstitial tissue present in the
intact total testis (4); this has been attributed to
cell damage caused by the dissection procedure.

Leydig cell suspensions (which also respond to LH
in vitro) can be obtained by collagenase treatment of
decapsulated testes (5) or simply by washing testes with
buffer solutions without collagenase treatment (6). The
Leydig cell preparations obtained by these methods also
contain cells from the seminiferous tubules. The different
cell types in the seminiferous tubules can be partially
separated from each other by collagenase treatment of
total testis tissue followed by unit gravity sedimentation
(Staput technique) (see (7) for references). Preparations
rich in Sertoli cells have been isolated by using tissues
from immature, cryptorchid or hypophysectomized rats in
which the other cells involved in spermatogenesis are
absent or present in low amounts (8).

3. EXPERIMENTAL MODELS FOR THE MECHANISMS OF LH AND FSH ACTION

For the regulation of steroidogenesis in the testis by
LH a model may be considered which is based on that
proposed for the mechanisms of ACTH action on the adrenal
gland (9) (Fig. 1). The sequence of events may be as
follows: 1. interaction of LH with its receptor in the
plasma membrane, 2. activation of adenylate cyclase to
form cyclic AMP, 3. activation of cyclic AMP dependent
protein kinase by cyclic AMP, 4. action of protein kinase
on protein synthesis to form a protein regulator, 5.
stimulation of steroidogenesis by the protein regulator.
A model to describe the action of FSH in the testis is
more difficult because the precise physiological function
of FSH is not clear. The induction of the androgen
binding protein, however, by this hormone (see section 7)
may be a possibility. The discussion that follows will
therefore mainly deal with the mechanism of LH and FSH
action in terms of the model proposed for LH.

4. LH AND FSH RECEPTORS

The action of hormones at their target tissues is
initiated by interaction with receptors to which they
are specifically bound with high affinity. It has been
shown that specific binding sites exist for trophic
hormones in the testis; LH and HCG bind specifically
with the leydig cells of the interstitial tissue (10,11)
and FSH binds with cells in the seminiferous tubules of
the rat testis (11,12,13). The cell type(s) which bind
FSH in the seminiferous tubules have not yet been
determined, although observations with immature testis
rich in sertoli cells may reflect that FSH binds to the
sertoli cells (12). Immunofluorescence studies have

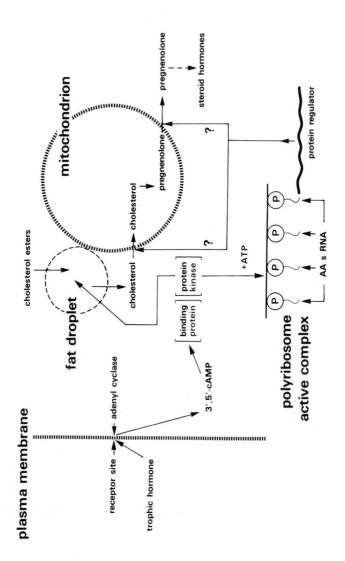

Figure 1. Scheme for control of steroidogenesis.

shown that LH may also bind to the peritubular myoid cells of the seminiferous tubules (11).

In agreement with studies with other trophic hormones it is thought that FSH and LH interact with receptors in the cell membrane because gonadotrophin binding has been found to be associated with membrane fragments during differential centrifugation of testis homogenates (12,14). In addition HCG covalently linked to sepharose (a molecule which does not enter the cell) still retains its biological activity of stimulating testosterone biosynthesis in rat testis tissues in vitro (15).

It has been demonstrated that LH is firmly bound to leydig cell tumours because removal of LH from the medium within 1 hour of incubation by washing the cells had no effect on the rate of steroid synthesis previously stimulated by LH (16,17). LH antiserum was required to reduce steroid synthesis (again indicating that LH has to be attached at a cell membrane receptor site to stimulate steroid production). Dufau et al. found that gonadotrophin can be removed from the receptor site in rat testis by eluting the incubated tissue containing bound ^{125}I-gonadotrophin with buffer at a low pH. The eluted gonadotrophin was still biologically active, in fact the activity was enhanced; this was attributed to affinity purification of the original hormone preparation by selective uptake at receptor sites. FSH bound to seminiferous tubules can also be recovered by elution of the tissue at acid pH and it retains its ability to activate protein kinase when added to fresh tissue (19).

There is apparently an excess of gonadotrophin receptor sites in rat testis because it has been shown that the capacity for gonadotrophin binding is 300 to 400 times greater than that required to stimulate maximally steroidogenesis during in vitro incubation. That these sites represent receptors rather than non-specific binding sites was shown by the parallel rise in cyclic AMP levels which accompanied the binding (20). Dufau & Catt (21) have solubilized the LH/HCG receptors in rat testis by treatment of membrane fragments of testes tissue containing broken interstitial cells, with Triton X-100. The solubilized receptors retained their ability to bind LH and HCG although the affinity was somewhat reduced. The properties of the receptor isolated were consistent with those of a highly asymmetric molecule, predominantly of protein nature, with a minor but functionally important phospholipid

component. Sucrose density gradient centrifugation
showed that the sedimentation constant of the free
receptor was 6.5 S, and that of the hormone-receptor
complex was 7.5 S. The molecular weights were calculated
to be 194,000 and 224,000 respectively (22). Further
studies by the same group revealed the presence of
several physical forms of the receptor depending on the
conditions and solubilizing agents used; e.g. dialysis
of the 7.5 S complex against detergent-free solutions
caused reversible conversion to an 8.8 S form of the
complex (23).

5. CYCLIC AMP AND TESTOSTERONE PRODUCTION

It has been shown that LH specifically stimulates in
vitro cyclic AMP production in interstitial tissue
obtained by wet dissection (4,8,24,25) and in leydig
cell preparations (5) whereas FSH specifically stimulates
cyclic AMP production in seminiferous tubules probably
in the sertoli cells (4,8,25,26). In initial studies
with seminiferous tubules little or no demonstrable
effect of FSH on cyclic AMP was obtained when tissue
from normal rats was used (24,26). It was found
necessary to hypophysectomize the animals first (26).
However, it is now realized that this apparent lack of
effect of FSH is because of the high phosphodiesterase
activity present in this tissue; if this enzyme is
inhibited then FSH stimulation of cyclic AMP production
can be demonstrated with tissue from normal rats (8,25).

It is well established that LH can stimulate
testosterone biosynthesis in the testis both in vivo
and in vitro (15,27). The site of testosterone
biosynthesis is the leydig cells in the testis
interstitial tissue (28,29,30) and it has been
demonstrated that LH but not FSH will stimulate
testosterone production in this tissue in vitro (4,5,31).
The intracellular mediator of LH action is thought to be
cyclic AMP (see review (32)).

There have been various reports (see (33) for
references) suggesting that the seminiferous tubules
may also form steroids from endogenous and/or added
substrates. However, endogenous production of steroids
has been found to occur almost exclusively (95-98%) in
intact cells and mitochondria from interstitial tissue
when compared to similar preparations of seminiferous
tubules (29,30). It has also been shown that LH added
with or without FSH to testis tissues causes 300 times
more testosterone to be formed in interstitial tissue

compared with the seminiferous tubules. The small
production of steroids which was found to occur in
seminiferous tubules may indicate steroid synthesis in
this testis compartment but at this low level
contamination by residual interstitial tissue could not
be ruled out (4).

It has been shown FSH does not stimulate
testosterone production in testis tissues in vitro and
that there is no synenergistic effect of FSH and LH (4,
15). However, there are several reports suggesting that
FSH potentiates the stimulating effect of LH in vivo.
This has been demonstrated both in the rabbit and in the
rat (35,36). Furthermore in cryptorchid boys it has been
shown that the higher the FSH plasma levels the higher
the testosterone production was after administration of
HCG (37). What the mechanism of this FSH effect is and
whether FSH works via the seminiferous tubules or the
leydig cells to produce this synenergistic effect remains
to be determined.

Finally there remains the question of the discrepency
between the amounts of trophic hormone required to
stimulate testosterone and cyclic AMP production. Several
groups have reported that approximately ten times more
LH is required to detect changes in cyclic AMP production
compared with that required to stimulate testosterone
production (5,20,31). This may, of course, imply that
with low levels of LH, cyclic AMP is not involved in the
intracellular action of this hormone. It is also possible
that small changes in cyclic AMP occurring with low
levels of gonadotrophins were not detected; that the
latter may be true is indicated by the stimulatory effect
of theophylline on testosterone release (but not on
detectable cyclic AMP) produced by low levels of HCG
(20).

6. PROTEIN KINASE

The cyclic AMP-dependence of protein kinases in rat
testis tissues has been demonstrated (19,38). Reddi et
al. (38) have reported that the soluble fractions of
testis homogenates are rich in the protein kinase enzyme
and that cyclic AMP markedly stimulated the enzyme using
various histones as substrates. An effect of
gonadotrophins on testicular protein kinase has been
described by Means et al. (19). They found that FSH
specifically stimulates protein kinase activity in
seminiferous tubules and that the stimulation was
accompanied by corresponding increase in cyclic AMP

production. The activation of the protein kinase depended
on the age of the animal and it disappeared when the
animals were 30 days old. The response could also be
observed in rats older than 30 days if phosphodiesterase
inhibitors were added to the incubation medium or by
using tissue from hypophysectomized rats. Their results
suggested that the appearance of an active
phosphodiesterase may be responsible for the decreased
response to FSH in the older rats; this also coincided
with the onset of spermatogenesis. Recent studies from
our laboratory have shown that cyclic AMP-dependent
protein kinases are also present in rat testis
interstitial tissue from adult rats and that LH
stimulates the protein kinase and causes parallel
increases in cyclic AMP. It was also found that when
0.5 M NaCl was added to the tissue before homogenization
(in order to overcome possible effects of dilution on the
association of the subunits of the protein kinase (40))
a marked reduction in the level of the cyclic AMP-
dependent protein kinase occurred. The same effect was
obtained when NaCl was added directly to the enzyme
preparation (105,000xg supernatant obtained after
centrifugation for 1 hour); these results suggest that
NaCl may inhibit or denature the protein kinase enzyme
or possibly activate a protein kinase inhibitor.

7. PROTEIN AND RNA SYNTHESIS

Irby & Hall (6) have studied the effect of LH on protein
synthesis in rat testis leydig cell preparations. They
found that little or no increase in protein synthesis in
these cells isolated after the hormone was administered
in vivo to normal rats. However, they did find that 5
days after hypophysectomy protein synthesis increased 5
hours after injection of the hormone.

More recent studies (40) have shown that although
changes in total protein synthesis could not be detected
after incubation of interstitial tissue from normal rats
with LH in vitro, inhibition of protein synthesis with
cycloheximide also inhibited the effect of LH on
testosterone synthesis. This suggests that a specific
protein could be involved in steroidogenesis in rat
testis interstitial tissue. Addition of cycloheximide
during superfusion of the tissue indicated that the
protein had a short half life (13 min). The specific
effect of cycloheximide on protein synthesis and not on
other mechanisms involved in steroidogenesis is suggested
by the parallel inhibition of protein synthesis and
steroidogenesis obtained with different doses of

cycloheximide (approximately 50% inhibition of both parameters was obtained with 0.25 μg/ml) and the lack of effect of this compound on LH induced cyclic AMP production. Moyle et al. (17) have also shown that cycloheximide (300 μg/ml) inhibits LH stimulated steroidogenesis in leydig cell tumours.

FSH has been shown to stimulate testicular protein synthesis in rat testis within 1 hour following administration to immature (20-day old) or mature hypophysectomized rats (41,42). The stimulation obtained in immature rats continued for at least 12 hours and occurred independent of amino acid transport or activation. An earlier effect of FSH was found on RNA synthesis; the testicular incorporation of ^{3}H-cytidine into rapidly labelled nuclear RNA occurred within 15 min and was inhibited by actinomycin D (43). FSH has also been shown to induce the production of an androgen binding protein (ABP) in the testis (44,45,46,47) which is secreted into the testicular fluid and concentrated in the caput epididymis. The protein is produced within the seminiferous tubules, since it is present in efferent duct fluid and completely absent from testicular lymph. The present evidence indicates that it is formed in the sertoli cells and may have important functions in spermatogenesis.

Recent observations have shown that dibutyryl cyclic AMP stimulates ABP production in sertoli cell cultures thus suggesting that cyclic AMP may also be involved in this action of FSH (48).

8. SUMMARY AND CONCLUSIONS

It is apparent from the foregoing discussion that evidence from studies with separated tissues and cells from the testis indicate that there are specific sites of action of LH and FSH as depicted in Fig. 2.

To summarize, the available evidence suggests that:
1. There are specific receptors for LH and FSH in the leydig cells and seminiferous tubules respectively and that they are situated in the cell plasma membranes.
2. LH and FSH specifically stimulate cyclic AMP production and protein kinase activity in the leydig cells and seminiferous tubules respectively.
3. LH specifically stimulates steroidogenesis in the leydig cells and FSH acts synergistically to increase testis steroidogenesis in vivo but not in vitro.
4. A specific protein is involved in the action of LH on

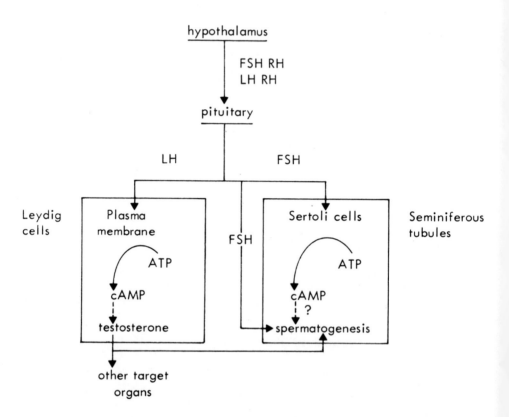

Figure 2.   Action of trophic hormones on the testis.

steroidogenesis in the leydig cells.
5. FSH stimulates RNA and protein synthesis and the production of ABP in the seminiferous tubules.

With respect to the action of LH on steroidogenesis there are many outstanding problems; one of the main ones being the establishment that a specific protein exists and subsequently the elucidation of the mechanism by which it is formed. The role of cyclic AMP in this respect is not clear although one might expect that the activation of the protein kinase will result in the phosphorylation of an essential intermediate. The actual mechanism by which steroidogenesis is stimulated is still unknown. Studies with leydig cell tumours (which contain an abnormally high percentage of esterified cholesterol) suggest that steroidogenesis is stimulated by increasing the hydrolysis of cholesterol esters in the lipid droplets to free cholesterol and subsequent uptake by mitochondria (49). The hydrolysis of the cholesterol esters may be under the control of cyclic AMP because it has been shown that in the rat adrenal cortex this nucleotide, via a protein kinase dependent phosphorylation reaction, stimulates cholesteryl esterase (50). The subsequent uptake of the cholesterol and/or the release of steroid intermediates from the mitochondria may be influenced by the proposed specific protein (Fig. 1). Until the precise physiological role of FSH is defined it is difficult to determine its mode of action. It is apparent that FSH is activating similar biochemical reactions to LH but what their relationship is to its effect on spermatogenesis remains to be elucidated.

REFERENCES

1. Christensen, A.K. & Mason, N.R. (1965) Endocrinology 76, 646-656
2. Van Doorn, L.G., De Bruijn, H.W.A., Galjaard, H. & van der Molen, H.J. (1974) Biology of Reproduction 10, 47-53
3. Rommerts, F.F.G., van Doorn, L.G., Galjaard, H., Cooke, B.A. & van der Molen, H.J. (1973) J. Histochem. Cytochem. 21, 572-579
4. Cooke, B.A., Rommerts, F.F.G., van der Kemp, J.W.C.M. & van der Molen, H.J. (1974) Molec. & Cell. Endocr. 1, 99-111
5. Moyle, W.R. & Ramachandran, J. (1973) Endocrinology 93, 127-134
6. Irby, D.C. & Hall, P.F. (1971) Endocrinology 89, 1367-1375
7. Loir, M. & Lanneau, M. (1974) Exptl. Cell Research 83, 319-327
8. Dorrington, J.H.& Fritz, I.B. (1974) Endocrinology 94, 395-403
9. Garren, L.D., Gill, G.N., Masui, H. & Walton, G.M. (1971) Recent Progr. Hormone Res. 27, 433-474
10. De Kretser, D.M., Catt, K.J. & Paulsen, C.A. (1971) Endocrinology 80, 332-337
11. Castro, A.E., Alonso, A. & Mancini, R.A. (1972) J. Endocrinology 52, 129-136
12. Means, A.R. & Vaitukaitis (1972) Endocrinology 90, 39-46
13. Bhalla, V.K. & Reichert, L.E. (1974) J. Biol. Chem. 249, 43-51
14. Catt, K.J., Tsurhara, T. & Dufau, M.L. (1972) Biochim. Biophys. Acta 279, 194-201
15. Dufau, M.L., Catt, K.J. & Tsurhara, T. (1971) Biochim. Biophys. Acta 252, 574-579
16. Moudgal, N.R., Moyle, W.R. & Greep, R.O. (1971) J. Biol. Chem. 246, 4983-4986
17. Moyle, W.R., Moudgal, N.R. & Greep, R.O. (1971) J. Biol. Chem. 246, 4978-4982
18. Dufau, M.L., Catt, K.J. & Tsuruhara, T. (1972) Proc. Nat. Acad. Sci. 69, 2414-2416
19. Means, A.R., MacDougall, E., Soderling, T.R. & Corbin, J.D. (1974) J. Biol. Chem. 249, 1231-1238
20. Catt, K.J. & Dufau, M.L. (1973) Nature New Biology 244, 219-221
21. Dufau, M.L. & Catt, K.J. (1973) Nature New Biology 242, 246-248
22. Dufau, M.L., Charreau, E.H. & Catt, K.H. (1973) J. Biol. Chem. 248, 6973-6982

23. Charreau, E.H., Dufau, M.L. & Catt, K.J. (1974) J. Biol. Chem. 249, 4189-4195
24. Cooke, B.A., van Beurden, W.M.O., Rommerts, F.F.G. & van der Molen, H.J. (1972) FEBS lett 25, 83-86
25. Braun, T. & Sepsenwol, S. (1974) Endocrinology 94, 1028-1033
26. Dorrington, J.H., Vernon, R.G. & Fritz, I.B. (1972) Biochem. Biophys. Res. Comm. 46, 1523-1528
27. Eik-Nes, K.B. (1971) Recent Progr. Hormone Res. 27, 517-535
28. Hooker, C.W. (1970) In: The Testis, Vol. I. Development, Anatomy and Physiology Eds. A.D. Johnson, W.R. Gomes and N.L. Van Demark (Academic Press, New York and London) p 493
29. Cooke, B.A., de Jong, F.H., van der Molen, H.J. & Rommerts, F.F.G. (1972) Nature New Biology 237, 255-256
30. Van der Vusse, G.J., Kalkman, M.L. & van der Molen, H.J. (1973) Biochim. Biophys. Acta 297, 179-185
31. Rommerts, F.F.G., Cooke, B.A., van der Kemp, J.W.C.M. & van der Molen, H.J. (1973) FEBS lett 33, 114-118
32. Rommerts, F.F.G., Cooke, B.A. & van der Molen, H.J. (1974) J. Steroid Biochem. 5, 279-285
33. Bell, J.B.G., Vinson, G.P. & Lacy, D. (1971) Proc. Roy. Soc. London B. 176, 433-443
34. Johnson, B.N. & Ewing, L.L. (1971) Science 173, 635-637
35. Swerdloff, R.S., Jacobs, H.S. & Odell, W.J., In Saxena, B.B., Beling, C.G. & Gandy, H.M. (eds) Gonadotropins, Wiley-Interscience, New York, (1972) p 546
36. Safoury, S.E. & Bartke, A. (1974) J. Endocrinology 61, 193-198
37. Sizonenko, P.C., Cuendet, A. & Paunier, L.(1973) J. Clin. Endocr. Metab. 37, 68-73
38. Reddi, A.H., Ewing, L.L. & Williams-Ashman, H.G. (1971) Biochem. J. 122, 333-345
39. Corbin, J.D., Soderling, T.R. & Park, C.R. (1973) J. Biol. Chem. 248, 1813-1821
40. Cooke, B.A., Clotscher, W.F., de Jong, C.M.M., Renniers, A.C.H.M. & van der Molen, H.J. (1974) J. Endocrinology 63, 17-18
41. Means, A.R. & Hall, P.F. (1967) Endocrinology 81, 1151-1160
42. Means, A.R. & Hall, P.F. (1968) Endocrinology 82, 597-602
43. Means, A.R. (1971) Endocrinology 89, 981-989
44. Ritzén, E.M., Dobbins, M.C., French, F.S. & Nayfeh, S.N. (1972) Excerpta Medica Int. Congress Series abstract no. 199, 256, p 79

45. Vernon, R.G., Dorrington, J.H. & Fritz, I.B. (1972)
    Excerpta Medica Int. Congress Series abstract no.
    200, 256, p 79
46. Hansson, V., Trygstad, O., French, F.S., McLean, W.S.,
    Smith, A.A., Trindall, D.J., Weddington, S.C.,
    Petrusz, P., Nayfeh, S.N. & Ritzen, E.M. (1974)
    Nature 250, 387-391
47. Vernon, R.G., Kopec, B. & Fritz, I.B. (1974) Molec.
    Cell. Endocr. 1, 167-187
48. Fritz, I.B., Rommerts, F.F.G., Louis, B.G. &
    Dorrington, J.H. (unpublished results)
49. Moyle, W.R., Jungas, R.L. & Greep, R.O. (1973)
    Biochem. J. 134, 407-413
50. Trzeciak, W.H. & Boyd, G.S. (1973) Eur. J. Biochem.
    375, 327-333

POSSIBLE ROLES OF CYCLIC NUCLEOTIDES IN THE REGULATION OF SMOOTH MUSCLE TONUS

Günter Schultz
Joel G. Hardman

Department of Pharmacology
University of Heidelberg
Heidelberg (Germany)

and

Department of Physiology
Vanderbilt University
Nashville, Tennessee, 37232 (USA)

Contents

INTRODUCTION

Within the last few years, our knowledge about the roles of cyclic nucleotides in some tissues has grown tremendously (17, 18). The role of cyclic nucleotides in smooth muscle, however, is still poorly understood, Smooth muscular tonus is affected by a variety of hormones and neurotransmitters that are known to affect cyclic nucleotide metabolism in mammalian tissues. In this paper we will discuss the effects of some physiological and pharmacological agents on cyclic nucleotide levels in smooth muscle and the possible importance of these changes for cellular functions.

CYCLIC AMP

The very large body of evidence suggesting a role for cAMP in the smooth muscle relaxing actions of β-adrenergic agents and other substances has been extensively reviewed by Somlyo and Somlyo (39), Andersson *et al.* (3) and more recently by Bär (5) and Prosser (26) and will be covered only briefly here. The satisfaction of several criteria (28) has been a suggested requirement for the implication of cAMP as the intracellular mediator of a certain hormone action. In brief these criteria are :

(a)   The hormone should increase the intracellular cAMP level in intact cells;

(b)   the hormone should increase adenylate cyclase activity in broken cell preparations;

(c)   exogenous cAMP should mimic the hormonal effect when added to intact cells;

(d)   phosphodiesterase inhibitors should potentiate or imitate the hormonal effect when added to intact cells.

To the above criteria, another might be added (this is adapted from a suggestion by Walsh and Ashby (48)):

(e)   cAMP should affect in cell free system processes known to be involved in the response of the intact cell to the hormone.

These criteria will serve as an outline to discuss the possible role of cyclic AMP in smooth muscle.

Hormonal Effects on Cyclic AMP Levels in Intact Tissues

β-adrenergic stimulation leads to an increase in the cyclic AMP content and to relaxation of most smooth muscular tissues (for references see : Phosphodiesterase inhibitors). In intestinal smooth muscle, relaxation caused by catecholamines involves both β *and* α-adrenergic receptors (10), but only the β-adrenergic effect is associated with increased cyclic AMP formation (3).

The C-terminal octapeptide of cholecystokinin causes relaxation and an increase in the cyclic AMP level in the sphincter of Oddi (2). While most prostaglandins cause contraction of smooth muscle, prostaglandin E_2 causes relaxation of bovine and canine veins accompanied by an increased cyclic AMP content (15), and prostaglandin E_1 causes relaxation and increases cyclic AMP levels in guinea pig tracheal rings (25).

Often the association between cAMP elevation and smooth muscle relaxation has not been carefully examined with regard to time courses and dose-response curves for both events. Furthermore, even the qualitative relation between the cyclic AMP level and the contractile response of a smooth muscle is not always clear. In a very careful study, Vesin and Harbon (47) have shown that prostaglandin E_1 and epinephrine both produce in rat myometrium cyclic AMP elevations that are indistinguishable in their rate of increase and maximum level reached. Moreover, the two agents appear to act on a single adenylate cyclase. The contractile responses to the two agents are opposite, however, prostaglandin E_1 produces contraction whereas epinephrine produces relaxation. Thus, the mere ability of a substance to increase the cAMP level in smooth muscle may not entirely account for the ability of the substance to produce relaxation of the muscle.

Hormonal Effects on Adenylate Cyclase Activity
in Cell-Free Systems

Adenylate cyclase has been studied only superficially in smooth muscle compared to other tissues (for references see : Phosphodiesterase inhibitors). It is not yet known whether the enzyme is restricted to plasma membranes or is also associated with other structures. Adenylate cyclase of some smooth muscular tissues has been reported to be stimulated by catecholamines; this effect was blocked by β-adrenergic blocking agents (46). Often, however, it has not yet been possible to demonstrate a β-adrenergic effect on adenylate cyclase activity in cell-free systems from smooth muscle (e.g. 31) despite the ability of these agents to increase cAMP levels in the intact tissue.

Effects of Exogenous Cyclic AMP and Its Dibutyryl Derivative on Smooth Muscle Tonus

Exogenous cAMP and its dibutyryl and other derivatives have been applied to many smooth muscular preparations (for references see : Phosphodiesterase inhibitors). Dibutyryl cAMP has produced relaxation of all preparations reported, and Somlyo *et al.* (39, 40) have shown that the hyperpolarizing effect of β-adrenergic agents in vascular smooth muscle can be mimicked by dibutyryl cyclic AMP.

Cyclic AMP itself, however, has produced inconsistent effects on the tonus of various smooth muscular tissues. In some preparations it has produced relaxation, but in others it has caused contraction or an augmentation of the effect of contracting agents (for references see : Phosphodiesterase inhibitors). In many studies involving effects of exogenous cAMP and its derivatives control experiments have been inadequate. The apparently para-doxical contracting effect of exogenous cAMP is probably non-speci-fic for the cyclic nucleotide with most if not all preparations, and the relaxing action of the cyclic nucleotide and its derivatives may also be non-specific in some cases. For example, low concen-trations of ATP and other nucleotides can cause either contraction or relaxation of many smooth muscles (9, 11), and these effects have not been shown to be related to changes in cAMP levels.

Effects of Cyclic AMP on Cellular Processes

Increased phosphorylation of proteins by cAMP-stimulated pro-tein kinases has been established in some tissues as an essential step in hormone actions involving increased formation of cAMP (21, 48). cAMP-stimulated protein kinase has been demonstrated in some smooth muscular tissues (29, 30), but the physiological role of the enzyme in smooth muscle is not yet known.

The possibility that hormones and drugs affect smooth muscle tonus by altering intracellular Ca^{++} distribution has been con-sidered for some time (19, 39). Some investigators have shown that cAMP (and, for unclear reasons, agents that affect cAMP meta-bolism) may increase Ca^{++} binding by microsomal fractions from intestinal (4) and vascular (6) smooth muscle.

Casnellie and Greengard (12) have recently reported that cAMP can stimulate the endogenous phosphorylation of three proteins associated with membranes of mammalian smooth muscle. The possible relation of this phosphorylation to altered Ca^{++}-binding or to other alterations in membrane properties has not been demonstrated.

Phosphodiesterase Inhibitors

Several drugs that are known to inhibit cyclic nucleotide phosphodiesterase *in vitro* have been shown to cause relaxation of smooth muscular tissues (for references see 5). However, for several reasons, it is not clear that the relaxant action of these compounds involves solely an inhibition of cAMP degradation :

a) Some of these drugs are apparently able to alter Ca^{++} distribution at least in skeletal muscle by phosphodiesterase-independent mechanisms (49).

b) Methylxanthines, the oldest known group of phosphodiesterase inhibitors, are capable of blocking purinergic agents at the receptor level (11) and of inhibiting renal trans-tubular transport of cAMP (13).

c) All phosphodiesterase inhibitors studied so far inhibit not only cAMP but also cGMP degradation when applied to cell-free systems (50) as well as to intact tissues (34, 43). For example, the phosphodiesterase inhibitor methylisobutylxanthine (SC-2964) relaxes the rat ductus deferens and causes an even greater relative increase in cGMP than in cAMP content (34).

d) It has recently been reported that papaverine, a potent phosphodiesterase inhibitor and smooth muscle relaxant may inhibit oxidative phosphorylation in astrocytoma cells (8), and this agent may also inhibit cAMP extrusion from avian erythrocytes (24). These effects do not appear to involve phosphodiesterase inhibition. Furthermore, stimulation of cyclic nucleotide phosphodiesterase from rat heart by papaverine has recently been reported (1).

Although most of these observations were made in cell types other than smooth muscle, they should be taken into consideration in general when using methylxanthines, papaverine and other phosphodiesterase inhibitors as tools in assessing a role for cAMP in a certain cell response. These and other findings indicate that potentiation or imitation of a hormonal effect by phosphodiesterase inhibitors should be used only very carefully as a criterion for establishing cAMP as an intracellular mediator of actions of that hormone.

CYCLIC GMP

There are now numerous findings to suggest a role for another naturally occurring cyclic nucleotide, cGMP, in the control of cellular functions (for review see : 17), and some observations indicate that this substance may be involved in the contractile response of smooth muscle to various agents. It has been suggested that cGMP and cAMP play opposing roles in the regulation of smooth muscle tone (15, 22). In discussing the possible role of cGMP in smooth muscle, we shall consider the same criteria

that were used in evaluating the role of cAMP. Although it may
be naive to look at the possible roles of cGMP and cAMP in the
same manner, there should be some value in examining the evidence
for a function for cGMP along these lines.

Hormonal Effects on Cyclic GMP Levels in Intact Tissues

Several agents that promote smooth muscle contraction have
been found to increase the intracellular content of cGMP. These
compounds and the tissues affected are summarized in Table I.

The effects of acetylcholine on cyclic nucleotide levels in
rat ductus deferens (under isotonic conditions) is shown in Figure
1 (34). The effect of cholinergic agents on the cGMP level is
blocked by the simultaneous or preceding addition of atropine (22,
34). This finding indicates that muscarinic cholinergic receptors

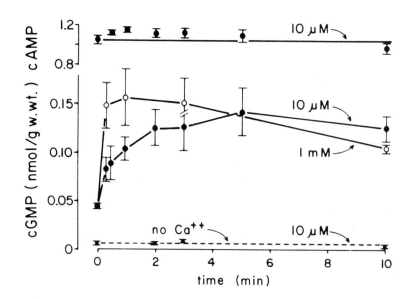

FIGURE 1. Effects of acetylcholine on cyclic nucleotide levels in
rat ductus deferens. Tissues were incubated under isotonic conditions in a balanced salt solution (35). After 30 min. of preincubation in the absence of Ca^{++} (dotted line) or in the presence of
1.8 mM Ca^{++} (solid lines), acetylcholine (10 µM,●, or 1 mM,○) was
added for various lengths of time. Cyclic nucleotides were determined by published procedures (35). Values are means of 5-25 samples,
and vertical lines are 2 SEM.w.wt., wet weight. Reproduced from
Schultz et al. (34).

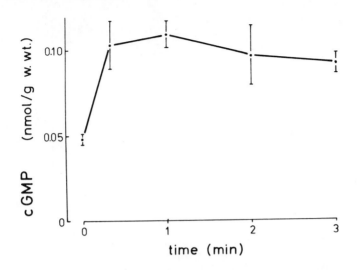

FIGURE 2. _Effect of potassium chloride on the cGMP level in rat ductus deferens. After preincubation for 30 minutes in a balanced salt solution, the tissue samples were transferred to medium containing 125 mM KCl but no NaCl for the times indicated. From data of Schultz et al. (34)._

are involved in the effect of acetylcholine and its derivatives on the cGMP level (as well as contraction) in smooth muscle.

Another compound that causes contraction and increases the cGMP level of the ductus deferens is potassium chloride. A depolarizing concentration of KCl increased the cGMP level 2-fold within 20 seconds (Figure 2) (34).

Catecholamines also increased the cGMP content in the ductus deferens (Figure 3) (35, 37). The effect of norepinephrine on cGMP was blocked by the α-adrenergic blocking agent, phentolamine, whereas the effect on cAMP was abolished by the β-adrenergic agent, propranolol. Atropine did not affect the norepinephrine-induced changes in cyclic nucleotide levels. The synthetic catecholamine derivative, phenylephrine, which has only a weak β-adrenergic stimulatory effect, increased cGMP but not cAMP. These findings indicate that α-adrenergic receptors are involved in the effect of catecholamines on cGMP levels in the ductus deferens.

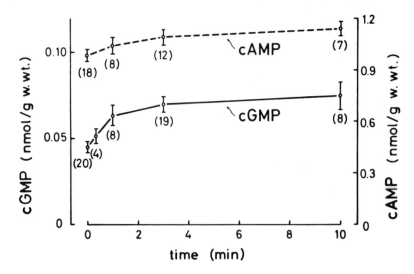

FIGURE 3. *Effects of norepinephrine on cyclic nucleotide levels in rat ductus deferens. After 30 minutes of preincubation, l-norepinephrine (10 μM) was added for various lengths of time. Modified from data of Schultz et al. (35). The number of tissue samples per group is given in parentheses.*

   In contrast to the increase in cGMP caused by acetylcholine, the effect of norepinephrine and phenylephrine on cGMP in the ductus deferens was observed only after contraction (as determined under isometric conditions) was fully developed (37). The car- bachol-induced increase in cGMP in guinea pig uterus and taenia coli also appears to occur after development of contraction (14). Moreover, carbachol-induced contractions of rat uterus are reported to occur without any change in the cGMP level (14), and some prostaglandin-induced contractions of human umbilical arteries occur without detectable changes in cGMP (see Vaughan et al. : these proceedings). Thus, although with several agents there appears to be a close association between stimulation of

contraction and elevation of cGMP levels, the change in the nucleotide concentration may not be a primary and necessary event in the
stimulation of contraction.

Guanylate Cyclase Activity in Cell-Free Systems

Guanylate cyclase has been studied only very superficially in
smooth muscle. As in other tissues, the enzyme occurs in both
particulate and soluble fractions (7). Effects of divalent cations
and of hormones or neurotransmitters on the enzyme activity in
smooth muscle have not been reported yet. A review of reported
effects of cations, neurotransmitters and hormones on guanylate
cyclase in various tissues can be found in the article in this
volume by Garbers *et al*.

Effects of Exogenous Cyclic GMP and Its Derivatives on Smooth Muscle Tonus

In smooth muscle, as in other tissues, there are only a few
reports indicating that hormonal effects involving increased
intracellular cGMP levels can be imitated by exogenously applied
cGMP. When cGMP or its dibutyryl or 8-bromo derivatives were
added to isolated smooth muscle preparations, relaxation was
observed with the guinea pig ileum (23) and trachea (23, 44).
Some investigators have observed a contraction that was blocked
by atropine, indicating that the action of the nucleotide was
indirect and involved the release of endogenous acetylcholine
(23, 27). Other observations indicate that under certain conditions
exogenous cGMP can promote smooth muscle contraction more directly.
In guinea pig ileum, dibutyryl cGMP has been reported by other
workers to cause a contraction that in most cases was not blocked
by atropine (45); K^+-depolarized tissue was said to be even more
sensitive to exogenous dibutyryl cGMP. However, as is the case
with studies involving effects of exogenous cAMP and its derivatives,
adequate nucleotide and butyrate controls are missing from most
studies of cGMP and its derivatives on intact tissues.

Effects of Cyclic GMP on Cellular Processes

There is very little information about molecular processes
affected by cGMP in smooth muscle as well as in other tissues.
Andersson *et al*. (4) have reported that cGMP in rather high concentrations inhibited the binding of Ca^{++} by "microsomal fractions"
from intestinal smooth muscle and antagonized the stimulatory
effect of cAMP on this process.

Casnellie and Greengard (12) have shown that cGMP in apparently physiological concentrations can stimulate the endogenous phosphorylation of two proteins in membrane fractions from various smooth muscular tissues. The phosphorylation of these two proteins was also stimulated by cAMP, but in concentrations about 10-fold higher than those of cGMP. Since the content of cAMP is usually 10-fold higher than that of cGMP in most tissues including smooth muscle, the endogenous phosphorylation system studied by Casnellie and Greengard could be equally sensitive to stimulation by physiological amounts of the two nucleotides.

Phosphodiesterase Inhibitors

As already mentioned, most or all known phosphodiesterase inhibitors decrease the hydrolysis of cGMP as well as cAMP. Where their effects on intact smooth muscular tissues have been examined, phosphodiesterase inhibitors have produced a proportionately greater increase in cGMP than in cAMP levels (14, 32, 34, 35, 43). Since these agents usually produce relaxation rather than contraction of smooth muscle, their effects do not furnish evidence for a role for cGMP in promoting smooth muscle contraction. It might be argued that when levels of both cyclic nucleotides rise, the effects of cAMP predominate over those of cGMP; however, this argument seems inadequate in view of the finding that a contraction-producing concentration of norepinephrine produces in the rat ductus deferens relative increases in cAMP and cGMP that are indistinguishable from those produced by a relaxation-producing concentration of the phosphodiesterase inhibitor SC-2964 (32, 37). It should be kept in mind, however, that it may be misleading to make comparisons of cyclic nucleotide changes that are made under conditions of basal tone with contraction changes that are made under conditions of prestimulated tone.

Importance of Ca^{++} for Hormonal Effects on Cyclic GMP Levels

Since most studies performed in other tissues have not revealed direct effects of acetylcholine and other agents on guanylate cyclase, we considered the possibility that hormonally-induced changes in ion permeability and distribution are primary to changes in cGMP levels in smooth muscle. We have shown that Ca^{++} is involved in the regulation of the basal cGMP levels and in the effects of several agents on these levels in smooth muscle (32, 33, 34, 37).

When segments of ductus deferens were incubated in Ca^{++}-free buffer, cGMP was decreased by about 85 % and was not increased by acetylcholine (Figure 1) (34), norepinephrine (37) or KCl (34).

In intestinal smooth muscle, there was a smaller decrease in basal cGMP following Ca^{++} removal, but the effects of acetylcholine, histamine, serotonin and KCl on cGMP levels were completely abolished in the absence of Ca^{++} (33). These findings suggest that hormone- or neurotransmitter-induced increases in cGMP levels in smooth muscle are secondary to increased cytoplasmic Ca^{++}. An apparently similar requirement for Ca^{++} in the regulation of cGMP levels seems to be the case in many other cell types (e.g. 16, 20, 34, 38). Andersson *et al.* (4) and Haslam *et al.* (18) have shown in intestinal and bronchial smooth muscle and in platelets, respectively, that agents that block prostaglandin synthesis reduce the basal cGMP level and reduce and retard its response to hormones. However, we have not found any effect of indomethacin pretreatment on the basal cGMP level or on the effect of acetylcholine to raise cGMP in the rat ductus deferens (Figure 4). Similarly, Stoner *et al.* (42) saw no effect of indomethacin on cGMP levels in lung fragments. Therefore, it remains to be proven that prostaglandins in addition to Ca^{++} play an important and general role in the regulation of cGMP levels.

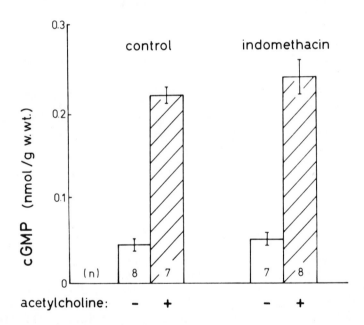

FIGURE 4. *Influence of indomethacin on the effect of acetylcholine on the cGMP level in rat ductus deferens. After 60 minutes of pre-incubation with or without 10 μM indomethacin, 100 μM acetylcholine was added for 3 minutes. The composition of the medium and the methods used were published elsewhere (35). (n) = number of determinations for each condition.*

TABLE I. Agents that cause contraction and raise the cyclic GMP level in smooth muscle.

AGENT	TISSUE
acetylcholine and other cholinergic agents	ductus deferus (14, 34, 35), uterus (14, 17), intestinal (4, 14, 22, 33) and tracheal (4, 25) smooth muscle
catecholamines (α-adrenergic component)	ductus deferens (37)
histamine	intestinal (33) and tracheal (4, 25) smooth muscle, coronary artery (43)
serotonin	uterus (17), intestinal smooth muscle (17)
oxytocin	uterus (17)
prostaglandin F_2	uterus (17), veins (15)
K^+	ductus deferens (34), intestinal smooth muscle (4, 33)

CONCLUDING REMARKS

There is substantial evidence that an increased level of cAMP is involved in the relaxing action of β-adrenergic stimulatory and perhaps other agents on smooth muscle. However, the criteria proposed by Sutherland and associates to establish the mediation of a hormonal effect by cAMP have been only partially fulfilled for cAMP as the primary and singular mediator of the smooth muscle relaxing action of hormones.

The role of cGMP in smooth muscle function is even more obscure. The increased formation of cGMP in smooth muscle is apparently secondary to an increased cytoplasmic Ca^{++} concentration that occurs in response to a number of agents that cause contraction. We have suggested that the increase in intracellular cGMP that has been observed under the influence of various contracting agents may be involved in the removal of the increased cytoplasmic free Ca^{++} (36). On the other hand, cGMP may act as a comediator with Ca^{++} in promoting the contractile process (4, 17, 36), or it may act to promote a greater increase in cytoplasmic Ca^{++} (4, 37). Establishing which, if any, of these possibilities is in fact correct obviously will require further study, but the probability seems high that cGMP in some way participates in the overall response of smooth muscle to some agents that alter contractility.

Acknowledgments

The authors' work has been supported by the Deutsche Forschungsgemeinschaft (Schu 2/5 and Schu 2/6) and by NIH grants GM-16811, HL-13996 and AM-07462.

REFERENCES

(1) AASS, H.J., OSNES, J.B., ØYE, I, (1974), Papaverine at low concentrations stimulates the cAMP phosphodiesterase activity of rat heart cytosol. Acta Pharm. Tox. 35, 56

(2) ANDERSSON, K.E., ANDERSSON, R., HEDNER, P., PERSSON, C.G.A., (1972) Effect of cholecystokinin on the level of cyclic AMP and on mechanical activity in the isolated sphincter of Oddi, Life Sci., 11, part I, 723

(3) ANDERSSON, R., LUNDHOM, L., MOHME-LUNDHOLM, E., NILSSON, K., (1972), Role of cyclic AMP and Ca^{++} in metabolic and mechanical events in smooth muscle, Adv. Cycl. Nucl. Res., 1, 213

(4) ANDERSSON, R., NILSSON, K., WIKBERG, J., JOHANSSON, S., LUNDHOLM, L., (1975), Cyclic nucleotides and contraction of smooth muscle. 2nd International Congress on Cyclic AMP, Vancouver 1974, Adv. Cycl. Nucl. Res., 5 (in press)

(5)   BÄR, H.P. (1974), Cyclic nucleotides and smooth muscle.
      Adv. Cycl. Nucl. Res., 4, 195

(6)   BAUDOUIN-LEGROS, M., MEYER, P., (1973) Effects of angio-
      tensin, catecholamines and cyclic AMP on calcium storage
      in aortic microsomes, Brit. J. Pharmacol., 47, 377

(7)   BÖHME, E., SCHULTZ, G., (unpublished observations)

(8)   BROWING, E.T., (1973), Metabolic effects of norepinephrine
      and papaverine in C-6 astrocytoma cells., Fed. Proc., 32,
      679 Abs.

(9)   BUEDING, E., BÜLBRING, E., GERCKEN, G., HAWKINS, J.T.,
      KURIJAMA, H., (1967), The effect of adrenaline on the
      adenosinetriphosphate and creatine phosphate content of
      intestinal smooth muscle. J. Physiol., 193, 187

(10) BÜLBRING, E., TOMITA, T. (1969), Suppression of spontaneous
      spike generation by catecholamines in the smooth muscle of
      the guinea-pig taenia coli., Proc. Roy. Soc. B., 172, 103

(11) BURNSTOCK, G., (1972), Purinergic receptors, Pharmacol. Rev.
      24, 509

(12) CASNELLIE, J.E., GREENGARD, P., (1974), Guanosine 3':5'-
      cyclic monophosphate-dependent phosphorylation of endogenous
      substrate proteins in membranes of mammalian smooth muscle.
      Proc. Nat. Acad. Sci. US, 71, 1891

(13) COULSON, R., BOWMAN, R.H. (1974), Excretion and degradation
      of exogenous adenosine 3',5'-monophosphate by isolated per-
      fused rat kidney. Life Sciences, 14, 545

(14) DIAMOND, J., HARTLE, D.K. (1974), Cyclic nucleotide levels
      during carbachol-induced smooth muscle contractions. Pharma-
      cologist, 16, 273

(15) DUNHAM, E.W., HADDOX, M.K., GOLDBERG, N.D. (1974), Alteration
      in vein cyclic 3':5' nucleotide concentrations during changes
      in contractility. Proc. Nat. Acad. Sci. US, 71, 815

(16) FERENDELLI, F.A., KINSCHERG, D.A., CHANG, M.M., (1973)
      Regulation of levels of guanosine cyclic 3',5'-monophosphate
      in the central nervous system: Effects of depolarising
      agents, Molec. Pharmacol., 9, 445

(17) GOLDBERG, N.D., O'DEA, R.F., HADDOX, M.K. (1973), Cyclic GMP.
      Adv. Cycl. Nucl. Res., 3, 155

(18) HASLAM, R.J., Mc CLENAGHAN, M.D. (1974), Effects of collagen
     and of aspirin on the concentration of guanosine 3':5'-cyclic
     monophosphate in human blood platelets: Measurement by a
     prelabelling technique. Biochem. J., 138, 317

(19) HURWITZ, L., SURIA, A. (1971), The link between agonist
     action and response in smooth muscle. Ann. Rev. Pharmacol.
     11, 303

(20) IGNARRO, L.J., CECH, S.Y., GEORGE, W.J. (1974), Mediation of
     lysosomal enzyme secretion from human neutrophils by guano-
     sine 3',5'-monophosphate: Requirement of calcium, and
     inhibition by adenosine 3',5'-monophosphate. Pharmacologist
     16, 309

(21) KREBS, E.G. (1972), Protein kinases, Curr. Top. Cell. Reg.
     (ed. by B.L. Horecker, E.R. Stadtman), 5, 99

(22) LEE, T.P., KUO, J.F., GREENGARD, P. (1972), Role of muscarinic
     cholinergic receptors in regulation of guanosine 3':5'-cyclic
     monophosphate content in mammalian brain, heart muscle, and
     intestinal smooth muscle. Proc. Natl. Acad. Sci. US, 69,
     3287

(23) LEWIS, A.J., DOUGLAS, J.S., BOUHUYS, A. (1973), Biphasic
     responses to guanosyl nucleotides in two smooth muscle
     preparations. J. Pharm. Pharmac., 25, 1011

(24) MAYER, S.E., KING, C.D. (1974), Inhibition of egress of
     cyclic AMP from pigeon erythrocytes, Abstract, 2nd Intern.
     Congr. on Cyclic AMP, Vancouver, 50

(25) MURAD, F., KIMURA, H., (1974) Cyclic nucleotide levels in
     incubations of guinea pig trachea, Biochim. Biophys. Acta,
     343, 275

(26) PROSSER, C.L. (1974), Smooth muscle, Ann. Rev. Physiol.,
     36, 503

(27) PUGLISI, L., BERTI, F., PAOLETTI, R., (1971) Antagonism of
     dibutyryl-Guo-3':5'-P and atropine on stomach muscle
     contraction. Experientia, 27, 1187

(28) ROBISON, G.A., BUTCHER, R.W., SUTHERLAND, E.W., (1971),
     Cyclic AMP, Academic Press, New York and London

(29) SANBORN, B.M., BHALLA, R.C., KORENMAN, S.G. (1973), The
     endometrial adenosine cyclic 3',5'-monophosphate dependent
     protein kinase. Distribution, subunit structure, and
     kinetics of adenosine cyclic 3',5'-monophosphate binding.
     J. Biol. Chem., 248, 3593

(30) SANDS, H., MEYER, A., RICKENBERG, U. (1973), Adenosine 3',
     5'-monophosphate-dependent protein kinase of bovine tracheal
     smooth muscle. Biochim. Biophys. Acta, 302, 267

(31) SCHÖNHÖFER, P.S., SKIDMORE, J.F., FORN, J., FLEISCH, J.H.,
     (1971), Adenyl cyclase activity of rabbit aorta, J. Pharm.
     Pharmac., 23, 28

(32) SCHULTZ, G., HARDMAN, J.G. (1975), Regulation of cyclic GMP
     levels in the ductus deferens of the rat. 2nd Internat.
     Congress on Cyclic AMP, Vancouver 1974, Adv. Cycl. Nucl.
     Res., 5 (in press)

(33) SCHULTZ, G., HARDMAN, J.G., HURWITZ, L., SUTHERLAND, E.W.,
     (1973), Importance of calcium for the control of cyclic GMP
     levels. Fed. Proc. 32, 773 Abs.

(34) SCHULTZ, G., HARDMAN, J.G., SCHULTZ, K., BAIRD, C.E.,
     SUTHERLAND, E.W. (1973), The importance of calcium ions for
     the regulation of guanosine 3':5'-cyclic monophosphate
     levels. Proc. Natl. Acad. Sci. US, 70, 3889

(35) SCHULTZ, G., HARDMAN, J.G., SCHULTZ, K., DAVIS, J.W.,
     SUTHERLAND, E.W.. (1973) A new enzymatic assay for guanosine
     3':5'-cyclic monophosphate and its application to the ductus
     deferens of the rat. Proc. Natl. Acad. Sci. US, 70, 1721

(36) SCHULTZ, G., HARDMAN, J.G., SUTHERLAND, E.W. (1973), Cyclic
     nucleotides and smooth muscle function. In: Asthma –
     Physiology, Immunopharmacology and Treatment. Ed. by K.F.
     Austen and L.M. Lichtenstein, 123, Acad. Press, New York
     and London

(37) SCHULTZ, G., SCHULTZ, K., HARDMAN, J.G. (1975) Effects of
     norepinephrine on cyclic nucleotide levels in the ductus
     deferens of the rat. Metabolism 24, 429

(38) SMITH, R.J., IGNARRO, L.J. (1974), Stimulation-secretion
     coupling in human neutrophils: Link between calcium influx
     and guanosine 3',5'-monophosphate accumulation in lysosomal
     enzyme secretion. Pharmacologist 16, 309

(39) SOMLYO, A.P., SOMLYO, A.V. (1970) Vascular smooth muscle.
     II. Pharmacology of normal and hypertensive vessels.
     Pharmacol. Rev. 22, 249

(40) SOMLYO, A.P., SOMLYO, A.V., SMIESKO, V. (1972), Cyclic AMP
     and vascular smooth muscle. Adv. Cycl. Nucl. Res., 1, 175

(41) SOMLYO, A.V., HAEUSLER, G., SOMLYO, A.P. (1970) Cyclic adeno-
     sine monophosphate: Potassium-dependent action on vascular
     smooth muscle membrane potential. Science 169, 490

(42) STONER, J., MANGANIELLO, V.C., VAUGHAN, M. (1973), Effects
     of bradykinin and indomethacin on cyclic GMP and cyclic AMP
     in lung slices. Proc. Natl. Acad. Sci. US, 70, 3830

(43) SUTHERLAND, C.A., SCHULTZ, G., HARDMAN, J.G., SUTHERLAND,
     E.W., (1973) Effects of vasoactive agents on cyclic nucleo-
     tide levels in pig coronary arteries. Fed. Proc., 32, 773
     Abs.

(44) SZADUYKIS-SZADURSKI, L., WEIMANN, G., BERTI, F. (1972)
     Pharmacological effects of cyclic nucleotides and their
     derivatives on tracheal smooth muscle. Pharmacol. Res. Comm.
     4, 63

(45) TAKAYANAGI, I., TAKAGI, K. (1973) The action of dibutyryl
     cyclic GMP (N^2-2'-O-dibutyryl cyclic guanosine-3',5'-mono-
     phosphate) on the ileum of guinea pig. Jap. J. Pharmacol.
     23, 573

(46) TRINER, L., NAHAS, G.G., VULLIEMOZ, Y., OVERWEG, N.I.A.,
     VEROSKY, M., HABIF, D.V., NGAI, S.H. (1971), Cyclic AMP and
     smooth muscle function. Ann. N.Y. Acad. Sci., 185, 458

(47) VESIN, M.F., HARBON, S. (1974), The effects of epinephrine
     prostaglandins, and their antagonists on adenosine cyclic
     3',5'-monophosphate concentrations and motility of the
     uterus. Molec. Pharmacol., 10, 457

(48) WALSH, D.A., ASHBY, C.D. (1973), Protein kinases: Aspects
     of their regulation and diversity. Rec. Progr. Horm. Res.,
     29, 329

(49) WEBER, A., (1968) The mechanism of the action of caffeine
     on sarcoplasmic reticulum. J. Gen. Physiol., 52, 760

(50) WELLS, J.N., BAIRD, C.E., HARDMAN, J.G. (1974) Inhibition
     of cyclic AMP and cyclic GMP phosphodiesterase activities
     from pig coronary arteries. Fed. Proc., 33, 480

THE REGULATION OF THYROID CELL METABOLISM

J.E. Dumont
J. Van Sande
F. Lamy
R. Pochet
F. Rodesch

Institut de Recherche Interdisciplinaire [1]
School of Medicine
University of Brussels and Biology Department
Euratom
1000 Brussels, Belgium

Contents

Thyroid cellular physiology
Methodology for the investigation of thyroid cellular metabolism
Framework for the investigation of the regulation of thyroid
 metabolism
Model of thyroid cell regulation
The cyclic 3',5'-AMP system
Regulation by iodite of the cyclic 3',5'-AMP system
Role of calcium
The cyclic 3',5'-GMP system
Conclusion
References

---

[1] The work from this laboratory which is reported in the present
review has been carried out under Contract of the Ministère de la
Politique Scientifique within the framework of the Association
Euratom – University of Brussels – University of Pisa and thanks
to grant of the Caisse Générale d'Apargne et de Retraite.

INTRODUCTION

The metabolism of the thyroid is principally regulated by the pituitary hormone thyrotropin. Other signals also influence this metabolism (see article included in this volume by Marshall), e.g. adrenalin, noradrenalin, acetylcholine, serotonin, etc. (1, 2) but their physiological role is still largely unknown. The action of thyrotropin on the thyroid has been reviewed recently (3). However, since that review, much new information has been provided on the intracellular regulatory circuits in this tissue. In this chapter the role of the cyclic nucleotides cAMP and cGMP, calcium and iodide will be considered. Aspects of these regulations which are peculiar to the thyroid or which may bear on other tissues but have not been considered yet will be emphasized. The role of prostaglandins (Jacquemin, see this volume) and of postaglandin, adrenergic agents, and immunoglobulins (Marshall, see this volume) in the regulation of the thyroid is analyzed in other chapters. Most of the results presented have been obtained in this laboratory.

THYROID CELLULAR PHYSIOLOGY

The thyroid is constituted mainly of follicles, in which follicular cells enclose a cavity, the colloid lumen, which is filled by colloid, i.e. mostly thyroglobulin. The gland contains about 80 % follicular cells, large numbers of fibroblasts and endothelial cells and at the periphery of follicles scarce thyrocalcitonin secreting parafollicular cells.

The function of the follicular cell is to concentrate iodide, to bind this iodide to the tyrosyl groups of thyroglobulin, thus forming iodotyrosyls to couple the iodotyrosines forming iodothyronines (the thyroid hormones) and to release the hormones from thyroglobulin by lysosomal digestion. The main steps of this metabolism are schematized in Figure 1. The basal pole of the cell faces the interfollicular-extracellular space; the apical pole covered by microvilli, is facing the colloid lumen. Iodide is actively transported (against the electrochemical gradient) at the basal membrane and concentrated in the lumen. Thyroglobulin, a heavy glycoprotein (M.W. 660,000) is synthesized by the membrane bound polyribosomes of the ergastoplasm, released in the cisternae, glycosylated by the smooth endoplasmic reticulum and the Golgi membranes, packaged in the Golgi, and secreted in the colloid. The mRNA(s) of the subunit(s) of this protein has (have) been recently isolated and characterized (4).

Iodide, in the lumen, is oxidized, presumably at the level of the apical membrane, i.e. the microvilli, and bound to the tyrosyl

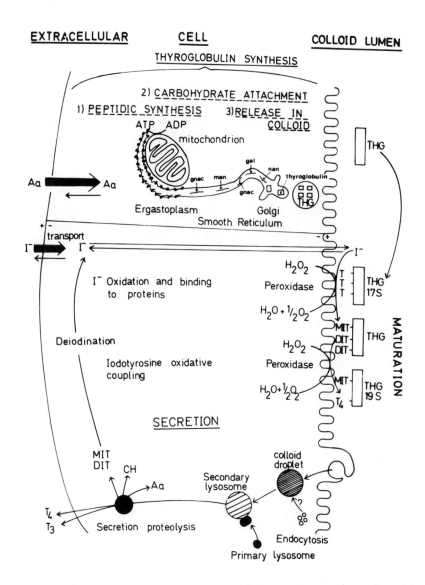

<u>FIGURE 1</u>. *Cell physiology of the thyroid. THG : thyroglobulin;*
MIT : monoiodotyrosine; DIT : diiodotyrosine; T_3 : triiodothyro-
nine; T_4 : thyroxine; CH : carbohydrate residues; Aa : aminoacids;
Gnac : acetylglucosamine; Man : mannose; Gal : galactose; Nan :
n-acetyl-neuraminic acid.

residues of thyroglobulin. The microvilli might be considered as
a cellular arrangement increasing the surface of the interface and
thus facilitating interface reactions such as thyroglobulin iodination. The enzymatic system involved in iodination is constituted
of a H_2O_2 generating system, poorly understood, the coenzyme of
which is NADPH, and a peroxidase which has recently been isolated
by Taurog (5) and Pommier *et al*. (6). The best known reducing
metabolic pathway for NADP in the thyroid cell is the pentose
phosphate cycle. The activity of this cycle is regulated mainly
by the level of $NADP^+$, i.e. of NADPH oxidation (3). The enzymatic
machinery which catalyzes iodide oxidation is also responsible for
the oxidative coupling of iodotyrosines to iodothyronines within
thyroglobulin (5).

In the secretory process, the colloid is ingested by the
follicular cell. After acute stimulation by TSH, this is mani-
fested as phagocytosis of the colloid. In other situations it is
possible that pinocytosis may occur (3, 7). The phagocytosis of
colloid requires the integrity of microtubules and microfilaments.
It is inhibited by agents which interfere with the stability or
the dynamic assembly-disassembly process of microtubules (colchicine, vinblastine, vincristine, D_2O, ethanol). It is also
depressed by cytochalasin B, which apart from its inhibitory
action on transport (e.g. hexose), also inhibits, in a manner as
yet unknown, the microfilaments (8, 9). After its endocytosis,
the colloid forms colloid droplets which are easily identified by
light and electron microscopy. The colloid droplets fuse with
lysosomes, thus forming secondary lysosomes in which thyroglobulin
is hydrolyzed, resulting in the release of aminoacids, carbohydrate
residues, iodotyrosines and iodothyronines. The iodothyronines are
thought to be released from the cells by a diffusion process whilst
the iodotyrosines are deiodinated by an iodotyrosine dehalogenase
with NADPH as coenzyme. The ATP supply of the dog thyroid cell
comes mostly from mitochondrial oxidative phosphorylation (> 80 %)
but glycolysis (20 %) also plays a role (10).

In the study of thyroid metabolism antithyroid drugs which
have specific inhibitory functions on metabolism are often used :
$NaClO_4$ or KSCN which block the trapping of iodide, methimazole and
propylthiouracil which inhibit the thyroid peroxidase.

TSH stimulates all facets of thyroid metabolism. On the basis
of kinetics, two types of effects can be distinguished : rapid
effects which correspond to a functional activation (e.g. activation of secretion, iodide binding to proteins, iodothyronine
formation, and of general metabolic pathways such as the pentose
phosphate cycle and mitochondrial respiration) and delayed effects
which correspond to growth or to an increased functional capacity
of the tissue (increased protein synthesis, RNA synthesis, etc.,

and thus increased volume of cells, RNA and protein contents of cells and number of cells). The kinetics of TSH action on iodide transport is clearly biphasic; it is depressed early (up to 1 to 2 hours) and greatly enhanced thereafter. In general all the rapid effects of TSH are not inhibited by protein or RNA synthesis inhibitors while the delayed effects which have been studied in this regard are inhibited by such agents. In the latter case, it is therefore believed that the hormone acts at the transcription level (3). There is some evidence that the immediate functional activation of thyroid cells requires lower TSH concentrations than the delayed growth promoting action of the hormone (11).

METHODOLOGY OF THE INVESTIGATION OF THYROID CELLULAR METABOLISM

Several systems have been used for the study of the regulation of thyroid metabolism. The most complex and physiological approach is the kinetic study of the morphology, secretion, or biochemical composition of the tissue after stimulation *in vivo*. This involves the use of small laboratory animals, the thyroids of which are very small, and an important interanimal variation. Although it is the experimental system which approaches the physiological norm most closely, its complexity makes the interpretation of dynamic studies with tracers or of pharmacological studies difficult. To obviate these difficulties, more direct methods have been used such as the study of the global metabolism of the tissue by venous and sometimes arterial catheterization. Long-term studies (more than a few hours) are precluded in these systems in which physiological nervous or interorgan regulations can still play a role (12). For methodological reasons, the perfusion of isolated thyroids has until now yielded little success. By far the most successful tool of thyroid investigation remains the thyroid slice incubated *in vitro*. The cells in this situation, for unknown reasons, appear to function well under carefully controlled incubation conditions. Their morphology (as studied by electron microscopy) remains normal; their energy charge is high (in fact almost all the nucleotides are in the form of triphosphates), their mitochondria remain tightly coupled, protein and RNA synthesis are linear for several hours, and the cells appear to trap and organify iodide, secrete iodothyronines, and respond to TSH in a manner expected from *in vivo* investigations (13). The use of dog thyroids (i.e. from laboratory rather than slaughterhouse animals) allows *in vivo* pretreatment of animal and affords the possibility of studying the kinetics of activation of a completely resting tissue.

More simplified *in vitro* intact cell systems have been used, such as trypsinized isolated cells (14) and cultured cells (15).

In the isolation of cells, tissue architecture, follicular organization and luminal colloid are lost : the variation from one sample to another from a given preparation is almost nil and the large bulk of colloid cannot interfere (as inactive space, amino-acid and iodide source, etc.) in tracer studies. However, the yield of such preparations is very low and their quality very variable from one day to another; they are a heterogeneous population of completely free non polarized cells and sheets of associated polarized cells (16); moreover, it is always difficult to exclude artefacts introduced by the trypsinization process *per se*. Thus apart from the interest of removing the colloid, such preparations offer little advantage over slices but have many disadvantages. When cultured, trypsinized cells may offer a relatively stable homogeneous system in which the association of cells into follicles (a process analogous to the formation *in vivo* of the architecture of the tissue), long-term effects of TSH and dedifferentiation can be studied very effectively (17). However, the yield of such preparations is also low and the physiological relevance of the findings should always be scrutinized. From this analysis it is easy to understand why three systems have been used with the greatest benefit : animals *in vivo, in vitro* incubated slices and cultured cells. Of course, great use has been made of acellular systems such as homogenates, purified plasma membranes, or purified enzymes. In such studies care should always be taken in the homogenization procedure, which, in a rather tough tissue may disrupt organelles and inactivate enzymes. Moreover, the thyroid is very rich in lysosomal enzymes.

Three general remarks should be made about these various systems :

1) As for other tissues, results are always easier to obtain and interpret in simpler systems but their relevance should always be checked in the more complex and more physiological systems (e.g. from membranes to slices, to *in vivo* animals).

2) In thyroid research the combined biochemical and morphological approach has always yielded much more information than either one alone.

3) The use of thyroids from large animals in order to get more biological material almost necessarily requires tissue from slaughterhouse animals. Even if the freshness of the tissue is ensured, the physiology and biochemistry of such thyroids may have been altered considerably by *in vivo* treatments unknown to the investigator, such as pretreatment with estrogens or antithyroid drugs. It has been the experience of several laboratories to fail for long periods to get any reproducible response to TSH from such glands. In laboratories

linked with Physiology Departments, the dog is a suitable compromise
between the contradictory requirements of thyroid size and controlled
biological material.

The data presented in the following part of this review have
mostly been obtained using the dog thyroid slices system. Generally,
thyroid glands from dogs pretreated for 3 days with thyroid extract
(100mg/dog/10kg) were sliced with a Stadie Riggs microtome (average
thickness $\pm$ 0.3mm), preincubated for one hour in Krebs Ringer
bicarbonate buffer supplemented with glucose (8mM) and albumin
(1mg/ml) under an atmosphere of 95% O_2, 5% CO_2. The slices are then
used for metabolic study in a second incubation (13, 18). Several
parameters of thyroid metabolism are usually studied :

a) cAMP and cGMP contents are measured by the method of Gilman
   (18, 19) and an adaptation of Murad's method (20, 21).

b) Protein phosphorylation (22) by measuring the incorporation of
   ^{32}P phosphate into various thyroid proteins. In such cases,
   the incubation medium contains no or 0.1mM phosphate.

c) The activity of the pentose phosphate pathway; in thyroid this
   activity is accurately measured by the $^{14}CO_2$ yield from $(1-^{14}C)$
   glucose minus the $^{14}CO_2$ yield from $(6-^{14}C)$ glucose (10). As, in
   short-term ($\pm$ 60 minutes) incubations, the latter is still low,
   glucose carbon 1 oxidation can be used as a semi-quantitative
   estimate of the activity of the pentose phosphate pathway. It
   is, however, useful to check glucose carbon 6 oxidation for any
   new agent studied. Although this is not proved, it is probable
   that a major part of the stimulation of this pathway by TSH is
   due to the activation of NADPH oxidation by the H_2O_2 generating
   system (3).

d) Iodide binding to proteins, i.e. the incorporation of ^{131}I iodide
   into the trichloroacetic precipitable material of the slices (23).
   This is measured at $10^{-5}M$ or $4.10^{-5}M$ iodide concentration, i.e.
   at concentrations at which the trapping is no longer the limiting
   step, but the binding of iodide to proteins is becoming saturated
   and thus limiting. As iodide binding rapidly depletes the medium,
   the action of stimulating agents is generally measured in short
   term ($\pm$ 45 minutes) incubations. The rate limiting factor of this
   reaction is probably the supply of H_2O_2.

e) Thyroid secretion. This is generally measured by the release of
   butanol soluble radioiodine (i.e. iodide + iodothyronines +
   iodotyrosines, but the latter are deiodinated in the cell and
   thus absent in the medium), from slices of dogs prelabelled *in
   vivo*. As the amount of labelled thyroglobulin in one slice
   depends mainly on the number and size of intact non-disrupted

follicles rather than on its weight, results are expressed as the
per cent of the total radioidine of the slice which is released
(13). The first step of secretion, phagocytosis can be evaluated
by observing the formation of pseudopods and intracellular colloid
droplets in the intact follicles of the slices (light or electron
microscopy) or by counting the pseudopods appearing on the surface
of open peripheral follicles of the slices - by scanning electron
microscopy. Although the two methods evaluate the same cellular
process, it should be kept in mind that in the first case, as in
the biochemical measurement of secretion, only the intact inner
follicles of the slice are studied, whereas in the latter case
(SEM) the open peripheral follicles are studied. The number of
intracellular colloid droplets reflects the rate of phagocytosis
and also the rate of thyroglobulin hydolysis.

Several other biochemical parameters have been studied using
slices (e.g. aminoacid, uridine incorporation, etc.) but their
modifications by all signals of thyroid regulation (TSH, prostaglandins, adrenergic and cholinergic drugs, etc.) have not been
systematically studied.

FRAMEWORK OF THE INVESTIGATION OF THE REGULATION OF THYROID METABOLISM

From the literature on hormonal and neurotransmitter action
available in 1969, one could distinguish the effects of such
signals from a physiological point of view by at least 2 criteria :
the delay of the action and the nature of the action (Figure 2).
The delays vary from milliseconds to days. The effect may be to
stimulate or inhibit an existing function, or to induce a new
function (i.e. to differentiate) in the target cell. The induction
of a new function obviously implies the formation of selective
units, these units being enzymes, organelles, etc. The stimulation
of a function may imply an increase in the number of units (growth)
or an activation of existing units. The primary biochemical
mechanisms involved in these actions may be very simple such as
changes of permeability (e.g. for Ca^{++}) or in membrane transport,
or the formation, or the release of allosteric effectors (e.g.
cyclic nucleotides). When new units are formed, the mechanisms
may operate at the translation and/or at the transcription level;
an induction, i.e. a differentiating action, would presumably
require an effect at the level of transcription. A probable point
of action of the signal in the cell may be proposed for each
mechanism (e.g. plasma membrane for effect on permeability, nucleus
for transcriptional events, etc.). It is obvious that an action
which requires prior synthesis of RNA and of protein will require
at least an hour and sometimes days whereas an effect on the membrane may be immediate. Similarly, effects which require RNA

synthesis will be blocked by inhibitors of transcription (e.g. Actinomycin) and translation (e.g. Puromycin, Cycloheximide, etc.). Thus from rather simple considerations a useful classification of hormone or signal effects may be proposed (Figure 2). For each type of action, closely investigated examples can now be found in the literature. Effects at one level can always cause effects at the subsequent levels, e.g. an activation of membrane transport could modify transcription. If an action at a given level causes one of the preceding types of effect, e.g. activation at the transcription level causing a change in membrane permeability, this effect acquires the characteristics of its cause (e.g. delay, sensitivity to inhibitors, etc.). However, it is conceivable that a signal may act independently at the different levels. In the case of tropic hormones acting on their target cells (such as TSH on thyroid tissue) one can find effects at all the levels. Thus, within this conceptual framework, the investigation of the regu-

	DELAY	INHIBITED BY ACTINO MYCIN	INHIBITED BY PURO MYCIN	POINT OF ACTION STRUCTURE	POINT OF ACTION FUNCTION	PHYSIOLOGICAL SIGNIFICANCE	PHYSIOLOGICAL SIGNIFICANCE INCREASE	EXAMPLES	DEPENDENT EFFECTS OF TSH
A	+ SEC	O	O	MEMBRANES	TRANSPORT PERMEABILITY : (EX: Ca++)	STIMULATION	ACTIVITY / UNIT	EPINEPHRINE INSULIN ACETYLCHOLINE	↗ UPTAKES (GLUCOSE Aa..) ↗ PBI FORMATION
B	+ + MIN	O	O	MEMBRANE CYTOPLASM	FORMATION OF ALLOSTERIC EFFECTORS (EX: 3'-5' AMP)	STIMULATION	ACTIVITY / UNIT	ACTH EPINEPHRINE β GLUCAGON	↗ PHAGOCYTOSIS ↓ ↗ ENERGETIC METABOLISM
C	+ + + MIN	O	+	CYTOPLASM	TRANSLATION (PROT. SYNTH.)	STIMULATION	N OF UNITS	INSULIN ACTH	?
D	++++++ HOURS	+	+	NUCLEUS	TRANSCRIPTION (RNA SYNTH.)	STIMULATION	N OF UNITS	ALDOSTERON ANDROGENS ESTROGENS	↗ IODIDE UPTAKE ↗ WEIGHT ↗ RIBOSOMES... ↗ MITOSES......
E	++++++ ++++++ DAYS	+	+	NUCLEUS	TRANSCRIPTION (RNA SYNTH.)	DIFFERENTIATION	PRODUCTION OF SELECTIVE UNITS	ERYTHROPOIETIN ECDYSON	APPEARANCE OF Tg SYNTHESIS I⁻ UPTAKE I⁻ OXIDATION FOLLICULAR STRUCTURE

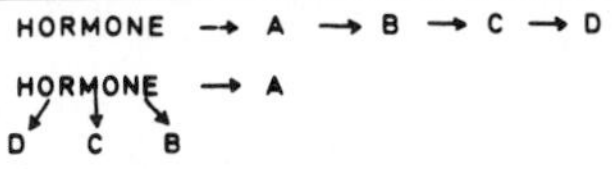

HORMONE → A → B → C → D

HORMONE → A
D C B

FIGURE 2. Conceptual framework of hormone action. Only stimulating processes have been considered, but the converse mechanisms might apply for depression or inhibitory actions. The "dependent effects of TSH" are examples of TSH effects on thyroid metabolism which may be caused by an action at the indicated level. A unit is any type of subcellular structure involved in a function : enzyme, cell organelle (e.g. ribosome), etc.
N = number.

lation of thyroid function should bear not on one but on several or
all the possible mechanisms.

MODEL OF THYROID CELL REGULATION

Our present working model of the regulation of thyroid cell
metabolism is outlined in Figure 3. This model is still largely
hypothetical but it provides a useful framework for understanding
recent results and for planning further research.

Three types of regulatory circuits have been demonstrated :
a) the cAMP system; b) the cGMP-Ca^{++} system; c) the iodide feedback loop (XI). In such a scheme continuous lines represent
chemical reactions while interrupted lines represent negative (-)
or postitive (+) controls, i.e. inhibition or activation. As can
be seen, TSH acts on the thyroid cell mainly through activation
of adenylate cyclase; cyclic 3', 5'-AMP formed by adenylate
cyclase is degraded by specific phosphodiesterases; it acts on
the cell metabolism through activation of cAMP dependent protein
kinases; phosphorylation of cellular proteins by the enzymes
activate or inactivate these proteins thus eliciting the hormonal
effects. This scheme is the direct application to TSH and thyroid
of the general Sutherland concept of hormonal action (24). The
cyclic 3',5'-AMP system is negatively controlled by the iodide
supply of the gland, this control being exerted by a postulated
oxidized derivative XI. The site of action of this compound
(adenylate cyclase, phosphodiesterases, cAMP efflux, etc.) is
unknown. As in other tissues, intracytoplasmic Ca^{++} also plays
a regulatory role. Its level presumably depends upon the balance
between passive influx through the plasma membrane or intracellular
stores (mitochondria ?), and conversely the active outflow through
the plasma membrane and uptake by the mitochondria. This level is
increased by a variety of agents or treatments (acetylcholine,
serotonin, KCl and possibly NaF some of which may have a physiological relevance. Ca^{++} mimics some effects of TSH (e.g. it
activates protein iodination and glucose carbon 1 oxidation) but
antagonizes some others (e.g. cAMP accumulation, secretion). The
level of intracellular Ca^{++} regulates cGMP accumulation; but it
is not known whether Ca^{++} acts through cGMP or whether cGMP
accumulation is just a side effect of an increase in Ca^{++} concentration.

The scheme presented does not account for some TSH effects
which are clearly not secondary to adenylate cyclase activation
(such as the acceleration of phosphatidylinositol turnover). It
makes no mention of the possible role of adrenergic agents, nor
of the possible role of prostaglandins or prostaglandin-like
agents as intermediates in TSH actions or as intercellular signals
(see the reviews of Jacquemin and Marshall - in this volume).

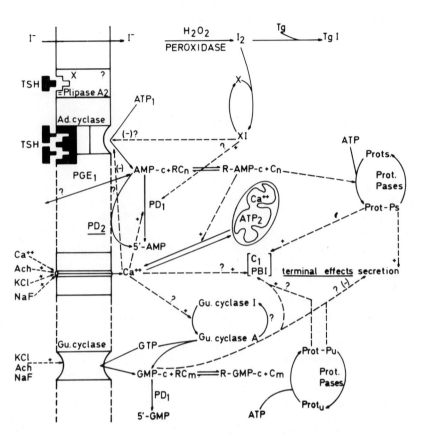

FIGURE 3.   A general working hypothesis for the regulation of dog
thyroid cell metabolism. ⟶ chemical reaction; − −► control
+ = stimulation; (−) = inhibition. Tg : thyroglobulin; Plipase
A_2 : phospholipase A_2; RCn : cyclic AMP dependent kinases
(according to the model, n may be equal to 1, 1/2, 2); RCm :
postulated cyclic GMP dependent kinase (m may be equal to 1, 1/2,
2, etc.); Prots : substrates of cyclic AMP dependent kinases;
Protu : substrates of the postulated cyclic GMP dependent kinases;
PD_1 : high Km cyclic nucleotide phosphodiesterase; PD_2 : postulated
low Km, membrane bound cyclic AMP phosphodiesterase; Pases : postulated protein phosphatases; ATP_1, ATP_2 : separate pools of ATP;
PBI : iodide binding to proteins; C_1 : oxidation of glucose carbon
1 (i.e. activity of the pentose phosphate pathway); Ach : acetylcholine; GMPc, AMPc : cyclic GMP and cyclic AMP; Ad cyclase :
adenylate cyclase.

THE CYCLIC AMP SYSTEM

It is now well accepted that most effects of TSH on the thyroid are secondary to the activation of thyroid adenylate cyclase by the hormone (3). However, it should be pointed out that the criteria proposed by Sutherland to validate this hypothesis (24) have only been fully satisfied for dog thyroids *in vitro* and for some effects of TSH, namely the activation of secretion, of glucose carbon 1 oxidation and of the binding of iodide to proteins. Only in this system and for these metabolic parameters, has it been shown that :

- TSH activates thyroid adenylate cyclase over the range of TSH concentrations which elicit the hormonal effects in intact cells.

- TSH enhances the accumulation of cAMP in the cells at concentrations which elicit the other effects of the hormones, and the rise of cAMP level precedes the faster effects of the hormone (e.g. pseudopod formation).

- The effects of TSH are mimicked by cAMP itself and by its analogue dibutyryl cyclic 3',5'-AMP but not by other nucleotides or butyrate.

- The effects of low concentrations of TSH are potentiated by inhibitors of cAMP phosphodiesterases such as caffeine (3).

The elements of the system have been fairly well studied. Some peculiar characteristics may be pointed out. Adenylate cyclase exhibits a negatively cooperative type of response to TSH. However, this pattern changes to positive cooperativity in the presence of ITP or GTP (25). This provides a mechanism by which the target cell may regulate its response to its activating signal. So far as they have been studied, phosphodiesterases and protein kinases seem to be similar to the corresponding enzymes in other tissues. The natural substrates of protein kinases have been studied by measuring the incorporation of ^{32}P phosphate in the proteins of resting and stimulated thyroid slices. The striking result of these studies was the fact that TSH does not markedly activate general protein phosphorylation in these cells. Thus most protein phosphorylation is independent of TSH and its induced rise in cAMP concentration. However, the phosphorylation of some specific proteins is greatly enhanced in stimulated tissue in particular f_1 histones and one contractile protein. The phosphorylation of f_1 histones is enhanced for concentrations of TSH greater than those required to elit functional activation effects (e.g. secretion, etc.) (22). It is known that hormonal concentrations required to elicit growth of the tissue are also greater than those required to activate secretion (11). Moreover, a role of f_1 histone phosphorylation in the activation of transcription has been postulated (26). For these reasons, and although stimulation of RNA synthesis is difficult to quantitate in this material (27), it has been suggested that this action of TSH might be related to RNA synthesis and growth promotion (22).

TSH also specifically enhances phosphorylation of a protein which belongs to a group of proteins having the solubility and electrophoretic properties of contractile proteins. This protein could be one of the components of troponin or tropomyosin. The relation of such a phosphorylation to the role of microfilaments and contractile proteins in phagocytosis is now under active investigation.

Quantitative aspects of cAMP metabolism in the thyroid have been rather well defined. The tissue does not significantly degrade its trophic hormone, TSH (28). In dog thyroid slices pre-labelled with ^{3}H-adenine the specific activity of cAMP is higher than that of its precursor ATP. This suggests that all the ATP of the tissue may not participate in cAMP synthesis (29.).

The kinetics of cAMP accumulation in slices after stimulation by TSH exhibit a relatively rapid rise (in $\pm$ 30 minutes) to a plateau which remains more or less stable for up to 2 hours (18). The delay in reaching this plateau may result from the diffusion of TSH in the slices, the delay in the activation of adenylate cyclase, and the kinetics of cAMP accumulation in each cell. The activation of adenylate cyclase is quasi immediate. Diffusion of TSH in the slices accounts for a part of the delay and this factor becomes the most important in thick slices (Figure 4). The kinetics in each cell depend on the absolute activities of the syn-thesizing and degrading enzymes (mostly of the latter). On the other hand, the level of the plateau of cAMP concentration depends on the ratio of the activities of adenylate cyclase and phospho-diesterases.

The relation between cAMP accumulation and TSH concentration has been studied in dog thyroid slices. When compared to the corresponding curve of adenylate cyclase activation, several differences may be observed (Figure 5) (30) :

- Adenylate cyclase activation appears more sensitive to TSH (it is activated at lower TSH concentrations, and the TSH concentration of half maximal activation is lower).

- Absolute stimulation is higher for cAMP accumulation than for adenylate cyclase activation.

- While the adenylate cyclase activation curve exhibits a pattern of negative cooperativity, cAMP accumulation curve exhibits a pattern of positive cooperativity (not shown).

Several models (e.g. the hypothesis of cAMP sequestration) fail to account for the apparent discrepancies. The concentration effect

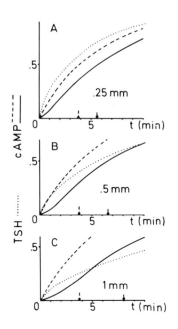

<u>FIGURE 4</u> *(see previous page)*

Simulation of the kinetics of cyclic AMP accumulation in dog thyroid slices of various thicknesses (0.25, 0.5 and 1 mm).

Three kinetics are represented :

1) the kinetics of TSH binding to receptors ....

2) the kinetics of cyclic AMP accumulation if the binding of TSH was immediately complete ------

3) the resulting kinetics of cAMP accumulation taking into account TSH penetration in the slice and the cyclic AMP metabolism in the cells ———

(from Swillens, S., unpublished data)

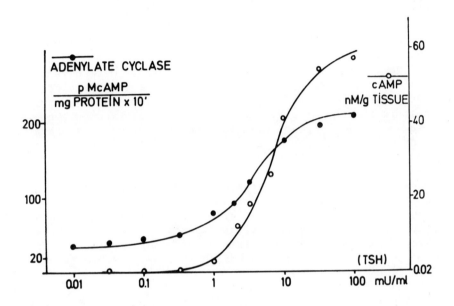

FIGURE 5. *Comparison of the concentration-response curves between TSH and adenylate cyclase activity in plasma membrane preparations (-o-) and of cyclic AMP accumulation in thyroid slices (-o-) from the same animal. Each point represents the mean of duplicate determinations. Equilibrium data have been obtained in both cases (from Boeynaems et al., 1974).*
Acknowledgement to J. Mol Cell Endocrinal.

curve for adenylate cyclase activation would however account for the curve of cAMP accumulation if 2 phosphodiesterases, one with a low Km and Vmax and another with higher Km and Vmax, were postulated. Such a situation applies to most tissues, and there is some evidence for the existence of 2 such phosphodiesterases in the thyroid. An important general conclusion may be derived from this theoretical analysis : the existence of 2 phosphodiesterases with different affinities for cAMP and different Vmax provides the cell with a potentially very powerful mechanism for the intracellular amplification of the hormonal signal (30).

REGULATION BY IODIDE OF THE CYCLIC 3', 5'-AMP SYSTEM

Iodide is the principal substrate of thyroid metabolism. However iodine is scarce in food and its intake is irregular. These factors are compensated by a very efficient iodide trapping mechanism in the thyroid, by the availability of excess thyroglobulin in the follicular lumen to bind iodine and by storage of this iodine in the thyroglobulin. All the biochemistry of the thyroid is geared to retain and make the most efficient use of iodine. It is therefore to be expected that regulatory mechanisms should exist to shift this pattern in case of excess iodine intake. Indeed, iodide at high concentrations inhibits its own binding to proteins in thyroid (the Wolff-Chaikoff effect), and decreases secretion and blood flow in activated glands. These properties have been widely used in the treatment of hyperthyroidism. The thyroid cyclic 3',5'-AMP system was an obvious possible target for iodide action.

Iodide *in vitro* inhibits the TSH enhancement of cAMP accumulation. Several indirect arguments have suggested a model to explain this action. Iodide (Figure 6) after its trapping by the follicular cell is oxidized by thyroid peroxidase and bound to thyroglobulin; part of the oxidized iodide is transformed to a compound XI which negatively controls cAMP accumulation by inhibiting adenylate cyclase, activating the phosphodiesterases or cAMP efflux from the cells (31). The identity of XI and its mechanism of action are unknown. Several predictions can be derived from such a model :

1) Iodide should decrease cAMP accumulation.

2) Iodide should inhibit the effects of TSH which are mediated by cAMP.

3) The inhibitory effects of iodide should be relieved by agents which inhibit uptake (e.g. $NaClO_4$) or iodide oxidation (e.g. methimazole, propylthiouracil).

All these predictions have been confirmed. The identity of XI is still unknown (31). Results showing that iodothyronines directly inhibit thyroid function (32) may suggest that the thyroid hormones themselves may be the negative feedback signals. However the rapid kinetics of the action of methimazole bears against this hypothesis.

ROLE OF CALCIUM

According to prevalent fashionable theories, tissues can be divided in two categories. In unidirectional systems the tissue is only submitted to positive control, i.e. to the action of one stimulatory signal. Examples of such systems may be the target tissues of pituitary tropic hormones, such as the thyroid or the adrenal. In bidirectional systems, the tissue is regulated both by positive and negative control, i.e. by stimulatory and inhibitory signals (37). Examples of such systems are the target cells of ortho- and parasympathetic control, such as the heart, where orthosympathetic stimulation by way of noradrenalin increases the heart rate and parasympathetic activation and acetylcholine decreases it. It has been proposed that in unidirectional systems cAMP on the one hand and cGMP and/or Ca^{++} on the other hand act in parallel, whereas signals in bidirectional systems would both be opposite (33).

The predominant role of Ca^{++} as a signal for muscle contraction in the excitation-contraction coupling and in the excitation-secretion coupling raised the question of a possible role of calcium in thyroid secretion or more generally in the regulation of thyroid metabolism (3, 34, 35). The first question that may be asked is whether calcium is necessary for TSH action. In experiments, designed to test this, thyroid slices were washed free from calcium by preincubation with EGTA then submitted to TSH stimulation *in vitro*. Contrary to expectations, while calcium depletion completely inhibited the activation of iodide binding to proteins and of glucose carbon 1 oxidation, it did not impair and may slightly increased thyroid secretion. Moreover, calcium depletion does not decrease the TSH induced accumulation of cAMP but blocks the activation of iodide organification and glucose oxidation by both 3',5'-cAMP and dibutyryl c3',5' cAMP. Thus, extracellular Ca^{++} is not necessary for the primary effect of TSH on thyroid, the increase of cAMP nor for one of its consequences, but is required for two other metabolic effects induced by this primary action (36).

If Ca^{++} is not necessary for TSH action, it could however either reinforce or antagonize it. One possible approach to investigate this question further was to define the consequences of a rise in Ca^{++} concentration in the cell. This can be achieved

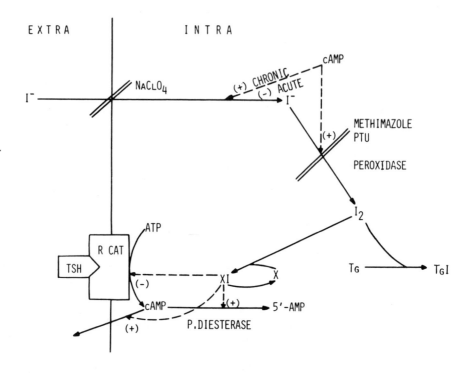

<u>FIGURE 6.</u>   Model of regulation by iodide of cyclic AMP
                metabolism in the dog thyroid cell.

⟶   chemical reaction;

- - - ⇢   action; + activation;

(-)   inhibition;
cAMP   cyclic AMP
PTU   propylthiouracil;
Tg   thyroglobulin;
R   regulatory unit of adenylate cyclase;
C   catalytic unit of adenylate cyclase;
Pdiesterase : cyclic AMP phosphodiesterase

(from Van Sande et al., 1975)

by the use of ionophores specific for divalent cations such as
A23187. Such ionophores tend to equilibrate cation levels on both
sides of membranes and thus to raise the low intracellular level
(10^{-7} – 10^5M) to concentrations closer to the extracellular level
(10^{-3}M). In such experiments, if it is the role of Ca^{++} *per se*
which is studied, the ionophore and Mg^{++} should remain constant
while only Ca^{++} concentration is varied. Under such conditions,
Ca^{++} in the thyroid considerably activated the binding of iodide
to proteins and glucose oxidation; it is necessary and sufficient
to elicit such activations. On the other hand, Ca^{++} not only
failed to increase cAMP accumulation and secretion but it also
depressed these variables (37). Thus Ca^{++} appears to have both
similar and opposite effects to TSH and cAMP.

It may be worthwhile at this point to ask whether TSH by
itself affects Ca^{++} levels in the cytosol of thyroid follicle
cells. A direct approach of this problem exists. In large muscle
cells, the fluorescence of Equorin in the presence of Ca^{++} permits
the estimation of free Ca^{++} concentrations. However this method
requires the injection of this protein into the cell, which appears
almost virtually impossible for follicular cells at the present
stage of methodology. Thus, this problem has to be approached by
use of tracer Ca^{++}, but the data obtained by this methodology are
difficult to interpret. The uptake of Ca^{++} in thyroid slices is
not markedly influenced by TSH; however, considering that the
cellular space represents at best 30% of the slice volume and that
much Ca^{++} is concentrated in the follicular lumen, such negative
evidence has little value. When slices are prelabelled at 0°C, a
compartment (A) is labelled which is rapidly discharged (20 minutes).
When the prelabelling is carried out at 37°C, the discharge involves
a first compartment, presumably A, which is rapidly discharged while
another (B) is emptied over 2 to 3 hours. Ionophore A23187 accelerates the discharge from compartment B but not from A. Our interpretation of these and other kinetic data is that while compartment
B is mostly intracellular, compartment A is mainly extracellular
bound Ca^{++}. This Ca^{++} is released much slower at 0° than at 37°C.
An experimental protocol, which involves the labelling of thyroid
slices followed by a first washing at 37°C (which depletes compartment A) allows one to measure, in a third incubation at 37°C, the
release of Ca^{++} from compartment B. This release is accelerated
by ionophore A23187, and antimycin, which may suggest a mitochondrial location. TSH, DBcAMP and acetylcholine were also found
to accelerate this release, which showed that TSH, by a cAMP
mediated action, caused a translocation of Ca^{++} in thyroid tissue
(38). This effect could correspond to an increased release of Ca^{++}
from an intracellular sequestrating site to the cytosol, with a
subsequent spill-over of this Ca^{++} out of the cells, but it could
also reflect an increase in the discharge of Ca^{++} from the cytosol
to the extracellular space. Thus, this cAMP mediated TSH action

could correspond to an increase or a decrease of cytosol Ca^{++} level. The simplest unifying explanation of all these findings would be that TSH and cAMP increase the cytosol calcium concentration by enhancing plasma membrane permeability and by releasing Ca^{++} from an intracellular store; the released Ca^{++} would in turn activate the binding of iodide to proteins and the pentose phosphate pathway.

THE CYCLIC 3',5'-GMP SYSTEM

Elements of the cGMP system have been identified in thyroid. This tissue contains cGMP (39) and a guanylate cyclase (40), and *in vitro* the cGMP levels are increased by acetylcholine and fluoride (39). In dog thyroid slices cGMP levels are enhanced by carbamylcholine (10^{-6} to 10^{-4}M), KCl (155 meq), serotonin (10^{-4}M) and NaF (5mM). In other tissues the three former agents are believed to enhance the concentration of free calcium in the cytosol (41). The action of carbamylcholine is inhibited by atropin (10^{-6}M). Under various experimental conditions TSH failed to enhance cGMP levels in this tissue.

It has been shown in the ductus deferens that intracellular cGMP levels depend on the level of extracellular Ca^{++} (42). In dog thyroid slices, whatever the stimulatory agent, no increase in cGMP level was observed in the absence of Ca^{++} in the medium. Thus, Ca^{++} appeared to be required to increase cGMP level in thyroid cells. In the presence of ionophore A23187, calcium *per se* (10^{-3}M) markedly enhanced cGMP concentration in dog thyroid slices. Thus, calcium appeared necessary and sufficient to raise or even maintain the intracellular cGMP level (21). Given that we may be beginning to understand the regulation of cGMP concentration in thyroid, the problem of its role remains unclear. According to the Ying-Yang hypothesis (33), cGMP could be expected to antagonize cAMP action if the thyroid is a bidirectional system, or to mimic cAMP action if the thyroid is a monodirectional system. In fact, all agents which raise cGMP levels in thyroid cells activate, as does TSH, the binding of iodide to proteins and the pentose phosphate pathway, but depress the stimulation of cAMP accumulation and of thyroid secretion induced by TSH. These effects are abolished in calcium depleted thyroid slices. Thus, the thyroid cell behaves neither as a unidirectional nor as a bidirectional system, but rather as a system with both types of properties.

The question may of course be raised whether *in vivo* the thyroid is a uni- or a bidirectional system. Classically, until now, the thyroid, like the adrenal, has been considered as a typically unidirectional system, being regulated by one positive signal (TSH, or ACTH respectively). However, the existence of cholinergic sensitive cGMP accumulation as well as of cholinergic nerve terminals

in some thyroids are compatible with the hypothesis of a negative
cholinergic regulation, i.e. with the concept of a bidirectional
control of this tissue.

Thus all the agents which increase cGMP concentration in the
thyroid tissue, also elicit certain metabolic effects : activation
of the binding of iodide to proteins, of the pentose pathway,
inhibition of cAMP accumulation and thyroid secretion. There is
good evidence that these effects are secondary to a rise of Ca^{++}
in the cytosol. It is however not clear whether they are caused
by Ca^{++} or by the rise in cGMP which is consequent to enhanced
calcium concentrations; the question remains whether the increased
cGMP accumulation is a necessary link between agents such as acetylcholine and their effects or is a mere by-product of this main
action. (Figure 7)

The mechanism by which Ca^{++} or cGMP negatively modulates cAMP
accumulation is not clear. This effect is not due to a depletion
of ATP, as the agents which enhance cGMP accumulation do not
decrease cellular ATP levels. Based on studies in other tissues,
several mechanisms could be postulated : inhibition by Ca^{++} of
thyroid adenylate cyclase, activation of cyclic AMP phosphodiesterase by calcium or by cGMP, etc. Preliminary studies suggest that
these biochemical mechanisms can be demonstrated for thyroid
enzymes but their real role in the regulation of cAMP level in
the intact cell remains to be elucidated.

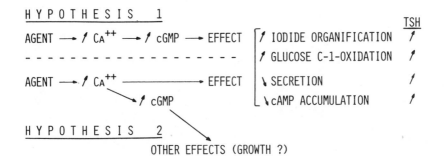

FIGURE 7. _Effect of calcium on thyroid metabolism. Hypotheses
concerning the role of cyclic GMP._

CONCLUSION

The regulation of the dog thyroid cell may thus be summarized as follows. The main regulatory circuit involves the activation of thyroid adenylate cyclase by TSH, cAMP synthesized by the enzyme acting as secondary intracellular messenger of TSH. On this first circuit are superimposed two negative regulatory systems. The first one involves a derivative of iodide, the main thyroid substrate, which decreases cAMP accumulation. The second loop involves intra-cytosol Ca^{++} and cGMP which also decrease cAMP accumulation. This scheme may not be entirely valid for all species. Several major questions remain unanswered. The role of Ca^{++} in the action of TSH is unclear. Calcium is required for some TSH effects, and by itself can reproduce these effects. On the other hand, TSH induces a translocation of calcium in the thyroid. All these data would be compatible with the hypothesis that cAMP releases sequest-rated Ca^{++} and thus increases Ca^{++} concentration in the cytosol. This in turn, would cause some of the hormonal effects. However, all the agents which increase Ca^{++} concentration in the cell also enhance cGMP levels and TSH has no such effect. Until now, it should therefore be postulated that Ca^{++} does not mediate any TSH or cAMP effect on thyroid metabolism although it may required for the expression of these effects. There is as yet almost no information about the role or action of cGMP.

The demonstration of acetylcholine and serotonin action on the dog thyroid, as well as the growing literature on the effects of prostaglandins and catecholamines on the metabolism of this tissue also raise many questions about the role of these trans-mitters as local or general intercellular signals in the regulation of thyroid function.

Acknowledgments

The authors would like to thank Prof. J.G. Hardman for helpful discussion and Mrs. Ch. Borrey for the preparation of the manuscript.

REFERENCES

(1) SÖDERBERG, V., (1959), Physiol. Rev., 39, 777

(2) MELANDER, A., ERISSON, L.E. and SUNDER, F., (1974) Life Sci., 14, 237

(3) DUMONT, J.E. (1971), Vit. Hormones, 29, 287

(4) VASSART, G., BROCAS, H., LECOCQ, R. and DUMONT, J.E., (1975) Europ. J. Biochem. 55, 15

(5) TAUROG, A., (1970), Rec. Progr. Horm. Res., 26, 189

(6) POMMIER, J., DE PRAILAUME, S., and NUNEZ, J. (1972), Biochimie, 54, 483

(7) PANTIC, V.R., (1974), Int. Rev. Cytol., 38, 153

(8) NEVE, P., WILLEMS, C., and DUMONT, J.E. (1970), Exptl. Cell Res., 63, 457

(9) WOLFF, J., and WILLIAMS, J.A., (1973), Rec. Progr. Horm. Res., 29, 229

(10) DUMONT, J.E., and TONDEUR-MONTENEZ, T. (1965), Biochim. Biophys. Acta, 3, 258

(11) BATES, R.W. and CONDLIFFE, P.G. (1960), Rec. Progr. Horm. Res., 16, 309

(12) DUMONT, J.E., and ROCMANS, P., (1964), J. Physiol. 174, 26

(13) DUMONT, J.E., WILLEMS, C., VAN SANDE, J. and NEVE, P., (1971) Ann. N.Y. Acad. Sci., 185, 291

(14) TONG, W. (1964), Endocrinology, 75, 527

(15) KERKOF, P.R.,LONG, P.J. and CHAIKOFF, I.L., (1964) Endocrinology, 74, 170

(16) NEVE, P., RODESCH, F and DUMONT, J.E., (1968), Exptl. Cell Res., 51, 68

(17) FAYET, G., PACHECO, H., and TIXIER, R., (1970), Bull. Soc. Chim. Biol., 52, 299

(18) VAN SANDE, J. and DUMONT, J.E., (1973) Biochim. Biophys. Acta, 313, 320

(19) GILMAN, A.G. (1970), Proceed. Natl. Acad. Sci. (US), 67,
      305

(20) MURAD, F., MANGANIELLO, V. and VAUGHAN, M. (1971), Proceed.
      Natl. Acad. Sci. (US), 68, 736

(21) VAN SANDE, J., DECOSTER, C. and DUMONT, J.E. (1975), Biochem.
      Biophys. Res. Comm., 62, 168

(22) LAMY, F. and DUMONT, J.E., (1974), Europ. J. Biochem., 45,
      171

(23) RODESCH, F., NEVE, P., WILLEMS, C. and DUMONT, J.E. (1968),
      Europ. J. Biochem. , 8, 26

(24) SUTHERLAND, E.W., ØYE, I and R.W. BUTCHER, (1965) Rec. Progr.
      Horm. Res., 21, 623

(25) POCHET, R., BOEYNAEMS, J.M. and DUMONT, J.E., (1974) Biochem.
      Biophys. Res. Comm., 58, 446

(26) LANGAN, T.A. (1969) Proceed. Natl. Acad. Sci. (US), 64,
      1276

(27) LAMY, F., WILLEMS, C., LECOCO, R., DELCROIX, C. and DUMONT,
      J.E., (1971), Horm. Metab. Res., 3, 414

(28) BOEYNAEMS, J.M., GOLSTEON-GOLAIRE, J. and DUMONT, J.E., (1975)
      Endocrinology, 93, 1227

(29) VAN SANDE, J. and DUMONT, J.E., (1975), Mol. Cell. Endocr.
      2, 289

(30) BOEYNAEMS, J.M., VAN SANDE, J., POCHET, R. and DUMONT, J.E.
      (1974) Mol. Cell. Endocr., 1, 135

(31) VAN SANDE, J., GRENIER, G., WILLEMS, C. and DUMONT, J.E.
      (1975), 96, 781

(32) SHIMIZU, T. and SHISHIBA, Y., (1975) Endocrinol. Japon, 22,
      55

(33) GOLDBERG, N.D., O'DEA, R.F. and HADDOX, M.K., (1973), Adv.
      Cycl. Nucl. Res. 3 155

(34) SELJELID, R. and NAKKEN, K.F., (1969), Scand. J. Clin. Lab.
      Invest. Suppl. 106, 125

(35)   WILLIAMS, J.A. (1972), Endocrinology, 90, 1459

(36)   WILLEMS, C., ROCMANS, P. and DUMONT, J.E., (1971) FEBS
       Letters, 14, 323

(37)   GRENIER, G., VAN SANDE, J., GLICK, D. and DUMONT, J.E.,
       (1974), FEBS Letters, 49, 96

(38)   RODESCH, F., BOGAERT, C. and DUMONT J.E., (1974) Cptes
       Rend. Acad. Sci. (Paris) 278, 931

(39)   YAMASHITA, K. and FIELD, J.B., (1972) J. Biol. Chem., 247,
       7062

(40)   BARMASCH, M., PISAREV, M.A. and ALTSCHULER, N.,
       (1973) Acta Endocr. Panam, 4, 19

(41)   DOUGLAS, W.W., (1968), Brit. J. Pharmacol., 34, 451

(42)   SCHULTZ, G., HARDMAN, J.G., SCHULTZ, K., BAIRD, C.E. and
       SUTHERLAND, E.W., (1973) Proceed. Natl. Acad. Sci., 70,
       3889

BEHAVIOR OF CULTURED FIBROBLASTS, THE CELL SURFACE AND CYCLIC AMP

Enrique Rozengurt

Imperial Cancer Research Fund Laboratories

P.O. Box 123, 44 Lincoln's Inn Fields, London WC2A 3PX

The availability of cell lines which grow and differentiate under controlled in vitro conditions offers an excellent opportunity to explore the factors involved in these important processes. Although it has not been rigorously proven that these model systems reproduce in full the physiological controls operating in vivo, the manifestations of some controls of proliferation and differentiation observed in tissue culture pose fundamental questions of regulation that can be attacked experimentally.

A useful in vitro model to study growth control is provided by stable lines of fibroblastic cells. It is possible that primary diploid cultures reflect more closely than the cell lines the controls that operate in vivo, but they are a heterogeneous population of cells and thus are not suitable for some biochemical studies. For this reason many experiments are carried out with stable cell lines which can be easily grown, cloned and transformed, i.e. stable changes in morphology, growth, surface properties and tumorigenicity are induced in vitro by oncogenic viruses and other carcinogens.

In the first part the behaviour of fibroblasts in culture will be discussed, particularly the manifestations of growth regulation observed in this system. The purpose of the second part will be to analyze the present evidence for a possible role of cyclic AMP in growth regulation of normal cultured fibroblasts.

711

Behaviour of Fibroblasts in Culture

Normal fibroblasts in vitro exist in two alternative growth states
one of active proliferation or one of reversible arrest (1). These
states are particularly evident in cultures of 3T3 cells, a mouse cell
line which has been selected for cessation of DNA synthesis at
confluency and against growth of spontaneous variants under
crowded culture conditions (2).

a) The growing state. In the growing state, animal cells
proceed from one mitosis to the next by a poorly understood
sequence of events. The interval between two successive mitosis
(the cell cycle) has been divided into four stages following the early
observation that DNA synthesis (S phase) takes place only during a
discrete part of the cell cycle. The G_1 phase is the period between
mitosis (M phase) and initiation of DNA synthesis; the G_2 phase is
the interval between completion of chromosome replication and
mitosis. Which events are crucial for the progress through the
cell cycle and particularly through G_1 and G_2 remain major
questions of cell biochemistry.

After division, i.e. in early G_1, a decision is made in the cell
either to proceed through G_1 toward DNA synthesis or to remain
in the resting state, called G_0. It is generally suspected that this
decision is a key point for the control of the initiation of the cell
cycle (3). The duration of G_1 is variable even in growing cultures,
indicating a loose coupling in the interval between division and S
phase. The nature of this variability is not clear. Smith and
Martin (4) propose that all the cells enter a G_0-like state called
A state from which they escape with constant probability per unit
of time; this model accounts for the variability of G_1. At a certain
point of G_1 (or according to a certain transition probability) the
cell becomes irreversibly committed to DNA synthesis and division.
Then it proceeds through the S, G_2 and M phases in a rather
constant length of time further suggesting that growth control is
exerted in the G_1 (G_0) phase of the cycle.

Studies on the regulation of the cell cycle usually require
synchronized populations of cells. They can be produced by blocking
the progression of the cycle reversibly at specific points, e.g. amin
acid (5) and serum (1, 6) starvation stops growth in G_1; compounds
that inhibit the synthesis of DNA precursors like hydroxyurea
arrest growth at the G_1/S boundary and alkaloids like colchicine
and vinblastine arrest the cell cycle at M(7). Inhibitors used for

producing synchronized populations of cells may have undesirable effects on cell metabolism; the use of various independent procedures largely circumvents this potential limitation.

Studies on synchronized populations of cells have revealed some marked biochemical alterations such as changes in the levels of some enzymes (8, 9), in the physical state of the chromatin (10), in histone phosphorylation and synthesis (11), in the concentration of precursors for DNA synthesis (11) etc. The majority of these changes take place during or shortly before the initiation of S and therefore they may be part of the deterministic sequence (S, G_2 and M). On the other hand, some striking membrane changes have been detected during M and early G_1. For example, growing cells exposed to lectins conjugated with fluorescein retain label only in M and early G_1 (12, 13). A similar pattern of expression was observed with other antigenic sites (14). In addition, mitotic cells release surface-bound heparansulfate (15), have an increased electrophoretic mobility (16) and become agglutinable by plant lectins (17). Further, the iodination of an external protein is reduced during M and increases in G_1 (18). Transport changes have been found also shortly after mitosis (19). All these results suggest that the cell membrane changes its configuration during M and early G_1. The primary event could be a change in the mobility of membrane proteins followed by a rearrangement of the surface, a release of substances attached to the cell surface, a preferential insertion of some antigenic sites during M and early G_1 or a combination of some or all these processes. It has been proposed that this transient change in membrane configuration is fundamental for the cell to proceed to the next cycle (3, 17, 20).

b) The resting state. In cultures of 3T3 cells, growth ceases with the formation of a confluent monolayer (1, 2). This phenomenon has been called density dependent inhibition of growth (21). In contrast, transformed cells usually continue to multiply long after they reach the confluent state and they form a multilayer sheet. The significance of density-dependent inhibition of growth resides in the possibility that it is an in vitro manifestation of an inherent growth regulatory mechanism, the loss of which may be factor contributing to malignancy. Indeed, loss of density-dependent inhibition of growth in vitro has been correlated with tumour-forming ability in vivo (22-25).

Why do non-transformed cells cease to divide at confluence? Two alternative hypothesis concerning this problem have evolved.

One holds that the restriction of growth is caused by a reduction
in the availability of components of the medium, i.e. growth
factors supplied by serum (20, 26). The other proposes that contact
between cells through specific receptors produces a negative signal
that inhibits the initiation of DNA synthesis (1, 27, 28).

Several lines of evidence support the first hypothesis: a) high
levels of serum can transitorily overcome the growth block in
resting 3T3 cells (20-26) b) in most cell lines of normal fibroblasts
the final saturation density is largely dependent upon the concentration of serum present in the medium; in low concentrations
of serum growth stops before confluence (29-32) and c) an inhibitory
role of cell-cell contract, as suggested by the classical wound-
healing experiment (29), seems unlikely because cell separation is
insufficient to stimulate the initiation of DNA synthesis (33) and
because inhibition of cell migration does not prevent the stimulation
of growth produced by serum in confluent cultures (34). Further,
Stoker (35) has emphasized that a diffusion barrier extremely close
to a confluent layer of cells may limit the uptake of critical nutrients
or growth factors from the medium. This phenomenon could account
for the very short-range topographical effects seen in wounded
cultures. All these experiments support the notion that contact or
proximity among cells may limit the utilization of growth factors,
perhaps by reducing their uptake from the medium. This possibility
becomes particularly evident if the combined effects of a diffusion
barrier (34), a partial depletion of medium components (30) and a
drop in transport rates for several small molecules (see below)
are considered together. In the framework of this hypothesis it is
conceived that transformed cells can grow under restrictive conditions because they have lower nutritional requirements. Indeed,
cancer cells in vitro are known to have a very low serum requirement for the initiation of DNA synthesis (27, 30-32) and a greater
ability to transport low molecular components from the medium
(see below).

Density inhibited cells are arrested in the G_0 (G_1) state. In
addition to cell density, cells stop at this point under many non-
optimal conditions like nutritional insufficiency (3), low pH(36),
lack of a proper substratum (31) or in the presence of some
polyanions like dextran-sulfate (37). Pardee (38) has proposed
that all these cultures are in a common resting state (R point)
irrespective of the non-optimal condition that blocks proliferation;
transformed cells which apparently do not stop in G_0 are proposed
to have lost their R-point control. The nature of the molecular

event that switches G_0 cells into growth is unknown but in the next
section I will briefly describe some of the experimental evidence
that strongly implicate the cell surface in the switching mechanism.

The Cell Surface and the Control of Growth

Many lines of evidence suggest that the plasma membrane plays
a central role in the control of cell proliferation (for review see
3, 17, 18, 20, 39); a) membrane glycoproteins, glycolipids and
phospholipids change markedly and the rate of transport of phosphate,
glucose and nucleosides is sharply reduced when mouse and chick
fibroblasts reached the confluent state, b) many of the agents that
stimulate resting cells to initiate DNA synthesis and cell division
may act on the cell membrane (some examples are listed in Table I),
and membrane changes are among the earliest events associated with
the re-initiation of growth, e. g. an increase in transport of
phosphate, uridine and glucose (40) can be detected within minutes
of serum addition c) marked surface changes take place during M
and early G_1 as mentioned before.   Transformation by oncogenic
virus dramatically alters the cell surface in several ways.   Transformed cells are agglutinated by some plant lectins more readily
than are the parental cells (17), partly because the lectin receptors
can move more freely in the plane of the membranes of transformed
fibroblasts than in those of normal cells (41).   Microtubules and
microfilaments have been proposed as internal anchoring points
for surface proteins (41) and a major external protein, absent in
transformed cells, has been suggested to play a similar role in the
outer part of the membrane of normal cells (18).   Transformation
appears also to increase the fluidity of the lipid phase of the
membrane (42-44) presumably through a decrease in the content
of cholesterol in at least some cells (43).   Transport rates for
small molecules (aminoacids and glucose) are also significantly
increased after transformation (45-47).

Many of the surface changes initially considered characteristic
of transformed cells are also detected in normal mitotic cells and
can be induced in normal fibroblasts in interphase by proteolytic
treatment.   In addition, transformed cells exhibit an enhanced
proteolytic activity (48).   Burger (17) suggested that both the
mitotic configuration of the membrane and the aberrant growth are
caused by the action of surface proteases.   However, addition of
inhibitors of proteolytic activity fails to restore density-dependent
inhibition of growth to some transformed cells (49, 50).   Clearly,

more experiments are required to define the contribution of
proteases to the phenotype of transformed cells.

All these results indicate that the cell surface plays a fundamental role in the control of cell proliferation. A basic question
is how the plasma membrane instructs the rest of the cell to elicit
an appropriate growth response. An attractive possibility initially
suggested by Burk (51) is that cyclic AMP constitutes a negative
signal that leads to the resting state. In recent years this hypothesis has been examined by different groups and some general
findings are emerging although the field is still fragmentary and
contradictory in some cases. In what follows I will describe some
of these results, point out the experimental pitfalls of some
interpretations and suggest future experiments. The role of
cyclic GMP as a positive signal in growth control is discussed
by Kram in another section of this volume. Transmembrane
communication not involving cyclic nucleotides has also been
suggested but will not be considered here (41).

Cell Behaviour and Cyclic AMP

a) Effect of cyclic AMP on cell morphology. The initial
approach followed by several groups consisted in examining different
parameters of cell behaviour after the addition to the culture medium
of cyclic AMP analogues or compounds which elevate its intracellular concentration. Addition of cyclic AMP analogues
dramatically changes the morphology of both normal and transformed
cells (52-54); within a few hours they induce a marked cell elongation.
The morphological change is readily reversible (52, 54), does not
depend on protein synthesis (55) and can be inhibited by agents like
colcemid and vinblastine which prevent assembly of microtubular
proteins (52, 54). Furthermore, dibutyryl cyclic AMP-treated cells
exhibit an increase in the number of microtubules and a change in
their distribution from a random to an ordered arrangement in
parallel to the long axis of the cell (56).

Prostaglandins, which activate the adenyl cyclase and elevate
the intracellular levels of cyclic AMP in fibroblasts (58-60) also
cause morphological changes (61). In addition, a temperature
sensitive mutant shows a fall in cyclic AMP levels and a parallel
rounding up when the cultures are shifted to a different temperature
(62). Although all these results suggest a role for cyclic AMP in
the regulation of cell shape modulating the organization of the

microtubules, recently Johnson et al. (63) reported that some N^6 derivatives of adenine rapidly and reversibly induce cell elongation without increasing the levels of cyclic AMP. These experiments suggest that the effect of dibutyryl cyclic AMP may be caused by substitutions in the N^6 position of the purine rather than by the cyclic moiety of the molecule. Undoubtedly, cell shape is a complex property presumably regulated at different levels and the N^6 derivatives of adenine might act at a site beyond cyclic AMP synthesis and degradation. However, the results stress that effects obtained by using only dibutyryl cyclic AMP should be interpreted with caution; other ways of changing the intracellular level of cyclic AMP are required to demonstrate cyclic AMP-mediated functions.

   b) Effect of cyclic AMP-elevating agents on cell growth. Addition of dibutyryl cyclic AMP decreases the rate of cell growth in a variety of cultured cells, e.g. neuroblastoma (64), adrenal (65), melanoma (66), hepatoma (67), myeloblastic (68, 69) and fibroblastic cell lines are affected.

   When 3T3 cells were treated with dibutyryl cyclic AMP, there was a significant reduction of the final saturation density (70). Since cell growth is inhibited independently of the cell density, cyclic AMP is thought to inhibit growth directly rather than by inducing the formation of surface receptors which become operative when cell-cell contact takes place. In contrast, the saturation density of several virus-transformed 3T3 cells is not decreased by cyclic AMP analogues which therefore do not restore the phenomenon of density-dependent inhibition of growth to transformed cells (70 and see below).

   An important question is whether or not cyclic AMP-elevating agents depress growth by acting selectively on a specific point of the cell cycle. This problem was approached in two ways. Normal growing cells were treated with dibutyryl cyclic AMP until significant depression or cessation of growth was attained. The compounds were removed, and the rate of DNA synthesis and cell numbers measured at frequent intervals. If the cells were reversibly arrested or delayed in a specific point of the cell cycle the removal of the inhibitors should have been followed by a synchronized wave of growth. Experiments of this type were carried out in CHO cells (71) and in secondary cultures of human diploid fibroblasts (72). In both cases the results were consistent with a cyclic AMP-sensitive point in early G_1.

The other approach was to test the inhibition of DNA synthesis and cell division produced by cyclic AMP-elevating agents in cultures released from $G_1(G_0)$ by trypsinization or by addition of serum. In cultures of 3T3 cells synchronized by trypsinization, dibutyryl cyclic AMP inhibited the initiation of DNA synthesis when added along with the trypsin but the cells became insensitive shortly after trypsinization (73, 74). However, the possibility that this cell-cycle sensitivity reflects changes in dibutyryl cyclic AMP uptake was not investigated.

Other studies have consistently shown that cyclic AMP-elevating agents added along with serum to $G_1(G_0)$ arrested cells, partly prevent or delay the initiation of DNA synthesis (71-73, 75-79). The inhibitors were effective when added in early G_1 but not in late G_1 or S (38, 72, 80).

A G_2-sensitive point has also been suggested on the basis that dibutyryl cyclic AMP added to 3T3 cells in S did not depress thymidine incorporation but inhibited cell division (62). However, it is not completely clear whether there was a complete block or a delay in G_2 since cell numbers determined at only one time were presented; more studies concerning effects of cyclic AMP-elevating agents on late events of the cell cycle are needed.

In contrast to the results obtained with normal cells, transformed cells exposed to dibutyryl cyclic AMP are not stopped at the G_1-sensitive point but they appear to accumulate in G_2 (81). This is an interesting result because it suggests that the inability of transformed cells to become quiescent in the G_1 phase of the cell cycle is not simply caused by a deficiency in the intracellular content of cyclic AMP. Transformed cells may have a defective response to cyclic AMP or alternatively transformation may alter the regulation of cell growth in ways which are non-dependent on cyclic AMP. A study of the cyclic AMP-dependent protein kinase activities present in normal and transformed cells should help in discriminating between these possibilities.

Before drawing final conclusions from the results summarized in this section, it must be kept in mind that a) the exact mechanism of action of dibutyryl cyclic AMP is still not clear; an advantage of this compound over cyclic AMP in crossing cell membranes has been challenged (82) and the demonstration that N^6-substituted adenines are biologically active (63) raises important questions concerning the specificity of the effects. In addition, the concentrations of dibutyryl cyclic AMP usually used to depress growth are very high, and non physiological: b) the possibility that the effects of dibutyryl cyclic AMP on the cell cycle merely reflect cell-cycle dependent changes in the uptake of the compound has not been carefully examined: c) in many studies, the effect of cyclic AMP-elevating agents on the initiation of DNA synthesis was monitored by measuring the incorporation of (H^3) thymidine into acid-insoluble material. However, an effect of these compounds on the induction of thymidine transport by serum, as was observed with cytochalasin B (34) was not rigorously ruled out.

The objections a) and b) are considerably weakened by the demonstration that PGE_1 blocks the initiation of DNA synthesis as measured by thymidine incorporation (38, 79). Furthermore, PGE_1 is more effective than $PGF_{2}\alpha$ in inhibiting the entry into S in serum-stimulated 3T3 cells and in increasing the endogenous levels of cyclic AMP (unpublished results).

We discussed before the likelihood that a fundamental event for the regulation of the cell cycle takes place in early G_1 or G_0. Results obtained by several groups provide evidence that clearly suggest that cyclic AMP may act at this stage of the cell cycle of normal cells but more experimental work is needed to fully evaluate this hypothesis. In the next section the changes in cyclic AMP concentration detected during the growth and cell cycle will be described. Obviously this division is arbitrary and was made for the organization of this presentation.

c) Variations in the intracellular level of cyclic AMP during the growth and cell cycle.

The concentration of cyclic AMP increases when 3T3 cells susceptible to density-dependent inhibition of growth have reached the confluent state (59, 83, 84). In addition, significant changes in cyclic AMP levels were found when the saturation density of WI 38 fibroblasts was altered by the pH of the medium (85). In normal rat-kidney cells, the increase in cyclic AMP levels correlates with an increase in the activity of the adenyl cyclase (86).

These results are consistent with the possibility that cyclic AMP is the intracellular mediator of or is associated in the density-dependent inhibition of growth.

The increase in cyclic AMP observed in confluent cultures

appears to be related to the concentration of serum in the medium rather than to cell-cell contact. Accordingly, 3T3 cells arrested before confluence by serum starvation exhibit a doubling in cyclic AMP level (87). Furthermore, revertants of transformed cells which require high serum to grow, accumulate cyclic AMP when serum is removed from the medium (88).

The levels of cyclic AMP are inversely correlated with the growth rates of a variety of cell lines and were found to be lower (2-3 fold) in transformed cells (77, 84, 85, 88, 89). Whether or not serum starvation increases the levels of cyclic AMP in virus-transformed 3T3 cells is not clear; while a several-fold increase in cyclic AMP levels is reported by Oey et al. (88), no changes were found by Kram et al. (77) in the same system. Further, the cyclic AMP content of serum-starved 3T6 cells did not change substantially (unpublished results). The reason for this discrepancy is unknown but it may be of interest that Oey and coworkers did not purify their extracts before the cyclic AMP-determinations.

Serum (59, 60, 72, 73, 77, 87, 89), trypsin (59, 73, 89) and insulin (59, 60, 89), the addition of which reinitiates DNA synthesis in resting fibroblasts, induce a rapid and transient fall in cyclic AMP concentration. Several groups (20, 59, 73, 77) proposed that this early change in cyclic AMP concentration may act as a signal that triggers the initiation of the reactions leading to DNA synthesis. Further, the demonstration that the level of cyclic AMP drops during mitosis and early G_1 (73, 90), is also consistent with the proposal that a transient decrease in cyclic AMP may signal the initiation of the cell cycle. An interesting prediction of this model that remains unproven, is that cyclic AMP should not drop during the mitotic period that precedes the shift to G_0.

It should be pointed out that a drop in cyclic AMP concentration, although necessary, may not be sufficient to induce DNA synthesis, since when cells were exposed to serum for only minutes, the serum did not stimulate DNA synthesis although it produced a fall in cyclic AMP (unpublished results). Thus, other factors are likely to be involved in the initiation of growth. As discussed before, there are extensive surface changes coinciding with variations in cyclic AMP levels and therefore a fundamental question is whether or not the changes in cyclic AMP trigger the subsequent events of the cycle or simply reflect the modifications of the membrane. An answer for this question requires to show how changes in cyclic AMP affect the progression of the cell cycle. The available evidence which suggests an inhibitory role in the initiation of DNA synthesis as well as the experimental objections to which it is still open have been discussed in the previous section.

In what follows, I will consider the role of cyclic AMP in the early membrane changes stimulated by serum in G_0-arrested cells.

d) Role of cyclic AMP in the early events stimulated by serum. Addition of serum to G_0-arrested cultures rapidly increases the rate of transport of glucose, phosphate and nucleosides and lowers the intracellular level of cyclic AMP. The co-ordinate development of these different changes suggests that they may be causally related to each other. An attractive unifying hypothesis of growth control and malignant transformation holds that cyclic AMP (72) and also cyclic GMP (92) modulate the expression of these initial membrane events and the synthesis of macromolecules (RNA and proteins) which is also stimulated by serum. According to this hypothesis the various effects of serum should be mediated by cyclic nucleo- tides. Based on studies concerning the role of cyclic AMP in the early transport changes a different view has evolved. The results indicated that the drop in cyclic AMP levels may be required for the early activation of nucleoside transport but not for the stimu- lation of phosphate uptake (60). In short, the results strongly suggest early cyclic AMP-independent processes of growth control. Further studies showed that serum addition increases phosphate transport as rapidly as it drops the level of cyclic AMP and that both changes precede the activation of uridine transport (91). In addition, cyclic AMP does not regulate the rapid activation of glucose transport produced by serum (40). All these results suggest that several specific transport systems which are stimulated by serum and associated with growth initiation are probably regulated independently of each other.

Previously it has been suggested that the membrane exists in at least two different states, called P and Q which regulate the ability of the cells to grow (20). The P state has been conceived as a membrane configuration productive for cells, it is present continuously in transformed cells and transiently during M and early G_1 in normal cells. The Q state is the membrane configuration of G_0-arrested cells. The nature of the molecular events involved in the transitions of state, remains undefined. However, it seems reasonable to suggest that a common underlying event in these transitions may be a change in the mobility of the membrane proteins (18, 41-44). This suggestion accounts for the dissociability

TABLE I

Agents that stimulate DNA synthesis in resting (G_0) fibroblasts.

Agent	Ref.
Serum	1, 6, 27-34
Insulin	37, 93, 94
Proteases	17, 18, 39
Neuraminidase	93
Heavy Metals	95
Colchicine	96
Phorbol myristate acetate	97
Fibroblastic growth factor	98

Factors from conditioned medium of cultured cells.

L	99
BHK	100
SV40 BHK	101
Hepatoma	102

of the early changes in membrane transport associated with the
initiation of growth. For instance, both the increase in phosphate
transport and the change in cyclic AMP may reflect a transition
in membrane state from O to P; afterwards, nucleoside transport
is activated presumably by the drop in cyclic AMP level. According
to this model even a single molecule can activate several membrane-
linked processes independently. Certainly, other possibilities can
be easily imagined, e. g. the presence of several different factors
in serum acting on specific functions of the cell membrane.

Not only may the membrane state influence the level of cyclic
AMP but conversely changes in cyclic AMP may modify the state
of the membrane. For instance, cyclic AMP appears to regulate
the organization of microtubules which, in turn, may provide
internal anchoring points for membrane proteins like transport
carriers, receptors and enzymes. If confirmed, these reciprocal
interactions between membranes state and cyclic AMP provide an
interesting regulatory circuit which might be of particular importance during G_2M and early G_1 when important processes - extensive
surface changes, reorganization of microtubular subunits, changes
in cyclic AMP, cell division and eventually the decision to stay in
G_0 or proceed to S - take place.

SUMMARY

Normal fibroblasts in vitro exist in two alternative states:
either growing or resting in early $G_1(G_0)$. In contrast, transformed
fibroblasts are fixed in the growing state. The transitions of growth
in normal cells are largely controlled by serum factors. A variety
of unrelated agents (see TableI), many of which may act on the cell
surface, stimulate DNA synthesis in resting cultures.

The interplay of surface and internal events appear to have a
fundamental role in the regulation of growth. There are extensive
changes in several surface properties during the cell cycle, when
the cells move into G_0 when resting cells are induced to recommence
DNA synthesis and after transformation (see Table II). Cyclic AMP
also changes under these transitional conditions. Many experiments
suggest a G_1 point more sensitive to changes in cyclic AMP levels,
but this interesting suggestion requires further experimental
verification.

There are early increases in membrane permeability associated

TABLE II

Changes in cell surface related properties of cells in different growth states

	Growing	Resting in $G_1(G_0)$	Resting + Serum	Mitotic	Transformed	Ref.
Transport						
Aminoacids	++	+/−	++	+/−	+++	19, 45, 46, 77
Glucose	+++	+	+++	N.D. a)	++++	40, 46, 47
Nucleoside	+++	+	+++	+	+++	19, 60, 104
Phosphate	+++	+	+++	N.D.	+++	60, 104
High M. W. Fucose glycopeptide	++	+	N.D.	+++	+++	103
Chain length of sugar glycolipids	+	+++	+++	N.D.	+	14, 105
Lectin agglutinability	+/−	+	++	+++	+++	17, 18, 39
Iodination of 250K protein	++	+++	+++±	+	−	18

a) N. D. = not determined

with the initiation of growth.   Some of the changes are under
cyclic AMP control but others are not, indicating early cyclic AMP-
independent processes of growth control.   The changes in cyclic
nucleotides and in transport rates for some substrates may reflect
a change in the state of the membrane.   It is suggested that there
are reciprocal influences between the membrane state and cyclic
AMP which might intervene in the control of processes taking
place in G_2, M and early G_1.

References

1) Todaro, G. , Lazar, G. K. and Green, H. (1965)
      J. Cell Physiol. 66, 325.

2) Todaro, G. and Green, H. (1963)
      J. Cell Biol. 17, 299.

3) Pardee, A. B. and Rozengurt, E. (1974) In, "Biochemistry of
      Cell Walls and Membranes" (ed. C. F. Fox) Medical and
      Technical Publ. Co. London, 155.

4) Smith, J. A. and Martin, L. (1973) Proc. Nat. Acad. Sci.
      70, 1263.

5) Tobey, R. A. (1973) Methods in Cell Physiol. 6, 67.

6) Bürk, R. R. (1970) Exp. Cell Res. 63, 309.

7) Taylor, E. W. (1973) In, "Drugs and the Cell Cycle" (eds)
      Zimmerman, A. M. , Padilla, G. M. and Cameron, J. L.
      Academic Press, New York, 11.

8) Turner, M. F. , Abrams, R. and Lieberman, I. (1968)
      J. Biol. Chem. 243, 3725.

9) Hogan, B. , Shields, R. and Curtis, D. (1974) Cell (in press).

10) Pederson, T. (1972) Proc. Nat. Acad. Sci. , U.S. 69, 2224.

11) Tobey, R. A. , Gurley, L. R. Hildebrand, C. E. , Ratcliff, R. L.
      and Walters, R. A. In, "Control of Proliferation in
      Animal Cells" (eds) B. Clarkson, and Baserga, R. ,
      Cold Spring Harbor Laboratory, 665.

12) Fox, T. O. , Sheppard, J. P. and Burger, M. M. (1971) Proc.
      Nat. Acad. Sci. , U. S. 68, 244.

13) Shoham, J. and Sachs, L. (1972) Proc. Nat. Acad. Sci. , U. S.
      69, 2479.

14) Wolf, B. A. and Robbins, P. W. (1974) J. Cell Biol. 61, 676.

15) Kraemer, P. M. and Tobey, R. A. (1972) J. Cell Biol. 55, 713.

16) Kraemer, P. M. (1967) J. Cell Biol. 33, 197.

17) Burger, M. M. (1973) Fed. Proc. 32, 91.

18) Hynes, R. O. (1974) Cell 1, 147.

19) Sander, G. and Pardee, A. B. (1972) J. Cell Physiol. 80, 267.

20) Pardee, A. B., Jimenez de Asua, L. and Rozengurt, E. (1974) In, Control of Proliferation in Animal Cells (eds) Clarkson, B. and Baserga, R., Cold Spring Harbor Laboratory, 547.

21) Stoker, M. G. P. and Rubin, H. (1967) Nature 213, 171.

22) Aaronson, S. A. and Todaro, G. (1968) Science 162, 1024.

23) Pollack, R., Green, H. and Todaro, G. (1968) Proc. Nat. Acad. Sci. 60, 126.

24) Pollack, R. and Teebor, G. W. (1969) Cancer Res. 29, 1770.

25) Martz, E. and Steinberg, M. (1972) J. Cell Physiol. 79, 189.

26) Holley, R. W. (1972) Proc. Nat. Acad. Sci. 69, 2840.

27) Dulbecco, R. (1970) Nature 227, 802.

28) Dulbecco, R., and Stoker, M. G. P. (1970) Proc. Nat. Acad. Sci., U.S. 66, 204.

29) Todaro, G. J., Matsuiya, Y., Bloom, S., Robbins, A. and Green, H. (1967) In, "Growth regulating substances for Animal Cells in Culture" (eds) Defendi, V. and Stoker, M. G. P. Wistar Institute Press, Philadelphia, 87.

30) Holley, R. W. and Kiernan, J. (1968) Proc. Nat. Acad. Sci., U.S., 60, 300.

31) Clarke, G. D., Stoker, M. G. P., Ludlow, A. and Thornton, M. (1970) Nature, 227, 798.

32) Dulbecco, R. and Elkington, J. (1973) Nature 246, 197.

33) Lipton, A., Klinger, I., Paul, D. and Holley, R. W. (1971)
    Proc. Nat. Acad. Sci., U.S. 68, 2799.

34) Brownstein, B., Rozengurt, E., Jimenez de Asua, L. and
    Stoker, M. G. P. (1975) J. Cell Physiol. (in press)

35) Stoker, M. G. P. (1973) Nature 246, 200.

36) Rubin, H. (1971) J. Cell Biol. 51, 686.

37) Clarke, G. D. and Stoker, M. G. P. (1971) In, "Growth Control
    in Cell Cultures" (eds) G. E. W. Wolstenholme and
    J. Knight, Churchill Livingstone, London, 17.

38) Pardee, A. B. (1974) Proc. Nat. Acad. Sci., U.S. 71, 1286.

39) Noonan, K. D. and Burger, M. M. (1974) Progress in Surface
    and Membrane Science 8, 245.

40) Jimenez de Asua, L. and Rozengurt, E. (1974) Nature, 251, 624.

41) Nicolson, G. L. (1974) In, "Control of Proliferation in Animal
    Cells" (eds) B. Clarkson and R. Baserga, Cold Spring
    Harbor Laboratory, 251.

42) Barnett, R. E., Furcht, L. T. and Scott, R. E. (1974) Proc.
    Nat. Acad. Sci., U.S. 71, 1992.

43) Inbar, M. and Shinitzky, M. (1974) Proc. Nat. Acad., Sci.,
    U.S. 71, 2128.

44) Barnett, R. E., Scott, R. E., Furcht, L. T. and Kersey, J. H.
    (1974) Nature 249, 466.

45) Foster, D. O. and Pardee, A. B. (1969) J. Biol. Chem. 244,
    2675.

46) Isselbacher, K. J. (1972) Proc. Nat. Acad. Sci., U.S. 69, 585.

47) Weber, M. J. (1973) J. Biol. Chem. 248, 2978.

48) Ossowski, L., Unkeless, J.C., Tobia, A., Quigley, J.P., Rifkin, D.B. and Reich, E. (1973) J. Exp. Med. 137, 112.

49) Chou, I.N., Black, P.H. and Roblin, R.O. (1974) Nature 250, 739.

50) Chou, I.N., Black, P.H. and Roblin, R.O. (1974) Proc. Nat. Acad. Sci., U.S. 71, 1748.

51) Burk, R.R. (1968) Nature 219, 1272.

52) Hsie, A.W. and Puck, T.T. (1971) Proc. Nat. Acad. Sci., U.S. 67, 358.

53) Hsie, A.W., Jones, C. and Puck, T.T. (1971) Proc. Nat. Acad. Sci., U.S. 68, 1648.

54) Johnson, G.S., Friedman, R.M. and Patstan, I. (1971) Proc. Nat. Acad. Sci., U.S. 68, 425.

55) Patterson, D. and Waldren, C.A. (1973) Biochem. Biophys. Res. Commun, 50, 566.

56) Porter, K.R., Puck, T.T., Hsie, A.W. and Kelley, D. (1974) Cell, 2, 145.

57) Peery, C.V., Johnson, G.S. and Pastan, I. (1971) J. Biol. Chem. 246, 5785.

58) Manganiello, V. and Vaughan, M. (1971) Proc. Nat. Acad. Sci., U.S., 69, 269.

59) Otten, J., Johnson, G.S. and Pastan, I. (1972) J. Biol. Chem. 247, 7082.

60) Rozengurt, E. and Jimenez de Asua, L. (1973) Proc. Nat. Acad. Sci., U.S. 70, 3609.

61) Johnson, G.S. and Pastan, I. (1971) J. Nat. Cancer Inst. 47, 1357.

62) Willingham, M.C., Carchman, R. and Pastan, I. (1973) Proc. Nat. Acad. Sci., U.S. 70, 2906.

63) Johnson, G. S. , D'Armiento, M. and Carchman, R. (1974)
        Exp. Cell Res. 85, 47.

64) Prasad, K. N. and Hsie, A. W. (1971) Nature New Biology,
        233, 141.

65) Masui, H. and Garren, L. D. (1971) Proc. Nat. Acad. Sci. ,
        U. S. 68, 3206.

66) Johnson, G. S. and Pastan, I. (1972) Nature New Biology
        237, 267.

67) Wijk, R. , Wicks, W. D. and Clay, K. (1972) Cancer Res.
        32, 1905.

68) Zalin, R. J. (1973) Exp. Cell Res. 78, 152.

69) Epstein, C. , Jimenez de Asua, L. and Rozengurt, E. (1975)
        J. Cell. Physiol. (in press)

70) Johnson, G. S. and Pastan, I. (1972) J. Nat. Cancer Inst.
        48, 1377.

71) Rozengurt, E. and Pardee, A. B. (1972) J. Cell Physiol.
        80, 273.

72) Froehlich, J. E. and Rachmeler (1972) J. Cell Biol. 55, 19.

73) Burger, M. M. , Bombik, B. M. , Breckenridge, B. M. and
        Sheppard, J. R. (1972) Nature New Biology 239, 161.

74) Willingham, M. C. , Johnson, G. S. and Pastan, I. (1972)
        Biochem. Biophys. Res. Comm. 48, 743.

75) Frank, W. (1972) Exp. Cell Res. 71, 238.

76) Bombik, B. M. and Burger, M. M. (1973) Exp. Cell Res. 80, 88.

77) Kram, R. , Mamont, P. and Tomkins, G. M. (1973) Proc. Nat.
        Acad. Sci. U. S. 70, 1432.

78) Schor, S. and Rozengurt, E. (1973) J. Cell Physiol. 81, 339.

79) Kurtz, M. J. , Polgar, P. , Taylor, L. , and Rutenburg, A. M. (1974) Biochem. J. 142, 339.

80) Hollengerberg, M. D. and Cuatrecasas, P. (1973) Proc. Nat. Acad. Sci. U. S. 70, 2964.

81) Smets, L. A. (1972) Nature New Biology 239, 123.

82) Ryan, W. L. and Durick, M. A. (1972) Science, 178, 1002.

83) Bannai, S. and Sheppard, J. R. (1974) Nature 250, 62.

84) Otten, J. , Johnson, G. S. and Pastan, I. (1971) Biochem. Biophys. Res. Comm. 44, 1192.

85) D'Armiento, M. , Johnson, G. S. and Pastan, I. (1973) Nature New Biology 242, 78.

86) Anderson, W. B. , Russell, T. R. , Carchman, R. A. and Pastan, I. (1973) Proc. Nat. Acad. Sci. , U. S. 70, 3802.

87) Seifert, W. and Paul, D. (1972) Nature 240, 281.

88) Oey, J. , Vogel, A. and Pollack, R. (1974) Proc. Nat. Acad. Sci. , U. S. 71, 694.

89) Sheppard, J. (1972) Nature New Biology 236, 14.

90) Sheppard, J. and Prescott, D. M. (1972) Exp. Cell Res. 75, 293.

91) Jimenez de Asua, L. , Rozengurt, E. and Dulbecco, R. (1974) Proc. Nat. Acad. Sci. , U. S. 71, 96.

92) Kram, R. and Tomkins, G. M. (1973) Proc. Nat. Acad. Sci. , U. S. 70, 1659.

93) Vaheri, A. , Ruoslahti, E. , Hovi, T. and Nordling, S. (1973) J. Cell Physiol. 81, 355.

94) Jimenez de Asua, L. , Surian, E. , Flawia, M. and Torres, H. (1973) Proc. Nat. Acad. Sci. , U. S. 70, 1388.

95) Rubin, H. and Koide, T. (1973) J. Cell. Physiol. 81, 387.

96) Vasiliev, J. M., Gelfand, I. M. and Guelstein, V. I. (1971)
     Proc. Nat. Acad. Sci., U.S. 68, 977.

97) Sivak, A. (1972) J. Cell. Physiol. 80, 167.

98) Gospodarowicz, D. (1974) Nature 249, 123.

99) Shodell, M. (1972) Proc. Nat. Acad. Sci., U.S. 69, 1455.

100) Stoker, M. G. P., Clarke, G. D. and Thornton, M. (1971)
      J. Cell. Physiol. 78, 345.

101) Bürk, R. R. (1973) Proc. Nat. Acad. Sci., U.S. 70, 369.

102) Dulak, N. C. and Temin, H. M. (1973) J. Cell. Physiol. 81, 153.

103) Glick, M. C. and Buck, C. A. (1973) Biochem, 12, 85.

104) Cunningham, D. D. and Pardee, A. B. (1969) Proc. Nat. Acad.
      Sci., U.S. 64, 1049.

105) Critchley, D. R. and Macpherson, I. (1973) Biochem. Biophys.
      Acta 296, 145.

CHROMATIN STRUCTURE AND THE ROLE OF HISTONE PHOSPHORYLATION IN

THE CELL CYCLE

Harry R. Matthews

Biophysics Laboratory, Department of Physics
Portsmouth Polytechnic, Gun House
Hampshire Terrace, Portsmouth, Hampshire, U.K.

Chromatin contains 3 major components at the molecular level:
DNA, histones and non-histones. RNA and, possibly, lipids are
present in smaller quantities. Histones are basic proteins
strongly bound to the DNA and they are currently thought to be
responsible for the overall structure of DNA in chromatin. Non-
histones are the other chromatin proteins and include structural
proteins, enzymes, putative specific controllers of gene
expression and RNA "packaging" proteins. DNA and histones are
normally present in approximately equal amounts but the proportion
of non-histones varies with the tissue and the preparation method.
In general, rather little is known about the non-histone component.
The histones from almost all organisms fall into five groups, F1,
F2A1, F2A2, F2B and F3, with some exceptions notably in the highly
repressed avian erythrocyte chromatin where F2C appears to replace
F1. The other common nomenclatures for histones are given in Table
1. The four histones, F2A1, F2A2, F2B, F3, are extremely similar
in different organisms, F2A1 in particular showing only minor
sequence differences between pea and calf. All the amino acid
sequences show a characteristic non-random distribution of residues,
giving rise to highly basic regions and hydrophobic regions. The
basic regions are thought to interact with DNA while the hydrophobic
regions take up highly specific folded structures which can interact
with other histones and, presumably, non-histones. There is a
considerable amount of physical chemical data to support this
view (1,2,3).

Nuclei, chromatin and deoxynucleohistone from a number of
sources produce a characteristic low angle X-ray diffraction
pattern with reflections corresponding to Bragg spacings of

TABLE 1

HISTONE NOMENCLATURE

VERY LYSINE RICH	F1	I	H1
LYSINE-ARGININE RICH	F2A2	IIB2	H2A
LYSINE RICH	F2B	IIB1	H2B
ARGININE RICH	F3	III	H3
ARGININE RICH	F2A1	IV	H4
LYSINE RICH	F2C	V	H5

approximately 11 nm, 5.5 nm, 3.7 nm, 2.7 nm and 2.2 nm. This
pattern indicates that chromatin possesses a regular repeating
structure (4,5). The form of the structure is unknown although
the early supercoil models are now being replaced by "bead on a
string" models following electron microscopy (6,7,8) and partial
nuclease digestion (9,10,11,12) experiments which have indicated
the presence of "particles" in chromatin containing up to 200 base
pairs of DNA and an amount of protein roughly equivalent to a subunit composition $(F2A1.F3)_2$ $F2B_2$ $F2A2_2$. Although F2A1 and F3
occur in a 1:1 ratio in all chromatins examined(13) and they can
be chemically cross linked in gently extracted histone (14) and F1
unlike the other histones has been shown to be unnecessary for the
regular chromatin structure (15) the above sub-unit composition,
and in fact, the sub-unit structure are still speculative. However,
neutron diffraction of chromatin in D_2O: H_2O mixtures shows great
promise of providing the data required for a solution to this
problem (16).

The structure is probably present throughout the normal nuclear
division cycle and the phenomena of DNA replication, transcription
and chromosome condensation may be due to other factors. F1 histone,
and particularly, its phosphorylation, have been linked to all three
of these processes. Unlike the other histones F1 shows a certain
amount of primary sequence heterogeneity in individual cells and
this heterogeneity is tissue and species-specific (17,18,19). All
the F1 subfractions show the general feature that the hydrophobic
amino acids are clustered in the region from approximately residue

40 to approximately residue 110 leaving very alanine, proline and
lysine rich N terminal (1 to 40) and C terminal (110 to 220)
regions. These histones can be enzymatically modified by
phosphorylation of serine and threonine residues and such
phosphorylation (at serine 37 and 106 in calf F1) has a very large
effect on the interaction of F1 with DNA in vitro (20). Three
separate phosphokinases which can phosphorylate F1 have been characterised by Langan (20,21). All three are present in the rapidly
dividing Ehrlich ascites tumour cells but only two of them, HK1 and
HK2, are present in non-dividing liver cells. The third kinase,
growth associated histone phosphokinase HKG, is probably common to
all dividing cells and has been characterised in cells arrested in
metaphase where activity was much greater than in interphase (22).

HK1 is a cyclic AMP dependent enzyme which phosphorylates
specifically serine 37 in mammalian F1 histone. In resting liver
this serine residue is not phosphorylated but after stimulation
with glucagon or cAMP about 1% of the F1 molecules were
phosphorylated specifically at site 37. Glucagon or cAMP were
effective both in the live rat and in isolated perfused rat liver
(23). Insulin also stimulated this phosphorylation in the live rat
but not in the isolated liver. It is suggested that this phosphorylation may be at least partly responsible for the change in template
activity of chromatin after stimulation. HK2 is a cyclic AMP
independent enzyme which phosphorylates calf F1 histone in vitro
specifically at serine 106. Phosphorylation of serine 106 has not
been observed in vivo so the function, if any, of this activity
is unknown (20). HKG is also a cAMP independent enzyme which
phosphorylates multiple sites of both serine and threonine in both
the N and C terminal regions of F1 molecules but not in the
hydrophobic segment (24). Similar sites of phosphorylation are
probably observed both in vivo and in vitro. Part of the multiplicity
of sites is probably due to differences between the various F1 sub
fractions (Langan, personal communication).

A great deal of work has been carried out on the phosphorylation
of histones in vivo, particularly using pulse-chase techniques or
synchronously growing cells. It is important to distinguish clearly
the kinds of information that can be obtained from the following
different types of experiment:

1. overall phosphate content

2. pulse label + chase (a) ^{3}H amino acid
                         (b) ^{32}P-phosphate

3. pulse label   (a) ^{32}P-phosphate
                         (b) ^{3}H amino acid

1. The overall phosphate content of Fl gives a measure of the number of phosphorylated residues in the histone population as a whole, i.e. not selected for old or newly synthesised histone. The best method of measurement is to separate histone into phosphorylated and non-phosphorylated forms and then estimate the amounts of histone in each form. Alternatively, alkali-labile phosphate can be measured chemically or steady-state radio-active labelling can be used. These methods give results which are independent of the overall level of phosphokinases and phosphatases, i.e. they ignore "turn-over" effects. Transfer of phosphate from one site to another on the same molecular species would not be observed. However, if histone function is structural then the overall level of phosphate content may be important.

2. The ^{3}H-amino acid is only incorporated into those histones synthesised during the pulse period. The chase then follows the fate of these particular molecules. Since histones are only synthesised in S phase some cell cycle data can be obtained from non-synchronised cells. In practice the method works well because histone turn-over is very slow and so long chase periods can be used. However, the pattern observed need not apply to the histone population as a whole and this can lead to a distinction between "old" and "newly" synthesised histone. Turnover of phosphate will not be observed if it occurs within a single molecular species.

^{32}P-phosphate is only incorporated into those histones phosphorylated during the pulse period. The chase then gives the life-time of these histone phosphates, so turn-over of histone phosphate will be observed. This label cannot be used for cell cycle studies in non-synchronised cells as the time of phosphorylation (except possibly for F3) is not located in a single short period of the cell cycle.

3. Pulse labelling with ^{32}P-phosphate also measures turn-over of histone phosphate. In the presence of phosphatases as well as phosphokinases ^{32}P incorporation during a pulse is not a good guide to possible changes in phosphate content in the histones. However, incorpoaration will be observed when phosphate is transferred from one site to another, by turn-over processes, even within the same molecular species. Most information can be obtained by looking at incorporation into specific sites. For cell cycle studies synchronised cells must be used.

Pulse labelling with ^{3}H amino acids can show whether newly synthesised histones are in the modified form or if the modification occurs well after synthesis. In synchronised cell cultures the time in the cycle when histone synthesis occurs can be determined.

When using the techniques involving ^{32}P labelling it is vital
to be sure that the label is in the histone being studied and not
in contaminating nucleic acid or non-histone protein. The best
way is to physically separate the phosphorylated species but counting of the histone bands after electrophoresis at low pH in
urea-polyacrylamide gels is also satisfactory.

Histone F2A1, studied by these techniques, does not appear to
be phosphorylated in mammalian cells but the N-terminal acetyl
serine in trout testis is phosphorylated soon after synthesis
and then loses it phosphate more slowly, over about 1 cell cycle
(25,26,27,28). Histone F2A2 shows a similar behaviour in trout
testis although the dephosphorylation occurs more quickly. In HTC
cells (hepatoma tunour cells) ^{32}P pulse label experiments show
incorporation only during S phase which is what would be expected
if it behaved in the same way as trout testis F2A2 and it has been
speculated that the phosphorylation of F2A2 is involved in the
process of DNA binding. In contrast, CHO cells (Chinese hamster
ovary) show a constant level of incorporation of a ^{32}P pulse
through the whole cycle. Histone F2B is not phosphorylated except
possibly, to a very small extent in trout testis. Histone H3 is
phosphorylated at mitosis in CHO cells and no phosphorylation is
seen in G1 or S phase in either CHO cells or HTC cells. Low
incorporation of ^{32}P is observed in trout testis. It has been
speculated that F3 phosphorylation is involved with chromosome
changes at mitosis.

In contrast to the other histones F1 phosphorylation has been
studied in some detail. It has been established that the proportion
of F1 in the phosphorylated form increases as cell growth rate increases in cancer cells as well as normal cells and implies that
F1 phosphorylation is involved in the process of cell growth (29).
Phosphorylation of F1 occurs in two parts of cell growth, S phase
and late G2 and M phases and the increased phosphorylation in
rapidly dividing cells reflects the higher proportion of the cycle
occupied by these phases. Pulse label experiments with ^{32}P have
shown significant incorporation in S phase in mammalian cells (26).
Long term radio-active labelling in Physarum polycephalum showed
no overall change in phosphate content in S phase (30). These
results are consistent if the S phase incorporation is assumed to
be due to histone synthesis and/or phosphate turn-over, as can be
seen by a mathematical transformation (21) of the long term
labelling experiments to show the expected results of pulse
labelling Figure 1.

The transform has not yet been checked experimentally. The
possible significance of the S phase phosphorylation has thus been
questioned. Moreover, recent inhibitor studies have shown that
histone phosphorylation and DNA synthesis are not inextricably
linked (27). This question is being pursued by a comparative study

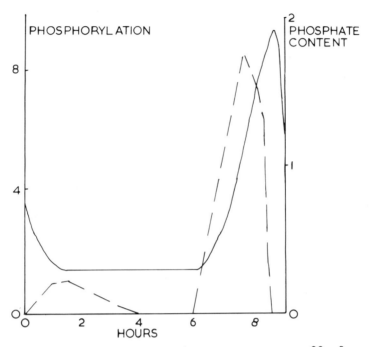

Figure 1: ——— measured histone phosphate content (^{32}P/^{3}H ratio)
            ---- simulated pulse label experiment.
^{32}P-phosphate and ^{3}H-lysine were added to a P.polycephalum plasmodium
immediately after fusion. The plasmodium was harvested at a known
time in the cycle, and histones isolated and fractionated on urea-
acrylamide gels[33]. The ^{32}P/^{3}H ratio in the lysine rich histone band
was plotted as a function of the time in the cycle when the histones
were isolated to show changes in the overall phosphate content per
molecule. The results of a simulated pulse label experiment were
obtained from the above data, the known time course of DNA synthesis
and the assumption that lysine rich histone synthesis closely follows
DNA synthesis (21,33).

of sites of phosphorylation in S phase and G2 phase because phosphorylation of a specific site in S phase would demonstrate a true
S phase correlation which is not simply due to histone synthesis.

    A much larger phosphorylation occurs in late G2 phase and M
phase of the mitotic cycle and this is accompanied by a large increase in the overall F1 phosphate content (30,31).Figure 1. This
massive phosphorylation has been observed in several mammalian cell
culture types and in the slime mould P. polycephalum and it appears
to be a universal phenomenon in dividing cells. The most detailed
studies have been carried out in P. polycephalum where the maximum

phosphate content occurs in prophase at the time when chromatin condensation becomes visible in the phase contrast microscope (30). There is considerable physical chemical data linking F1 with chromosome condensation in vitro (32) and it has been proposed that phosphorylation of F1 histone in vivo causes initiation of chromosome condensation in prophase (30). This proposal has received support from other groups in the field (25,27) but the evidence for it is still largely circumstantial.

Work on the control of F1 phosphorylation has been carried out on the true slime mould P.polycephalum. This organism has now become a classic tool for cell cycle studies in higher eukaryotes, partly because of its naturally synchronous nuclear division cycle in the acellular plasmodium and partly because its nuclear behaviour is in many respects very similar to that of higher eukaryotes rather than lower eukaryotes (33,34,35). These advantages make P.polycephalum suitable for analytical studies rather than comparative studies, in contrast to a number of other non-mammalian systems. In the division cycle synchronous metaphases in 10^8 nuclei occur within 5 min of one another in a division cycle time of 9h. Many other nuclear processes, notably DNA synthesis, are also highly synchronised and this degree of synchrony can probably be maintained indefinitely. (It has been demonstrated for 5 complete consecutive cycles (34)). This allows very detailed studies of cell cycle events to be made over the whole cycle and in the absence of the potentially disturbing effects of artificial synchronisation processes. Culture methods are straightforward, closely resembling standard bacterial handling procedures and groups are already in existence in most Western countries (36,37). In the last 10 yrs many detailed studies aimed at describing the processes controlling the cell cycle have been reported. In particular, ,attempts have been made to alter the time of a mitosis relative to a previous mitosis by adding extracts of plasmodia prepared at various times in the cycle. In some cases a shortening of the intermitotic time has been observed specifically using G2 phase extracts (38,39). However, several experienced workers have failed to obtain statistically significant results over many such experiments and so these techniques have not been successfully used as an assay system for purifying putative mitogenic factors. More general acceptance has been gained for experiments in which different plasmodia are allowed to fuse together. The fusion results in rapid cytoplasmic mixing including the diffusion of nuclei from one cytoplasm to another. In fused plasmodia the nuclei divide synchronously at a time intermediate between the division times in the homogeneous controls unless one of the fused plasmodia was close to division in which case nuclei from this plasmodium are not affected by the fusion, ie. a "point of no return" is reached in G2 phase about 0.14 of a generation time before metaphase. These experiments, together with data on the effect of mild heat shock, ultraviolet irradiation,

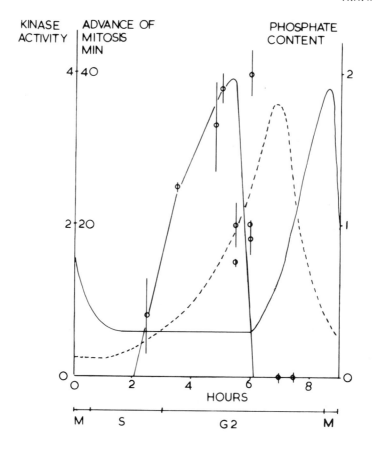

Figure 2: Synchronous plasmodia of P.polycephalum were prepared by
fusion of microplasmodia on filter paper. At a known time between
mitosis 2 (the second mitosis after fusion) and mitosis 3, the
filter paper was cut into quarters and transferred to petri dishes.
Each culture constituted a complete experiment with its own control,
conducted in duplicate. Duplicates of the same plasmodium divided
within 5 minutes of each other. Plasmodia were treated by carefully
pipetting on their surface 0.1 ml of solution. Enzyme solutions,
containing approximately 1.5 mg/ml protein, had been dialysed
overnight against 0.02M Tris-HCl buffer pH 7.2. The time of the
3rd mitosis was determined by microscopic examination of glycerol/
ethanol fixed smears under phase contrast. Advancement of mitosis
by Fl phosphokinase is shown as a function of the time in the cycle
when the enzyme was added,————————·————————, with the errors calculated from the differences between duplicates as in Table 5.For
comparison, the level of endogenous enzyme activity --- and Fl phosphate content————are also shown together with the timing of the
main events in the P.polycephalum mitotic cycle.

TABLE 2: P.Polycephalum histone kinase activity
(P.Campbell, unpublished)

Incubation mixture*	Units enzymic activity* per mg DNA				
	no added protein	+F1	+F1 +cAMP	+F1 +cGMP	+F1 +cAMp & cGMP
Source					
Nuclei	44	75	96	76	92
Cytoplasm	--	3	24	10	21

* 1 unit activity = 1 nmole $^{32}P/20$ min
+ Incubation mixture contained 10 μmoles Tris-HCl pH 7.2 +
1 μmole $MgCl_2$ + 0.15 μmole $\gamma^{32}P$-ATP (20,000 to 60,000 cpm/nmole)
+ up to 50μg enzyme protein in 0.15 ml.
+F1: 0.375 mg F1 histone was added
+ cAMP: $10^{-5}M$ cAMP added
+ cGMP: $10^{-5}M$ cGMP added

TABLE 3: Comparison with plasmodial fusion data

Unfused control time to mitosis	Unfused time difference between plasmodia	Observed stimulation of mitosis ± .04	Calculated stimulation of mitosis
0.49	0.34	0.21	0.22
0.51	0.30	0.22	0.19
0.67	0.40	0.26	0.27
0.58	0.31	0.20	0.20
0.42	0.13	0.09	0.07
0.38	0.06	0.05	0.03
0.47	0.17	0.10	0.10

Times are given as fractions of one cycle time.

TABLE 4: Comparison with mitotic stimulation data

Stage of donor plasmodium h before mitosis	fraction of generation time	Acceleration of mitosis h.	Phosphorylating activity moles ATP per nucleus x 10^{-21}
7.00	0.82	0.42	30
4.50	0.56	0.42	100
3.00	0.35	1.08	210
1.25	0.15	0.92	110
0.33	0.04	0.67	50

TABLE 5 – CONTROL EXPERIMENTS

Treatment begun h. before expected MIII	treatment Segments A	Segments B	Advancement of A before B min	Error due to differences[1] between duplicates min ±
3.4	Fl phosphokinase	Buffer	15	0
3.0	Fl phosphokinase	0.1 x phosphokinase	40	3
5.5	Fl phosphokinase	Fl phosphokinase inactivated by freezing and thawing	25	0
4.2	Fl phosphokinase	Fl phosphokinase inactivated by dialysis & storage	33	6
3.0	Fl phosphokinase	Fl phosphokinase inactivated by dialysis and storage	20	0
3.0	Fl phosphokinase	creatine phosphokinase	18	2
4.0	Fl phosphokinase	albumin	38	2

[1]This error is obtained as $[(\text{difference between mitosis times of A segments})^2 + (\text{difference between mitosis times of B segments})^2]^{\frac{1}{2}}$

X-ray treatment, cycloheximide and actinomycin provide a background on the expected behaviour of the unknown biochemical mechanisms that control the initiation of mitosis (33).

In order to follow up the histone phosphate content data in P.polycephalum the nuclear histone phosphokinase activity was measured. Preliminary data on the characteristics of the P.polyceph-alum histone phosphokinase activities are given in Table 2.The nuclear activity was cAMP independent but it was assayed through the mitotic cycle in the presence of 1μM cAMP using isolated sonicated nuclei as the source of enzyme activity and excess added calf F1 histone as substrate, Figure 2.

A very large peak of activity was observed in late G2 phase preceding the increase in histone phosphate content. This immediately suggested that the histone phosphate content is controlled by the histone kinase activity and reinforced the suggestion that chromosome condensation was initiated by histone phosphorylation. Even more interesting, however, was a detailed comparison of the variation of enzyme activity with the behaviour of the putative "mitotic trigger" expected from other experiments on plasmodial fusion, Table 3, and the effects of mild heat shock or plasmodial extracts, Table 4. The comparison showed that histone kinase behaves exactly like the "mitotic trigger" and it was concluded: that phosphorylation of F1 initiates chromosome condensation (which is then completed by a second process); that this phosphorylation is controlled by F1 kinase activity; and that these processes are the two main steps in the initiation and con- trol of initiation of mitotic cell division (40). In a direct test of these proposals Ehrlich ascites growth associated histone kinase, HKG, was added to growing plasmodia of P.polycephalum.Enzyme added during the normal rise in endogenous kinase activity produced a highly significant acceleration of initiation of mitosis, Figure 2. Inactivated enzyme preparations were without effect as were several other control substances, Table 5, but these experiments are subject to the reservation that no direct evidence is yet available that the added enzyme actually reached the nucleus and that the preparation used was not pure (21). Work is in progress to test these points using a fluorescent labelled anti-body and pure enzyme. It is also intended to study the correlation of histone kinase, phosphate content and mitosis in plasmodia treated so as to alter the normal intermitotic period.

Acknowledgements

The work reported is being pursued in Dr.E.M.Bradbury's laboratory in collaboration with Drs. R.J.Inglis and H.Molgaard, Mrs. J.McNaughton and Mrs. N. Sarner and with technical assistance from Miss S.L.Miller, Mrs. J.Robinson and Mrs. S. Nettell. Generous support was received from the Cancer Research Campaign and the Science Research Council.

REFERENCES

1. "Histone and Nucleohistones" ed. D.M.P.Phillips, Plenum Publishing Co.Ltd., London 1971.
2. "The structure and biological functions of histones", L.S. Hnilica, C.R.C.Press.Cleveland, 1972.
3. Bradbury E.M., Cary P.D., Crane-Robinson C., and Rattle,H.W.E. (1973). Ann.N.Y.Acad.Sci. 222, 226.
4. Bram.S. and Ris M.(1971) J.Mol.Biol. 55, 325.
5. Pardon G.F. and Wilkins M.H.F. (1972) J.Mol.Biol. 68, 115.
6. Olins, A.D., and Olins D.E.(1973) J.Cell.Biol. 59, 252a.
7. Woodcock C.L.F. (1973) J.Cell.Biol. 59, 368a.
8. Olins A.D. and Olins D.E. (1974) Science 183, 330.
9. Rill R. and Van Holde K.E. (1973) J.Biol.Chem.248.1080.
10. Sahasrabuddhe C.G. and Van Holde K.E. (1974) J.Biol.Chem.249, 152.
11. Hewish D.R. and Burgoyne L.A. (1973) Biochem.Biophys.Res.Comm. 52, 504.
12. Burgoyne L.A., Hewish D.R., and Mobbs J. (1974) Biochem.J. in press.
13. Bradbury E.M. (1974) CIBA Symposium, London.
14. Kornberg R.D. and Thomas J.D. (1974) Science 184, 865.
15. Bradbury E.M., Molgaard H.V., Stepehens R.M., Bolund L.B. and Johns E.W. (1972) Eur.J.Biochem. 31, 474.
16. Baldwin J.P., Boseley P.G., Bradbury E.M. Bram S., and Ibel K. (1975) Nature 253, 245.
17. Bustin M. and Cole R.D. (1969) J.Biol.Chem. 244 5286.
18. Kinkade J.M. (1969) J.Biol.Chem. 244 3375.
19. Bustin M. and Cole R.D. (1968) J.Biol.Chem. 243 4500.
20. Langan T.A. (1971) Ann.N.Y.Acad.Sci. 185, 166.
21. Bradbury E.M., Inglis R.J., Matthews H.R., and Langan T.A. (1974). Nature 249, 553.
22. Lake R.S. (1973) J.Cell.Biol. 58, 317.
23. Mallette L.E. Neblett M., Exton J.H., and Langan T.A.(1973). J.Biol.Chem. 248, 6289.
24. Langan T.A. and Hohman P. (1974) Fed.Proc.Abstract 2111.p.1597
25. Gurley, L.R., Walters R.A. and Tobey R.A. (1974) J.Cell.Biol. 60, 356.
26. Balhorn R., Bordwell J., Sellers L., Granner D. and Chalkley R.(1972) Biochem.Biophys.Res.Comm. 46, 1326.

27. Marks D.B., Paik W.K., and Borun T.W.(1973) J.Biol.Chem. 248, 5600.
28. Louie A.J., Sung M.T., and Dixon G.H (1973) J.Biol.Chem. 248, 3335.
29. Balhorn R., Balhorn M., Morris H.P. and Chalkley R.(1972) Cancer.Res. 32, 1775.
30. Bradbury E.M., Inglis R.J., Matthews H.R., and Sarner N., (1973) Eur.J.Biochem. 33, 131.
31. Gurley L.R., Walters R.A. and Tobey R.A. (1973) Biochem. Biophys.Res.Comm. 50, 744.
32. Bradbury E.M., Carpenter B.G., and Rattle H.W.E. (1973) Nature 241, 123.
33. Rusch H.P. (1971) Adv.in Cell.Biol. 1, 297.
34. Mohberg J., (1974) in "The Cell Nucleus" ed. H.Busch vol.1 p.187,Academic Press.N.Y.
35. "Physarum polycephalum" ed. A.Hutterman, 1973 G.Fischer Stuttgart.
36. Guttes E. and Guttes S. (1964) in "Methods in Cell Physiology" ed. D.M.Prescott, Academic Press. N.Y. p.43.
37. Daniel J.W.and Baldwin H.H. ibid, p.9.
38. Oppenheim A. and Katzir N. (1971) Exp.CellRes. 68, 224.
39. Blessing J. (1974) Abst.Europ.Physarum Meet.
40. Bradbury E.M. Inglis R.J. and Matthews H.R. (1974) Nature 247, 257.

CYCLIC NUCLEOTIDES AND CELL ADHESION

Robert Shields*

Biochemistry Group, School of Biological Sciences
University of Sussex
Falmer, Brighton, Sussex, U.K.

CONTENTS

Introduction
Methods
Results
Discussion

INTRODUCTION

Cell-cell and cell-substrate associations play an important role in many processes including morphogenetic movements in the embryo, cell recognition preceding myoblast fusion, cell locomotion and contact inhibition of cell movement. So called normal cells (i.e. those that do not form tumours when injected into animals) are "anchorage dependent" [1], require a solid surface in order to attach and grow and exhibit contact inhibition of movement. Tumour cells on the other hand do not exhibit these properties and are more easily detached from the culture dish and will often grow in suspension [2]. These results suggest that cell-substrate and cell-cell interactions may be altered in oncogenic transformation.

I have examined the adhesion of cells to the culture dish as a model system, but there is strong evidence from electron microscopy, the effects of temperature and divalent cations that cell-substrate adhesions and cell-cell adhesions are

---

*Present Address: Imperial Cancer Research Fund, Lincoln's Inn
                   Fields, London WC2A 3PX, U.K.

similar [3], so observations of adhesions in cultured cells may be relevant to intact tissues and to processes such as metastasis.

I looked at cell substrate adhesion by detaching cells in the presence of the calcium chelating agent EGTA [4]. Although adhesion and de-adhesion may be converse processes [3], I studied detachment as it takes place over a shorter time period and so is less complicated by processes such as membrane turnover.

METHODS

The cells used in this study BHK 21/13, and its transformed derivatives PyJ1 BHK, PyY1 BHK and freshly transformed ts3 Py BHK were obtained from The Imperial Cancer Research Fund, London and cultured in Dulbecco's medium containing 10% serum.

Cell detachment was performed as described [4]. Briefly cells were incubated at 37° in Ca++ Mg++ free buffer containing EGTA. At the end of the incubation the culture plates were rocked and detached cells counted and expressed as a percentage of the total cells present (detached and attached).

RESULTS

Fig.1 shows that about fivefold higher concentrations of EGTA are necessary to detach BHK cells than their polyoma transformed derivatives, demonstrating the greater adhesion of normal cells described by others [5]. Since the cells used in this experiment have been in culture for some time, and the original isolation of transformed cells depended on their ability to grow in suspension, it seemed possible that the difference in adhesion observed between BHK and Py BHK cells might have arisen by selection of non-adhesive cells in culture rather than being property of transformed state. To test this, I made use of BHK cells transformed by the temperature sensitive mutant of polyoma virus ts3 [6]. Cells transformed by this virus show the transformed pheno-type at 32°C but have a more normal behaviour at 39°C. Fig.2 shows that cells transformed by this virus are temperature sensitive for adhesion, although at 39°C the adhesion is still rather less than that observed in untransformed BHK cells. The results show that at least some of the differences in adhesion between normal and transformed cells is due to the presence of the tumour virus genome and does not arise through natural selection in culture.

Recently a great deal of interest has been generated by the idea that a major difference between growing normal and

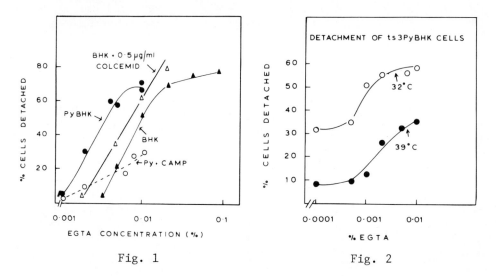

Fig. 1   Fig. 2

Fig. 1. Effect of different concentrations of EGTA on the detachment of BHK and Py BHK cells. When colcemid or dibutyl cyclic AMP was used it was present in a one hour preincubation in complete medium at 37°C as well as in the EGTA buffer. The cells were allowed to detach for 30 mins. ●——● Py BHK; ○——○ Py BHK + 0.5 mM dibutyl cyclic AMP + 1 mM theophylline; ▲——▲ BHK; △——△ BHK + colcemid 0.5 g/ml.

Fig. 2. The effect of different concentrations of EGTA on the detachment of ts3 Py BHK cells at 32°C and 39°C. ts3 Py BHK cells were grown at 32°C and seeded out into dishes, one set of which was incubated at 39°C. 24 hours later cell detachment on the cells was done at 37°C.

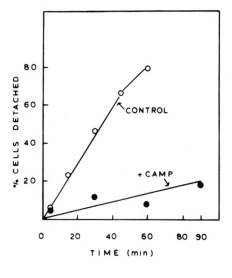

Fig. 3. Time course of detachment of BHK cells. The cells were detached in 0.01% EGTA in buffer. ○——○ BHK control; ●——● BHK + 0.5 mM dibutyl cyclic AMP + 1 mM theophylline.

Table 1. The Effect of Various Additions on
          the Detachment of BHK Cells

Additions	% cells detached
None	38
1mM dibutyl cyclic AMP	16
1mM theophylline	32
1mM dibutyl cylic AMP + 1mM theophylline	5
1mM 5'AMP	38
1mM IBMX[1]	3
1mM butyric acid	23
1mM RO20 1724[2]	20
1mM 5'GMP	18
1mM 8-bromo cyclic GMP	4

The cells were preincubated for one hour at 37°C in complete medium with the relevant addition. Cells were then
detached for 30 minutes in 0.01% EGTA in buffer containing
the additions.

[1]IBMX is 1-methyl-3-isobutyl Xanthine.
[2]RO20 1724 is 4-(3-butoxy-4 methyoxy benzyl)-2-imidazol-
 idinone.

transformed cells might be that normal cells have elevated levels of cyclic AMP. When cyclic AMP is added to tumour cells or generated endogenously after prostaglandin E_1 addition, many of the cell's properties such as growth rate, adhesion and morphology are altered towards those of normal cells [7]. Accordingly I tested the effects of dibutyl cyclic AMP on Py BHK cells. Their growth rate was altered (unpublished observations) and Fig.1 shows that much higher levels of EGTA were now required to detach them. Fig.3 shows that dibutyl cyclic AMP also has a marked effect on the adhesion of untransformed BHK cells.

I believe that the increase in adhesion of cells with dibutyl cyclic AMP is due to a direct effect of the cyclic nucleotide for a number of reasons. Firstly, the effect of dibutyl cyclic AMP is potentiated by phosphodiesterase inhibitions such as theophylline and IMBX (a theophylline analogue), and these compounds are active by themselves (Table 1). Secondly, the increase in adhesion cannot be mimicked by 5'AMP and only partly by butyric acid at high concentrations and thirdly cyclic AMP generated endogenously by the addition of prostaglandin E_1 also increases cell adhesion [5, and unpublished observations]. Furthermore the analogue 8-bromo cyclic AMP is also active (not shown), so the increased adhesion is probably not due to the effects of the N^6 substituted adenines [8].

Recently it has been shown that cyclic GMP might play a role in the control of cell growth and that its level in the cell varies inversely with cyclic AMP [9]. It has also been reported that exogenously added cyclic GMP reverses some of the effects of cyclic AMP on cellular processes such as membrane transport [10]. If this were the case it might be expected that cyclic GMP would decrease the adhesion of BHK cells as cyclic AMP increased it. Accordingly I examined the effect of 8-bromo cyclic GMP (a cyclic AMP analogue more resistant to phosphodiesterase) on the adhesion of BHK cells. Table 1 shows that 8-bromo cyclic GMP actually increases the adhesion of BHK cells.

The morphological changes induced by dibutyl cyclic AMP in CHO as well as other cells are reversed by agents that disrupt microtubules [11,12]. I used colcemid to examine the role microtubules play in cyclic AMP induced cell adhesion. Fig.4 shows that 0.5 µg/ml of colcemid will completely overcome the effect of dibutyl cyclic AMP and will also reduce the adhesion of untreated cells (Fig.1), suggesting that microtubules may play a role in normal as well as induced cell adhesion. Vinblastin at 0.1 µg/ml was also effective (not shown). Cytochalasin B as well as colcemid has been reported

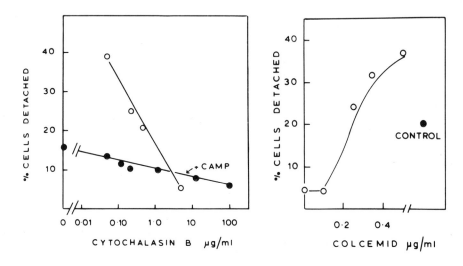

Fig. 4   Fig. 5

Fig. 4.   The effect of colcemid on BHK cells treated with dibutyl
cyclic AMP and theophylline.   BHK cells were preincubated with 0.5 mM
dibutyl cyclic AMP and 1 mM theophylline and the appropriate concentrations of colcemid for one hour.   Detachment was performed in 0.01%
EGTA for 30 minutes with the appropriate concentration of dibutyl
cyclic AMP, theophylline, and colcemid.   The control is the % cells
detaching without any additions.

Fig. 5.   The effect of cytochalasin B on cell adhesion.   Cells were
preincubated in the presence of cytochalasin B and dibutyl cyclic
AMP + theophylline were appropriate for one hour.   Detachment was
for 30 minutes.   o——o BHK; ●——● BHK + 0.5 mM dibcAMP + 1 mM
theophylline.

to overcome the morphological effects induced in CHO cells by
dibutyl cyclic AMP [13]. I examined the effect of this drug
on BHK cells and found that it increased rather than decreased
cell adhesion (Fig.5).

Examination of detaching cells under phase-contrast showed
some interesting effects. EGTA alone causes the cells to round
up with only a hint of polar asymmetry and these cells are then
easily detached with gentle agitation (Fig.6a). However, as the
cells treated with dibutyl cyclic AMP (Fig.6b) or 8-bromo cyclic
GMP (Fig.6c) round up they leave behind a network of processes
radiating from the cell body. These processes contain microtubules and are probably responsible for the increased adhesion
of the nucleotide treated cells, for if colcemid is added the
processes 'dissolve' in situ leaving behind bubbles of cytoplasm
(Fig.6d and 6e) and the cells detach early. Cytochalasin B
(1 µg/ml) has no effect on these processes.

                            DISCUSSION

I would like to suggest a model for cell adhesion and
locomotion which is consistent with our results and those of
others. Firstly, fibroblasts are known to adhere to the
substratum only over a very limited area of their undersurface
[14,15,16]. In the electron microscope most of the cell appears
to be 60 nM from the substrate but in certain regions, e.g.
behind the leading lamella the membrane approaches very close
to the substratum [14,17]. These are probably the points of
adhesion. The existence of these points of adhesion behind
the leading ruffling membrane has been elegantly confirmed by
scanning electron microscopy [16]. I propose that these small
areas are rich in "adhesion proteins" which float in the cell
membrane and are organized at the cell-substratum interface
into "adhesion patches" corresponding to limited contact areas.
We ebvisage that these "adhesion patches" are analogous to
patches of antigens formed on the membranes of mouse lymphocytes
treated with anti-mouse immunoglobin [18]. These antigen-
antibody patches will only form if the antibody is divalent and
probably results from the crosslinking of the antigen by the
antibody [19]. These patches of antigens then become linked
through the cell membrane to the cytoplasmic contractile system
containing microfilaments and microtubules and this leads to
the formation of a "cap" of antigen-antibody complex at one end
of the cell [18].

"Adhesion patches" would also be formed from adhesion
proteins by crosslinking, but in this case the substratum plays
the role of the multivalent antibody. These "adhesion patches"

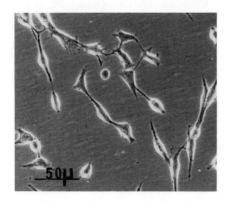

6a

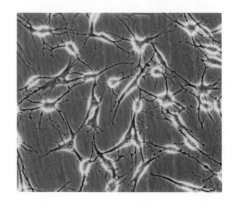

6b

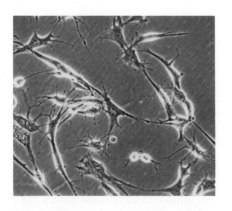

6c

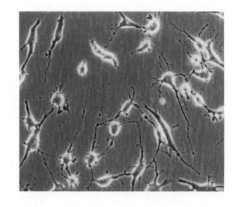

6d

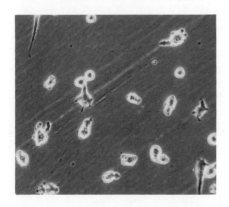

6e

Fig. 6.   See p. 755 for
          legend.

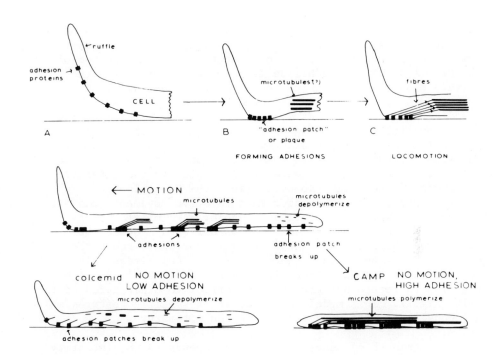

Fig. 7. Proposed model for cell adhesion and locomotion. For explanation see text.

Fig. 6. Detachment of BHK cells observed by phase contrast. Where appropriate, cyclic nucleotides were added to the cultures one hour before detachment was started. Cells were detached with 0.01% EGTA with the relevant additions. a) Control, 35 minutes in EGTA; b) with 0.5 mM dbcAMP + 1 mM theophylline, 25 minutes; c) with 1 mM 8-BrcGMP, 30 minutes; d) with 0.5 mM dbcAMP + 1 mM theophylline at 48 minutes, 0.5 g/ml colcemid added at 30 minutes; e) as d at 64 minutes, 0.5 µg/ml colcemid added at 30 minutes.

are probably identical to the electron dense "plaques" observed
in close proximity to the substratum behind the lamellipodia of
chick heart cells [14]. Similar plaques have been seen at the
points of cell-cell contact [20] again emphasizing the
similarities of cell-substrate and cell-cell interactions. Very
soon after the formation of such plaques filaments are observed
running obliquely from the plaque towards the dorsal area of the
cell and away from the advancing lamellipodia [14]. Further
evidence for the relationship between the fibrillar system of
the cell and the cell adhesion is provided by examining the
culture dish after mechanical detachment of the cells.
Occasionally the underside of the cell will be left attached to
the dish and the fibrillar system can be clearly made out [16].
We believe that the joining of these plaques to the cell's
contractile machinery is exactly analogous to the linking of
antigen-antibody patches to this system and that in both cases
the patches are moved backwards with respect to the internal
framework of the cell. However, since the "adhesion patches"
are attached to the substratum this relative movement leads to
forward movement of the cell as a whole. A similar analogy
between cap formation and cell motion has been proposed before
[18]. What happens when these "adhesion patches" reach the end
of the cell is not clear; there could be local disassembly of the
cell's contractile machinery leaving the individual adhesion
proteins to return by membrane counterflow to other parts of the
cell (Fig.7). This model has a number of specific features which
are consistent with many results in the literature.

(1) The strength of adhesion of cells depends on the integrity
of the "adhesion patches". If these adhesion patches break up,
although the total number of adhesive contacts may be the same,
they may be broken individually by the constant application of a
small force and so the cell detaches. However, if the adhesive
contacts are organized into patches a much larger force is
necessary to break the adhesion.

(2) In a moving cell the adhesion patches are undergoing constant,
ordered assembly and disassembly. The relative proportions of
assembled and disassembled "adhesion patches" govern the strength
of adhesion and the rate of cell movement. This is a possible
explanation for the commonly observed inverse relationship between
cell adhesion and cell motion [21].

(3) The adhesion patches once formed are stabilized by linking
to contractile machinery within the cell. This includes
apparatus sensitive to colcemid (probably microtubules) and
possibly microfilaments or tonofilaments [22]. The integrity
of the adhesion patches depends in turn on the state of assembly
of this contractile apparatus. Agents that promote the assembly

or prevent the disassembly of the contractile machinery such as cyclic AMP and cyclic GMP will enhance "adhesion patch" integrity and hence promote adhesion and decrease locomotion [5]. Conversely agents that destabilize the contractile apparatus, such as colcemid, will lower adhesion and lead to random motion. The importance of the integrity of contractile machinery in promoting stability of proteins grouped in the cell membrane in the form of caps has recently been demonstrated [23].

Thus our model can account for the increased cell adhesion and decreased locomotion in cells treated with cyclic nucleotides.

Several possible explanations can be advanced for the greater adherence of normal rather than tranformed cells. One is that normal cells have more polymerized microtubules, possibly because of higher levels of cyclic AMP or cyclic GMP or other factors; the actual "stickiness" of the adhesion proteins may be altered in transformation and the fluidity of the cell membrane may also play a role [4].

ACKNOWLEDGMENTS

I wish to thank Karen Pollock for skilled technical assistance. The work was supported by the Medical Research Council. RS was a Beit Memorial Fellow.

Figs. 1-6 are reproduced by kind permission of the editors and publishers of Cell.

REFERENCES

1) Stoker, M.G.P., O'Neill, C., Berryman, S. & Wasman, V. (1968)
   Int. J. Cancer 3, 683
2) Clarke, G.D., Stoker, M.G.P., Ludlow, A. & Thornton, M. (1970)
   Nature 227, 798
3) Curtis, A.S.G. (1967) in The Cell Surface, p.125. Academic
   Press, New York
4) Shields, R. & Pollock, K. (1974) Cell 3, 31
5) Johnson, G.S. & Pastan, I. (1972) Nat. New Biol. 236, 247
6) Dulbecco, R. & Eckhart, W. (1970) Proc. Natl. Acad. Sci. U.S.
   67, 1775
7) Johnson, G.S. & Pastan, I. (1972) J. Natl. Cancer Inst. 48,
   1377
8) Johnson, G.S., D'Armiento, M. & Carchman, R.A. (1974)
   Exp. Cell Res. 85, 47
9) Seifert, W.E. & Rudland, P.S. (1974) Nature 248, 138
10)Kram, R. & Tomkins, G.M. (1973) Proc. Natl. Acad. Sci. U.S.
   70, 1659
11)Hsie, A.W. & Puck, T.T. (1971) Proc. Natl. Acad. Sci. U.S.
   68, 358
12)Johnson, G.S., Friedman, R.M. & Pastan, I. (1971) Proc.
   Natl. Acad. Sci. U.S. 68, 425
13)Puck, T.T., Waldren, C.A. & Hsie, A.N. (1972) Proc. Natl.
   Acad. Sci. U.S. 69, 1943
14)Abercrombie, M., Heaysman, J.E.M. & Pegrum, S.M. (1971)
   Exp. Cell Res. 67, 359
15)Harris, A. (1973) Devel. Biol. 35, 97
16)Revel, J.P., Hoch, P. & Ho, D. (1974) Exp. Cell Res. 84, 207
17)Harris, A. (1973) in Locomotion of Tissue Cells, Ciba Foundation
   Symposium, 14, 20
18)De Petris, S. & Raff, M.C. (1973) in Locomotion of Tissue Cells,
   Ciba Foundation Symposium, Elsevier, Amsterdam, Vol. 14,
   pp. 27-40
19)Edelman, G.M., Yahara, I. & Wang, J.L. (1973) Proc. Natl. Acad.
   Sci. U.S. 70, 1442
20)Heaysman, J.E.M. & Pegrum, S.M. (1973) Exp. Cell Res. 78, 71
21)Gail, M.H. & Boone, C.W. (1972) Exp. Cell Res. 70, 33
22)Goldman, R.D. & Knipe, D.M. (1973) Cold Spring Harbor
   Symposia on Quantitative Biology, 37, 523
23)De Petris, S. (1974) Nature 250, 54

CYCLIC AMP AND CANCER

J. Otten

Institut de Recherche Interdisciplinaire
School of Medicine
University of Brussels (Belgium)

Contents

INTRODUCTION

Fibroblasts grown in monolayer on Petri dishes display various characteristics some of which help one to differentiate normal from malignant cells. For example, malignant fibroblasts, also called "transformed" cells, usually grow faster than their normal counterpart, they do not show density-dependent inhibition of growth, they move more rapidly, adhere less to the substratum, etc. Considering that cAMP mediates the regulation of numerous functions in all kinds of cells, mostly those functions which are

Abbreviations

cAMP = 3',5' cyclic adenosine monophosphate
Bt_2cAMP = N^6,O^2-dibutyryl cyclic AMP
CEF = chick embryo fibroblasts
RSV = Rons sarcoma virus
RSV-Ts = temperature sensitive mutant of Rons sarcoma virus

759

characteristic of the differentiated state of a cell line, it
was reasonable to hypothesize that cAMP was involved in the expression of those properties in cultured fibroblasts which distinguish normal from malignant cells.

This hypothesis has been checked by 3 kinds of experiments :

1) Studies where the addition of cAMP (or cAMP analogues) to the
   culture medium of transformed cells has been shown to "nor-
   malize" these cells, i.e. to reverse their properties from
   those of transformed cells.

2) cAMP concentration, adenylate cyclase and phosphodiesterase
   activities have been compared in normal and transformed cells.

3) The changes in cyclic AMP metabolism have been studied during
   transformation of normal cells by oncogenic viruses.

The greatest part of the work reviewed in this paper has been
carried out in Pastan's laboratory at the National Institutes of
Health, Bethesda.

EFFECT OF CYCLIC AMP ANALOGUES ON MALIGNANT FIBROBLASTS

Morphology

Normal fibroblasts grown on a plate are usually spread out,
have long processes and when they become confluent tend to
become spindly and to orient in parallel arrays. By contrast,
transformed cells are rounder, have less processes and after
confluency is reached they pile up on each other. Many transformed fibroblast lines, when treated with $\pm$ 1.2 mM Bt_2cAMP *
recover a normal morphology. They produce very long processes
and tend to become parallel at confluency (1-3). This effect is
specific for cAMP or its analogues, is usually visible within 3
hours and is reversible if cyclic AMP is removed from the medium.

Growth Rate

Bt_2cAMP in the presence of 1mM theophylline inhibits the
growth of many transformed mouse fibroblasts, as shown in Figure 1
for SV40 and Polyoma virus transformed cells (4). The effect of
Bt_2cAMP is not a toxic one as the cells rapidly resume a normal
growth after removal of the nucleotide from the medium and maintain a normal viability. As transformed cells usually grow faster
than normal cells, the inhibition of growth by Bt_2cAMP could be
considered as a normalization of the growth properties of these

* N^6,O^2-dibutyryl cyclic AMP

cells. Some prostaglandins, which increase the endogenous levels
of cAMP, also inhibit the growth of several fibroblast lines (5).

Motility

Transformed cells move faster on the substratum than normal
cells. By using time-lapse cinematography, it is possible to
measure the displacements of individual cells over a definite time
and to check the response to effectors on the velocity of these
cells.

In Figure 2, the effect of Bt_2cAMP (1.2 mM) on the motility
of L-929 cells is evident. Each line represents the displacements
of one L-cell over a 150 minute time-lapse. Control cells (left
side of the figure) move much faster than cells treated with
Bt_2cAMP (right side) (6). This effect is also readily reversible
and has been reproduced by addition of prostaglandin E_1.

The observation that in the presence of Bt_2cAMP transformed
cells recover several properties of normal cells, including also
adhesion to substratum (7) and agglutination by Concanavalin A (8),
suggests that malignant cells contain less cAMP than normal cells
and that their inability to maintain high levels of cAMP is directly
related to their abnormal characteristics.

CYCLIC AMP LEVELS IN TRANSFORMED CELLS

Sheppard (9) and Otten (10) showed that transformed fibroblasts contain less cAMP than the original untransformed cells.
Moreover, there is an inverse correlation between the growth rate
and the cAMP content of the cells, i.e. cells which grow faster
contain less cAMP than cells which grow slowly (Figure 3). This
observation suggests that cAMP directly controls the proliferation
of fibroblasts, and that the lower levels of cAMP in transformed
cells allows these cells to grow more rapidly.

cAMP concentration rises at confluency in several contact
inhibited cell lines while it decreases in non-contact inhibited
cultures (10). This observation has later been confirmed in
Pastan's laboratory (11) and by Paul (12) but Kram (13) and
Sheppard (9) found no change in cAMP content in confluent contact-
inhibited cell lines.

The discrepancies between the results from different laboratories could depend on the peculiarities of the cell lines under
study or to differences in the culture and feeding conditions.

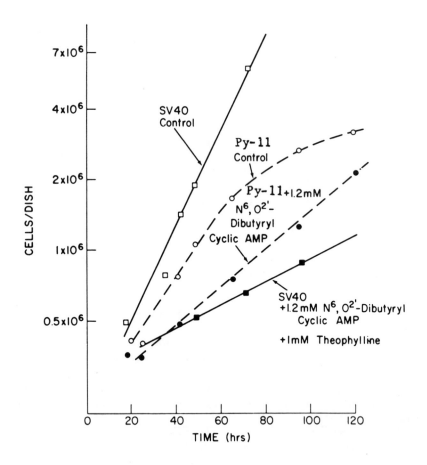

<u>FIGURE 1</u>. *Growth of control and treated 3T3 Py-11 and 3T3 SV C X cells. 3T3 Py-11 cells were planted at 3 x 10⁵ cells/50-mm dish (1.5 x 10⁴ cells/cm²), and 3T3 SV C X cells were planted at 4 x 10⁵ cells/dish (2 x 10⁴ cells/cm²). Each point represents the average of 2 determinations. (See reference (4))*

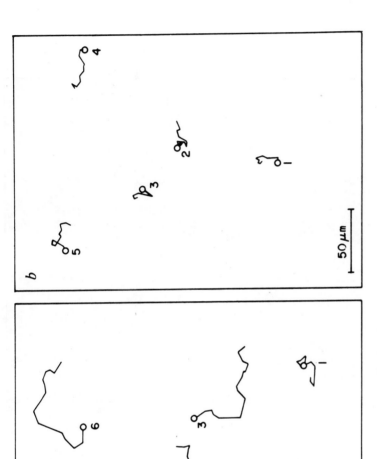

FIGURE 2. a. Migration of untreated L-929 fibroblasts over 150 minutes. The analysis was begun about 20 minutes after addition of fresh medium. The migration rate ranged from 0.3 μm/ minute to 1 μm/minute. Individual cell paths have been arbitrarily oriented to avoid overlapping lines.
b. Migration of L-929 fibroblasts treated with 1.2 mM dbc-AMP over 150 minutes. Migration analysis was begun about 20 minutes after addition of fresh medium containing the dbc-AMP. The migration rate was 0.2 μm/minutes to 0.25 μm/minute. (Reference (6))

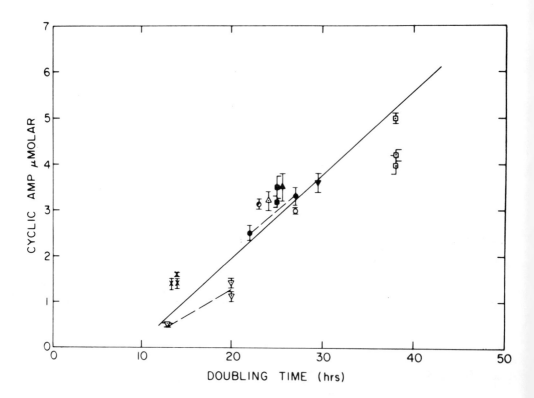

FIGURE 3. Comparison of cAMP levels with the growth rate of fibroblasts. Each value of cAMP is the mean ± S.E. of the mean. The
values in the Py-3T3 and SV40-3T3 were determined over a two-month
interval. □, 3T3; ▼, MSV/MuLV; ●, Py11; ○, SV-Py11; ▲, SVT2;
■, MEF; △, L-929; ◑, 3T6; ▽, SV40; ×, XC. The dashed lines
connect those cells which have changed their doubling time.
(Reference (10))

The results of Otten *et al.*(10) suggest that in some cell
lines at least, high levels of cAMP are necessary for contact-
inhibition of growth to occur and that the loss of growth control
in malignant cells at high density is related to their inability
to maintain high levels of cAMP.

CYCLIC AMP DURING TRANSFORMATION

The studies reviewed above have been done on established cell
lines, i.e. cells which were transformed a long time ago and have
been continuously subcultured. Such cells may alter their properties with time and changes in cAMP metabolism might result from
long maintained artificial conditions of life. Therefore, it was
important to check whether the metabolism of cAMP is altered in
freshly transformed cells or during the very process of transformation.

Otten *et al.* (14) studied the role of cAMP in viral oncogenesis
by making use of secondary chick embryofibroblasts (CEF) freshly
transformed by the Bryan high-titer strain of the Rous sarcoma
virus (RSV) or by a temperature-sensitive mutant of this virus
(RSV-ts). This mutant, developed by Bader (20), transforms CEF
only when the cells are grown at 36°. CEF infected by the mutant
RSV-ts and kept at 40.5°C are morphologically and biochemically
normal, but when shifted to 36°C, they acquire the characteristics
of cells infected by the wild type RSV.

Figure 4 shows a typical aspect of RSV-ts infected CEF at 36°.
These cells are not distinguishable from those transformed by the
wild type. They are rounded up and contain many vacuoles. If
these cells are treated by But$_2$cAMP (1 mM) before the temperature
is shifted down from 40.5°C to 36°C, they remain morphologically
similar to untransformed CEF (Figure 5). They remain spindly and
do not contain visible vacuoles.

The inhibition of transformation by But$_2$cAMP suggests that
endogenous levels of cAMP must be low in order for transformation
to occur.

Normal CEF indeed contain much more cAMP than transformed
cells (Figure 6). In RSV-ts infected cells, the cAMP content is
similar to that of normal CEF at 40.5. By contrast, at 36°, i.e.
the permissive temperature, the cAMP content is very low.

Kinetic studies have shown that the cAMP content of these
RSV-ts infected CEF has fallen by 40 % 10 minutes after the temperature shift down, which is well before the appearance of the first
morphological characteristics of transformation. Anderson *et al.*
investigated the mechanism of this fall in cAMP concentration (15).

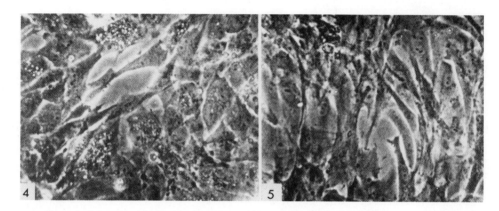

FIGURES 4 AND 5.   *Effects of Bt_2-cAMP and theophylline on morphology of chick embryo fibroblasts transformed by RSV-Ts.*

Figure 4 : chicken embryo fibroblasts (RSV-Ts) incubated at 36°;

*Figure 5 : chicken embryo fibroblasts (RSV-Ts) incubated at 36°
            with 1.2 mM Bt_2-cAMP and 1 mM theophylline.*

*Cells infected with RSV-Ta were grown at 40.5° and previously
treated with control medium or medium with Bt_2-cAMP and theophylline for 2 hours at 40.5°. The cells in Fig. 4 and 5 were then
incubated at 36° for 12 hours. Cells were grown in Eagle's minimal
essential medium supplemented with d-glucose (1 g per liter),
sodium pyruvate (5 mM), 5 % fetal bovine serum, 10 % tryptose phosphate broth, penicillin (50 units per ml), streptomycin (50 μg per
ml), and tylosine (50 μg per ml). (Reference (5))*

Cells	Growth temperature	
	40.5°	36°
	pmoles cAMP per mg nucleic acid	
CEF	207 ± 13	214 ± 22
CEF (RSV)	39 ± 3	34 ± 3
CEF (RSV-Ta)	197 ± 15	< 20

FIGURE 6. Cyclic AMP content of chick embryo cells in culture. Cells were grown at 40.5° and half of the plates were shifted to 36° 12 hours before cyclic AMP was extracted. Cyclic AMP was extracted and assayed as previously described (10). The values shown are the mean ± S.E. of mean. CEF = chick embryo fibroblasts.

They showed that it could be related to a decrease in adenylate cyclase activity in the transformed cells. In their first experiments however, using high ATP concentrations (3 mM) in the adenylate cyclase assay, they could not find any difference in the activity of normal and wild type RSV-transformed CEF. By contrast, at low ATP concentration (0.3 mM), the enzyme activity was much lower in transformed cells. A kinetic analysis of adenylate cyclase activity in these cells revealed that transformation by the wild-type RSV or by RSV-ts was associated with a decrease in the affinity of the enzyme for ATP. The Km of adenylate cyclase for its substrate increased from 0.25 mM in normal cells to 1.0 mM in transformed cells (Figure 7). Moreover, stimulation of the enzyme activity by Mg^{++} was much less in the preparation from transformed cells.

Later, Anderson *et al.* showed that in CEF transformed by the Schmidt-Ruppin strain of RSV, the fall in cAMP is related to a decrease in the maximal velocity of adenylate cyclase, the affinity of which for ATP and Mg^{++} remains unchanged.

In the past, several authors have compared adenylate cyclase activity in normal and transformed cell lines, but no clear-cut pattern has emerged from these studies, the activity being higher

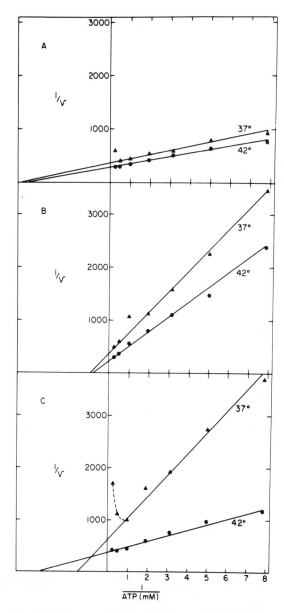

FIGURE 7. The effect of ATP concentration on the adenylate cyclase activity of (A) CEF cells; (B) RSV-BH-infected cells; and (C) RSV-BH-Ta-infected cells all grown at either (▲) 37° or (●) 42°. Enzyme activity was determined under the conditions described in Methods with 5 mM Mg^{++}. Velocity, V, is expressed at pmol of cAMP formed per 10 minutes per mg of protein.

in some transformed cells and lower in others (17-19). In addition, there was sometimes a discrepancy between cAMP levels and adenylate cyclase activity. This could perhaps be accounted for by changes in phosphodiesterase activity or release of cAMP from the cells into the medium. Anderson's work shows that in order to validly compare adenylate cyclase activities from different cell lines, the kinetic properties of the enzymes must be studied.

Bader has shown that inhibitors of DNA, RNA and protein synthesis do not prevent the transformation resulting from the temperature shift in RVS-ts infected cells. This led him to postulate that the transformation factor is a protein present in the virus. This viral product could induce an alteration in the structure of the plasma membrane and secondarily decrease the activity of adenylate cyclase, thereby reducing the cAMP content of the cell and allowing the expression of some at least of its malignant characteristics.

CONCLUSION

cAMP regulates many properties which distinguish normal from transformed fibroblasts in culture : growth rate, morphology, motility, adhesiveness, agglutinability by plant lectins, etc.

The different behaviour of malignant fibroblasts can at least in part be ascribed to their inability to maintain high intracellular levels of cAMP.

In some cases this metabolic defect was directly linked to the effect of an oncogenic virus factor. It does not follow that all the properties which define a cell as malignant result from the alteration in the adenylate cyclase cAMP system, nor that these data could be extrapolated to other kinds of cells or to situations *in vivo*.

The effect of oncogenic virus products on the adenylate cyclase system provides a tool for the isolation and further study of the factors which possibly mediate viral transformation of fibroblasts.

REFERENCES

(1) JOHNSON, G.S., FRIEDMAN, R.M., and PASTAN, I. (1971) Ann. N.Y. Acad. Sci., 85, 413

(2) JOHNSON, G.S., FRIEDMAN, R.M., and PASTAN, I., (1971), Proceed. Natl. Acad. Sci. (USA) 68, 425

(3) HEIDRICK, M.L., and RYAN, W.L. (1971), Cancer Res., 31, 1313

(4) JOHNSON, G.S. and PASTAN, I. (1972), J. Natl. Cancer Inst., 48, 1377

(5) OTTEN, J., JOHNSON, G.S., and PASTAN, I. (1972), J. Biol. Chem., 247, 7082

(6) JOHNSON, G.S., and PASTAN, I (1972), Nature, New Biol., 235, 54

(7) JOHNSON, G.S., and PASTAN, I (1972), Nature, New Biol., 236, 247

(8) HSIE, A.W., JONES, C. and PUCK, T.T. (1971) Proc. Natl. Acad. Sci. (USA), 68, 1648

(9) SHEPPARD, J.R. (1972), Nature, New Biol., 236, 14

(10) OTTEN, J., JOHNSON, G.S., and PASTAN, I (1971) Biochem. Biophys. Res. Comm., 44, 1192

(11) CARCHMAN, R.A., JOHNSON, G.S., PASTAN, I., and SCOLNICK, E.M., (1974), Cell. 1, 59

(12) PAUL, D. (1970), Nature, New Biol., 240, 179

(13) KRAM, R. et al. (in this volume)

(14) OTTEN, J., BADER, J., JOHNSON, G.S., and PASTAN, I. (1972) J. Biol. Chem., 247, 1632

(15) ANDERSON, W.B., LOVELACE, E., and PASTAN, I. (1973), Biochem. Biophys. Res. Comm., 52, 1293

(16) ANDERSON, W.B., JOHNSON, G.S., and PASTAN, I. (1973) Proceed. Natl. Acad. Sci. (USA), 70, 1055

(17) BÜRK, R.R. (1968), Nature, 219, 1272

(18) MAKMAN, M.H. (1971) Proceed. Natl. Acad. Sci. (USA), 68, 2127

(19) PERRY, C.V., JOHNSON, G.S., and PASTAN, I. (1971) J. Biol. Chem., 246, 5785

(20) BADER, J.P., and BROWN, N.R. (1971), Nature, New Biol., 234, 11

CYCLIC NUCLEOTIDES AND CELL GROWTH

Raphaël Kram
William Moens
Alain Vokaer

Free University of Brussels
Department of Molecular Biology
67, rue des Chevaux
1640 Rhode-Saint-Genese (Belgium)

Contents

INTRODUCTION

Recent speculation concerning the role of cyclic nucleotides in the control of cell proliferation centres on mechanism in which cyclic AMP and cyclic GMP have opposing regulatory actions. (Hadden *et al.*, (1); Kram and Tomkins, (2); Goldberg *et al.*, (3)). According to this model, cyclic AMP and cyclic GMP act as intracellular signals, respectively negative and positive, for cell growth in response to changes occurring in the environment. This hypothesis was developed independently as the result of personal investigations on the role of cyclic AMP and cyclic GMP as mediators of the "pleiotypic control" of cell growth proposed by Tomkins and

co-workers, and of the work in Goldberg's laboratory on the "Yin
Yang or dualism hypothesis" of biological control through opposing
actions of cyclic AMP and cyclic GMP.

THE PLEIOTYPIC CONTROL

This hypothesis is based on the assumption that a common
mechanism underlies the growth-promoting or growth-inhibiting properties of different specific stimuli in different tissues.
Indeed, the induction of cell growth by serum in quiescent cultured
fibroblasts is preceded by a sequential series of regular steps.
(Hershko *et al.*, (4)). These sequential steps include the stimulation of some transport systems (4, 5) protein synthesis (4),
ribosomal and t-RNA synthesis (4, 6), inhibition of protein degradation (4) and eventually the induction of DNA synthesis
followed by cell division (7, 8). The same set of reactions is
regulated, in many other tissues, following stimulation or inhibition of growth by different, chemically unrelated, specific
effectors. For example, androgens, estrogens, glucocorticoids, or
phytohemagglutinin influence, in their target cells, the same
general biochemical functions which are controlled by serum in
fibroblasts. Therefore, Hershko *et al.* proposed a regulatory programme designated as the "pleiotypic control", because of the
diversity of the biochemical parameters which respond coordinately
to external stimuli affecting cell growth. They proposed that the
ultimate mechanism for control of cell proliferation is unique and
involves changes either in the concentration or in the responsiveness
to the levels of common pleiotypic mediators. Since, in transformed
fibroblasts, the rates of growth and of the pleiotypic reactions
are relatively insensitive to factors which control proliferation
of normal fibroblasts, they suggested that cancer cells could be
viewed as "relaxed" variants of pleiotypic controlled cells (4).

Further work by Kram, Mamont and Tomkins (9) indicated that
increasing the intracellular cyclic AMP content in 3T3 fibroblasts
by various means inhibits uridine and leucine transport, slows the
overall rates of RNA and protein synthesis and enhances the rate of
protein degradation (Figure 1). These pleiotypic effects of cAMP
on a number of biochemical processes related to cell growth, can
account for the inhibitory role which cyclic AMP appears to play in
the proliferation of fibroblasts. Contributions from different
laboratories in this field are discussed in the preceding lectures
and should be referred to for a more detailed description of the
subject. On one hand, the intracellular concentrations of cyclic
AMP are high in resting cell cultures (9 - 11) and fall after a
brief exposure to a variety of mitogenic agents which include serum
factors, insulin, somatomedin and proteases (9 - 16). On the other
hand, exogenous addition of high concentrations (10^{-4} to 10^{-3}M) of
dibutyryl cyclic AMP to the culture medium causes a partial inhibi-

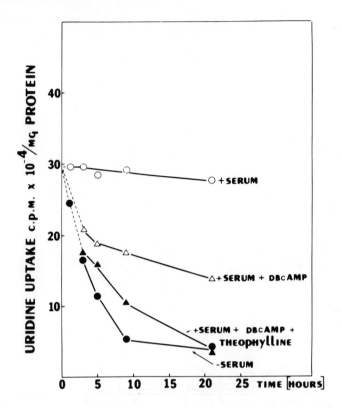

Figure 1. The effect of dibutyryl cyclic AMP, theophylline and serum starvation on rates of uridine transport in 3T3 mouse fibroblasts. Experiments were performed with sparse cultures (3 x 10⁵ cells per 25 cm² dish) growing in complete medium, i.e. supplemented with 10 % calf serum. At time 0, the media were removed and the cells were further incubated in medium with and without serum, and containing, as indicated, 0.5 mM dibutyryl cAMP alone or in combination with 1 mM theophylline. From R. Kram et al., Proc. natl. Acad. Sci. USA 70, 1432 (1973)

tion of growth response (9, 17, 18) (Figures 2 and 3). Moreover, the lack of regulation of the pleiotypic functions in malignant cells (4) is consistent with the finding of alterations in the metabolism (11, 13, 19), or in the action of cAMP (20) in these cells.

As in the case of cyclic AMP-mediated hormonal effects on metabolic functions (21), the inhibitory pleiotypic effects of cAMP seem to be exerted by activation of protein kinases. Indeed, cyclic AMP-resistant variants of lymphoma cells have been selected for

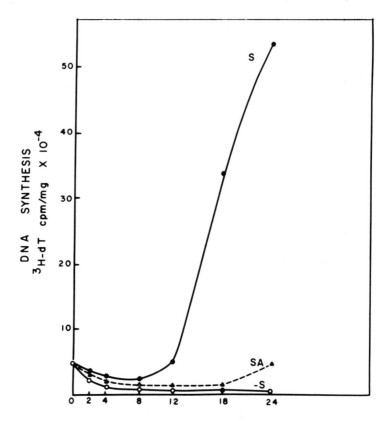

Figure 2. *Inhibition by dibutyryl cyclic AMP (0.2 mM) and theo-*
phylline (1 mM) of serum-stimulated thymidine incorporation into
DNA. After serum deprivation for 16 hours, 3T3 cells were, from
time 0, further incubated in either medium without serum (-S),
medium with serum (S), or medium with serum containing dibutyryl
cyclic AMP and theophylline (SA). From R. Kram et al., Proc. natl.
Acad. Sci. USA 70, 1432 (1973).

in Tomkin's laboratory. The resistant population has a faster
doubling time and grows to higher densities than the parent sensitive population. The intracellular actions of cyclic AMP in the
resistant cells are blocked and this defect is accompanied by
reduced activity of the cyclic AMP-activated protein kinases (20).

Whereas cyclic AMP acts as a negative pleiotypic mediator,
cyclic GMP functions as a positive pleiotypic mediator in fibro-

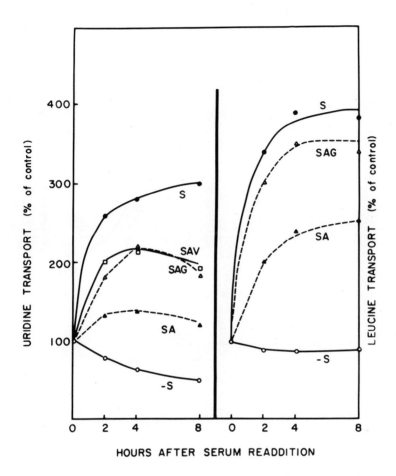

Figure 3. Antagonistic effects of cyclic AMP and cyclic GMP on the serum-stimulated rates of uridine and leucine transport in 3T3 fibroblasts. After serum deprivation for 16 hours, the cells were, from time 0, further incubated in either medium without serum (-S), or medium plus 10 % calf serum (S), with or without the following additions symbolized as follows : A : dibutyryl cyclic AMP (0.2 mM) and theophylline (1 mM); G = cyclic GMP (1 mM). V refers to the addition of vinblastine at 0.01 µg/ml : note that microtubules inhibitors also antagonize the transport inhibition caused by cyclic AMP. From R. Kram and G.M. Tomkins, Proc. natl. Acad. Sci. USA, 70, 1659 (1973)

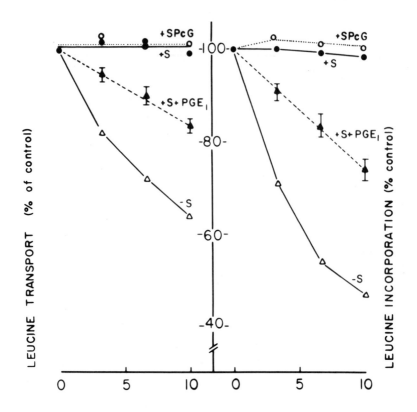

<u>Figure 4</u>.   *Reversal by cyclic GMP of the inhibition by prostaglandin*
E₁ of leucine transport and incorporation into proteins.   Sparse
cultures of mouse 3T3 fibroblasts growing in medium supplemented
with 10 % calf serum were further incubated, from time 0, in medium
without serum (-S), or medium plus serum (+ S) with, as indicated,
the addition of 5 µg/ml of protaglandin E₁ (P) alone or in com-
bination with 1 mM cyclic GMP (cG).   From R. Kram and G.M. Tomkins,
Proc. natl. Acad. Sci. USA 70, 1659 (1973)

blastic cells in tissue culture. Kram and Tomkins showed that
cGMP counteracts the inhibitory effects of cAMP on the pleiotypic
reactions, whether the inhibition was caused by dibutyryl cyclic
AMP or prostaglandin E₁ (2) (Figures 3 and 4). Moreover, additions
of the same high, non-physiological (10^{-4} – 10^{-3} M) concentrations
of cGMP can induce substantial increases in DNA synthesis in
quiescent fibroblasts (23). The recent demonstrations of a transient increase in intracellular cGMP after growth induction by
serum in these cells lend support to the physiological relevance
of these observations (23, 24).

THE YIN YANG OR DUALISM HYPOTHESIS OF BIOLOGICAL CONTROL
THROUGH CYCLIC AMP AND CYCLIC GMP

The information obtained by the Goldberg group (25, 26) with
respect to the role of cyclic GMP in cell proliferation has emerged
as the logical consequence of their numerous contributions on the
subject of the regulation of biological processes by cyclic GMP and
of the recent advances implicating cyclic AMP in the control of
cell growth. Their work originated from a challenge, on both
theoretical and experimental grounds, against the "unitary" concept
of "bidirectional" control through changes in the levels of cyclic
AMP alone. According to this unitary concept, bidirectional changes
(i.e. increases and decreases) in only intracellular cyclic AMP
concentrations can provide for both the positive and negative regulatory influences in systems that appear to be modulated by opposing
biological effectors : e.g. epinehrine versus acetylcholine on
heart function and smooth muscle contractility. In contrast, the
"dualism" hypothesis proposes that responses antagonistic to those
produced in such bidirectionally controlled systems by an increase
in cyclic AMP are initiated by an active signal, represented by an
elevation of cellular cyclic GMP concentration, rather than by a
passive one, represented by a lowering of the cyclic AMP concentration. The data in favour of this dualism derive from experiments
on a number of different biological systems where hormones and
other substances, which generate respectively increased levels of
cyclic AMP and cyclic GMP, promote opposing responses in the same
tissues. This concept is symbolized by the term Yin Yang, an
oriental philosophy based on a dualism between two opposing natural
forces (25, 26).

In contrast to these bidirectionally controlled systems,
Goldberg designates as "monodirectional" those which appear to be
susceptible to only one type of regulatory influence, i.e. a
positive or stimulatory one, e.g. steroidogenesis in the adrenal
cortex. In these systems, it might be possible that the two
cyclic nucleotides mediate the actions of different stimulatory
effectors or promote different steps of the same processes. This
view could explain similar effects produced by cholinergic drugs
and agents that elevate cyclic AMP, as in the thyroid (27, 28)
and in pancreatic islets (29).

Within the framework of the "Yin Yang Hypothesis", Goldberg
and his co-workers have proposed that an elevation of cyclic GMP
rather than a decreased concentration of cyclic AMP (11, 16)
represents the signal for the initiation of cell proliferation.
Indeed, the first observation implicating cyclic GMP in this
process was the finding by Hadden *et al.* (1) of a striking increase of this nucleotide in circulating lymphocytes within 20
minutes of stimulation by phytohemagglutinin (PHA). The levels of
cyclic AMP were unaltered when a purified preparation of PHA with
minimal agglutinating activity was used.

EXPERIMENTAL EVIDENCE IN DIFFERENT CELL TYPES

Fibroblasts

The growth of non-transformed fibroblasts in tissue culture is regulated by serum factors and cell-to-cell contact. Transition from a growing state to a resting state occurs upon depletion or removal of the serum and upon cell confluence. The data from different laboratories agree on the fact that intracellular cyclic AMP concentrations increase in serum-restricted cultures (9-11, 13). In contrast, the mediation by cyclic AMP of density-dependent inhibition of growth remains controversial, since some (11), but not other investigators (12, 13, 24) observe a rise in cyclic AMP as cells approach confluence.

Mouse fibroblasts transformed by simian virus 40 (SV373 cells) are characterized by cyclic AMP and cyclic GMP levels, respectively, about half (11-13) and twice (24) those found in growing untransformed 3T3 cells (Table 1).

Table 1. Cyclic nucleotide concentrations in growing [*] and serum-restricted [**] fibroblast cultures

Cell line	Serum concentration	Cyclic nucleotide concentrations (pmoles/mg protein)[**]	
		cAMP	cGMP
3T3	10 %	23	0.44
3T3	0.5 %	49	0.06
SV - 3T3	10 %	10	0.82
SV - 3T3	0.5 %	20	0.32

[*] *All assays were performed on sparse cultures (about 1.5 x 10^6 cells per 75 cm^2 plate, at time of harvesting) growing in medium supplemented with 10 % serum or after 1 day of serum-restriction in medium + 0.5 % serum.*

[**] *Levels measured in separate experiments did not usually deviate from the reported mean values by more than ±3 pmoles/mg protein and ± 0.05 pmoles/mg protein for cAMP and cGMP respectively. The procedure for purification and assays of cyclic nucleotides are described in reference 24.*

The levels of cyclic GMP are greatly reduced in sparse cultures of normal but not in SV 40-transformed 3T3 cells cultured in medium with reduced serum concentration (24) (Table 1). The cellular concentrations of cyclic GMP have also been found to be much greater during log phase growth than at confluency in cultured chick embryo fibroblasts (3); however, since these experiments were performed without change of medium over a 5-day period, the data are only indicative of decreased cyclic GMP concentrations in quiescent cultures. We have followed cyclic GMP levels with regular changes of medium in the mouse fibroblast lines 3T3, SV 40-transformed 3T3 and density-restricted revertant lines derived from SV 40-3T3 by Vogel *et al*. (30, 31). The cellular cyclic GMP levels fall gradually as the cell density increases in the density-dependent cell lines (Figure 5). On the contrary, in SV 40-transformed 3T3 fibroblasts the levels remain constant over the same range of cell population until the transformed cells reach their saturation density, at which point the cyclic GMP concentrations start suddenly to decrease (24) (Figure 6).

Proliferation of resting fibroblasts in culture can be induced by a variety of mitogenic agents including serum, insulin and pro-teases. Exposure to these agents is followed by a rapid drop (2 to 3 fold) of the intracellular concentration of cAMP (11-16), whereas cyclic GMP rises by a factor of approximately tenfold within a few minutes after serum addition to quiescent cultures (23, 24) (Figure 7). Recent experiments with a new polypeptide hormone, fibroblast growth factor (FGF) isolated from bovine piputary glands, lend support to Goldberg's hypothesis that cell proliferation is initiated by an active signal, i.e. increased cyclic GMP concentra-tions, rather than by a passive one, represented by decreased cyclic AMP levels. FGF, in combination with hydrocortisone and a non-specific carrier protein such as bovine serum albumin, can complete-ly replace animal serum and produces in 3T3 fibroblasts the same transient increase in cellular cyclic GMP with little or no altera-tions in cyclic AMP levels (32). Furthermore, Rudland *et al*. have demonstrated a direct stimulation by FGF of plasma-membrane bound guanyl, but not adenyl cyclase (32). Increases in cyclic GMP, similar to those produced by serum, have also been reported by Goldberg and co-workers (3) to occur after insulin treatment of confluent monolayers of 3T3 cells. With high, non-physiological concentrations of insulin (10^{-7}M to 10^{-6}M), Rudland *et al*. obtained increases in DNA synthesis and in cyclic GMP which were only 40 % of those observed with FGF. Although the concentration dependence for the cyclic GMP response and for the stimulation of DNA synthesis are roughly parallel, the decrease in cyclic AMP occurs at much lower insulin concentrations, in the physiological range (10^{-10}M to 10^{-9}M). Whereas hydrocortisone alone in the absence of serum fails to initiate DNA synthesis, the glucocorticoid hormone exerts its permissive effect on the growth response and the changes in both

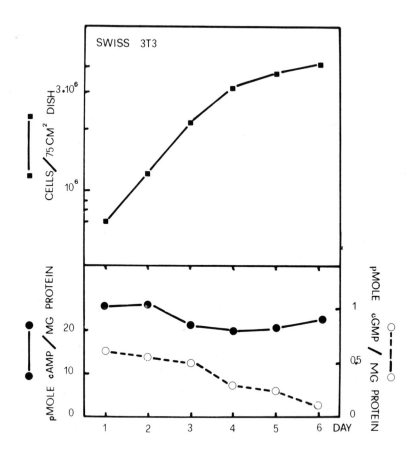

Figure 5. *Response of cyclic nucleotide levels to
density-dependent inhibition of growth in 3T3 fibroblasts. Cultures were grown to confluence, in 10 %
serum, with replacements of fresh medium every other
day to prevent changes in cyclic nucleotide concentrations due to serum depletion. From W. Moens
et al., Proc. natl. Acad. Sci. USA 72, 1063 (1975)*

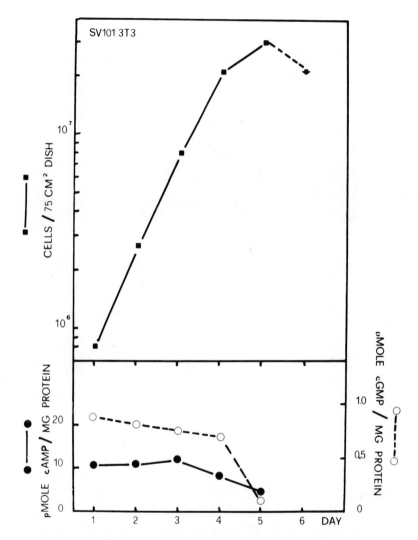

Figure 6. Response of cyclic nucleotide levels to cell density restriction in SV3T3 fibroblasts. Growth conditions were as described under Figure 5. From W. Moens et al., Proc. natl. Acad. Sci. USA 72, 1063 (1975)

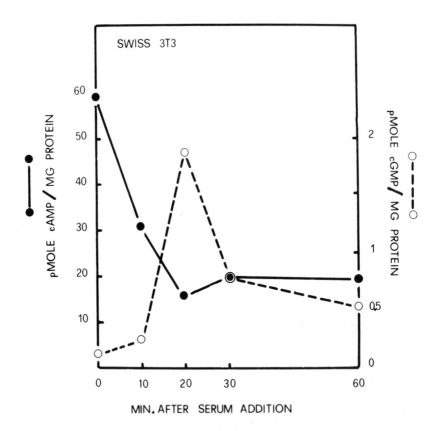

Figure 7.   *Kinetics of cyclic nucleotide responses to serum readdition to 3T3 fibroblasts. Sparse cultures (1.5 x 10⁶ cells per 75 cm² plate) had been maintained for 24 hours in 0.5 % serum before shifting up (at zero time) serum concentration to 20 %.   From W. Moens et al., Proc. natl. Acad. Sci. USA 72, 1063 (1975)*

cyclic nucleotide levels produced by FGF and insulin. These results might explain an earlier observation that physiological levels of glucocorticoids can initiate DNA synthesis and division in density-inhibited 3T3 and early-passage human diploid fibroblasts (33).

Finally, another observation relating increased cyclic GMP concentrations with proliferation in fibroblasts arises from studies with phorbol myristate acetate (PMA), a tumor promoter isolated from croton oil. PMA produces an increase in confluent density of a wide variety of cell types including 3T3 fibroblasts (34). Unlike the former mitogenic agents that increase cyclic GMP concentration in fibroblasts, PMA produces an increase in cyclic GMP that is maximal (tenfold) within the first minute and returns to control levels by 3 minutes (35).

Lymphocytes

The lymphocyte is normally a quiescent cell, but it can be activated upon exposure to antigen. Certain plant lectins, such as phytohemagglutinin (PHA) and concanavalin A (Con A) are also potent mitogens which, unlike antigens, stimulate a large population of predominantly thymus-derived lymphocytes. Early in this process, there occurs an activation of diverse transport systems and of macromolecular synthesis which mimics the activation of the pleiotypic programme in quiescent fibroblasts upon exposure to mitogenic agents (4).

Smith *et al.* (36) have reported that PHA produces early (within 1 to 2 minutes) increases (25 - 300 %) in cyclic AMP levels. However, the question arises as to whether cyclic AMP's role in lymphocyte stimulation is inhibitory or stimulatory since exogenous cyclic AMP or pharmacological agents, that stimulate its generation, inhibit mitogen-induced proliferation (37). This discrepancy is probably accounted for by the observation that the elevation of cyclic AMP is associated with the agglutinating activity and does not occur when a purified preparation of PHA, with minimal agglutinating activity is used (1). The evaluation of the role of cyclic AMP in lymphocyte proliferation is furthermore complicated by various results obtained by Whitfield, Mac Manus and co-workers. They have shown that epinephrine and prostaglandins A_1 and E_1 stimulate thymic lymphocyte adenylate cyclase with resultant increases in the intracellular level of cyclic AMP and the rate of cell proliferation (38, 39). Physiological levels (10^{-8} to 10^{-6}M) of cyclic AMP also promote DNA synthesis and mitotic activity in suspension cultures of rat thymocytes whereas higher concentrations of cyclic AMP inhibit cell growth (40). However these results were obtained with a tissue culture medium containing low concentrations of calcium (0.6 m M), since higher calcium concentrations would themselves maximally stimulate mitotic activity. The same investigators have subsequently found that exogenous cyclic AMP concentrations, which are stimulatory in low-calcium medium, block the stimulation of lymphoblast proliferation (41) in the presence of higher (1.5 m M), but more physiological, calcium concentrations. Therefore, in my opinion, cyclic AMP is more likely an inhibitor of lymphocyte proliferation, especially in view of the fact that cyclic AMP and hormones which raise its intracellular levels slow the growth and ultimately kill mouse lymphoma cells in culture. Biochemical investigations on variant clones, resistant to the killing action of the cyclic nucleotide, have indicated that this effect involves activation of protein kinases (20).

With respect to cyclic GMP, Hadden *et al.* (1) have shown that addition of PHA or Con A to preparations of human lymphocytes results in a dramatic rise in cyclic GMP levels within twenty minutes of lectin addition. Phorbol myristate acetate is also a potent mitogen for lymphocytes. Although in the latter case cyclic GMP was not measured, the rapid and important increases in its levels associated with its mitogenic action on fibroblasts and its stimulation of platelet aggregation suggest that the effect of PMA on lymphocyte proliferation may be mediated by cyclic GMP (35). The addition of dibutyryl cyclic GMP (10^{-4} to 10^{-3} M) to mouse spleen lymphocytes in serum-free medium also results in a ten-fold increase in the rate of DNA synthesis and it further enhances the stimulation of DNA synthesis and purine biosynthesis produced by Con A. Dibutyryl cyclic AMP inhibits both the effects of Con A and dibutyryl cyclic GMP on both processes (42). These studies have also demonstrated an activation by cyclic GMP of the phosphoribosyl pyrophosphate synthetase activity, an enzyme central to purine and pyrimidine biosynthesis, which is induced upon stimulation of lymphocytes by Con A.

Epithelial cells

Several lines of evidence indicate that tropic hormones (pituitary hormones, steroids such as estrogens) are involved in the control of mammalian cell proliferation *in vivo*. However, practical difficulties inherent in *in vivo* experiments have limited the understanding of hormone-dependent tissue growth. On the other hand, the development of cultured epithelial cells retaining physiological growth responses to hormones has unfortunately proved to be very difficult. Sata and co-workers have recently established in culture a line of ovarian cells responsive to gonadotropin and glucocorticoids (43) and a line of mammary cells responsive to glucocorticoids (44). In the mammary cells, the intracellular levels of cyclic AMP are 2 to 10 times higher in the absence of hydrocortisone than in the presence of physiological concentrations of the hormone.

Hydrocortisone, however, has no effect on cyclic GMP levels whereas it markedly enhances the increase in cyclic GMP generated in resting fibroblasts by a pituitary fibroblastic growth factor (44, 32). Since these mammary cells are not "quiescent" but continue to grow, *albeit* slowly, in the absence of the hormone, these results suggest that cyclic GMP might be involved in the transition from a "resting" to a "proliferative" cellular state. Unfortunately, the cyclic nucleotide levels have not yet been measured in the ovarian cell line which has an absolute requirement for an ovarian growth factor (OGF), which contaminates some impure preparations of LH and TSH. This OGF is a protein, which has recently been purified from bovine pituitary glands (45). It is different from LH and FSH, which do not trigger the growth of this ovarian cell line when highly purified preparations of the gonadotropins are used.

Further investigations along this line might help to solve the contradiction between the fact that all pituitary tropic hormones increase cyclic AMP levels in their target tissues and the fact that cyclic AMP has inhibitory effects on the growth of other cells. These tissues might represent monodirectional systems (25). Alternatively, the possibility that an increase in the level of cyclic AMP might not mediate the growth-promoting action of these tropic hormones is suggested by an observation of Masui and Garren on functional adrenal tumor cells in culture. ACTH and cyclic AMP, which stimulate steroidogenesis in this system, do, on the contrary, inhibit cell proliferation (46).

Another paradoxical observation, from this point of view, was provided by the stimulatory effect of isoproterenol on DNA synthesis in the parotid gland of rodents (47). Recent investigations, with a number of catecholamine analogues, have in fact demonstrated a clear lack of correlation between effects on cyclic AMP levels and adenylate cyclase activity and the stimulation of DNA synthesis (48). Thus, an increase in cyclic AMP is not involved in this mitogenic response. Obviously, it will be interesting to learn the results of investigations which are in progress to test the correlation with respect to cyclic GMP levels.

Recent data indicate that cyclic GMP might be involved in the response of the uterine tissue to estrogens. When ovariectomized rats are treated with estradiol or diethylstilbestrol, cyclic GMP levels in the endometrium increase while cyclic AMP concentrations drop. The cyclic nucleotide levels were also monitored in the uterus at each stage of the estrous cycle of the rat : cyclic GMP concentrations were found to be highest and cyclic AMP concentrations lowest during proestrus when plasma estrogen levels are at a peak. Clomiphene, an antiestrongenic compound, blocks the estrogen-induced accumulation of cyclic GMP (49).

Finally, unbalanced levels of cyclic AMP and cyclic GMP have been found in a proliferative skin disease. The epidermis of psoriasis is characterized by excessive cell proliferation, reduced differentiation and glycogen accumulation. When uninvolved and involved epidermis of the same patient are compared, cyclic AMP is decreased and cyclic GMP increased in the epidermis of the psoriasis lesion. In addition, the epidermal mitogens tetradecanoyl-phorbol acetate and histamine produce rapid elevation of cyclic GMP in epidermal slices (50).

Bacterial Growth

Goldberg and co-workers have also found a relationship between cyclic GMP and bacterial growth (51). In the two strains which they investigated, cyclic GMP levels are highest during exponential growth in glucose-containing media and fall to about 10 % to 20 % of the initial level when the cultures approach the stationary phase of growth. Significantly lower concentrations of cyclic GMP are also found when glucose is replaced by glutamate or succinate which support a slower rate of growth. In one strain (E. coli), the cyclic AMP concentrations vary in a direction opposite to those of cyclic GMP. Cyclic AMP was not detected in the other strain (B. licheniformis).

The role of calcium in cell proliferation

Evidence has been accumulating recently that calcium plays an important role in regulating cell proliferation. Calcium has a profound influence on the proliferation of rat thymocytes (41) and is required for the initiation of cell cycling in normally resting lymphocytes stimulated by phytohemagglutinin (52), phorbol myri-state acetate (53) and allogeneic lymphocytes (54). PHA signifi-cantly stimulates calcium uptake within minutes after treatment (3, 55). Calcium is also involved in controlling the proliferation of normal but not virally-transformed fibroblasts (56).

Thus cell proliferation like each of the cellular processes that have been shown to be linked to an accumulation of cellular cyclic GMP (3) appears to have a dependence on calcium. This concept is consistent with recently demonstrated biochemical effects of calcium on cyclic nucleotide metabolism. On one hand, calcium inhibits the activation of adenylate cyclase by epinehrine and glucagon (57), and on the other hand, calcium is required for acetylcholine-promoted accumulation of cyclic GMP (58). However, a role for calcium, independent of these mechanisms, is also possible.

CONCLUSION

In a number of cell types, the induction of cell proliferation by different specific stimuli is associated with early increases in cyclic GMP and/or decreases in cyclic AMP. These findings suggest that cyclic AMP and cyclic GMP may serve as intracellular signals, respectively negative and positive, which mediate the response to external growth-regulating influences. This hypothesis originates mainly from studies on fibroblastic and lymphoid cells. Its validity in the case of epithelial cells can be questioned in view of the fact that, *in vivo*, some tropic hormones raise intracellular cyclic AMP in their target tissues. However, it can be argued against this objection on the basis of (a) cellular heterogeneity in these organs, (b) the recent isolation from pituitary glands of new growth factors : a fibroblastic growth factor which elevates cyclic GMP and an ovarian growth factor that is distinct from LH and FSH, (c) studies with catecholamine analogues, which indicate a clear lack of correlation between increased cyclic AMP and the induction of DNA synthesis by isoproterenol in the parotid gland of rodents.

Whether the changes in the intracellular concentrations of cyclic nucleotides following exposure to mitogenic substances represent the or one among other initiating events, or whether they represent a secondary facet of the complex growth response is the important issue for further investigations. Exogenous additions of the cyclic nucleotides have already been shown to be effective in some systems, although high, non-physiological concentrations are usually required. This suggests that other factors may be needed for full expression of the response to the mitogenic signal. Calcium could be one of these important partners. Some observations lend support to a further speculation that increased cyclic GMP concentration is involved in the transition from a resting to a proliferative state, whereas cyclic AMP modulates the rate of cell growth. It will be important in this regard to establish the steps which are controlled by the cyclic nucleotides during progression in the cell cycle.

REFERENCES

(1)   HADDEN, J.W., HADDEN, E.M., HADDOX, M.K. and GOLDBERG, N.S. (1972) Proc. Nat. Acad. Sci. USA, 69, 3024

(2)   KRAM, R. and TOMKINS, G.M. (1973) Proc. Nat. Acad. Sci. USA, 70, 1659

(3)   GOLDBERG, N.D., HADDOX, M.K., DUNHAM, E., LOPEZ, C. and HADDEN, J.W. (1974) in "Cold Spring Harbor Symposium on Regulation of Cell Proliferation in Animal Cells (BASERGA, R. and CLARKSON, B. eds) 609, Academic Press, New York

(4) HERSHKO, A., MAMONT, P., SHIELDS, R. and TOMKINS, G.M. (1971)
Nature New Biol. 232, 206

(5) CUNNINGHAM, D.D. and PARDEE, A.B. (1969) Proc. Nat. Acad. Sci.
US, 64, 1049

(6) RUDLAND, P.S. (1974). Proc. Nat. Acad. Sci. USA, 71, 750

(7) HOLLEY, R.W. and KIERNAN, J.A. (1968). Proc. Nat. Acad. Sci.
USA, 60, 300

(8) DULBECCO, R. (1970) Nature 227, 800

(9) KRAM, R., MAMONT, P. and TOMKINS, G.M. (1973) Proc. Nat. Acad.
Sci. USA, 70, 1432

(10) SEIFFERT, W. and PAUL, D. (1972). Nature New Biol. 240, 281

(11) OTTEN, J., JOHNSON, G.S. and PASTAN, I. (1972). J. Biol. Chem.
247, 7082

(12) SHEPPARD, J. (1972) Nature New Biol. 236, 14

(13) OEY, J., VOGEL, A. and POLLACK, R. (1974). Proc. Nat. Acad.
Sci, USA, 71, 694

(14) BURGER, M., BOMBIK, B., BRECKENRIDGE, B. and SHEPPARD, J.
(1972), Nature 239, 161

(15) DE ASUA, L.J., SURIAN, E.S., FLAVIA, M.M. and TORRES, H.N.
(1973). Proc. Nat. Acad. Sci. USA, 70, 1388

(16) TELL, G., CUATRECASAS, P., VAN WYK and HINTZ, R. (1973).
Science 180, 312

(17) FROEHLICH, J. and RACHMELER, M. (1972). J. Cell Biol. 55, 31

(18) FRANK, W. (1972). Expl. Cell. Res. 71, 238

(19) PASTAN, I., ANDERSON, W.B., CARCHMAN, R.A., WILLINGHAM, M.C.,
RUSSEL, T.R. and JOHNSON, G.S. (1974) in "Cold Spring Harbor
Symposium on Regulation of Cell Proliferation in Animal Cells"
(Baserga, R. and Clarkson, B. eds) 563, Academi Press, New
York

(20) DANIEL, V., LITWACK, G. and TOMKINS, G.M. (1973) Proc. Nat.
Acad. Sci. USA, 70, 76

(21) SUTHERLAND, E.W. (1972). Science 177, 401

(22) KRAM, R. and TOMKINS, G.M. (1973). Proc. Nat. Acad. Sci. USA
      70, 1659

(23) SEIFFERT, W.E. and RUDLAND, P.S. (1974). Nature 248, 138

(24) MOENS, W., VOKAER, A. and KRAM, R. Proc. Nat. Acad. Sci. USA
      72, 1063 (1975)

(25) GOLDBERG, N.D., O'DEA, R.F. and HADDOX, M.K. (1973). Cyclic
      GMP in "Recent Advances in Cyclic Nucleotide Research"
      (Greengard, P. and Robison A.G. eds.) Vol. 3, 155, Raven Press,
      New York

(26) GOLDBERG, N.D. (1974). Hospital Practice, 9, 127

(27) PASTAN, I., HERRING, B., JOHNSON, P. and FIELD, J.B. (1961)
      J. Biol. Chem. 236, 340

(28) ALTMAN, M., OKA, H. and FIELD, J.B. (1966). Biochim. Biophys.
      Acta 116, 586

(29) BURR, I.M., TAFT, H.P., STAUFFACHER, W. and RENOLD, A.E.
      (1971). Ann. N.Y. Acad. Sci. 185, 245

(30) VOGEL, A., RESSER, R. and POLLACK, R. (1973) J. Cell Physiol.
      82, 181

(31) VOGEL, A. and POLLACK, R. (1973) J. Cell Physiol. 82, 189

(32) RUDLAND, P.S., GOSPODAROWICZ, D. and SEIFERT, W. (1974)
      Nature 250, 741

(33) THRASH, C.R. and CUNNINGHAM, D.D. Nature, 242, 399

(34) SIVAK, A. (1972) J. Cell Physiol. 80, 167

(35) ESTENSEN, R.D., HADDEN, J.W., HADDEN, E.M., TOURAINE, F.,
      TOURAINE, J.L., HADDOX, M.K. and GOLDBERG, N.V. (1974) in
      "Gold Spring Harbor Symposium on Control of Proliferation in
      Animal Cells" (Baserga, R. and Clarkson, B. eds.), 627,
      Academic Press, New York

(36) SMITH, J.W., STEINER, A.L., NEWBERRY, W.M. and PARKER, C.W.
      (1971). J. Clin. Invest. 50, 432

(37) SMITH, J.W., STEINER, A.L. and PARKER, C.W. (1971) J. Clin.
      Invest. 50, 442

(38) MacMANUS, J.P., WHITFIELD, J.F. and YOUDALE, T. (1971).
      J. Cell Physiol 77, 103

(39) FRANKS, D.J., MacMANUS, J.P. and WHITFIELD, J.F. (1971)
      Biochem. Biophys. Res. Commun. 44, 1177

(40) MacMANUS, J.P., and WHITFIELD, J.F. (1969) Exptl. Cell Res.
      58, 188

(41) WHITFIELD, J.F., MacMANUS, J.P. and GILLAN, D.J. (1973) J.
      Cell Physiol. 81, 241

(42) CHAMBERS, D.A. and MARTIN, D.W. and WEINSTEIN, I., Cell, 3,
      375 (1974)

(43) CLARK, J.L., HONES, K.L., GOSPODAROWICZ, D. and SATO, G.H.
      (1972) Nature New Biol. 236, 180

(44) ARMELIN, H.A., NISHIKAWA, K. and SATO, G.H. (1974) in
      "Cold Spring Harbor Symposium on Control of Proliferation
      in Animal Cells" (Baserga, R. and Clarkson, B eds.), 97,
      Academic Press, New York

(45) GOSPODAROWICZ, D., JONES, K.L. and SATO, G.H. (1974) Proc.
      Nat. Acad. Sci. US, 71, 2295

(46) MASUI, H. and GARREN, L.D. (1971) Proc. Nat. Acad. Sci. US,
      68, 3206

(47) BARKA, T (1965) Exptl. Cell Res. 39, 355

(48) DURHAM, J.P., BASERGA, R. and BUTCHER, F.R. (1974) in "Cold
      Spring Harbor Symposium on Control of Proliferation in
      Animal Cells", 595, Academic Press, New York

(49) KUEHL, F.A., HAM, E.A., ZANETTI, M.E., SANFORD, C.H.,
      NICOL, S.E. and GOLDBERG, N.D. (1974) Proc. Nat. Acad. Sci.
      US, 71, 1866

(50) VOORHEES, J.J., COLBURN, N.H., STAWISKI, M., DUELL, E.A.,
      HADDOX, M. and GOLDBERG, N.D. (1974) in "Cold Spring
      Harbour on Control of Proliferation in Animal Cells"
      (Baserga, R. and Clarkson, B. eds). 635, Acadmic Press,
      New York

(51) BERNLOHR, R.W., HADDOX, M.K. and GOLDBERG, N.D. (1974) J.
      Biol. Chem. 249, 4329

(52) WHITNEY, R.B. and SUTHERLAND, R.M. (1972), J. Cell Physiol.
      80, 329

(53) WHITFIELD, J.F., MacMANUS, J.P. and GILLAN, D.J. (1973).
J. Cell. Physiol. 82, 151

(54) WHITNEY, R.B. and SUTHERLAND, R.M. (1972). J. Immunol. 108,
1179

(55) WHITNEY, R.B. and SUTHERLAND, R.M. (1973). J. Cell Physiol.
82, 9

(56) BALK, S.D. (1971) Proc. Nat. Acad. Sci. US, 68, 271

(57) BIRNBAUMER, L., POHL, S.L. and RODBELL, M. (1969). J. Biol.
Chem. 244, 3468

(58) SCHULTZ, G., HARDMAN, J.G., SCHULTZ, K., BAIRD, C.E. and
SUTHERLAND, E.W. (1973) Proc. Nat. Acad. Sci. US 70, 3889

CYCLIC AMP AND MYOBLAST DIFFERENTIATION

Rosalind J. Zalin

School of Biological Sciences
University of Sussex, Falmer
Brighton, Sussex, England

INTRODUCTION

Cell differentiation in the embryo occurs in at least two distinct stages. The first involves a gradual loss in omnipotence of the cells which become 'covertly' committed to a particular developmental path. The second is an expression of this newly acquired commitment, a process involving changes in cell morphology and the appearance of specialised cell products characteristic of the particular cell type. Examination of this second stage in differentiation of cells cultured in vitro has revealed that the extent of expression of the differentiated state depends upon a number of external factors. Manipulation of culture conditions for example can often push cells toward differentiation or to continual proliferation (1) and if initially kept under culture conditions which promote proliferation, cells can often still be made to differentiate when placed in more appropriate culture conditions (2,3). Thus it seems that cells can retain the 'knowledge' of their commitment to a particular cell type, the expression of the differentiated state involving a complex interaction between the undifferentiated but committed cells and their environment. It is the nature of this interaction in primary cultures of differentiating chick skeletal muscle cells which is the general concern of the work presented here.

Myoblasts, if cultured under conditions which promote differentiation, cease proliferation and begin a phase of cell fusion which eventually gives rise to the large multinucleate fibres characteristic of the mature muscle tissue. At the same time the contractile proteins and enzymes specific to muscle function begin

795

to accumulate.   Muscle differentiation is thus a process which is accompanied by an abrupt cessation of DNA synthesis and change in growth pattern.   Both these events are very sensitive to culture conditions.   Medium composition and, in particular, the serum and embryo extract used, affect both the time of onset and the extent of differentiation (3).   In addition it has been shown that the culture medium changes whilst in contact with the myoblasts in such a way as to promote expression of the differentiated state (4,5).

Interest in the possible involvement of cyclic AMP in muscle differentiation was initially aroused by reports in the literature that cyclic AMP was able to regulate cell growth in normal and transformed fibroblasts (6) and induce differentiated function in neuroblastomas (7).Evidence has since accumulated, derived largely from work with normal and transformed cells in culture, of a funda- mental regulatory role of cyclic AMP in both the growth and diffe- rentiation of eukaryotic cells.   An inverse correlation has been found to exist between the intracellular level of cyclic AMP in a cell line and its growth rate (8) and of particular interest in relation to differentiation, are indications that cyclic AMP is in- volved in the expression and maintenance of several differentiated functions of cultured cells.   Dibutyryl cyclic AMP stimulates axon formation in neuroblastoma cells (9), collagen synthesis in chinese hamster ovary cells (10) and the synthesis and secretion of sulphated acid polysaccharides in transformed fibroblasts (11).

The following sections describe a series of experiments in which the relationship of cyclic AMP levels to myoblast differen- tiation has been investigated.   The results are discussed in relation to the role that the intracellular cyclic AMP levels of the myoblasts may play in the control of expression of the cell's differentiated state.

RESULTS AND DISCUSSION

Our initial finding in relation to cyclic AMP and muscle dif- ferentiation was that when either 0.1 mM dibutyryl cyclic AMP or 1 mM 3-isobutyl-1-methylxanthine (a specific inhibitor of phospho- diesterase) were added to myoblast cultures 24 hours after plating, there was a marked delay in the onset of cell fusion (12).   Under the experimental conditions adopted, in which the cells were pla- ted out at a density of 2×10^6 in 85 mm plates (12), fusion nor- mally began at approximately 44 hours of culture (Fig. 1).   Di- butyryl cyclic AMP prevented any equivalent increase in multi- nucleate cells until 52 hours and the theophylline derivative on its own or in addition to dibutyryl cyclic AMP delayed fusion until approximately 60 hours of culture.   In each case the effect of the reagent was temporary and once fusion began it proceeded at

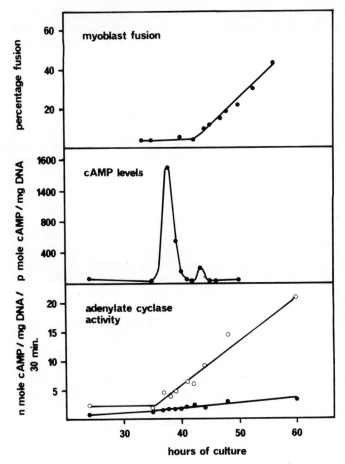

<u>Fig. 1</u>

Time course of fusion, intracellular cyclic AMP, and adenylate cyclase activity in primary cultures of chick myoblasts.

Abscissa: hours of culture; ordinate: myoblast fusion expressed
as the percentage of total cell nuclei in myotubes; intracellular
cyclic AMP levels expressed as the pmoles of cyclic AMP/mg of
cell DNA; adenylate cyclase activity expressed as the nmoles
of cyclic AMP formed/mg of cell DNA/in 30 min; basal enzyme
activity (● - ●), enzyme activity in the presence of 10^{-4}M NaF
(o - o).

a rate comparable to that found under control conditions, yielding
similar final percentages of cells fused. The absence of any
effect of 5' - AMP upon the cells and the marked delay in fusion
obtained after the addition of the theophylline derivative suggest

that it is an increase in intracellular cyclic AMP which is causing the delay in onset of myoblast fusion.   In addition, the marked effect of 3-isobutyl-1-methylxanthine implies the presence of an active adenylate cyclase and phosphodiesterase in the differentiating myoblasts.

An inhibition of fusion was also obtained by Wahrmann, Luzzati & Winand (13) after the addition of either dibutyryl cyclic AMP or theophylline to a rat myoblast cell line.   In their study, however, the inhibition was a permanent one, an anomaly, which is difficult to explain unless it reflects a difference in response of the two types of muscle cells used.   Both sets of findings suggest that an increase in cyclic AMP inhibits myoblast fusion, one of the main parameters of muscle differentiation.   This result appears to conflict with a number of other reports, in which the addition of dibutyryl cyclic AMP promoted the expression and maintenance of differentiated function of cultured cells (10,11). In both the present study and that of Wahrmann et al. (13), the reagents were added during the phase of myoblast proliferation in the cultures and well before the start of fusion.   Thus it is not possible to distinguish between an effect of cyclic AMP upon some critical cellular event prior to the onset of fusion (for example a reduction in the rate of growth of the cells) or a direct effect upon fusion itself.   Two further observations suggest that a direct effect upon the fusion process is the more likely explanation.   First, a delay in myoblast fusion was also obtained when either 0.1 mM dibutyryl cyclic AMP or 1.0 mM 3-isobutyryl-1-methyl xanthine were added at 44 hours of culture, to coincide with the onset of cell fusion in the cultures (unpublished findings). Under these conditions an inhibition of fusion was observed within as little as one hour.   Secondly, when added at 24 hours of culture, dibutyryl cyclic AMP had no observable effect upon the growth rate of the cells during the proliferation phase of culture (12).

Creatine phosphokinase was chosen as the second parameter of muscle differentiation because of its special function in adult muscle and the marked increase in its activity which occurs during muscle differentiation (4,14).   Enzyme activity was examined from 24 hours after plating, when the dibutyryl cyclic or theophylline derivative were added, until the end of the rapid phase of cell fusion in the cultures.   In contrast to their effects upon myoblast fusion neither reagent had any observable effect upon the time course of appearance of creatine phosphokinase activity. The lack of any inhibition in expression of this second parameter of muscle differentiation again suggests that the elevated cyclic AMP level is not inhibiting differentiation per se but having a specific effect upon the process of cell fusion.

To obtain further information of the effects of cyclic AMP

levels upon the differentiating cells, the intracellular cyclic
AMP levels of the myoblasts were measured.   In particular, we
wished to examine the possibility that the observed effects of
dibutyryl cyclic AMP and the theophylline derivative are due to
perturbations in the levels of cyclic AMP normally existing in
the differentiating cells.   Cyclic AMP was measured in samples
of cells obtained from between the 2nd and 50th hours of culture.
Samples of cell homogenates were acidified and purified by elution
from Dowex - 50 columns, before analysis of cyclic AMP content by
the saturation method described by Brown, Albano, Ekins & Sgherzi
(15).   Approximately 95% of the cyclic AMP measured using this
procedure was lost after treatment with phosphodiesterase.

     There was very little overall increase of cyclic AMP in the
myoblasts during the time examined which included the prefusion
period of culture and the first phase of the fusion process.   However, there was a transient 10-15 fold increase in intracellular
cyclic AMP (Fig.1), which lasted for less than 1 hour and occurred
at about 38 hours of culture (16).   In all the cultures examined,
the cyclic AMP consistently appeared in the cells 5-6 hours before
the onset of fusion, suggesting a link between the two events.

     In search of some explanation for the rapid generation and
disappearance of the cyclic nucleotide in the differentiating myoblasts, the activities of both adenylate cyclase and phosphodiesterase were examined over the same period of culture.   Phosphodiesterase activity was measured in both the soluble and particulate fractions obtained after centrifugation of cell homogenates
at 17,500 x g.   The enzyme activity in these fractions was then
assessed by the rate of hydrolysis of cyclic-(^{3}H)-AMP to 5'-(^{3}H)-
AMP, after conversion of the latter to (^{3}H)-adenosine by 5'-nucleo-
tidase (17).   Kinetic analysis of the activity present revealed
a pH optimum of between 7.5 and 8.5 and two apparent Km values
for cyclic AMP of approximately 1 M and 10 M respectively (Fig. 2).
The 2 Kms suggest the presence of two enzyme activities, a finding
which is in agreement with a number of similar studies on mammalian tissues (17-19).   The time course of enzyme activity (Fig.3)
revealed very little change in phosphodiesterase activity except
for a small transient increase in the low Km enzyme of the soluble fraction, and suggests it is not a change in phosphodiesterase activity which is responsible for the observed transient
increase of cyclic AMP.

     In contrast, adenylate cyclase activity changed in two pos-
sibly significant respects, over the same period of cell culture
(Fig. 1).   At approximately 35 hours of culture a gradual increase in basal enzyme activity was observed and this had associated with it a more marked increase in the enzyme's sensitivity
to NaF.   The latter changed from a 2-fold effect at 35 hours of

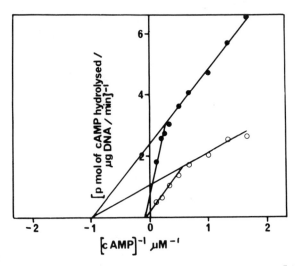

<u>Fig. 2</u>

Effect of substrate concentration on the rate of cyclic AMP hydrolysis by the phosphodiesterase in primary cultures of chick myoblasts; in the soluble fraction (●-●); in the particulate cell
fraction (o-o).

Abscissa: 1[-cyclic AMP-] (μM^{-1});   ordinate: [pmoles of cyclic
AMP hydrolysed/μg of DNA/min]$^{-1}$

culture to a 5 fold one at 60 hours.   In view of the close correlation between the onset of these changes in adenylate cyclase activity and the peak of cyclic AMP in the cells (38 hours), it
seems probable that it is an increase in this enzyme's activity
which is the cause of the elevated cyclic AMP.   There is ample
evidence that external agents and in particular hormones modulate
adenylate cyclase activity (20,21) and examples exist where the
effect is temporary as in the present study (22).   Thus it is
tempting to suggest that the increase in the sensitivity of the
enzyme to NaF reflects a change in adenylate cyclase which, in
turn, is responsible for the peak in cyclic AMP.   A similar
increase in NaF stimulation was found to occur in the adenylate
cyclase of developing rat liver (23) where the increases in adenylate cyclase activity were also correlated with an increase of
cyclic AMP in the liver.   These authors found a 2-fold NaF stimulation of enzyme activity during the early stages of development
which increased to a 6-fold stimulation coincidental with the
appearance of hormone sensitivity in the liver.   Such a finding
raises the possibility of a similar link between the increase in
NaF stimulation of the myoblast adenylate cyclase and the appearance of a sensitivity in the enzyme to a hormone or other external factor.

A possible explanation for the very rapid disappearance of the
high level of the intracellular cyclic AMP is its rapid loss into
the culture medium.   It has been assumed that cyclic AMP, like
other organic phosphates, crosses biological membranes only with
difficulty.   However, it appears that some cells can release
intracellular cyclic AMP (24,25) and evidence now exists of a rapid and extensive loss of cyclic AMP from fibroblasts after hormonal increase of their intracellular cyclic AMP level (26).   To
examine this possibility⌐ in the differentiating myoblasts, samples of medium obtained from cells cultured for between 15 and
44 hours were collected and after the addition of theophylline (to
a final concentration of 1mM) to prevent further cyclic AMP breakdown, were placed in a boiling water bath for 5 min.   The resulting precipitate was then removed and the samples lyophilised to
reduce their volume before preparation for cyclic AMP estimation

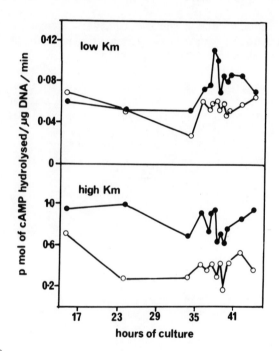

<u>Fig. 3</u>

Time course of phosphodiesterase activity in differentiating myoblasts.   Mean values obtained from 3 experiments;   activity in
the soluble cell fraction (● - ●);   activity in the particulate
cell fraction (o - o).

Abscissa: hours of culture;   ordinate: phosphodiesterase activity expressed as pmoles of cyclic AMP hydrolysed/μg of
DNA/min.)

as described above.   This procedure yielded recoveries of between 55 and 60%.

The cyclic AMP content of the medium remained the same through-out the time analysed, no increase occurring to correspond to the transient peak found inside the cells (Table 1). This finding may reflect the absence of much leakage from the cells or the rapid breakdown of cyclic AMP once it has entered the culture medium.   To examine these two alternatives the rate of turnover of cyclic AMP in the medium was measured.   A trace amount of cyclic-(8-^{3}H)-AMP was added to the myoblast cultures at 34, 38 and 42 hours after plating and samples removed for cyclic-(8-^{3}H)-AMP recovery 0, 15, 30 and 60 min. later.   The preparation procedure for cyclic-(^{3}H)-AMP was the same as that for the estimation of the cyclic AMP con-tent of the medium and the cyclic-(8-^{3}H)-AMP separated from other labelled products by its elution from Dowex-50 columns.

The results demonstrate a rapid turnover of cyclic AMP at the concentrations found in the medium (Fig. 4), with half lives at all three times analysed of approximately 20 min.   Since the con-centration of cyclic AMP in the medium remains constant (Table 1) it follows that cyclic AMP is entering the medium from the cells at a rate equal to its rate of breakdown within the culture medium. Such a high rate of cyclic AMP turnover probably explains its lack

TABLE 1

Time of culture hours	cyclic AMP in cells p/mole/mg DNA[1*]	cyclic AMP in medium p/mole/plate[2*]
24	0	1.1
34	-	2.0
35	67	-
36	-	2.2
37	43	1.2
37.5	-	0.6
38	300	1.3
38.5		1.1
39	1000	1.1
39.5		1.4
40	190	2.0
42	182	1.2
44	156	2.6

[1*] results of a typical experiment

[2*] mean values from 4 experiments

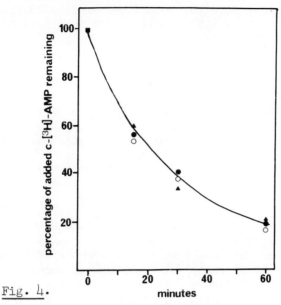

Fig. 4.

Rate of disappearance of cyclic-[^{3}H]-AMP from the culture medium.
Mean values of 4 experiments;   cyclic-[^{3}H]-AMP present at 34
hours (● - ●), 38 hours (o - o) and at 42 hours (▲ - ▲) respectively.

Abscissa: minutes after the addition of cyclic-[^{3}H]-AMP;
ordinate: percentage of added cyclic-[^{3}H]-AMP remaining.

of accumulation, and also suggests that the increased intracellular
cyclic AMP is unlikely to have any function once it has passed into the medium, its primary site of action being inside the cell in
which it is generated.

    What effects the transient increase in cyclic AMP has upon the
cell are as yet not known.   However, it seems unlikely that the
increase is an artifact of in vitro culture conditions, since a
temporary increase in cyclic AMP has also been observed in chick
skeletal muscle tissue during its embryological development (27).
Analyses of muscle tissue taken from chick embryos after different
periods of incubation revealed a temporary increase in muscle cyclic AMP levels at a stage in development which corresponded to
the onset of cell fusion in the tissue.   Stronger evidence of a
link between the cyclic AMP peak in the myoblast cultures and expression of the cell's differentiated state has been obtained in
experiments where the intracellular cyclic nucleotide levels have
been examined under culture conditions in which differentiation is
prevented.   5-Fluorodeoxyuridine has been shown to block DNA syn-

thesis in chick myoblast cultures and as a result to prevent the
onset of differentiation (28). When added to myoblast cultures
24 hours after plating, the reagent not only prevented the onset
of cell fusion but also the transient increase in intracellular
cyclic AMP (unpublished results). Although the author is unaware
of any other examples of such a transient increase in cyclic AMP
correlated with expression of the differentiated state, there are
reports of temporary increases in the cyclic nucleotide during
embryological development (23, 29) which, in the case of the mammary gland were found to be due to specific hormonal changes in
the developing tissue (30). Finally, it is worth noting that
the elevation of cyclic AMP levels in response to hormonal stimulation in many cells and tissues has been found to be transient
(31-33).

Marked fluctuations in cyclic AMP have also been found during
the cell cycle (34) and it has been proposed that lower levels of
cyclic AMP at a specific point in the cell cycle of normal cells
may trigger the cell cycle (35). Conversely increasing the level
of cyclic AMP has been shown to inhibit either the onset of mitosis
or DNA synthesis in human lymphoid cells (36), the specificity of
inhibition being a function of when the increase occurred during
the cell cycle. The relationship between the cell cycle and myo-
genesis has been studied in some detail (37) and it has been suggested that there is a "critical" cycle of DNA synthesis and subsequent mitosis in the myoblasts, which places the cells in a distinct postmitotic state preparatory to fusion (38). In view of
the small time interval between the observed transient increase in
cyclic AMP and the onset of myoblast fusion, the peak of cyclic AMP
must be occurring at some point in the final cell cycle before differentiation. Finally, a link between DNA synthesis and the cyclic AMP peak is suggested by the effects of adding 5-fluorodeoxy-
uridine to the cultures. Since the effect that the reagent has
upon DNA synthesis and cell division is correlated with marked effects upon differentiation and the transient cyclic AMP increase.

In view of the observed changes in adenylate cyclase in the
muscle cultures prior to the appearance of the cyclic AMP peak, it
is tempting to suggest that one of the events during the myoblasts
'critical' cycle of DNA synthesis and cell division is that which
gives rise to an adenylate cyclase which is more sensitive to external factors. This would then give rise to the increase in cyclic AMP which once produced could trigger an event or events inside the myoblasts required for the expression of their differentiated state.

ACKNOWLEDGEMENT

This work was supported by a grant from the Muscular Dystrophy
Group of Great Britain.

REFERENCES

1. Coon, H.C. and Cahn, R.D. (1966) Science, 153, 1116
2. Yaffe, D. (1969) Curr.Top.Devel.Biol. 4, 37
3. Yaffe, D. (1971) Exptl. Cell Res. 66, 33.
4. Hauschka, S.D. (1968) In 'The Stability of the Differentiated State' H.Ursprung, ed. (Berlin: Springer-Verlag), p.37
5. Konigsberg, I.R. (1971) Dev.Biol. 26, 133
6. Johnson, G.S., Friedman, R.M. and Pastan, I. (1971) Proc.Natl. Acad.Sci. USA 63, 425
7. Furmanski, P., Silverman, D.J. and Lubin, M. (1971) Nature 233, 413.
8. Otten, J., Johnson, G.S. and Pastan, I. (1971) Biochem.Bio-phys.Res.Communs. 53, 982
9. Prasad, K.M. and Hsie, A.W. (1971) Nature New Biol. 233, 141
10. Hsie, A.W., Jones, C. and Puck, T.T. (1971) Proc.Natl.Acad. Sci. 68, 1648
11. Goggins, J.F., Johnson, G.S. and Pastan, I. (1972) J.Biol. Chem. 247, 5759
12. Zalin, R.J. (1973) Exptl. Cell Res. 78, 152.
13. Wahrmann, J.P., Luzzati, D. and Winand, R. (1973) Nature New Biol. 245, 112
14. Shainberg, A., Yagil, G. and Yaffe, D. (1971) Dev.Biol. 25, 1
15. Brown, B.E., Albano, J.D., Ekins, R.P. and Sgherzi, A.M. (1971) Biochem.J. 121, 561.
16. Zalin, R.J. and Montague, W. (1974) Cell 2, 103
17. Beavo, J.A., Hardman, J.G. and Sutherland, E.W. (1970) J.Biol. Chem. 245, 5649
18. Brooker, G., Thomas, L.J. and Applaman, M.M. (1968) Biochemi-stry 7, 4177
19. Daniel, V., Bourne, H.R. and Tomkins, G.M. (1973) Nature New Biol. 244, 167
20. Tomasi, V., Réthy, A. and Trevisani, A. (1973) In "The Role of Cyclic Nucleotides in Carcinogenesis". Shultz and Gratzner eds. (Acad. Press) p.127
21. Birnbaumer, L. (1973) Biochim.Biophys.Acta 300, 129
22. Franklin, T.J. and Foster, S.J. (1974) Nature New Biol. 246, 119.
23. Christoffersen, T., Mørland, J., Osnes, J.B. and Øye, I.(1973) Biochim.Biophys.Acta 313, 338
24. Broadus, A.E., Northcutt, R.C., Hardman, J.G., Kaminsky, N.I., Sutherland, E.W. and Liddle, G.W. (1969) Clin.Res. 17, 65
25. Broadus, A.E., Kaminsky, N.I., Northcutt, R.C., Hardman, J.G., Sutherland, E.W. and Liddle, G.W. (1970) J.Clin.Invest. 49, 2237
26. Franklin, T.J. and Foster, S.J. (1974) Nature New Biol. 246, 146
27. Zalin, R.J. and Montague, W. (accepted for publication in Exptl. Cell Res.)
28. Bischoff, R. and Holtzer, H. (1970) J.Cell Biol. 44, 134

29. Novák, E., Drummond, G.I., Skála, J. and Hahn, P. (1972)
    Arch. Biochem. Biophys. 150, 511
30. Sapag-Hagar, M. and Greenbaum, A.L. (1973) Biochem. Biophys.
    Res.Commun. 53, 982
31. Ho, R.J. and Sutherland, E.W. (1971) J.Biol.Chem. 246, 6822
32. Robison, G.A., Butcher, R.W., Oye, I., Morgan, H.W. and
    Sutherland, E.W. (1965) Molec. Pharmac. 1, 168
33. Kuo, J.F. and De Renzo, E.C. (1969) J.Biol.Chem. 244, 2252
34. Abell, C.W. and Monahan, T.M. (1973) J.Cell Biol. 59, 549
35. Burger, M.M., Bombik, B.M., Breckenridge, B.McL. and Sheppard,
    J.R. (1972) Nature New Biol. 239, 161
36. Millis, A.J.T., Forrest, G.A. and Pious, D.A. (1974) Exptl.
    Cell Res. 83, 335
37. Holtzer, H.(1972) In "Cell Differentiation" Harris, Allin
    and Viza, ed. (Munksgaard), p.33
38. Bischoff R. and Holtzer, H. (1969) J.Cell Biol. 41, 188

DISEASES INVOLVING CYCLIC AMP

Georges Van den Berghe [1]

Laboratoire de Chimie Physiologique
International Institute of Cellular and Molecular
 Pathology
Université de Louvain
Avenue Hippocrate, 75
B-1200 Brussels, Belgium

Contents

[1] "Bevoegdverklaard Navorser" of the "National Fonds voor Weten-
schappelijk onderzoek"

INTRODUCTION

In view of the wide variety of physiological functions in which cAMP plays a crucial role, it is not surprising that the metabolism of the cyclic nucleotide is involved in several diseases. In this lecture, the studies of the cAMP system that have been performed in a certain number of endocrinopathies and other disorders will be reviewed. Most of the data presented will concern human pathology but occasional reference will be made to animal experiments that have provided fundamental understanding of the disease process. The eventual role of cAMP in cancer has been covered in detail in other lectures of this series. Since much of the knowledge concerning the pathology of cAMP has been gathered from the analysis of plasma and especially urine, a survey of the data concerning the concentration of the cyclic nucleotide in these body fluids will be given first. The diseases involving the metabolism of cAMP will be classified into those in which a decreased formation of cAMP has been described, and those in which an increased production of the cyclic nucleotide has been reported.

THE CYCLIC NUCLEOTIDES IN PLASMA AND URINE

Basal Values

<u>Plasma</u>. The concentrations of cAMP which have been determined in most extracellular fluids, with the exception of semen, milk, and urine, are in the 10^{-8} M range. This is 10-100 times lower than the concentration of the cyclic nucleotide in most tissues (for a review, see (1). Although in general the measurements of cyclic nucleotides are simpler to perform in extracellular fluids than in tissues, special precautions must be taken when handling blood samples because of the presence of phosphodiesterase activity in plasma, which is probably due to damage to the cellular elements of blood. A convenient method to correct for the potential error caused by the degradation of cyclic nucleotides has been described by Broadus <u>et al</u>. (2). The freshly drawn, heparinized whole blood sample is added to a chilled tube containing a tracer amount of the radioactive cyclic nucleotide and eventually inhibitors of phosphodiesterase : methylxanthines or EDTA. The plasma is immediately separated by centrifuging at 6000-8000 g for 3-6 minutes, and an aliquot is pipetted directly into perchloric acid at the final concentration of 0.3 N. After centrifugation and neutralization, the protein-free perchloric extract can be purified and used for the assay of the cyclic nucleotide or stored frozen for several months. Distribution of the tracer into the cellular elements of

blood is not detectable, so that the level of the cyclic nucleotide
in the plasma can be calculated from the volume of blood withdrawn
and the hematocrit.

The basal level of cAMP in the plasma of normal man is 10-25
nmol/1 and is slightly higher than the level of cGMP (2-16 nmol/1)
(3). The precise origin of plasma cyclic nucleotides in basal
conditions is not known.

Urine. The presence of cAMP in human urine was described by
Butcher and Sutherland (4). cGMP was initially discovered in urine
(5). Both nucleotides constitute the only organic phosphorus compounds that have been identified with certainty in urine (6).
Since a normal adult excretes important quantities of cAMP in
basal condition (Table I), the measurement of the concentration
of the cyclic nucleotide in the urine is easy to perform. When a
sensitive assay is used the sample must be diluted several fold
and purification is not necessary. Urine samples that have been
frozen rapidly after voiding can be used as such. The addition
of 10 ml of glacial acetic acid with 0.75 % thymol has been recom-
mended as a preservative for 24-hour urine collections. Occasional
losses of cAMP have been observed in frozen samples of rat urine
stored for long periods (Hardman et al., cited by Broadus et al.
(1).

The question how best to express the urinary excretion of
cyclic nucleotides deserves discussion. Since the excretion of
cAMP is proportional to the excretion of creatinine (7), the ratio:
nmol of cAMP/mg of creatinine is used most often because it cor-
rects for the variable dilution of the urine. This expression is
very useful in serial urine collections from a single subject,
but involves the assumption of proportionality to both muscle mass
and glomerular filtration rate when comparing different individuals
and is therefore subjected to certain limitations. In young
children, higher values of urinary cAMP expressed as nmol/mg of
creatinine have been reported (8, 9). This finding is explained
by the lower excretion rate of creatinine per kg body weight in
children (10). The increased cAMP/creatinine ratios reported in
patients with hyperthyroidism (11) were shown to reflect a decreased creatinine excretion (12). In azotemic renal disease a
decreased cAMP/creatinine ratio can be calculated, which is due
to a proportionally more important reduction of the excretion of
the cyclic nucleotide (13). The expression of cAMP excretion as
μmoles/24 hours has proven useful for certain diagnostic purposes
that will be discussed later. When the urinary excretion of cAMP
is expressed as μmoles/24 hours/m^2 of body surface area the age-
related pattern is not seen any more (9).

The origin of the cyclic nucleotides in normal human urine has been studied in detail (3, 2, 7). From the finding that the renal clearance of infused cAMP {^{3}H} was almost identical to the clearance of inulin, whereas the clearance of endogenous cAMP exceeded the clearance of inulin with a factor of approximately 1.5, (3) concluded that plasma cAMP is cleared by glomerular filtration and that about 1/3 of the urinary cAMP is added directly to the urine by the kidneys. As the clearance of both exogenous and endogenous cGMP were identical to the clearance of inulin it appeared that virtually all of the cGMP in the urine is derived from plasma by glomerular filtration. The study of the effect of several hormones on the plasma and urinary levels of cAMP (2, 7) has provided further insight into the origin of urinary cyclic nucleotides. This will be discussed in the following section.

Rather narrow limits for the normal urinary excretion of cAMP have been reported by some laboratories, in contrast to the wider range which has been found by other investigators (Table I) and has also been our experience. The values reported for the urinary excretion of cGMP are somewhat lower than those for cAMP and range from 0.4 to 3 μmoles/day (6, 3, 7).

TABLE 1.   Basal Values of cAMP Excretion in Normal Adults

Cyclic AMP		Reference
μmol/24 hours	nmol/mg creatine	
2 - 7		Butcher and Sutherland (4)
4.2 - 6.1		Takahashi et al. (14)
1.1 - 8.6 (*)	3 - 4.5	Chase et al. (16)
1.4 - 3.2		Abdulla and Hamadah (161)
1.8 - 9 (*)	1.5 - 5	Broadus et al. (3)
5.6 ± 0.7		Paul et al. (162)
3.5 ± 0.2		Taylor et al. (13)
3.2 ± 0.2	2.5 ± 0.1	Murad and Pak (17)
6.5 ± 0.3	4.1 ± 0.2	Neelon et al. (34)

(*) extrapolated values

The influence of several factors on the basal values of
urinary cAMP has been studied. It has been claimed that the
excretion of cAMP was decreased by a water load (14). However,
Broadus et al. (1) and Owen and Moffat (15) have been unable to
demonstrate a consistent effect of the degree of hydratation on
the excretion rate of cAMP in man over a 60-fold range of urine
flow. The existence of a circadian rhythm of cyclic nucleotide
excretion is controversial. Chase et al. (16) and Broadus (1)
did not find any diurnal variation in the excretion of cAMP in
small series. However, Murad and Pak (17), Sagel et al. (18)
and Holmes et al. (19) report circadian rhythms. Two patterns
were found : the majority of the subjects showed a maximal
excretion of cAMP in the morning; a minority showed a peak in
the afternoon. Exercise has been shown to increase the 24-hour
excretion of the cyclic nucleotide (20). In women, a distinct
variation of the urinary excretion of cAMP during the menstrual
cycle with a peak associated with ovulation has been reported
(13). This variation was not seen any more in women receiving oral
contraceptives or during pregnancy (21). A progressive rise in
cAMP excretion from 12th - 36th week of gestation followed by a
plateau sustained until delivery has been described (13).

A decreased excretion of the cyclic nucleotide, to half of
the value in normal pregnancy, has been reported in late untreated
toxaemia (22).

Hormonal Influences on the Concentration of Cyclic Nucleotides in Plasma and Urine

The study of the effects of pharmacological doses of hormones
on the concentration of cAMP in plasma and urine has provided
interesting data concerning the origin of the cyclic nucleotide in
these body fluids. Table 2 gives a summary of these effects.
Parathyroid hormone (PTH) provokes up to 50-fold increases of the
urinary excretion of cAMP but only modest rises of the plasma
level of the cyclic nucleotide. Under these conditions the cAMP :
inulin clearance ratio can go up as high as 15, indicating that
almost all of the increase of urinary cAMP is of renal origin
(7). The observation that in anephric subjects PTH provokes little
or no increase of plasma cAMP indicates that apparently all of the
observed PTH-induced cAMP is of renal origin (see also : (23)).
The findings that suppression of endogenous PTH secretion by Ca^{++}
infusion decreases, and that stimulation of the secretion of the
hormone by infusion of the Ca^{++} chelator EDTA increases the cAMP :
inulin clearance ratio indicates that the portion of urinary cAMP
that is added directly by the kidney may be under control of PTH.

Glucagon infusion provokes up to 30-fold increases of the
urinary excretion of cAMP and, in contrast with PTH, parallel rises
of the plasma level of the cyclic nucleotide. The cAMP inulin
clearance ratio is not modified, indicating that the increased
cAMP excretion is entirely a consequence of the increased filtered
load of the nucleotide (2). The fact that the response of cAMP to
the hormone is not affected by parathyroidectomy or by nephrectomy
(7) indicates that neither PTH nor the kidney are involved in the
effect of glucagon. The finding that an infusion of glucagon in
a hepatectomized dog produced no increase in cAMP concentration
in plasma or urine points out to the liver as the major source
of the cAMP released into the circulation in response to glucagon.

TABLE II. Hormonal Influences on the Level of cAMP in Plasma
           and Urine of Normal Man

Hormone	Plasma cAMP (nmol/1)	Urine cAMP (nmol/min)	Clearance ratio cAMP inulin
No	10 - 25	1 - 6	1.2 - 2.1
PTH (2.5-160 mU/kg/min)	up to 80	up to 150	up to 15
+ nephrectomy	no increase	-	
Glucagon (50-200 ng/kg/ min)	up to 800	up to 100	1.2 - 2.1
+ nephrectomy	nl increase	-	
+ parathyroidectomy	nl increase	nl increase	
+ hepatectomy (*)	no increase	no increase	

(*) animal experiment

After Broadus et al. (3, 2) and Kaminsky et al. (7).

Epinephrine causes only modest increases of plasma and urinary levels of cAMP (2). The stimulation of the secretion of insulin by a glucose tolerance test does not cause significant changes of the excretion of the cyclic nucleotide during the hyperinsulinaemic phase, but a slight increase in cAMP excretion has been reported during the hypoglycemic phase (2). The influence of antidiuretic hormone on the urinary excretion of cAMP is very controversial and will be discussed later.

DISORDERS WITH DECREASED FORMATION OF cAMP

Pseudohypoparathyroidism and Related Diseases

The action of parathormone (PTH), the hormone of calcium and phosphorus homeostasis, has been shown to be mediated by cAMP (for a review, see (24)). Pseudohypoparathyroidism is a complex hypocalcaemic genetic disorder which is clinically very similar to idiopathic hypoparathyroidism. Albright et al. (25) made the observation that patients with pseudohypoparathyroidism did not show the characteristic phosphaturic response to parathyroid extract, and proposed that the pathophysiology of this disorder could be attributed to refractoriness of the receptor tissues to the action of PTH. This hypothesis has been confirmed by the demonstration of high concentrations of biologically active (26) and immunologically reactive (27) PTH in pseudohypoparathyroidism.

Chase et al. (16) investigated the effect of PTH on the urinary excretion of cAMP in patients with pseudohypoparathyroidism. They found that the 30-50 fold increase of the excretion of the cyclic nucleotide which is seen in normal subjects after the administration of 300 U of PTH was nearly completely abolished in these patients. In contrast, patients with idiopathic or surgical hypoparathyroidism and pseudopseudohypoparathyroidism (a syndome with physical and roentgenographic findings similar to pseudohypoparathyroidism but normal calcaemia) responded in the normal range. This finding very strongly suggested that the refractoriness to the hormone in patients with pseudohypoparathyroidism was due to a defect of the PTH-responsive adenylate cyclase of the renal cortex, resulting in a deficient formation of cAMP. The observation by Bell et al. (28) that patients with pseudohypoparathyroidism showed a phosphaturic response to dibutyryl cAMP was a further support of this hypothesis. However, post-mortem assay of adenylate cyclase in the renal cortex of a single patient with pseudohypoparathyroidism showed a normal response to PTH (29).

This result indicates that the hormone receptor and the catalytic unit of the enzyme are present in pseudohypoparathyroidism.
A possible explanation proposed by these authors may be that an
abnormal hormone receptor is inaccessible to PTH in vivo, but that
disruption of the cell structures, due to freezing of the tissue
prior to the assay, may have given access to the hormone in vitro.
Although the exact mechanism of the refractoriness to PTH in
pseudohypoparathyroidism remains unsettled and deserves further
investigation, the measurement of the urinary excretion of cAMP
after the administration of the hormone has proven a very valuable
diagnostic test. The phosphaturic response to PTH is indeed often
difficult to evaluate due to wide daily variations in basal phosphate excretion and the relatively slight effect in normal subjects.
In a number of syndromes, considered refractory to PTH on the basis
of the phosphaturic response, a normal increase of the urinary
excretion of cAMP after the administration of the hormone has been
found (30). A child with increased basal excretion of cAMP,
elevated serum concentration of PTH and a marked rise in urinary
cAMP but no increase of urinary phosphate nor serum calcium in
response to the administration of PTH has been described (31).
This disorder has been attributed to a deficient action of cAMP
and named pseudohypoparathyroidism type II.

The observation that about 1/3 of the cAMP excreted in the
urine in control conditions is added directly by the kidney,and
may be under control of PTH (see previous section) has led to the
study of the basal excretion of the cyclic nucleotide in hyperparathyroidism have been reported to excrete more cAMP than normal
subjects (32, 7, 13). The increase was shown to be more marked in
hypercalcaemic patients than in normocalcaemic hyperparathyroidism,
and when normalized for the amount of creatinine (17). Considerable
overlap with normal values has, however, been observed (33) and has
led Neelon et al. (34) to develop a discriminant function to
segregate normal values from pathological ones. A decreased
excretion of cAMP has been reported in patients with hypoparathyroidism (16, 32, 13, 17). Chase et al. (16) have reported that
the values of urinary cAMP were lower only when expressed in μmoles/
24 hours, but Murad and Pak (17) have observed that the lower excretion also appears when expressed on a creatine basis. The usefulness of the determination of the basal excretion of cAMP to
evaluate subtle degrees of parathyroid gland dysfunction is thus
not yet established.

Nephrogenic Diabetes Insipidus

There is ample evidence from in vitro experiments that the
effect of vasopressin or antidiuretic hormone (ADH) on the permeability of a number of epithelial membranes to water is mediated

by cAMP (35). Vasopressin-resistant or nephrogenic diabetes
insipidus is a hereditary disease characterized by polyuria and
an inability of the kidneys to respond to ADH with a decrease of
urine output and an increase of urine osmolality (36, 37). The
pathogeny of the disease is thus analogous to the one of pseudohypoparathyroidism and the studies of Chase et al. (16) in the
latter disorder have prompted similar investigations in nephrogenic diabetes insipidus. Unfortunately, the effect of ADH on the
urinary excretion of cAMP is very controversial : Takahashi et al.
(14), Pawlson et al. (38) and Taylor et al. (13) have claimed that
vasopressin induces a significant increase of the urinary excretion
of the cyclic nucleotide in normal human subjects; numerous other
investigators have, however, not been able to reproduce their
results (16, 7, 39, Van den Berghe and Proesmans, unpublished
results). The reports of Fichman and Brooker (40) and of Bell et
al. (41) that there is a deficient response of urinary cAMP to
ADH in patients with vasopressin-resistant diabetes insipidus, in
comparison with normal subjects, should thus await further confirmation. The study of the effect of cAMP on urine osmolality
has not provided further insight in this problem. An antidiuretic
effect of cAMP has been shown in normal individuals (42) and in
patients with vasopressin responsive diabetes insipidus (41). In
patients with nephrogenic diabetes insipidus, cAMP had no effect
on urine osmolality (41) but dibutyryl cAMP had a paradoxical
diuretic effect (43). The vasopressin-resistant concentrating
defect observed in Bartter's syndrome (44) has been shown to respond with antidiuresis to both cAMP and its dibutyryl derivative
(45).

Bronchial Asthma

     The smooth musculature of the bronchi is under adrenergic
control : stimulation of α-receptors provokes contraction, whereas
stimulation of β-receptors induces relaxation. The normal balance
between the two classes of receptors appears to favour the β-
adrenergic response, relaxation, to circulating epinephrine. For
most types of smooth muscle, there is good evidence that relaxation
in response to stimulation of the β-receptor - which has even been
tentatively identified with adenylate cyclase (46) is mediated by
an increase of the intracellular level of cAMP. The role of cAMP
in bronchial smooth muscle relaxation has been established by Moore
et al. (47), Vulliemoz et al. (48) and Ross and Oppelt (49).
Bronchial asthma is characterized by breathing difficulties caused
by an obstructive process in the bronchial tree, in which, besides
edema and hypersecretion of mucus, smooth muscle spasm plays a predominant role. The asthmatic episode is triggered by a large
variety of factors : allergens, infection, psychic stimuli. The
hypothesis that bronchial asthma might be due to a deficiency of

the cAMP system was proposed by Szentivanyi (50) in his so-called
"β-adrenergic theory of atopic abnormality". The theory postulates
that in bronchial smooth muscle of asthmatic patients, the β-
receptor should have an inherited or acquired diminished sensitivity
to catecholamines. This would result in a decreased concentration
of cAMP, a predominance of the α-receptors, and a shift of the balance of the response to the catecholamines towards bronchocon-
striction.

The theory is based on a series of clinical and experimental
findings which have been described in detail by its author and can
be summarized as follows : 1° β-adrenergic blockade in asthmatic
patients as well as in experimental models (pertussis sensitized
animals) increases the sensitivity to the factors that trigger the
asthmatic episode. 2° The sensitivity to epinephrine is decreased
in patients with asthma in comparison with normal subjects;
besides bronchial relaxation, other β-adrenergic responses like
eosinopenia are also impaired. 3° The therapeutic effectiveness
of antiasthmatic drugs is related to their capacity to either by-
pass or restore β-adrenergic action; the sensitivity of asthmatic
patients to aminophylline and other methylxanthines is usually
normal and can be related to the capacity of these drugs to increase
the level of cAMP by inhibition of phosphodiesterase; the corticosteroids in addition to their anti-inflammatory activity might
increase the sensitivity of the β-receptor to catecholamine.
4° The large variety of stimuli that trigger asthmatic episodes
suggests that an unusually broad messenger system operates through
a final common pathway. By assuming that adenylate cyclase may be
deficient in different tissues, the theory also explains why some
allergic patients have asthma, whereas others have rhinitis or
eczema (atopic dermatitis).

Direct arguments in favour of the β-adrenergic theory in
asthma have not been given up to now, probably because of the difficult to study bronchial muscle of asthmatic patients. Indirect
data in favour of the hypothesis have, however, been provided.
Smith and Parker (51), Falliers et al. (32) and Gillespie et al.
(53) have reported that the stimulation of leukocyte adenylate
cyclase by isoproterenol was decreased to various extents in
asthmatic individuals, and Logsdon et al. described that the stimulation could be restored by steroid therapy. Bernstein et al.
(55) showed that epinephrine induced a prompt rise of the excretion
of cAMP in normal children, but not in asthmatic children. In
full-thickness skin biopsies of lesions of atopic dermatitis,
adenylate cyclase was found normal (56), but stimulation of the
enzyme by catecholamines could not be demonstrated in normal skin
by this technique (57). Duell et al. (58), however, using broken
cell preparations of epidermis, could demonstrate a stimulation of
adenylate cyclase by isoproterenol. Much work remains thus to be
done to verify the β-adrenergic theory.

Hypertension

The adrenergic control of vascular smooth muscle is similar
to the one of bronchial muscle : α-adrenergic receptor stimulation
results in contraction and β-adrenergic agents provoke relaxation.
Evidence has also been obtained for vascular smooth muscle that
relaxation in response to β-adrenergic agonists is mediated by an
increased level of cAMP (59). The hypothesis that essential hypertension might be due to a deficient formation of cAMP in vascular
muscle has received support from animal experiments. Amer (60)
has reported significantly lower concentrations of cAMP in the
aortas from rats with spontaneous or stress-induced hypertension.
In the hypertensive animals, adenylate cyclase was less responsive
to stimulation by isoproterenol and the activity of the low Km
phosphodiesterase was increased. Clinical studies, on the contrary, have shown an increased urinary excretion of cAMP associated
with the upright position in patients with labile hypertension
(62). This type of hypertension is, however, characterized by a
normal or even decreased peripheral resistance. An increased
urinary excretion of cAMP, correlated with an increased secretion
of catecholamines has also been reported in myocardial infarction
(63). This report is difficult to reconcile with the finding that
children with catecholamine-secreting neuroblastoma, had a normal
urinary excretion of cAMP (64).

Psoriasis

Psoriasis is a genetic skin disease with typical lesions that
are characterized, as compared with uninvolved epidermis, by
1° marked glycogen accumulation; 2° increased rate of tissue
proliferation and 3° decreased tissue differentiation. The hypothesis that psoriasis might be caused by a deficient formation of
cAMP has been proposed by Voorhees and Duell (163). It is based
on the well-documented function of the cyclic nucleotide in the
stimulation of glycogen degradation in various tissues, and on the
finding that epidermal cell division has been shown to be inhibited
by epinephrine (65) and by dibutyryl cAMP (66). The presence of
adenylate cyclase (57, 58), protein kinase (67, 68), phosphorylase
kinase (69) and phosphorylase (70) has been demonstrated in the
skin. Although stimulation of adenylate cyclase by catecholamines
has been observed in normal epidermis (58, 71), there is no certainty as to the physiological control of the concentration of
cAMP in epidermal cells. Catecholamines perhaps play a primary
role (72) so that the β-adrenergic theory may apply to psoriasis
as well. The intracellular level of cAMP might also be controlled
locally by chalones (73). These tissue specific, species non-
specific molecules exert a negative feed-back on cell mitosis (for
a review, see (74)).

Direct arguments in favour of a deficient formation of cAMP in psoriasis have been given. Voorhees et al. (66) have shown a markedly decreased concentration of cAMP in psoriatic lesions as compared with uninvolved skin areas. Hsia et al. (75) have reported that adenylate cyclase in psoriatic skin slices has a lower basal activity, is less responsive to stimulation by epinephrine and unresponsive to NaF. It is interesting to mention that recent research by Voorhees et al. (76) has shown that the decreased skin levels of cAMP are associated with increased concentrations of cGMP, lending thus further support to Goldberg's application of the "Ying-Yang" or dualism hypothesis of biological regulation (77). The therapeutically very important verification that increasing the concentration of cAMP decreases glycogen accumulation and inhibits cell division in psoriatic lesions has however not yet been obtained. Local treatment of psoriatic lesions with cAMP, its dibutyryl derivative and theophylline, has given poor results in comparison with classical therapy, which may be attributed to an insufficient penetration in the cells of the substances used (78, 24).

Growth Hormone Deficiency

Growth hormone has been postulated to exert a facilitating effect on the production of cAMP under the influence of other hormones, by increasing the synthesis of adenylate cyclase (79, 80). More recently, it has been proposed that the lipolytic action of human growth hormone may be mediated by the cyclic nucleotide (81). In normal subjects, the infusion of growth hormone did not alter the urinary excretion of cAMP (13). In children with hypopituitary dwarfism, the administration of 5 mg of human growth hormone for five consecutive days was also without effect on the excretion of cAMP (Van den Berghe and Vanderschueren-Lodeweyckx, unpublished observations). This may be due to the opposing inhibitory action of somatomedin on adenylate cyclase which has been reported in various tissues (82).

Evidence is also accumulating that the action of growth hormone releasing hormone may be mediated by cAMP (83, 84, 85, 86). cAMP and dibutyryl cAMP have been shown to increase the plasma level of growth hormone in normal humans (87, 88). In children with hypopituitary dwarfism, dibutyryl cAMP had no effect on the level of plasma growth hormone, but one patient has been reported, where a low-normal level of growth hormone could be observed after the administration of the nucleotide but not after the classical stimuli of growth hormone release, such as insulin, arginine and glucagon (89). This observation raises the possibility of hypophyseal defects of the formation of cAMP or of a decreased sensitivity to the nucleotide of the growth hormone releasing mechanism.

Hereditary Fructose Intolerance

In patients with this rare inborn error of metabolism, the ingestion of fructose provokes a profound hypoglycaemia (90) which does not respond to the administration of glucagon (91). This problem has been investigated in detail by clinical and animal studies (8). It could be shown that in children with hereditary fructose intolerance, the approximately 10-fold increase in the urinary excretion of cAMP induced by a single subcutaneous injection of glucagon, was almost completely abolished by the prior administration of fructose. This diminished capacity to form cAMP provoked by fructose, did not appear, however, to be the cause of the absence of response to glucagon, since the administration of dibutyryl cAMP during a fructose-induced hypoglycaemia, was also without effect on blood glucose. From animal experiments it could be concluded that the diminished production of cAMP in response to glucagon after the administration of fructose was caused by the ATP-depleting effect of this ketose, which has been described by Mäenpää (92). The absence of glycogenolytic response to glucagon and cAMP was shown to be due to an inhibition of phosphorylase a by the accumulation of ketose 1-phosphate (93). This study demonstrates that there is not necessarily a causal relationship between a deficient formation of cAMP and the absence of hormonal effect.

Depression and Mania

Paul et al. (162, 164) and Abdulla and Hamadah (161) have reported that the excretion of cAMP was below normal in depressed psychotics and above normal in manic patients. A marked elevation of urinary cAMP was also described on the day of rapid switch from a depressed into a manic state in subjects with manic-depressive illness (94). These data have not been confirmed by others (95, 147). The causal relationship of these observations with the psychotic symptoms has also been challenged (96) on the basis that the variations of the urinary excretion of cAMP may result from changes in physical activity, as confirmed by Eccleston et al. (20). The report by Robison et al. (97) that the concentration of cAMP in the cerebrospinal fluid of patients with affective disorders was not modified, is a further argument against the involvement of cAMP in the aetiology of depression and mania.

DISORDERS WITH INCREASED PRODUCTION OF cAMP

Cholera

Infection with Vibrio cholerae provokes a fulminant, life-threatening diarrhea, which is due to a massive loss of fluid throughout the small intestine. This loss has been shown to be

caused by a stimulation by the bacterial exotoxin of an active
secretion of chloride and possibly bicarbonate, with isoosmotic
transport of water (for a review, see Field (98)). Recent reserve
has provided substantial evidence that the action of cholera exotoxin is mediated by cAMP (see also Vaughan, this volume). In the
ileal mucosa, cAMP and theophylline provoke a reversal of the
direction of chloride flux from a net absorption to a net secretion
(99, 100). Elevated concentrations of cAMP have been demonstrated
in the isolated dog ileal mucosa in vitro upon addition of a cell
free filtrate of a Vibrio cholerae culture (101). A marked increase
of the activity of mucosal adenylate cyclase has been described in
rabbit ileal loops (102) after in vivo exposure to cholera toxin,
and in jejunal biopsies from patients with cholera (103). The
activity of adenylate cyclase during cholera was increased more than
two-fold in comparison with the convalescent period. It should be
noted that, whereas the effects of cAMP and theophylline on net
chloride flux are almost immediate, the response to the enterotoxin
occurs only after about 30 minutes. The effects of the toxin on
the level of cAMP and on the activity of adenylate cyclase require
a similar time lag to become manifest. Furthermore, stimulation
of the enzyme is observed only when the toxin is administered in
vivo or to intact cells. The total amount of adenylate cyclase is
not modified, indicating that cholera toxin does not induce the
synthesis of new enzyme (104). The suggestion that the effect of
the toxin on cAMP metabolism may be mediated by locally synthesized
prostaglandins (105) has also been ruled out (106). The observation
that adenylate cyclase does not seem to be a normal constituent of
the brush border, but is localized instead in the plasma membrane
of the basal and lateral sides of the epithelial cells (107) raises
the question of the way through which cholera toxin reaches the
adenylate cyclase and may be related to the lag period reported.
Binding of the cholera toxin to liver and fat cell membranes has
been shown to be increased by monoganglionsides (108), providing
the hypothesis that transfer of the toxin from the brush border to
the plasma membrane might occur in association with gangliosides.

     Stimulation of intestinal adenylate cyclase may also play a
role in the pathogenesis of other diarrheic syndromes. Stimulation of the enzyme by Escherichia Coli enterotoxin has been
reported (104, 110). Prostaglandins have also been shown to
stimulate adenylate cyclase in human jejunal mucosal cells (104).
The diarrhea associated with medullary carcinoma of the thyroid
(111) and tumors of neural crest origin (112) both of which release
prostaglandins, may be due to this mechanism.

                         Diabetes

     A role for cAMP in the pathogenesis of diabetes mellitus has
been proposed at two levels : 1° in the pancreatic β-cell,

deficient production of the cyclic nucleotide has been postulated
to be the cause of a defective release of insulin; 2° in the liver,
evidence has been found that many of the metabolic abnormalities
due to insulin deficiency may result from an increased concentration of cAMP. These two aspects will be discussed separately.

    The hypothesis that diabetes might be caused by a reduced
ability of the pancreatic β-cell to produce cAMP was proposed by
Cerasi and Luft (113, 114) and is based on the finding that in
prediabetic subjects, the reduced rate of insulin release in response to the infusion of high concentrations of glucose can be
improved by the injection of theophylline. The stimulation of the
secretion of insulin by various hormones, phosphodiesterase
inhibitors, and cAMP (115, 116, 117) indicates a role for the
cyclic nucleotide in the insulin-releasing process (see Montegue
and Robison in this volume). Cerasi and Luft's proposal has
triggered several investigations of the effect of glucose, the
principal physiological effector of insulin release, on the cAMP
system in pancreatic islets. These have, however, given mostly
negative results. Glucose had no effect on cAMP concentrations
in mouse or rat pancreatic islets (118, 119). The activities of
adenylate cyclase (120, 121, 122, 123, 165) phosphodiesterase
(124, 125, 126) and protein kinase (127, 128) were not modified
by glucose. Elevated levels of cAMP in rat pancreatic islets
during acute glucose stimulation were, however, reported by
Charles et al. (129) and by Grill and Cerasi (130). The administration of glucose in vivo for several hours to rats has been
shown to increase the activity of islet adenylate cyclase (131)
suggesting that long-term regulatory effects of glucose on insulin
release may be mediated by the cAMP system.

    It has been objected against Cerasi and Luft's hypothesis
that theophylline influenced the insulin response to glucose
only in prediabetics, but not in overt diabetics or normal
subjects. These observations could perhaps be explained by the
assumptions that cAMP is not rate-limiting in normal subjects and
that in advanced diabetes, adenylate cyclase is too defective to
allow correction of the concentration of cAMP by inhibitors of
phosphodiesterase.

    The hypothesis that many of the metabolic abnormalities
observed in diabetes are caused by an increased concentration of
cAMP is based on several lines of evidence.

1°   cAMP has been shown to increase the hepatic output of glucose
     by stimulating glycogenolysis and gluconeogenesis; the cyclic
     nucleotide also enhances the production of ketone bodies by a
     direct stimulation of hepatic ketogenesis, as well as by
     increasing the mobilisation of fatty acids in adipose tissue
     (for a review, see Sutherland and Robison (133)).

2° Increased concentrations of cAMP have been measured in the liver
    of rats made diabetic by the administration of anti-insulin
    serum (134) alloxan (134, 135, 136) or streptozotocin (137).

3° Insulin treatment of alloxan-diabetic rats decreases the hepatic
    concentration of cAMP (134) with a time course similar to the
    reduction of the glucose output (136).

It should be mentioned that the increased hepatic levels of cAMP
during insulin deficiency have been reported only in rats. The
absence of increase observed in the liver of the pancreatectomized
dog (138) might be due to the simultaneous deficiency of the antagonistic hormone glucagon. In mice treated with anti-insulin serum
or alloxan, the hepatic concentration of cAMP was not significantly
modified (Table III). Normal levels of cAMP in adipose and hepatic
tissue in human diabetics have been reported (139). The output of
cAMP from the liver, which has been shown in experiments with the
perfused rat liver to be the most sensitive index of alterations
of the tissue level of the cyclic nucleotide (140, 141) was not
increased in hepatic venous blood of human diabetics (142). The
report by Tucci et al.(143) of an increased urinary excretion of
cAMP in patients with uncontrolled diabetes mellitus that could be
lowered by treatment with insulin is in contradiction with these
findings.

The increased concentration of hepatic cAMP in experimental
diabetes in the rat has been attributed to an increased sensitivity
of adenylate cyclase to epinephrine or glucagon. The experimental
results are, however, contradictory. An increased response to
epinephrine of the hepatic adenylate cyclase of alloxan or streptozotocin treated rats has been reported (144). An increased sensitivity of adenylate cyclase to glucagon in vitro was found in
streptozotocin treated mice (145) but not in similarly treated or
alloxanized rats (144). As shown in Figure 1, the levels of cAMP
observed in the liver of alloxan-treated mice 1 minute after the
administration of two different doses of glucagon in vivo, were not
different from those observed in control animals. A diminished
accumulation of cAMP in response to glucagon in diabetes has been
shown in isolated rat liver cells (146) and in perfused rat liver
(137). It is possible that the decreased sensitivity of rat
liver adenylate cyclase to glucagon may be compensated by the
inappropriately high concentration of the hormone which has been
found in diabetes (149, 150).

The mechanism whereby insulin lowers the concentration of
cAMP is even more controversial. Hepp (145) and Illiano and
Cuatrecases (151) have reported that insulin in vitro inhibits
adenylate cyclase in rat and mouse liver. This finding has not

TABLE III. Influence of Experimental Diabetes on the Concentration of cAMP in the Liver

EXPERIMENT	CONTROL GROUP	EXPERIMENTAL GROUP
Unanaesthetized mice		
alloxan – 8 days	0.60 + 0.04	0.65 + 0.04
A.I.S. – 1 H	0.80 + 0.05	0.97 + 0.05
A.I.S. – 2 H		0.97 + 0.10
Anaesthetized mice		
alloxan – 48 H	0.98 + 0.09	0.99 + 0.10
Anaesthetized rats		
alloxan – 48 H	0.44 + 0.05	1.44 + 0.07

The results are expressed as nmol/g liver + the standard error of the mean. There were 4–7 animals per group. Alloxan was administered at the dose of 70 mg/kg and anti-insulin serum (A.I.S.) at the dose of 25 U/kg. Anaesthesia was induced by the injection of pentobarbital at the dose of 75 mg/kg. cAMP in the unanaesthetized mice was determined as described in Van den Berghe et al. (147) and according to Gilman (148) in the anaesthetized animals (Van Den Berghe, unpublished experiments).

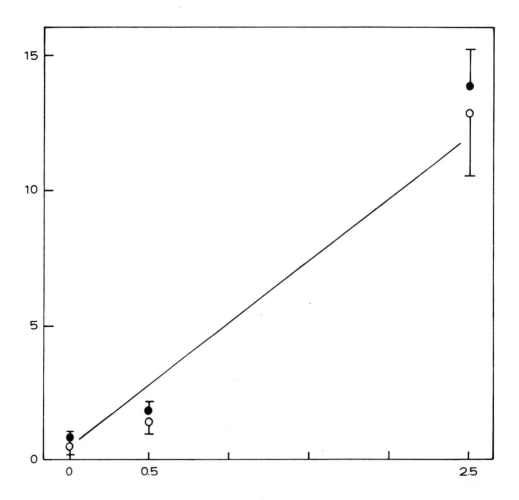

FIGURE 1.   Influence of glucagon on the hepatic level of cAMP in
             alloxan-treated and in control mice.

Alloxan was administered at the dose of 70 mg/kg intravenous and
the animals were used after 8 days. Glucagon was injected via a
tail vein, at the dose indicated, to unanaesthetized animals which
were killed 1 minute later. cAMP was determined according to Van
den Berghe et al. (147). Vertical bars represent ± the standard
error of the means (5 animals per experimental point). 0, control;
●, alloxan treated (Van den Berghe, unpublished experiments).

been confirmed by Pohl et al. (152), Rosselin and Freychet (153) and Pilkis et al. (137). In 1966, Schultz et al. (154) reported that insulin increased the activity of phosphodiesterase in muscle and liver of alloxan-diabetic rats. This observation could initially not be confirmed by several authors (155, 156) but the identification of two phosphodiesterase activities in several tissues with different Km values (157) has allowed further investigations. Loten and Sneyd (158) reported that insulin increases the activity of the low Km phosphodiesterase in adipose tissue, and Pilkis et al. (137) demonstrated that the activity of the low Km enzyme was decreased in liver plasma membranes from diabetic rats and was increased by insulin treatment of the rats in vivo.

Although as discussed by Park et al. (166), not all of the effects of insulin on the liver appear to be mediated by a decrease of the concentration of the cyclic nucleotide, the studies of the cAMP system in experimental diabetes have provided further insight in the pathogeny of the disease. The failure to demonstrate increased levels of cAMP in diabetic mice and humans might be due to the difficulty to measure small variations of the free cyclic nucleotide against a large background of bound cAMP. It should be kept in mind, however, that the history of the study of the mechanism of action of insulin contains many oversimplifications and misinterpretations.

Conclusion

The discovery of the cAMP system has provided new outlooks and original approaches to several problems in pathology, besides useful diagnostic tests. As is apparent from this lecture, abnormalities of the formation of cAMP have been postulated to explain the pathophysiology of numerous diseases. Although certain of the hypotheses outlined have received confirmation, other ones still lack direct support. Furthermore, it should be emphasized that, whereas several abnormalities of the metabolism of the cyclic nucleotide have been found, the causal relationship of these findings with the pathogeny of the disorder has been established only in very few cases and remains hypothetical or has even been ruled out in other instances. Up to now, very few examples of a deficient mechanism of action of cAMP have been reported. A case of glycogen storage disease (159) and a familial defect of triglyceride breakdown (160) have been attributed to a defect at the level of protein kinase, although no assays of this enzyme were performed. The role of cAMP in pathology will thus probably remain a very active field of research in future years.

REFERENCES

(1) BROADUS, A.E., HARDMAN, J.G., KAMINSKY, N.I., BALL, J.H.,
     SUTHERLAND, E.W. and LIDDLE, G.W. (1971), Ann. N.Y., Acad.
     Sci., 185, 50

(2) BROADUS, A.E., KAMINSKY, N.I., NORTHCUTT, R.C., HARDMAN, J.G.,
     SUTHERLAND, E.W. and LIDDLE, G.W. (1970b), J. Clin. Invest.,
     49, 2237

(3) BROADUS, A.E., KAMINSKY, N.I., KARDMAN, J.G., SUTHERLAND,
     E.W. and LIDDLE, G.W. (1970a) J. Clin. Invest., 49, 2222

(4) BUTCHER, R.W. and SUTHERLAND, E.W. (1962) J. Biol. Chem.,
     237, 1244

(5) ASHMAN, D.F., KIPTON, R., MELICOW, M.M. and PRICE, T.D.
     (1963), Biochem. Biophys. Res. Commun., 11, 330

(6) PRICE, T.D., ASHMAN, D.F. and MELICOW, M.M. (1967), Biochem.
     Biophys. Acta, 138, 452

(7) KAMINSKY, N.I., BROADUS, A.E., HARDMAN, J.G., JONES, D.J.,
     BALL, J.H., SUTHERLAND, E.W. and LIDDLE, G.W. (1970), J.
     Clin. Invest. 49, 2387

(8) VAN DEN BERGHE, G., HUE, L. and HERS, H.G. (1973), Biochem.
     J., 134, 63

(9) AUGUST, G.P. and HUNG, W. (1973), J. Clin. Endocrinol. Metab.
     37, 476

(10) O'BRIEN, D. and IBBOTT, F.A., (1964) Laboratory Manual of
     Pediatric Micro- and Ultramicro-Biochemical Techniques,
     3rd Edn, Hoeber, Harper and Row, New York

(11) ROSEN, O.M. (1972) N. EngL. J. Med. 287, 670

(12) LIN, T., KOPP, L.E. and TUCCI, J.R. (1973) J. Clin. Endo-
     crinol. Metab., 36, 1033

(13) TAYLOR, A.L., DAVIS, B.B., PAWLSON, L.G., JOSIMOVICH, J.B.
     and MINTZ, D.H. (1970) J. Clin. Endocrinol., 30, 316

(14) TAKAHASHI, K., KAMIMURA, M., SHINKO, T. and TSUJI, S. (1966)
     Lancet ii, 967

(15) OWEN, P. and MOFFAT, A.C. (1973) Lancet ii, 1205

(16)   CHASE, L.R., MELSON, G.L. and AURBACH, G.D. (1969), J. Clin.
       Invest., 48, 1832

(17)   MURAD, F. and PAK, C.Y.C. (1972) N. Engl. J. Med. 286, 1382

(18)   SAGEL, J., COLWELL, J.A., LOADHOLT, C.B. and LIZARRALDE, G.
       (1973) J. Clin. Endocrinol. Metab. 37, 570

(19)   HOLMES, H., HAMADAH, K., HARTMAN, G.C. and PARKE, D.V. (1974)
       Biochem. Soc. Trans., 2, 456

(20)   ECCLESTON, D., LOOSE, R., PULLAR, I.A. and SUGDEN, R.F.
       (1970) Lancet ii, 612

(21)   HAMADAH, K., HOLMES, H., STOKES, M.L., HARTMAN, G.C. and
       PARKE, D.V. (1974) Biochem. Soc. Trans. 2, 461

(22)   RAIJ, K., HÄRKÖNEN, M., CASTREN, O., SAARIKOSKI, S. and
       ADLERCREUTZ, H. (1974) Scand. J. Clin. Lab. Invest., 32, 193

(23)   TOMLINSON, S., BARLING, P.M., ALBANO, J.D.M., BROWN, B.L. and
       O'RIORDAN, J.L.H. (1974), Clin. Sci. 47, 481

(24)   AUERBACH, R. (1974), J. Am. Med. Assoc., 227, 326

(25)   ALBRIGHT, F., BURNETT, C.H., SMITH, P.H. and PARSON, W.
       (1942) Endocrinology, 30, 922

(26)   TASHJIAN, A.H., Jr., FRANTZ, A.G., and LEE, J.B. (1966) Proc.
       Natl. Acad. Sci. USA, 56, 1138

(27)   LEE, J.B., TASHJIAN, A.H., Jr. STREETO, J.M. and FRANTZ, A.G.
       (1968) N. Engl. J. Med., 279, 1179

(28)   BELL, N.H., AVERY, S., SINHA, T., CLARK, C.M., Jr. ALLEN, D.O.
       and JOHNSTON, C.Jr. (1972) J. Clin. Invest., 51, 816

(29)   MARCUS, R., WILBER, J.F. and AURBACH, G.D. (1971) J. Clin.
       Endocrinol., 33, 537

(30)   AURBACH, G.D., MARCUS, R., WINICKOFF, R.N., EPSTEIN, E.H., Jr.
       and NIGRA, T.P. (1970) Metabolism, 19, 799

(31)   DREZNER, M., NEELON, F.A. and LEBOVITZ, H.E. (1973) N. Engl.
       J. Med., 289, 1056

(32)   ESTEP, H., FRATKIN, M., MOSER, A. and ROBISON, G.A. (1970)
       Clin. Res. 18, 358

(33) DOHAN, P.H., YAMASHITA, K., LARSEN, P.R., DAVIS, B., DEFTOS,
      L. and FIELD, J.B. (1972) J. Clin. Endocrinol. Metab., 35,
      775

(34) NEELON, F.A., DREZNER, M., BIRCH, B.M. and LEBOVITZ, H.E.
      (1973), Lancet i, 631

(35) ORLOFF, J. and HANDLER, J. (1967) Am. J. Ned., 42, 757

(36) WARING, A.J., LASLOW, K. and TAPPAN, V. (1945), Amer. J. Dis.
      Child., 69, 323

(37) FORSMAN, H. (1956) Acta Med. Scand., 121, Suppl., 159, 1

(38) PAWLSON, L.G., TAYLOR, A., MINTZ, D.H., FIELD, J.B. and
      DAVIS, B.B., (1970) Metabolism, 19, 694

(39) WILLIAMS, R.H., BARISH, J. and ENSINCK, J.W. (1972) Proc.
      Soc. Exptl. Biol. Med. 139, 447

(40) FICHMAN, M.P. and BROOKER, G. (1972) J. Clin. Endocrinol.
      Metab. 35, 35

(41) BELL, N.H., CLARK, C.M., Jr., AVERY, S., SINHA, T.,
      TRYGSTAD, C.W., and ALLEN, D.O. (1974), Pediat. Res., 8, 223

(42) LEVINE, R.A. (1968a) Clin. Sci. 34, 253

(43) AVERY, S., CLARK, C.M., Jr., TRYSTAD, C. and BELL, N.H. (1971)
      J. Clin. Invest., 50, 3a

(44) BARTTER, F.C., PRONOVE, P., GILL, J.R., Jr. and MacCARDLE,
      R.C. (1962) Am. J. Med., 33, 811

(45) PROESMANS, W., EGGERMONT, E. and EECKELS, R. (1973) J.
      Pediatr., 82, 538

(46) ROBISON, G.A., BUTCHER, R.W. and SUTHERLAND, E.W. (1967)
      Ann. N.Y., Acad. Sci., 139, 703

(47) MOORE, P.F., IORIO, L.C. and McMANUS, J.M. (1968) J. Pharm.
      Pharmacol., 20, 368

(48) VULLIEMOZ, Y., VEROSKY, M., NAHAS, G.G. and TRINER, L. (1971)
      Pharmacologist, 13, 256

(49) ROSS, W. and OPPELT, W.W. (1973), Res. Commun. Chem. Pathol.
      Pharmacol., 5, 817

(50)   SZENTIVANYI, A. (1968), J. Allergy, 42, 203

(51)   SMITH, J.W. and PARKER, C.W. (1970), J. Lab. Clin. Med., 76, 993

(52)   FALLIERS, C.J., DE A. CARDOSO, R.R., BANE, H.N., COFFEY, R.G., and MIDDLETON, E., Jr. (1971), J. Allergy, 47, 207

(53)   GILLESPIE, E., VALENTINE, M.D. and LICHTENSTEIN, L.M. (1974) J. Allergy Clin. Immunol., 53, 27

(54)   LOGSDON, P.J., MIDDLETON, E., Jr., and COFFEY, R.G. (1972) J. Allergy, Clin. Immunol., 50, 45

(55)   BERNSTEIN, R.A., LINARELLI, L., FACKTOR, M.A., FRIDAY, G.A., DRASH, A.L. and FIREMAN, P. (1972), J. Lab. Clin. Med. 80, 772

(56)   MIER, P.D. and URSELMANN, E. (1970b), Br. J. Derm. 83, 364

(57)   MIER, P.D. and URSELMANN, E. (1970a) Br. J. Derm., 83, 359

(58)   DUELL, E.A., VOORHEES, J.J., KELSEY, W.H., and HAYES E. (1971), Arch. Derm., 104, 601

(59)   TRINER, L., NAHAS, G.G., VULLIEMOZ, Y., OVERWEG, N.I.A., VEROSKY, M., HABIF, D.V. and NGAI, S.H. (1971), Ann. N.Y. Acad. Sci., 185, 458

(60)   AMER, M.S., (1973), Science, 179, 807

(62)   HAMET, P., KUCHEL, O. and GENEST, J. (1973), J. Clin. Endocrinol., Metab. 36, 218

(63)   STRANGE, R.C., VETTER, N., ROWE, M.J. and OLIVER, M.F. (1974), Eur. J. Clin. Invest., 4, 115

(64)   SMITH, J.L., HELSON, L. and BALIS, M.E. (1971), J. Lab. Clin. Med., 77, 445

(65)   BULLOUGH, W.S. and LAURENCE, E.B. (1964), Exptl Cell Res., 33, 176

(66)   VOORHEES, J.J., DUELL, E.A., and KELSEY, W.H. (1972a) Arch. Derm., 105, 384

(67)   KUMAR, R., TAO, M. and SOLOMON, L.M. (1971) J. Invest. Derm. 57, 312

(68) MIER, P.D., and VAN DEN HURK, J. (1972) Br. J. Derm., 87,
      571

(69) MIER, P.D., and SUTORIUS, A.H.M. (1972) Br. J. Derm., 86, 49

(70) HALPRIN, K.M. and OHKAWARA, A. (1966), J. Invest. Derm., 46,
      43

(71) HSIA, S.L., WRIGHT, R., MANDY, S.H., and HALPRIN, K.M. (1972)
      J. Invest. Derm., 59, 109

(72) VOORHEES, J.J., DUELL, E.A., BASS, L.J., POWELL, J.A. and
      HARRELL, E.R., (1972b) J. Invest. Derm., 59, 114

(73) VOORHEES, J.J., DUELL, E.A., BASS, L.J. and HARRELL, E.R.
      (1973a) Natl. Cancer Inst. Monogr., 38, 47

(74) HOUCK, J.C. and HENNINGS, H. (1973) FEBS Letters, 32, 1

(75) VOORHEES, J.J., DUELL, E.A., BASS, L.J., POWELL, J.A. and
      HARRELL, E.R. (1972c) Arch. Derm., 105, 695

(76) VOORHEES, J.J., STAWISKY, M., DUELL, E.A., HADDOX, M.K. and
      GOLDBERG, N.D. (1973b) Life Sci., 13, 639

(77) GOLDBERG, N.D., O'DEA, R.F. and HADDOX, M.K. (1973) Advan.
      Cyclic Nucl. Res., 3, 155

(78) LAUGIER, P., POSTERNAK, T., ORUSCO, M., CEHOVIC, G. and
      POSTERNAK, F. (1973) Bull. Soc. Franç. Dermat. Syphill., 80,
      632

(79) GOODMAN, H.M. (1970) Endocrinology, 86, 1064

(80) MOSKOWITZ, J. and FAIN, J.N. (1970), J. Biol. Chem., 245,
      1101

(81) RAMACHANDRAN, J., LEE, V. and LI, C.H. (1972) Biochem.
      Biophys. Res. Commun., 48, 274

(82) TELL, G.P.E., CUATRECASAS, P., VAN WYK, J.J. and HINTZ, R.L.
      (1973) Science, 180, 312

(83) SCHOFIELD, J.G. (1967), Nature, 215, 1382

(84) ZOR, U., KANEKO, T., SCHNEIDER, H.P.G., McCANN, S.M., LOWE,
      I.P., BLOOM, G., BORLAND, B. and FIELD, J.B. (1969) Proc.
      Natl. Acad. Sci. USA, 63, 918

(85) MacLEOD, R.M. and LEHMEYER, J.E. (1970), Proc. Natl. Acad.
      Sci. USA, 67, 1172

(86) STEINER, A.L., PEAKE, G.T., UTIGER, R.D., KARL, I.E. and
      KIPNIS, D.M., (1970), Endocrinology, 86, 1354

(87) LEVINE, R.A. (1968b) J. Clin. Invest., 47, 62a

(88) LEVINE, R.A. (1970) Clin. Pharmacol. Ther., 11, 238

(89) VANDERSCHUEREN-LODEWEYCKX, M., VAN DEN BERGHE, G., PROESMANS,
      W., CORBEEL, L., EGGERMONT, E. and EECKELS, R. (1974) Acta
      Paediatr. Scand., 63, 364

(90) FROESCH, E.R., PRADER, A., LABHART, A., STUBER, H.W. and
      WOLF, H.P. (1957), SCHWEIZ, Med. Wochenschr., 87, 1168

(91) CORNBLATH, M., ROSENTHAL, I.M., REISNER, S.H., WYBREGT, S.H.
      and CRANE, R.K. (1963) N. Engl. J. Med., 269, 1271

(92) MÄENPÄÄ, P.H., RAIVIO, K.O. and KEKOMÄKI, M.P. (1968) Science
      161, 1253

(93) VAN DEN BERGHE, G., HUE, L. and HERS, H.G. (1974), Pediat.
      Res., 8, 910

(94) PAUL, M.I., CRAMER, H. and BUNNEY, W.E., Jr. (1971) Science
      171, 300

(95) BROWN, B.L., SALWAY, J.G., ALBANO, J.D.M., HULLIN, R.P. and
      EKINS, R.P. (1972), Brit. J. Psychiat., 120, 405

(96) BERG, G.R. and GLINSMANN, W.H. (1970) Lancet i, 834

(97) ROBISON, G.A., COPPEN, A.J., WHYBROWn P.C. and PRANGE, A.J.
      (1970), Lancet ii, 1028

(98) FIELD, M. (1971a) N. Engl. J. Med. 284, 1137

(99) FIELD, M. (1971b) Am. J. Physiol., 221, 992

(100) FIELD, M., FROMM, D., AL-AWQUATI, Q. and GREENOUGH, W.V. III
      (1972) J. Clin. Invest. 51, 796

(101) SCHAFER, D.E., LUST, W.D., SIRCAR, B. and GOLDBERG, N.D.
      (1970), Proc. Natl. Acad. Sci. USA, 67, 851

(102) SHARP, G.W.G. and HYNIE, S. (1971) Nature, 229, 266

(103) CHEN, L.C., ROHDE, J.E. and SHARP, G.W.G. (1971) Lancet i, 939

(104) CHEN, L.C., ROHDE, J.E. and SHARP, G.W.G. (1972), J. Clin. Invest. 51, 731

(105) BENNETT, A. (1971) Nature, 231, 536

(106) KIMBERG, D.V., Field, M., GERSHON, E. and HENDERSON, A. (1974) J. Clin. Invest., 53, 941

(107) PARKINSON, D.K., EBEL, H., DIBONA, D.R. and SHARP, G.W.G. (1972), J. Clin. Invest., 51, 2292

(108) CUATRECASAS, P. (1973), Biochemistry, 12, 3567

(109) EVANS, D.J., Jr., CHEN, L.C., CURLIN, G.T. and EVAN, D.G. (1972) Nature, 236, 137

(110) KANTOR, H.S., TAO, P. and GORBACH, S.L. (1974), J. Infect. Dis., 129, 1

(111) WILLIAMS, E.D., KARIM, S.M.M. and SANDLER, M. (1968) Lancet i, 22

(112) SANDLER, M., KARIM, S.M.M. and WILLIAMS, E.D. (1968) Lancet ii, 1053

(113) CERASI, E. and LUFT, R. (1969), Horm. Metab. Res., 1, 162

(114) CERASI, E. and LUFT, R. (1970), Nobel Symposium, 13, 17

(115) SUSSMAN, K.E., VAUGHAN, G.D. and TIMMER, R.F. (1966) Diabetes 15, 521

(116) MALAISSE, W.J., MALAISSE-LAGAE, F., MAYHEW, D. (1967) J. Clin. Invest., 46, 1724

(117) TURTLE, J.R., LITTLETON, G.K. and KIPNIS, D.M. (1967) Nature, 213, 727

(118) KIPNIS, D.M. (1970) Acta Diabetolog. Lat., 7, Suppl. 1, 314

(119) MONTAGUE, W. and COOK, J.R. (1971), Biochem. J. 122, 115

(120) ATKINS, T. and MATTY, A.J. (1971) J. Endocrinol., 51, 67

(121) DAVIS, B. and LAZARUS, N.R. (1972) Biochem. J. 129, 373

(122) MILLER, E.A., WRIGHT, P.H. and ALLEN, D.O. (1972) Endo-
      crinology, 91, 1117

(123) HOWELL, S.L. and MONTAGUE, W. (1973) Biochim. Biophys.
      Acta, 320, 44

(124) ASHCROFT, S.J.H., RANDLE, P.J. and TÄLJEDAL, I.B. (1972)
      FEBS Letters, 20, 263

(125) BOWEN, V. and LAZARUS, N.R. (1972), Biochem. J., 128, 97P

(126) SAMS, D.J., and MONTAGUE, W., (1972) Biochem. J. 129, 945

(127) MONTAGUE, W. and HOWELL, S.L. (1972) Biochem. J. 129, 551

(128) STEINER, D.F. (1972) Biabetes, 21, Suppl. 2, 571

(129) CHARLES, M.A., FANSKA, R., SCHMID, F.G., FORSHAM, P.H. and
      GRODSKY, G.M. (1973), Science, 179, 569

(130) GRILL, V. and CERASI, E. (1974) J. Biol. Chem., 249, 4196

(131) HOWELL, S.L., GREEN, I.C. and MONTAGUE, W. (1973), Biochem.
      J., 136, 343

(133) SUTHERLAND, E.W. and ROBISON, G.A. (1969) Diabetes, 18, 797

(134) JEFFERSON, L.S., EXTON, J.H., BUTCHER, R.W., SUTHERLAND,
      E.W. and PARK, C.R. (1968), J. Biol. Chem., 243, 1031

(135) GOLDBERG, N.D., DIETZ, S.B. and O'TOOLE, A.G. (1969) J.
      Biol. Chem., 244, 4458

(136) EXTON, J.H., HARPER, S.C., TUCKER, A.L. and HO, R.J. (1973)
      Biochim. Biophys. Acta, 329, 23

(137) PILKIS, S.J., EXTON, J.H., JOHNSON, R.A. and PARK, C.R.
      (1974), Biochim. Biophys. Acta, 343, 250

(138) BISHOP, J.S., GOLDBERG, N.D. and LARNER, J. (1971) Am. J.
      Physiol., 220, 499

(139) SUTHERLAND, E.W., ROBISON, G.A. and HARDMAN, J.G. (1970)
      Nobel Symposium, 13, 137

(140) EXTON, J.H., LEWIS, S.B., HO, R.J., ROBISON, G.A. and PARK,
      C.R., (1971), Ann. N.Y. Acad. Sci., 185, 85

(141) EXTON, J.H., LEWIS, S.B., HO, R.J., and PARK, C.R. (1972)
      Advanc. Cyclic Nucl. Res. 1, 91

(142) LILJENQUIST, J.E., BOMBOY, J.D., LEWIS, S.B., SINCLAIR-
      SMITH, B.C., FELTS, P.W., LACY, W.W., CROFFORD, O.B. and
      LIDDLE, G.W. (1974), J. Clin. Invest., 53, 198

(143) TUCCI, J.R., LIN, T. and KOPP, L. (1973), J. Clin. Endo-
      crinol. Metabl., 37, 832

(144) BITENSKY, M.W., GORMAN, R.E. and NEUFELD, A.H. (1972)
      Endocrinology, 90, 1331

(145) HEPP, K.D. (1972), Eur. J. Biochem., 31, 266

(146) INGEBRETZEN, W.R., Jr., MOXLEY, M.A., ALLEN, D.O. and
      WAGLE, S.R. (1972), Biochem. Biophys. Res. Commun., 49,
      601

(147) HULLIN, R.P., SALWAY, J.G., ALLSOPP, M.N.E., BARNES, G.D.,
      ALBANO, J.D.M. and BROWN, B.L. (1974), Brit. J. Psychiat.
      125, 457

(148) GILMAN, A.G. (1970), Proc. Natl. Acad. Sci. USA, 67, 305

(149) UNGER, R.H., AGUILAR-PARADA, E., MULLER, W.A. and EISENTRAUT,
      A.M., (1970), J. Clin. Invest., 49, 837

(150) MULLER, W.A., FALOONA, G.R. and UNGER, R.H. (1971) J. Cnin.
      Invest., 50, 1992

(151) ILLIANO, G. and CUATRECASAS, P. (1972) Science, 175, 906

(152) POHL, S.L., BIRNBAUMER, L. and RODBELL, M. (1971),J. Biol.
      Chem., 246, 1849

(153) ROSSELIN, G. and FREYCHET, P. (1973), Biochim. Biophys.
      Acta, 304, 541

(154) SCHULTZ, G., SENFT, G. and MUNSKE, K. (1966) Naturwissen-
      schaften, 20, 529

(155) MÜLLER-OERLINGHAUSEN, B., SCHWABE, U., HASSELBLATT, A. and
      SCHMIDT, F.H. (1968), Life Sci., 7, 593

(156) MENAHAN, L.A., HEPP, K.D. and WIELAND, O. (1969), Eur. J.
      Biochem., 8, 435

(157) BEAVO, J.A., HARDMAN, J.G. and SUTHERLAND, E.W. (1970) J.
      Biol. Chem., 245, 5649

(158) LOTEN, E.G. and SNEYD, J.G.T. (1970), Biochem. J., 120, 187

(159) HUG, G., SCHUBERT, W.K. and CHUCK, G. (1970), Biochem. Biophys. Res. Commun., 40, 982

(160) GILBERT, C., GALTON, D.J. and KAYE, J. (1973) Brit. Med. J. i, 25

(161) ABDULLA, Y.H. and HAMADAH, K. (1970), Lancet i, 378

(162) PAUL, M.I., DITZION, B.R. and JANOWSKY, D.S. (1970a) Lancet i, 88

(163) VOORHEES, J.J. and DUELL, E.A. (1971), Arch. Derm., 104, 352

(164) PAUL, M.I., CRAMER, H. and GOODWIN, F.K. (1970b) Lancet i, 996

(165) KUO, W.N., HODGINS, D.S. and KUO, J.F. (1973), J. Biol. Chem., 248, 270

(166) PARK, C.R., LEWIS, S.B. and EXTON, J.H. (1972) Diabetes 21, Suppl. 2, 439

I N D E X